PM&R
SECRETS

BRYAN O'YOUNG, MD

Instructor
Department of Physical Medicine and Rehabilitation
Johns Hopkins University School of Medicine
Baltimore, Maryland

MARK A. YOUNG, MD

Assistant Professor
Department of Physical Medicine and Rehabilitation
Johns Hopkins University School of Medicine
Baltimore, Maryland

STEVEN A. STIENS, MD, MS

Assistant Professor
Department of Rehabilitation Medicine
University of Washington School of Medicine
Staff Physician, Spinal Cord Injury Unit
VA Puget Sound Health Care System
Seattle, Washington

HANLEY & BELFUS, INC./ Philadelphia

Publisher: **HANLEY & BELFUS, INC.**
Medical Publishers
210 South 13th Street
Philadelphia, PA 19107
(215) 546-7293; 800-962-1892
FAX (215) 790-9330

Library of Congress Cataloging-in-Publication Data

PM&R Secrets /   [edited by] Bryan J. O'Young, Mark A. Young, Steven Stiens.
     p.   cm. – (The Secrets Series®)
   Includes bibliographical references and index.
   ISBN 1-56053-155-X (paper : alk. paper)
   1. Physical therapy–Examinations, questions, etc.   2. Medical rehabilitation-
rehabilitation–Examinations, questions, etc.   I. O'Young, Bryan J., 1962-.
  II. Stiens, Steven, 1959-.   III. Series.
    [DNLM: 1. Physical Medicine–examination questions.   2. Rehabilitation-
examination questions.   WB 18.2 P738 1996]
RM701.6.P56 1996
615.8' 2' 076–dc20
DNLM/DLC
for Library of Congress   96-32242
                                                    CIP

PM&R SECRETS   ISBN 1-56053-155-X

Last digit is the print number: 9   8   7   6   5   4   3   2

DEDICATIONS

To my beloved parents, Te See and Merla, for their lifelong love and inspiration

To my siblings, Andrew, Crosby, Dorene, and Eldred, for their support and encouragement

To my mentor Keith Sperling, M.D., who instilled in me a valuable clinical ethic: "Treat each patient as though he/she is the most important person in the world."

Bryan J. O'Young, M.D.

In memory of my beloved parents, Michael and Rowena, who during their lifetime and beyond inspired me to strive for academic excellence and always to provide quality and compassionate care to my patients in the process

To my loving wife, Marlene Malka, my children, Michelle, Michael and Jennifer, and my brother, Evan, who have supported me every step of the way

To Professor Heinz Lippmann, M.D., my earliest Physiatry residency mentor and a very special friend, whose example has imparted an unwavering commitment to teaching, scholarship, and patient care

Mark Allen Young, M.D.

To my wife, Beth, and children, Hanna and Duffy, for the love they keep in our "nest."

To my beloved and respected parents, Jean and Bill, for their devotion to meaningful work and their lifelong nurturing of my personhood

To my brothers, Scott and Doug, for their humor and creativity

To my first medical mentor, Gustav Eckstein, M.D., from the University of Cincinnati College of Medicine, who taught me "the body does have a head!"

Reference: Eckstein Gustav: The Body Has a Head. New York, Harper and Row, 1970.

Steven Andrew Stiens, M.D., M.S.

DEDICATION

This book is fondly dedicated to the memory of Arthur A. Siebens, M.D. (1921–1996), the founder of the Department of Physical Medicine and Rehabilitation at the Johns Hopkins University. His first office at the Johns Hopkins Hospital was situated in an old flower shop. He cultivated an interest in rehabilitation that has since blossomed. His exuberance and sensitivity, which nurtured faculty, students, and patients alike, have an enduring presence in all of us.

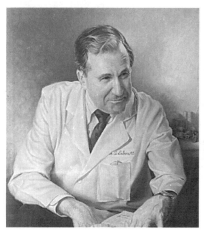 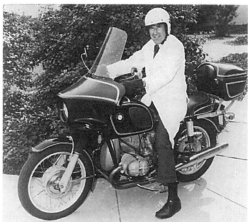

CONTENTS

CONTRIBUTORS

James C. Agre, M.D., Ph.D.
Professor and Chair, Department of Rehabilitation Medicine, University of Wisconsin Medical School, Madison; University of Wisconsin Hospital & Clinics, Madison, Wisconsin

J. Michael Anderson, M.D.
Assistant Professor, Department of Rehabilitation Medicine, Sinai Hospital of Baltimore, Baltimore, Maryland

Linda Jean Anderson, O.T.R.
Occupational Therapist, Owings Mills, Maryland

Elizabeth Augustine, P.T., M.S.
Oncology Services Coordinator, Department of Rehabilitation Medicine, Clinical Center, National Institutes of Health, Bethesda, Maryland

John R. Bach, M.D.
Professor and Vice Chairman, Department of Physical Medicine and Rehabilitation, University of Medicine and Dentistry of New Jersey—New Jersey Medical School, Newark, New Jersey

Jeffrey R. Basford, M.D., Ph.D.
Associate Professor, Department of Physical Medicine and Rehabilitation, Mayo Medical School, Mayo Clinic, Rochester, Minnesota

Norman Berger, B.S., M.S.
Clinical Professor (Retired), Department of Orthopaedic Surgery, New York University Medical Center, New York, New York

Daniel Blanke, Ph.D.
Director and Assistant Professor, School of Health, Physical Education, and Recreation, University of Nebraska at Omaha, Omaha, Nebraska

Michael L. Boninger, M.D.
Assistant Professor, Department of Orthopaedic Surgery, Division of Physical Medicine and Rehabilitation, University of Pittsburgh School of Medicine, Pittsburgh, Pennsylvania; University of Pittsburgh Medical Center, Pittsburgh, Pennsylvania

Marvin M. Brooke, M.D., M.S.
Associate Professor and Chair, Department of Physical Medicine and Rehabilitation, Tufts University School of Medicine, Boston; New England Medical Center, Boston; Sinai Hospital, Stoughton, Massachusetts

Scott E. Brown, M.D.
Department of Rehabilitation Medicine, Sinai Hospital of Baltimore, Baltimore, Maryland

Ann Burkhardt, M.A., O.T.R./L.
Assistant Director of Occupational Therapy, Department of Rehabilitation Medicine, Columbia-Presbyterian Medical Center, New York, New York; Clinical Instructor, Programs in Occupational Therapy, Columbia University College of Physicians and Surgeons, New York, New York

Rene Cailliet, M.D.
Professor Emeritus, Department of Physical Medicine and Rehabilitation, University of Southern California School of Medicine, Los Angeles, California; Santa Monica–UCLA Hospital, Santa Monica, California

Charles Cannizzaro, M.D., P.T.
Orthopaedic, Sports and Industrial Medicine Center of Dublin, Dublin, Georgia

Diana D. Cardenas, M.D.
Professor, Department of Rehabilitation Medicine, University of Washington School of Medicine, Seattle; University of Washington Medical Center, Seattle, Washington

Nancy A. Carlson, M.S., O.T.R./L.
Doctoral Candidate, Department of Human Development, University of Maryland, College Park, Maryland

Thomas J. Cava, M.D.
Director, Department of Physical Medicine and Rehabilitation, PC Rehabilitation Medicine, West Orange, New Jersey; Attending Physician, Mountainside Hospital and Montclair Community Hospital, Montclair, New Jersey

Leighton Chan, M.D., M.P.H.
Acting Assistant Professor, Department of Rehabilitation Medicine, University of Washington, Seattle, Washington

James R. Christensen, M.D.
Assistant Professor, Department of Physical Medicine and Rehabilitation and Department of Pediatrics, The Johns Hopkins University School of Medicine, Baltimore; Johns Hopkins Hospital and The Kennedy Krieger Institute, Baltimore, Maryland

Gary S. Clark, M.D.
Clinical Associate Professor, Department of Rehabilitation Medicine, State University of New York at Buffalo, Buffalo; Head, Department of Rehabilitation Medicine, Buffalo General Hospital, Buffalo, New York

Daniel M. Clinchot, M.D.
Assistant Professor, Department of Physical Medicine and Rehabilitation, The Ohio State University College of Medicine, Columbus, Ohio

Andrea S. Coladner, D.O.
Clinical Instructor, Department of Rehabilitation Medicine, Albert Einstein College of Medicine, Bronx; Associate Director, Physical Medicine and Rehabilitation, Southside Hospital, Bayshore, New York

Jeffrey L. Cole, M.D.
Clinical Associate Professor of Rehabilitation Medicine, Department of Surgery, Cornell Medical College, New York, New York; The New York Hospital Center of Queens, Flushing, New York

Paul J. Corcoran, M.D., M.S.
Lecturer, Department of Physical Medicine and Rehabilitation, Harvard Medical School, Boston; Staff Physiatrist, Spaulding Rehabilitation Hospital, Boston, Massachusetts

Lisa Marie Daley, M.D.
Attending Physician/Clinical Instructor, Department of Physical Medicine and Rehabilitation, New York University School of Medicine, New York, New York; Coler Memorial Hospital, Roosevelt Island, New York

Jacquelyn Dayton, M.S.W., C.S.W.
Social Worker, Rehabilitation Medicine, Columbia-Presbyterian Medical Center, New York, New York

Joel A. DeLisa, M.D., M.S.
Professor and Chairman, Department of Physical Medicine and Rehabilitation, University of Medicine and Dentistry of New Jersey–New Jersey Medical School, Newark, New Jersey; Kessler Institute for Rehabilitation, West Orange, New Jersey; University Hospital, Newark, New Jersey; Saint Barnabas Hospital, Livingston, New Jersey

Nancy M. DeSantis, D.O.
Assistant Professor, Department of Physical Medicine and Rehabilitation, Wayne State University School of Medicine, Detroit; Medical Director, Spinal Cord Injury Unit, Rehabilitation Institute of Michigan, Detroit, Michigan

Nasser Eftekhari, M.D.
Clinical Assistant Professor, Department of Orthopedics and Rehabilitation, University of Miami School of Medicine, Miami; Acting Chief, Physical Medicine and Rehabilitation Service, Veterans Administration Hospital, Miami, Florida

Eli D. Ehrenpreis, M.D.
Staff Gastroenterologist, Department of Gastroenterology, Cleveland Clinic Florida, Ft. Lauderdale, Florida

Susan R. Ehrenthal, M.D.
Attending Physician, Department of Physical Medicine and Rehabilitation, Spaulding Rehabilitation Hospital, Boston, Massachusetts

Maury Ellenberg, M.D.
Associate Professor, Department of Physical Medicine and Rehabilitation, Wayne State University School of Medicine, Detroit, Michigan

Frank J. E. Falco, M.D.
Clinical Assistant Professor, Department of Physical Medicine and Rehabilitation, Temple University School of Medicine, Philadelphia, Pennsylvania; Taylor Hospital, Lester, Pennsylvania; St. Francis Hospital, Wilmington, Delaware; Union Hospital, Elkton, Maryland

Gerald Felsenthal, M.D.
Chief, Department of Rehabilitation Medicine of Sinai Hospital; Clinical Professor, Department of Epidemiology and Preventive Medicine, University of Maryland School of Medicine; Associate Professor, Department of Physical Medicine and Rehabilitation, The Johns Hopkins University School of Medicine, Baltimore, Maryland

Gary J. Fisher
Lantek, Inc., Omaha, Nebraska

Steven V. Fisher, M.D., M.S.
Associate Professor, Department of Physical Medicine and Rehabilitation, Hennepin County Medical Center, University of Minnesota School of Medicine; Chief of Physical Medicine, Hennepin County Medical Center, Minneapolis, Minnesota

Paul S. Fishman, M.D., Ph.D.
Associate Professor, Department of Neurology, University of Maryland School of Medicine, Baltimore; University of Maryland Hospital, Baltimore; Veterans Administration Medical Center, Baltimore, Maryland

Sally S. Fitts, Ph.D.
Research Assistant Professor, Department of Rehabilitation Medicine, University of Washington School of Medicine, Seattle, Washington

Lisa P. Fugate, M.D., M.S.
Assistant Professor, Department of Physical Medicine and Rehabilitation, The Ohio State University College of Medicine, Columbus, Ohio

Fae H. Garden, M.D.
Assistant Professor, Department of Physical Medicine and Rehabilitation, Baylor College of Medicine, Houston; Assistant Chief of Service, Rehabilitation Medicine, St. Luke's Episcopal Hospital, Houston, Texas

Steve R. Geiringer, M.D.
Associate Professor, Department of Physical Medicine and Rehabilitation, Wayne State University, Detroit; Rehabilitation Institute of Michigan, Detroit, Michigan

Theresa A. Gillis, M.D.
Assistant Professor, Department of Physical Medicine and Rehabilitation, Baylor College of Medicine, Houston; Medical Director, Rehabilitation Services, and Chief of Physical Medicine and Rehabilitation Section, The University of Texas M.D. Anderson Cancer Center, Houston, Texas

John Giusto, M.D.
Resident, Department of Physical Medicine and Rehabilitation, Stanford University School of Medicine, Palo Alto, California

Lance L. Goetz, M.D.
Spinal Cord Injury Fellow, Department of Rehabilitation Medicine, Puget Sound Veterans Affairs Medical Center, Seattle, Washington

Kurt V. Gold, M.D.
Immanuel Rehabilitation Center, Omaha, Nebraska

Gary Goldberg, M.D.
Director, Electrodiagnostic Center, Moss Rehabilitation Hospital, Philadelphia; Associate Professor, Department of Physical Medicine and Rehabilitation, Temple University School of Medicine, Philadelphia, Pennsylvania

Stephen Goldberg, M.D.
Associate Professor, Department of Cell Biology and Anatomy, University of Miami School of Medicine, Miami, Florida

Barry Goldstein, M.D., Ph.D.
Assistant Professor, Spinal Cord Injury Service and Department of Rehabilitation Medicine, Department of Veterans Affairs, Puget Sound Health Care System and University of Washington School of Medicine, Seattle, Washington

Peter H. Gorman, M.D.
Assistant Professor, Department of Neurology, University of Maryland Medical System, Baltimore; Chief, Physical Medicine and Rehabilitation Service, Veterans Affairs Maryland Health Care System, Baltimore, Maryland

Carl V. Granger, M.D.
Professor, Department of Rehabilitation Medicine, University of Buffalo School of Medicine, Buffalo; Consulting Physician, Buffalo General Hospital, Erie County Medical Center, Buffalo Veterans Administration Hospital, Buffalo, New York

Bertram Greenspun, D.O.
Clinical Associate Professor, Department of Rehabilitation Medicine, Jefferson Medical College of Thomas Jefferson University, Philadelphia, Pennsylvania; Medical Director, Center for Rehabilitation at Wilmington Hospital, Wilmington, Delaware

Rochelle V. Habeck, Ph.D.
Professor, Department of Counseling, Educational Psychology, and Special Education, Michigan State University, East Lansing, Michigan

Eugen M. Halar, M.D.
Professor, Department of Rehabilitation Medicine, University of Washington School of Medicine, Seattle; Chief, Physical Medicine and Rehabilitation Service, Department of Veterans Affairs, Puget Sound Health Care System, Seattle, Washington

Margaret C. Hammond, M.D.
Associate Professor, Department of Rehabilitation Medicine, University of Washington School of Medicine, Seattle; Chief, SCI Service, Department of Veterans Affairs, Puget Sound Health Care System, Seattle, Washington

Robert L. Harmon, M.D., M.S.
Associate Professor, Department of Physical Medicine and Rehabilitation, Medical College of Ohio, Toledo; Medical College Hospitals, Toledo, Ohio

Richard F. Harvey, M.D.
Executive Vice President, Medical Services, Marianjoy Rehabilitation Hospital and Clinics, Wheaton, Illinois

Joseph M. Helms, M.D.
Founding President, American Academy of Medical Acupuncture, Berkeley, California

John E. Hewett, Ph.D.
Professor of Statistics and Internal Medicine, Department of Statistics, University of Missouri, Columbia, Missouri

Jeanne E. Hicks, M.D.
Deputy Chief, Department of Rehabilitation Medicine, National Institutes of Health, Bethesda, Maryland; Associate Professor of Rehabilitation Medicine, Department of Orthopedics, Georgetown University Medical Center, Washington, D.C.; Associate Professor, Department of Internal Medicine, George Washington University Medical Center, Washington, D.C.

Steven Russell Hinderer, M.D., M.S., P.T.
Assistant Professor, Department of Physical Medicine and Rehabilitation, Wayne State University, Detroit; Rehabilitation Institute of Michigan/Detroit Medical Center, Detroit, Michigan

Howard J. Hoffberg, M.D.
Associate Medical Director, Rehabilitation & Pain Management Associates, Towson, Maryland

Joseph C. Honet, M.D., M.S.
Professor, F.T.A., Department of Physical Medicine and Rehabilitation, Wayne State University School of Medicine, Detroit; Chairman, Department of Physical Medicine and Rehabilitation, Sinai Hospital, Detroit, Michigan

Lawrence J. Horn, M.D.
Coghlin Chair and Professor, Department of Physical Medicine and Rehabilitation, Medical College of Ohio, Toledo; Medical College Hospitals, St. Vincent's Medical Center, Toledo, Ohio

David S. Hungerford, M.D.
Professor, Department of Orthopaedics, The Johns Hopkins University School of Medicine, Baltimore; Good Samaritan Hospital, Johns Hopkins Hospital, Baltimore, Maryland

Edward A. Hurvitz, M.D.
Assistant Professor, Department of Physical Medicine and Rehabilitation, University of Michigan Medical Center, Mott Children's Hospital, Ann Arbor, Michigan

Martin Zelig Kanner, M.D.
Adjunct Assistant Professor, Department of Neurology, University of Maryland School of Medicine, Baltimore, Maryland; Chief, Division of Rehabilitation Medicine, Northwest Hospital Center, Randallstown, Maryland

Richard T. Katz, M.D.
Associate Professor of Clinical Medicine, Physical Medicine & Rehabilitation, St. Louis University School of Medicine; Medical Director and Vice President of Medical Affairs, SSM Rehabilitation Institute, St. Louis, Missouri

D. Casey Kerrigan, M.D., M.S.
Assistant Professor, Department of Physical Medicine and Rehabilitation, Harvard Medical School, Boston; Spaulding Rehabilitation Hospital, Boston, Massachusetts

Dennis Dae-Joo Kim, M.D.
Associate Professor, Department of Rehabilitation Medicine, Albert Einstein College of Medicine, Bronx, New York; Montefiore Medical Center, Bronx, New York

R. Lee Kirby, M.D.
Professor and Head, Division of Physical Medicine and Rehabilitation, Department of Medicine, Dalhousie University, Halifax; Physiatrist-in-Chief, Nova Scotia Rehabilitation Centre, Halifax, Nova Scotia, Canada

Mark D. Klaiman, M.D.
Consultant, Department of Rehabilitation Medicine, National Institutes of Health, Bethesda; Suburban Hospital, Bethesda, Maryland

Stanley H. Kornhauser, Ph.D.
Chief Operating Officer, Queens Surgi-Center, Queens, New York

Marilyn F. Kraus, M.D.
Assistant Professor of Psychiatry, Neuropsychiatry Program, Western Psychiatric Institute and Clinic, University of Pittsburgh School of Medicine, Pittsburgh, Pennsylvania

Francis P. Lagattuta, M.D.
Assistant Clinical Professor, Department of Orthopedics, Section of Rehabilitation, Loyola University of Chicago Stritch School of Medicine, Maywood, Illinois; Glen Oaks Medical Center, Glendale, Illinois

Richard W. Latin, Ph.D.
Professor of Physical Education and Exercise Science, School of Health, Physical Education, and Recreation, University of Nebraska at Omaha, Omaha, Nebraska

Jeffrey Alan Lehman, M.D.
Attending Physiatrist, Sinai/Johns Hopkins Physical Medical and Rehabilitation Residency Training Program, Baltimore, Maryland

Justus F. Lehmann, M.D.
Professor, Department of Rehabilitation Medicine, University of Washington School of Medicine, Seattle, Washington

James W. Leonard, D.O., P.T.
Assistant Professor, Department of Rehabilitation Medicine, University of Wisconsin Hospitals and Clinics, Madison, Wisconsin

Stephen F. Levinson, M.D., Ph.D.
Assistant Professor, Department of Physical Medicine & Rehabilitation, University of Rochester, Rochester; Strong Memorial Hospital, Rochester, New York

Charles E. Levy, M.D.
Assistant Professor, Department of Physical Medicine and Rehabilitation, The Ohio State University College of Medicine, Columbus, Ohio

Janet C. Limke, M.D.
Assistant Professor, Department of Physical Medicine and Rehabilitation, University of Cincinnati, Cincinnati; University Hospital, Drake Center, Cincinnati, Ohio

Heinz I. Lippmann, M.D.
Professor (Emeritus-Active), Department of Rehabilitation Medicine, Albert Einstein College of Medicine of Yeshiva University, New York, New York; Montefiore Hospital, Jack D. Weiler Hospital, Abraham Jacobi Hospital, New York, New York

Saul Liss, Ph.D.
President, C.E.O., MEDI Consultants, Inc., Paterson, New Jersey

James W. Little, M.D., Ph.D.
Associate Professor, Department of Rehabilitation Medicine, University of Washington, Seattle; Assistant Chief, Spinal Cord Injury Service, Department of Veterans Affairs, Puget Sound Health Care System, Seattle, Washington

Constantine G. Lyketsos, M.D., M.H.S.
Assistant Professor, Department of Psychiatry and Mental Hygiene, The Johns Hopkins University School of Medicine, Baltimore, Maryland

Ruth Torkelson Lynch, Ph.D.
Associate Professor, Department of Rehabilitation Psychology and Special Education, Department of Rehabilitation Medicine, University of Wisconsin–Madison, Madison, Wisconsin

Edgar L. Marin, M.D.
Assistant Professor, Department of Rehabilitation Medicine, Albert Einstein College of Medicine of Yeshiva University, Bronx, New York; Director, Physical Medicine and Rehabilitation, Southside Hospital, Bay Shore, New York

Richard S. Materson, M.D.
Professor of Physical Medicine and Rehabilitation, Department of Neurology, George Washington University School of Medicine, Washington, D.C.; Senior Vice President of Medical Affairs and Medical Director, National Rehabilitation Hospital, Washington, D.C.

David G. McDonald, Ph.D.
Professor, Department of Psychology, University of Missouri, Columbia, Missouri

Edward G. McFarland, M.D.
Director of Sports Medicine and Shoulder Surgery, Department of Orthopaedic Surgery, The Johns Hopkins University School of Medicine, Baltimore, Maryland

Arun J. Mehta, M.B.
Associate Clinical Professor, Division of Physical Medicine and Rehabilitation, Department of Medicine, University of California, Los Angeles, School of Medicine, Los Angeles; Assistant Chief, Physical Medicine and Rehabilitation, Veterans Affairs Medical Center, Sepulveda, California

Stuart D. Miller, M.D.
Attending Surgeon, Department of Orthopaedic Surgery, Union Memorial Hospital, Baltimore, Maryland

Susan M. Miller, M.D.
Assistant Professor of Neurology (Rehabilitation Medicine), George Washington University, Washington, D.C.; National Rehabilitation Hospital, Washington, D.C.

Michael A. Mont, M.D.
Associate Professor, Department of Orthopaedics, The Johns Hopkins University School of Medicine, Baltimore; Good Samaritan Hospital, Johns Hopkins Hospital, Baltimore, Maryland

Subhadra L. Nori, M.D.
Assistant Professor, Department of Rehabilitation Medicine, Albert Einstein College of Medicine of Yeshiva University, Bronx; Montefiore Medical Center, Bronx, New York

Kevin O'Connor, M.D.
Assistant Professor, University of Medicine and Dentistry of New Jersey–New Jersey Medical School, Newark, New Jersey; Staff Physiatrist, Kessler Institute for Rehabilitation, West Orange, New Jersey

Abna A. Ogle, M.D.
Assistant Professor, Department of Rehabilitation Medicine, University of Kansas School of Medicine, Kansas City; Dwight D. Eisenhower Veterans Administration Medical Center, Kansas City, Kansas

Theresa Oswald, M.D.
Rehabilitation Physicians of Northeast Wisconsin, Green Bay, Wisconsin

Bryan O'Young, M.D.
Instructor, Department of Physical Medicine and Rehabilitation, The Johns Hopkins University School of Medicine, Good Samaritan Hospital, The Johns Hopkins Hospital, Baltimore, Maryland

Jerry C. Parker, Ph.D.
Chief, Psychology Service, Harry S. Truman Memorial Veterans Hospital, Columbia, Missouri

Jaywant J. P. Patil, M.B.B.S., F.R.C.P.C.
Assistant Professor, Department of Medicine, Division of Pulmonary Medicine and Rehabilitation, Dalhousie University, Halifax; Active Staff, Queen Elizabeth II Health Sciences Centre, Nova Scotia Rehabilitation Centre, Halifax, Nova Scotia, Canada

Inder Perkash, M.D.
Professor, Department of Urology and of Physical Medicine and Rehabilitation; Paralyzed Veterans of America Professor of Spinal Cord Injury Medicine, Stanford University School of Medicine; Chief, Spinal Cord Injury Service, Department of Veterans Affairs Medical Center, Palo Alto, California

Frank S. Pidcock, M.D.
Assistant Professor, Department of Physical Medicine and Rehabilitation, Department of Pediatrics, The Johns Hopkins University School of Medicine, Baltimore; Johns Hopkins Hospital and the Kennedy Krieger Institute, Baltimore, Maryland

Tim L. Popovitch, M.S., R.D., L.D.
Chief Clinical Dietician, Department of Nutritional Services, Cleveland Clinic Florida, Ft. Lauderdale, Florida

Joel M. Press, M.D.
Clinical Assistant Professor, Department of Physical Medicine and Rehabilitation, Northwestern University Medical School, Chicago, Illinois

Michael M. Priebe, M.D.
Assistant Professor, Department of Physical Medicine and Rehabilitation, Baylor College of Medicine, Houston; Assistant Chief, Spinal Cord Injury Service, Veterans Affairs Medical Center, Houston, Texas

Kristjan T. Ragnarsson, M.D.
Dr. Lucy G. Moses Professor, Department of Rehabilitation Medicine, Mount Sinai School of Medicine, New York, New York; Chairman, Rehabilitation Medicine, Mount Sinai Medical Center, New York, New York

Rajiv R. Ratan, M.D., Ph.D.
Assistant Professor, Department of Neurology, Harvard Medical School, Boston; Beth Israel Hospital, Boston, Massachusetts

John B. Redford, M.D.
Professor, Department of Rehabilitation Medicine, University of Kansas School of Medicine, Kansas City, Kansas; University of Kansas Hospital, Kansas City, Kansas

Leon Reinstein, M.D.
Associate Professor, Department of Rehabilitation Medicine, The Johns Hopkins University School of Medicine; Clinical Professor, Department of Epidemiology and Preventive Medicine, University of Maryland School of Medicine; Associate Medical Director, Sinai Rehabilitation Center, Baltimore, Maryland

James K. Richardson, M.D.
Assistant Professor, Department of Physical Medicine and Rehabilitation, University of Michigan Medical School; Medical Director, Inpatient Rehabilitation Unit, University of Michigan Medical Center, Ann Arbor, Michigan

Mary Richardson, Ph.D., M.H.A.
Associate Professor, Department of Health Services, University of Washington, Seattle, Washington

Elizabeth A. Rivers, O.T.R., R.N.
Clinical Instructor in Rehabilitation, University of Minnesota Medical School, Minneapolis; Burn Rehabilitation Specialist, St. Paul-Ramsey Burn Center, St. Paul, Minnesota

Richard C. Robinson, M.D.
Assistant Professor, Department of Rehabilitation Medicine, University of Kansas Medical Center; Dwight D. Eisenhower Veterans Administration Medical Center, Kansas City, Kansas

Arthur A. Rodriquez, M.D.
Professor, Department of Rehabilitation Medicine, University of Wisconsin Medical School, Madison; University of Wisconsin Hospital & Clinics, Madison, Wisconsin

Richard A. Rogachefsky, M.D.
Assistant Professor, Department of Orthopedics, University of Miami; Jackson Memorial Medical Center, Miami, Florida

Norman B. Rosen, M.D.
Medical Director, Rehabilitation and Pain Management Associates of Baltimore, Baltimore, Maryland

Elliot J. Roth, M.D.
Professor and Chairman, Department of Physical Medicine and Rehabilitation, Northwestern University Medical School; Medical Director, Rehabilitation Institute of Chicago, Chicago, Illinois

Melinda-Ann Baker Roth, M.D.
Medical Director of the Women's Rehabilitation Center of Pomona and Private Practice, Owings Mills, Maryland

Jason Rudolph, M.D.
Chief Resident, Department of Orthopaedic Surgery, Monmouth Medical Center, Long Branch, New Jersey

Anthony S. Salzano, M.D.
Medical Director, Department of Physical Medicine, Westchester Square Medical Center, Bronx, New York; Clinical Assistant Professor, Department of Rehabilitation Medicine, Albert Einstein College of Medicine of Yeshiva University, Bronx, New York

Francisco H. Santiago, M.D.
Assistant Clinical Professor, Department of Rehabilitation Medicine, Albert Einstein College of Medicine of Yeshiva University, Bronx, New York; Assistant Medical Director, Department of Physical Medicine and Rehabilitation, Flushing Hospital Medical Center, Flushing, New York

Jay Schechtman, M.D.
Instructor, Department of Rehabilitation Medicine, Mount Sinai Medical School, New York, New York

Carson D. Schneck, M.D., Ph.D.
Professor, Department of Anatomy and Cell Biology, Temple University School of Medicine, Philadelphia, Pennsylvania

Lew C. Schon, M.D.
Attending Surgeon, Department of Orthopedic Surgery, The Union Memorial Hospital, Baltimore, Maryland

Michael L. Schwartz, M.D.
Assistant Professor, Department of Radiology, Wayne State University School of Medicine, Detroit, Michigan

Jay P. Shah, M.D.
Medical Officer/Staff Physiatrist, Department of Rehabilitation Medicine, National Institutes of Health, Bethesda, Maryland

Aaron Shamberg, M.L.A.
Abilities OT Services, Baltimore, Maryland

Shoshana Shamberg, O.T.R./L.
Abilities OT Services, Baltimore, Maryland

C. Norman Shealy, M.D., Ph.D.
Professor, Department of Psychology, Forest Institute of Professional Psychology; Director, Shealy Institute, Springfield, Missouri

Joseph A. Shrader, P.T., C.Ped.
Senior Staff Physical Therapist, Department of Rehabilitation Medicine, National Institutes of Health, Bethesda, Maryland

Arthur A. Siebens, M.D. (deceased)
The Richard Bennett Darnall Professor of Rehabilitation Medicine, The Johns Hopkins University School of Medicine; Former Director of the Department of Rehabilitation Medicine, The Johns Hopkins University, The Johns Hopkins Hospital, and The Good Samaritan Hospital of Maryland; Director of Pharyngology Research at the Milton Dance Center at Greater Baltimore Medical Center, Baltimore, Maryland

Kenneth H. C. Silver, M.D.
Associate Professor, Department of Neurology, University of Maryland School of Medicine, Baltimore; Director, Outpatient Rehabilitation Services, Kernan Hospital; Assistant Chief, Baltimore Veterans Affairs Medical Center, Baltimore, Maryland

Warren Slaten, M.D.
Associate Medical Director, Capitol Rehabilitation Clinic, Milwaukee, Wisconsin

Richard M. Smith, Ph.D.
Senior Research Scientist, Rehabilitation Foundation, Inc., Wheaton, Illinois

John Speed, M.B.B.S.
Associate Professor, Division of Physical Medicine and Rehabilitation, University of Utah School of Medicine, Salt Lake City; University of Utah Health Sciences Center, Salt Lake City, Utah

Neil Spiegel, D.O.
Center for Physical Medicine and Rehabilitation, Rockville; Medical Director, Department of Physical Medicine and Rehabilitation, Shady Grove Adventist Hospital, Rockville, Maryland

Barry David Stein, M.D.
Clinical Assistant Professor, Department of Epidemiology and Preventive Medicine, University of Maryland School of Medicine, Baltimore, Maryland

Steven A. Stiens, M.D., M.S.
Assistant Professor, Department of Rehabilitation, University of Washington School of Medicine, Seattle; Staff Physician, SCI Service, VA Puget Sound Health Care System, University Hospital, Seattle, Washington

Jay V. Subbarao, M.D., M.S.
Clinical Professor and Chief, Division of Physical Medicine and Rehabilitation, Department of Orthopaedics, Loyola University of Chicago Stritch School of Medicine, Maywood, Illinois; Director, Comprehensive Rehabilitation Service, Associate Chief of Staff, Hines Veterans Affairs Hospital, Hines, Illinois

W. Stephen Tankersley, M.D.
Fellow, Department of Orthopaedics, The Johns Hopkins University School of Medicine, Baltimore; Good Samaritan Hospital, Johns Hopkins Hospital, Baltimore, Maryland

Kay Thigpen, Ph.D.
Executive Director, Texas Orthopaedic and Sports Medicine Institute, San Antonio, Texas

Mark A. Thomas, M.D.
Assistant Professor, Department of Rehabilitation Medicine, Albert Einstein College of Medicine of Yeshiva University, Bronx; Attending Physiatrist, Montefiore Medical Center, Bronx, New York

Denise W. Thrope, M.S., C.C.C./A.
Clinical Audiologist, Northwest ENT Associates, Baltimore; Sinai Hospital of Baltimore, Baltimore, Maryland

Donna Clark Tippett, M.P.H., M.A., C.C.C.-S.L.P.
Senior Speech-Language Pathologist, Department of Communication Sciences and Disorders, University of Maryland Medical System, Baltimore; Instructor, Department of Physical Medicine and Rehabilitation, The Johns Hopkins University School of Medicine, Baltimore, Maryland

Brian M. Torpey, M.D.
Clinical and Academic Instructor, Department of Orthopaedic Surgery, Monmouth Medical Center, Long Branch, New Jersey

David Tostenrude, C.T.R.S.
Recreation Therapist, Department of Physical Medicine and Rehabilitation, Spinal Cord Injury Unit, Department of Veterans Affairs, Puget Sound Health Care System, Seattle, Washington

Ramon Vallarino, Jr., M.D.
Chief Resident, Department of Physical Medicine and Rehabilitation, Albert Einstein College of Medicine, Bronx, New York

Stanley F. Wainapel, M.D., M.P.H.
Associate Professor, Department of Rehabilitation Medicine, Albert Einstein College of Medicine, Bronx; Clinical Director, Rehabilitation Medicine, Jacobi Medical Center, Bronx, New York

Elizabeth T. Walz, M.D.
Assistant Professor, Department of Neurology, The Ohio State University College of Medicine, Columbus, Ohio

Steven B. Weinfeld, M.D.
Fellow, Foot and Ankle Service, Department of Orthopaedic Surgery, Union Memorial Hospital, Baltimore, Maryland

Ruth K. Westheimer, Ed.D.
Adjunct Professor, Department of Continuing Education, New York University, New York, New York

Raymond E. Wright, Ph.D.
Senior Research Scientist, Rehabilitation Foundation, Inc., Wheaton, Illinois

Jeffrey L. Young, M.D.
Assistant Professor, Department of Physical Medicine and Rehabilitation, Northwestern University Medical School, Chicago, Illinois

Mark A. Young, M.D., F.A.C.P.
Assistant Professor, The Johns Hopkins University School of Medicine; Attending Physician, The Johns Hopkins Hospital and Good Samaritan Hospital; Director of Inpatient Physiatry Consultative Services, The Johns Hopkins Hospital; Assistant Program Director–Hopkins Campus, The Sinai-Hopkins Physical Medicine and Rehabilitation Residency Training Program, Baltimore, Maryland

Cynthia Perry Zejdlik, R.N.
Rehabilitation Consultant, Bellingham, Washington

PREFACE

"To learn, you must ask the right questions so the answer will always remain with you."

– Confucius

Questions and answers drive the relationship of student and mentor through didactic dialogue. Their context reveals the process of clinical thought through reflection on experience and science. It is evident that such exchanges promote the student's formulation of questions as new clinical challenges are confronted. It is "the question" that leads the clinician to the vast variety of contemporary medical literature in search of answers. Should no answer be found, the question may provide the hypothesis for research.

Answers can be derived from many knowledge sources. *PM&R Secrets* emphasizes academic interaction and the thought processes of rehabilitation. It, therefore, does not replace a comprehensive text but acts as a bridge to interactive learning. Traditional texts offer students rediscovery of knowledge by building from anatomy to physiology then presenting pathology, pathokinesiology, evaluation and treatment. In practice, solutions for patients are accomplished through multifaceted physiatric interventions directed at multiple system levels and the effects are measured within varied outcome domains. Educational materials that respond to these challenges of practice are needed. The Socratic technique in *PM&R Secrets* assembles knowledge through answers to clinically pertinent questions, thereby complementing existing PM&R knowledge sources.

The authors of *PM&R Secrets* have crafted a book that skillfully uses techniques of classical philosophy to maintain the academic and medical traditions of bedside teaching. These logical sequences of questions and answers are expected to enrich rehabilitation by driving the clinician to the traditional texts, the primary references, and the laboratory!

Justus F. Lehmann, M.D.
Professor
Department of Rehabilitation Medicine
University of Washington School of Medicine
Seattle, Washington

INTRODUCTION: SOCRATIC LEARNING OF PM&R

"A physician is obligated to consider more than a diseased organ, more even than the whole person; the physician must view patients in their world."

— *Harvey Cushing*

1. Why the Socratic method of PM&R education?

This book emphasizes learning "in context." We have used the Socratic method because this is how knowledge is tested and applied in medical interchanges on the ward, at the bedside, in the conference room, and in oral examinations. These questions are questions you may ask yourself, patients may ask, or you may hear them from a colleague or an attending. The questions are designed to be thought-provoking and to develop the topic in stages with an emphasis on study.

2. What is the Socratic method of learning and how does it relate to medicine and rehabilitation?

Socrates was a Greek philosopher and moralist who focused primarily on the thinker and on methods for knowing rather than the knowledge itself. The Socratic method of learning requires an engaging dialogue with questions and answers between the teacher and student that brings the student from "the complacent dogmatic slumber of an unexamined opinion to a state of humility and perplexity."[3] It is a process of debunking pretensions and assumes that ignorance is a pedagogically useful device.

This dialectic educational model is particularly potent because it explicitly focuses on immediate patient problem-solving and implicitly educates the audience by answering questions they have regarding the management rationale. Furthermore, the exercise teaches students and staff members interaction techniques that bring forth critical rehabilitation issues for discussion and resolution.

3. What is "pimping"?

Pimping occurs when a medical "teacher" riddles the trainee with a series of difficult questions. Sir William Osler was reported to fire such questions at residents like a Gatling gun on the wards of the Johns Hopkins Hospital.[1] The tradition is celebrated to this day in rehabilitation education when residents present the intricate details of patients' diagnoses, disablement, environment, and personhood to the scrutiny of master clinicians.[5] Such a lively event is educational and humorous if orchestrated sensitively and received without pretention. This Socratic exercise builds effective physiatrists, nurses, therapists, prosthetists/orthotists, and other rehabilitationists.

4. How does one learn rehabilitation medicine?

The foundation of effective practice is applied knowledge of anatomy, physiology, kinesiology, and the social sciences. Prerequisites include a reflective awareness of one's own personal development and empathic regard for the individual priorities of others. The practice of Physical Medicine and Rehabilitation is an extension of general, disease-focused medical intervention. The biomedical model emphasizes diagnosis of illness and focused treatment as a mechanism for patient life enhancement. The rehabilitation process requires questioning of patients to determine the goals that will enhance their personal effectiveness despite the effects of illness or injury. Clinical data are derived through an exploration of the chief complaint that goes beyond diagnosis to include the secondary effects on the patient. The side effects can be categorized as related to the interactive Hierarchy of Natural Systems organization levels as described in the Biopsychosocial Model: subatomic particles, atoms, molecules, organelles, cells, tissue, organ system, nervous system, [person], two-person, family, community, culture–subculture, society–nation, biosphere.[2]

Learning through the practice of rehabilitation requires an ongoing commitment to understanding a patient's personal goals and integrating scientifically sound interventions to achieve them. Rehabilitation, therefore, is learned one patient at a time as unique combinations of interventions are orchestrated to produce unique solutions for particular persons.

5. How does the rehabilitation problem list guide learning?

In reviewing a patient, the focus of Socratic dialogue logically progresses from diagnosis confirmation through secondary effects by system level, with the problem list as an agenda. The problem list should be organized first to include the primary diagnoses followed by secondary effects as guided by the Hierarchy of Natural Systems. Discussion of each problem produces educational objectives for the clinician that are focused on the immediate care of a particular patient.

6. How should I use this book to improve my rehabilitation practice?

The chapter titles are organized for the sequential development of rehabilitation knowledge as related to specific problems or interventions. In practice the text is best used "in context." The book is meant to be part of the clinic, ward work, library research, and home study. Patient problems should generate questions to be answered. The text attempts to anticipate questions and provide answers. Review of these questions and answers provides a springboard for group discussions and should generate new sets of questions and answers that can be sought using problem-based learning techniques.[6]

7. What do you mean when you say this book is a developmental textbook?

PM&R Secrets offers the learner information that meets his or needs through all stages of rehabilitation medicine practice development. As such, the book is as useful to a beginner as it is to an established practitioner and educator in rehabilitation. For the novice student of rehabilitation, clear definitions and outlines of the rehabilitation process are provided. For the resident, specific evaluation techniques and questions are provided as a means to complement the resident's established medical knowledge and expand and integrate the functional approach to illness. For the rehabilitation educator, new questions are offered to carry on the Socratic tradition. Share it and enjoy!

REFERENCES

1. Brancati FL: The art of pimping. JAMA 262(1):89–90, 1989.
2. Engel GL: The clinical application of the biopsychosocial model. Am J Psychiatry 137:535–544, 1980.
3. Pekarsky D: Socratic teaching: A critical assessment. J Moral Educ 23:119–134, 1994.
4. Sherman RS: Is it possible to teach socratically? Thinking 6:28–36, 1986.
5. Stolov WC, Hays RH: Evaluation of the patient. In Kottke FS, Lehmann JF (eds): Krussen's Handbook of Physical Medicine and Rehabilitation, 4th ed. Philadelphia, W.B. Saunders, 1990, pp 1–20.
6. Albanese MA, Mitchell S: Problem-based learning: A review of literature on its outcomes and implementation issues. Acad Med 68:52–81, 1993.

Steven A. Stiens, M.D., M.S.
Bryan O'Young, M.D.
Mark A. Young, M.D.

ACKNOWLEDGMENTS

We would like to thank our patients, who provided us with the motivation for this volume. We appreciate their evocative questions which often lead to unique rehabilitation goals and research ideas.

The Editors wish to graciously acknowledge the following editorial consultants who have provided or reviewed selected materials for this textbook.

Michael Bokulich, Charles Cannizzarro, M.D., P.T.; Gloria Eng, M.D.; Charles Enzer, M.D.; George Engel, M.D.; George Kraft, M.D.; Justus Lehmann, M.D.; Richard Lehneis, Ph.D.; Heinz Lippmann, M.D.; David Jesse Peters, M.D., Ph.D.; Deborah McLeish, M.D.; Lawrence Robinson, M.D.; Keith Sperling, M.D.; and Donna C. Tippett, M.P.H., M.A., C.C.C.-S.L.P.

We are indebted to our publisher, Linda Belfus, for her practicality and expertise.

The Editors also which to extend special thanks to our colleagues and residents at the Johns Hopkins University and the University of Washington who have provided us with the academic inspiration and scholarly support to make this project a reality.

This book would not be in print without the creative, congenial, and diligent support from Debra Roberts, who revised manuscripts; Mia Hannula and other VA library staff, who researched topics; Karna McKinney, who created figures; and the staff of the VA Medical Media Department.

I. Fundamentals of PM&R

1. THE PERSON, DISABLEMENT, AND THE PROCESS OF REHABILITATION

Steven A. Stiens, M.D., Bryan O'Young, M.D., and Mark A. Young, M.D.

1. How are the person and personhood relevant to rehabilitation?

The **person** is a particular living human being with characteristic genetic, physical, mental, social, and spiritual dimensions. He or she is guided by past experience, changes through development, and is self-determining through life decisions made with free will.

The person therefore is the "real self," the subject of rehabilitation intervention. As such, **personhood** is the dynamic process of being and becoming the self. Awareness of the patient's self-understanding is critical to rehabilitation success. The person has the right of choice in problem-solving and is an essential contributor to health goal-setting.

2. What is health? Illness? Disease?

Health is the optimum condition of a person: physical, mental, and social well-being. Health is not merely the absence of disease or infirmity. An **illness** is the patient's unique subjective experience of "unwellness," distress or failed function. Illness is not only a biologic state but can be an existential transformation that affects trust in the body and reliance on the future. A **disease** is the medical construct that diagnoses a disorder as characterized by a set of symptoms, signs, and pathology, and attributable to infection, diet, heredity, or environment.

3. What is a patient? Case? Client?

A **patient** is a person who is affected by injury, illness, or disease and is under active medical treatment to return to better health. Working with a person as a patient implies an active medical relationship with expectations beyond that of a case, client, or customer. A **case** is an instance of disease or injury with its attendant circumstances as abstracted from the person for scientific study or education. A **client** is one for whom services are rendered, a patron, and does not require the person's participation in the relationship. Things are done for clients. A **customer** merely buys good or services.

4. What are the five responsibilities of the physician in the physician–patient relationship?

The practice of medicine requires the physician–patient relationship, within which the physician does five things:

1. **Suspension of judgment** means respect for the patient's personal values and priorities without imposing your own. Through empathy the physician seeks the patient's perspective.

2. **Evaluation** requires acquiring knowledge of the patient as a person, the manifestations of their disease or illness, and their unique experience of disablement.

3. **Diagnosis** requires an integration of many symptoms, signs, findings, and test results and deduction to a cause or syndrome.

4. In **reporting**, the physician interprets the diagnosis and prognosis of the condition for the patient and provides the education required for informed choices.

5. **Treatment** requires a formulation, prescription, or plan which is then offered for the patient's informed consent.

5. How does the understanding of suffering contribute to patient care?

Suffering must be differentiated from pain: **pain** is the psychophysiologic process of perception in response to nociceptive stimuli, whereas **suffering** is the perception of a threat to the intactness of personhood (i.e., the person's perception of his or her lived past, present, and future, the family, culture and societal roles, and others). Suffering can include physical pain but is not limited to it. Suffering can be relieved when the perception of threat is reinterpreted into a positive meaning. For example, childbirth can be excruciatingly painful, yet considered rewarding. The perceived meaning of pain influences the amount of medication required to control it. For example, a patient who believed that her pain was caused by sciatica could control it with small doses of codeine, but when she discovered that it was caused by malignant disease, a much greater amount of medication was required for relief.

6. How can the effects of the disease on the person be practically classified?

The World Health Organization published the International Classification of Impairments, Disabilities, and Handicaps (ICIDH) as a conceptual scheme for the consequences of disease. These collective consequences of disease on the health of the person, or **disablement**, can be conceptualized within three related system domains: (1) the **organ** or system, (2) the **person**, and (3) **society**. Limitations or deficits within these domains lie in three respective dimensions: impairment (organ domain), disability (person domain), or handicap (societal domain).

7. Define impairment.

An **impairment** is any loss or abnormality of a psychological, physiologic, or anatomic structure or function. Examples include loss of limb, weakness, sensory deficit, and facial disfigurement.

8. Define disability.

A **task** is a purposeful activity that requires engagement of the whole person. A disability is any restriction or lack (resulting from an impairment) of a person's ability to perform a task or activity within the range considered normal for a human. An example is an inability to perform activities of daily living, such as dressing, driving, shopping, or cooking.

9. How is handicap defined in the relationship of the person to society?

Handicap results from the interaction of the person (including impairments and disabilities) with the immediate environment (physical, psychological, and social). The resultant handicap is the disadvantage for a given individual, stemming from impairments and/or disabilities, in performing a role otherwise normal (age/sex-appropriate) for an individual.

10. What is rehabilitation?

In contrast to classic medical therapeutics, which emphasizes diagnosis and treatment directed against a pathologic process, rehabilitation produces multiple simultaneous interventions addressing both the cause and secondary effects of injury and illness (**Biopsychosocial Model**). Traditionally, medical science has directed treatment at the cause of disease (**Biomedical Model**), neglecting the secondary effects of illness. The very nature of rehabilitation includes assessment of the individual's personal capacities, role performance, and life aspirations.

Rehabilitation has been defined as the development of a person to his or her fullest physical, psychological, social, vocational, avocational, and educational potential, consistent with his or her physiology or anatomic impairment and environmental limitations. **Comprehensive rehabilitation** can be further considered to require five necessary and sufficient subcomponents:

1. Unique patient-centered plan, formulated by the patient and rehabilitation team
2. Goals derived and prioritized through an interdisciplinary process
3. Patient participation required to achieve the goals
4. Results in improvement in the patient's personal potential
5. Outcomes demonstrate reduction in impairments, disabilities, and handicaps

11. How did the specialty of Physical Medicine & Rehabilitation originate?

The specialty first grew out of organizations such as the American Congress of Physical Therapy founded by the AMA in 1921. Later, in 1936, Frank H. Krusen, M.D., started the first residency training program in "physical medicine" at the Mayo Clinic and proposed the term *physiatrist—fiz-ee-at'-rist*—for the graduates. The American Board of Physical Medicine was recognized in 1947 and the name was changed to the American Board of PM&R to recognize and include physicians within the specialty that practiced and promoted holistic rehabilitation.

12. What is the multidisciplinary practice of patient care? How does it differ from interdisciplinary practice?

Multidisciplinary teams consist of various professionals treating the patient separately, with discipline-specific goals. Patient progress with each discipline is communicated through documentation or at meetings for information exchange.

In the interdisciplinary collaborative practice model, each distinct profession evaluates the patient separately and then interacts together at team meetings, where they share assessments and long-term and short-term goals. The goals of each discipline are coordinated into a unified plan through the synergistic interaction of the team. The whole outcome therefore is more than the sum of the component parts. In addition, the team collaboratively participates in problem-solving and decision-making as the plan is carried out.

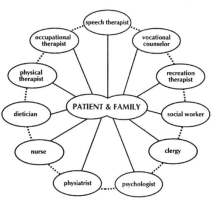

Interdisciplinary team interaction. (From Mumma CM, Nelson A: Models for theory-based practice of rehabilitation nursing. In Hoeman SD (ed): Rehabilitation Nursing: Process and Application. St. Louis, Mosby, 1995, with permission.)

13. What 9 conditions maximize the success of interdisciplinary rehabilitation teams?
1. Allegiance to a mission statement (i.e., person-centered rehab in the least restrictive setting)
2. Specifically delineated roles for each discipline
3. Balance of participation by each professional
4. Agreement on and implementation of ground rules for interaction
5. Clear and effective communication and documentation
6. Scientific approach to patient problems
7. Clearly defined, measurable goals
8. Working knowledge of group process
9. Expedient procedures for coming to consensus and decision-making

14. How does a transdisciplinary team interact?

Transdisciplinary teams are designed through cross-training of members and procedure development to allow **overlap of responsibilities** between disciplines. This overlap allows flexibility in problem-solving and produces closer interdependence of team members. Leadership may differ for each patient served by the team. Disciplines with extensive involvement with the patient may become **case managers** and coordinate team efforts.

15. Describe the phases in the rehabilitation process.

Phase I (Evaluation) requires knowledge of the patient's personal life tasks, roles, and aspirations. The individual effects of disablement (impairment, disability, and handicap) on the person are quantified. The person's unique characteristics—mediators that allow for adaptive capacity—limiting disablement severity are identified and targeted as foci for therapy. **Phase II** emphasizes treatment to arrest the pathophysiologic processes causing tissue injury. **Phase III (Therapeutic Exercise)** focuses on enhancement of organ performance. **Phase IV (Task Reacquisition)** emphasizes total person adaptive techniques. **Phase V (Environmental Modification)** directs efforts toward environmental enhancement (physical, psychological, social and political) to reduce handicap.

These phases approximate the emphasis of the team's interventions during a continuum that guides the patient out of acute treatment of the injury (or disease) and into reintegration into the community. The rehabilitation problem list is a sequence of diagnoses, impairments, disabilities, and handicaps that guide goal setting. Members of the rehabilitation team derive goals from their encounters with the patient as a whole person. The patient drives the process by demonstrating his or her particular predicament with disablement. Adaptation is achieved by enhancing the patient's personal characteristics that mediate or limit the disablement. The overall goal is the fullest personal enablement and action toward fulfillment of life roles.

BIBLIOGRAPHY

1. Bagley EM: An introduction to the concepts and classifications of the international classification of impairments, disabilities, and handicaps. Disabil Rehabil 15(4):161–178, 1993.
2. Cassell EJ: The nature of suffering and the goals of medicine. N Engl J Med 306:639–645, 1982.
3. Emanuel EJ, Emanuel LL: Four models of the physician-patient relationship. JAMA 267:2221–2226, 1992.
4. Granger CV, Gresham GE: International classification of impairments, disabilities, and handicaps (ICIDH) as a conceptual basis for stroke outcome research. Stroke 21(suppl II):II-66–II-67, 1990.
5. Rogers CR: A theory of therapy, personality and interpersonal relationships as developed in the client-centered framework. In Koch S (ed): A Study of Science: Vol III. Formulation of the Person and the Social Context. New York, McGraw HIll, 1959, p 184.
6. Stiens SA, Haselkorn JK, Peters DJ, Goldstein B: Rehabilitation intervention for patients with upper extremity dysfunction: Challenges of outcome evaluation. Am J Ind Med 29:590–601, 1996.

2. FUNCTIONAL OUTCOME MEASUREMENTS

Gary S. Clark, M.D., and Carl V. Granger, M.D.

1. Why is functional assessment and outcome so important suddenly?

Rehabilitation services are labor-intensive (involving many health professionals on the rehab team) and relatively expensive, at least in the short-term. This makes rehabilitation a likely target for cost-cutting under a managed-care health system, unless the cost-effectiveness of these services is documented objectively. To accomplish this goal requires that we be able to measure—and show—improvement in function (functional assessment) as a result of the rehabilitation intervention (functional outcome).

2. How can functional assessment help to establish cost-effectiveness of rehabilitation services?

The goal of rehabilitation intervention is to maximize functional independence such that an individual is able to function without needing assistance from others. That person's quality of life is thereby improved, avoiding a significant (up to lifelong) "burden of care" that otherwise would be needed to provide for his or her needs. By minimizing or eliminating this costly "burden of care," the up-front investment in rehabilitation services proves to be cost-effective in the long run.

3. What is functional assessment?

According to Lawton, functional assessment includes "any systematic attempt to measure objectively the level at which a person is functioning, in any of a variety of areas such as physical health, quality of self-maintenance, quality of role activity, intellectual status, social activity, attitude toward the world and self, and emotional status."

4. Please translate that!

In the context of rehabilitation, functional assessment has typically been applied to measuring what an individual is able to do for himself or herself, most commonly in self-care (activities of daily living, or ADL) and mobility. Other areas of function frequently assessed include homemaking skills (e.g., cooking, cleaning, laundry) and related instrumental ADL (IADL) skills, also referred to as community survival skills (e.g., using a telephone, managing a checkbook, shopping).

5. What self-care skills do the ADLs include?

Eating, grooming (e.g., brushing teeth, combing hair, shaving, applying makeup), bathing, dressing, and personal hygiene (e.g., toileting). Bathing and dressing can be divided into upper-body and lower-body management.

6. But what about mobility?

A variety of types of mobility can be assessed. **Bed mobility** includes sitting up and lying down in bed, as well as turning side-to-side. **Transfers** refer to moving between bed, chair (or wheelchair), toilet, and bathtub. Other forms of mobility include propelling a wheelchair (**wheelchair mobility**), actual walking (**ambulation**), as well as negotiating stairs, curbs, and uneven surfaces (e.g., sidewalks, ramps, gravel, grass).

7. How is function measured if someone needs help to perform an activity?

Most functional assessment scales include an indicator of level of function, or degree of assistance needed to complete a particular task. Someone who is able to complete a task with no outside input or assistance is considered independent. Another individual may demonstrate modified independence, as result of needing an assistive device (such as a cane or long-handled reacher). An individual performs an activity with supervision if he or she needs verbal cueing, coaxing, or set-up, without physical contact. The need for physical assistance ranges from contact guard (touching for balance only), to minimal assist, moderate assist, maximal assist, or dependent (depending on the amount of assistance required).

8. Are there other types of function, besides physical function, that can be measured?

Assessment strategies have been developed for a variety of other domains, including **mental functioning** (cognition, emotional, or affective state), **social functioning** (social contacts and relationships, social roles, activities), and **quality of daily living**. Attempts have also been made to combine multiple domains in global or multidimensional measures. By the same token, more focused (unidimensional) scales have also been developed (e.g., for aphasia).

9. Why do we need to measure function? Why not just describe it?

Standardized measurements of function improve on a clinician's observation and narrative description by providing objective, uniform data in a format useful for clinical decision-making. Functional assessment measurements can provide a baseline against which changes in function can be detected and monitored over time. These data may be useful in determining the effectiveness of a particular intervention (e.g., medication, bracing, therapy). Functional assessment instruments have been studied in different health care settings (inpatient rehab, outpatient, long-term care), demonstrating their ability to detect functional, cognitive, affective, and continence dysfunctions unrecognized on clinical examination.

10. If functional assessment is so helpful, why doesn't everyone use it?

There is no one assessment instrument that can measure everything that may be necessary or useful clinically. Many measures were developed for a specific purpose or in a particular setting but may not be generalizable to other settings or purposes. The more comprehensive an instrument, the more cumbersome it is: more time is required for clinicians to learn to administer it properly, and it takes longer to complete (and analyze).

While there is general agreement that a particular diagnosis (e.g., stroke, arthritis) does not connote the degree of functional impairment, it is equally true that functional assessment instruments cannot be used to reach a medical diagnosis. However, once a diagnosis has been established, functional assessment can provide an indication of the impact on the individual's ability to live and function independently (degree of disability).

11. What is the difference between impairment, disability, and handicap?

An **impairment** is a physical (or psychological) abnormality, which is usually a manifestation of a disease process or injury (tissue or organ level). Examples include painful limited range of joint motion due to arthritic inflammation or muscle weakness poststroke.

Disability is the resulting loss of ability to perform a particular activity or function, such as buttoning a shirt for the arthritis patient or ambulating for the stroke patient (whole-person level). There is clearly neither a one-to-one nor fixed relationship between impairment and disability: the arthritis patient's joint inflammation may be improved with medication, enabling him or her to regain function, or an adaptive device may be used to compensate for the impairment.

An individual who is unable to fulfill a usual role or life activity as a result of an impairment or disability now has a **handicap**. This could occur for a stroke patient if he or she is unable to get out of a nonaccessible house because of stairs. The handicap might be reversed by installing a chair-glide or elevator, without changing the patient's underlying impairment or disability.

12. So how do you measure functional status?

A number of functional assessment "instruments" (or scales) have been developed over the last several decades, beginning with Rankin in 1957. These measurements vary in their purpose, scope, detail, and often the type of patient or patient care setting for which they were developed.

Another variable is the method used to obtain information about patients. Self-report scales involve completion of a questionnaire by the patient. Observer-report scales are similar, but rely on a proxy to complete the questionnaire (usually a family member living with the patient or a health care professional working with the patient). Discrepancies may occur between these two measures, as patients frequently rate their function higher than observers do.

Advantages of interviewer-administered scales include ensuring that a complete data set is obtained and the ability to explore identified problem areas further. Disadvantages involve the time and cost to conduct the interview and the potential for interviewer bias in recording responses. Finally, the direct observation method requires a trained examiner/observer who rates the ability of a patient to perform various functional tasks. While more precise and accurate, these instruments are time-consuming.

13. What are the characteristics of an ideal functional assessment scale?

Validity, reliability, and sensitivity to change are probably the most important variables to consider first. The **validity** of an instrument refers to whether it actually measures what it is intended to measure. *Face validity* involves the appearance of measuring the desired characteristic, while *criterion validity* is determined by comparing the instrument to a commonly accepted "gold standard." Comparing two scales which purportedly measure the same characteristics provides *concurrent validity*, while *construct validity* is tested by comparing a scale's performance with other scales measuring similar but not identical functions.

Reliability relates to the reproducibility of findings from the instrument, including *interrater reliability* (same results when given by different raters) and *test-retest reliability* (consistency of findings on serial evaluation). Analysis of correlations between similar items on the scale and between individual items and the entire instrument yields *internal reliability*. The ideal measure is also reliable across differing educational, racial, and socioeconomic backgrounds.

Finally, the instrument must show **sensitivity** to change, such that clinically significant changes in functional ability can be detected, quantified, and monitored.

14. What problems can occur with functional assessment scales?

Several issues may affect the use and interpretation of functional assessment instruments. Depending on the method of test administration, the scale may reflect potential capacity rather than actual performance. Disparities can occur between performance and capacity due to poor motivation, intercurrent illness, or depression.

Another pitfall is the tendency to use summary scores for overall function, which may hide significant changes occurring in individual variables. Furthermore, some scales score certain variables more heavily than others, with proportionately greater impact on the summary score. Caution is advised when interpreting summary scores, particularly in regard to clinical decision-making.

15. Name some of the older functional assessment scales.

PULSES Profile (1957 and 1979)—A global scale that provides a measure of general functional performance, including overall mobility and self-care ability, as well as medical status and psychosocial factors. The scale rates physical condition (P), upper limbs (U), lower limbs (L), sensory status (S), excretory management (E), and psychosocial status (S), with scoring ranging from 6 (fully independent, medically stable) to 24 (dependent, requiring extensive medical/nursing care).

Katz Index of ADL (1963)—Developed from studies of geriatric patients with various disabilities. It rates six ADLs: bathing, dressing, toileting, transfers, continence, and feeding. Each area is rated as independent or not, with functional status graded from A (totally independent) to G (totally dependent). The Katz Index has practical utility but is mainly a descriptive, not a quantitative, instrument.

Kenny Self-Care Evaluation (1965)—Rates patients from 0 (dependent) to 4 (independent) in six categories of self-care: bed activities, transfers, locomotion, dressing, personal hygiene, and feeding. With a score ranging from 0 to 24, this scale has proven to be one of the most sensitive to change in functional ability.

Barthel Index (1965)—One of the best known and most frequently used functional assessment scales. It rates 10 aspects of function, using different relative weights for each variable based on the authors' clinical experience, with a score ranging from 0 (totally dependent) to 100 (totally independent). The original Barthel Index, as well as the adapted version, has been extensively studied, showing its high degrees of validity and reliability, sensitivity to changes in function over time, and ability to use across many types of physical disability.

16. Which functional assessment instruments are used most commonly today?

In a continuing quest to improve sensitivity, validity, and reliability of functional assessment, a national task force sponsored by the American Academy of Physical Medicine & Rehabilitation and the American Congress of Rehabilitation Medicine used a professional consensus process to develop the **Functional Independence Measure** (FIM[SM]). The FIM instrument consists of 18 categories of function (subgrouped under self-care, sphincter control, mobility, locomotion, communication, and social cognition), each scored on a scale from 1 (dependent) to 7 (independent). The FIM instrument incorporates components of the Barthel Index but is more sensitive and inclusive.

Another functional assessment instrument developed by a multidisciplinary team is the **Patient Evaluation and Conference System** (PECS), which tracks function (also using a 1–7 scoring range) among medical, physical, psychological, and social behaviors. PECS also tracks rehabilitation team goals, providing feedback on frequency of goal achievement by patients (program evaluation).

17. How does case-mix affect functional assessment?

Case-mix measures are used to classify patients into groups based on use of resources or outcomes of care and have been applied to payment mechanisms for both hospitals, with diagnosis-related groups (DRGs), and nursing homes, with resource utilization groups (RUGs). However, these case-mix measures do not accurately predict resource utilization or cost of inpatient rehabilitation services. Functional status, on the other hand, has been found to be a better predictor of length of stay and resource utilization. A new case-mix measure, unique to inpatient rehabilitation, is being developed that incorporates FIM data into function-related groups (FIM–FRGs). FIM–FRGs may provide a basis for prospective payment for inpatient rehabilitation, as well as for interfacility comparisons of resource utilization and patient outcomes.

BIBLIOGRAPHY

1. Applegate WB, Blass JP, Williams TF: Instruments for the functional assessment of older patients. N Engl J Med 322:1207–1214, 1990.
2. Granger CV, Albrecht GL, Hamilton BB: Outcome of comprehensive medical rehabilitation: Measurement by PULSES profile and Barthel index. Arch Phys Med Rehabil 60:145–154, 1979.
3. Granger CV, Cotter AC, Hamilton BB, Fiedler RC: Functional assessment scales: A study of persons after stroke. Arch Phys Med Rehabil 74:133–138, 1993.
4. Granger CV, Gresham GE (eds): Functional Assessment in Rehabilitation Medicine. Baltimore, Williams & Wilkins, 1984.
5. Granger CV, Gresham GE (eds): New developments in functional assessment. Phys Med Rehabil Clin North Am 4(3):417–611, 1993.
6. Guide for the Uniform Data Set for Medical Rehabilitation (Adult FIM[SM]), ver. 4.0. Buffalo, NY, State University of New York at Buffalo, 1993.
7. Hamilton BB, Granger CV, et al: A uniform national data system for medical rehabilitation. In Fuhrer MJ (ed): Rehabilitation Outcomes: Analysis and Measurement. Baltimore, Brookes Publishers, 1987, pp 137–147.
8. Kane RA, Kane RL: Assessing the Elderly. Lexington, MA, Lexington Books, 1981.
9. Seltzer GB, Granger CV, Wineberg DE: Functional assessment: Bridge between family and rehabilitation medicine within an ambulatory practice. Arch Phys Med Rehabil 63:453–457, 1982.
10. Stineman MG, Escarce JJ: Analysis of case mix and the prediction of resource use in medical rehabilitation. Phys Med Rehabil Clin North Am 4(3):451–461, 1993.

3. THE FUNDAMENTALS OF FUNCTIONAL OUTCOME ANALYSIS

Richard F. Harvey, M.D., Richard M. Smith, Ph.D., and Raymond E. Wright, Ph.D.

1. What is wrong with depending on my recollection of the outcomes?

Science depends on results that are objective, replicable, and generalizable. Simple recollections of events suffer from a number of problems. Recent events often predominate recollection. Unusual cases are recalled more readily. The typical case is often lost in its usualness. It is important to gather data in a systematic fashion, including all variables that might have potential interest.

2. Why can't I just summarize my cases?

Summarization of cases, although more systematic than simple recollection of outcomes, has several drawbacks:

1. The summarization process may actually change over time. Variables of interest at the beginning may not be of interest at the end, and new variables may have emerged.

2. Individualistic predisposition to certain variables may affect the review process. Two persons reviewing the same set of cases may produce two different summaries.

3. Usually, not all cases will contain the same pieces of information. The way that missing data are handled may greatly impact the results.

4. Data from the summarization process may have very limited generalizability and lack the mathematical property necessary to calculate means and standard deviations.

3. What are the four levels of measurement used to collect data?

Nominal—There are differences of kind but no implied order from less to more for the categories.

Ordinal—There is an implied order to the categories, but the distances between the categories are not equal.

Interval—The distances between the categories are equal throughout the scale, but there is no natural zero.

Ratio—There are equal intervals and a natural or absolute zero.

4. What is wrong with categorical (ordinal) scores?

Collecting information using defined score categories that represent more or less of the variable of interest is an improvement over recollections or summarizations of case records. Unfortunately, the simple rankings on scales, usually scored 1, 2, 3, 4, etc., are still flawed.

- Although the score categories look like numbers, they cannot be added or subtracted, and any attempt at doing arithmetic with these values could result in an answer that has no relationship to the true state of the variable. To solve this problem, one could use only statistical methods that are designed for ordinal data, such as nonparametric statistics, but these are less readily available and less powerful than the parametric statistics designed for interval data. The second solution would be to transform the ordinal data into interval data by way of a psychometric model, such as the Rasch models.
- When each variable is measured with only one item, the standard error associated with that observation is very large, so that even if two persons have different scores, the likelihood of their being statistically different from each other is very small. This problem can be solved only by increasing the replications of each observation, using 8–10 items that ask about the person's performance rather than just one measurement.

5. Why can't we just sum the raw (ordinal) scores for the items?

1. The sum, like the individual scores, is an ordinal scale and, as such, cannot be used to create gain scores (the difference between initial and discharge evaluation on the item or total scale).

2. In order to sum across item scores, the items must constitute a common theme, commonly called a **variable**. If all of the items measure the same theme, the scale is said to be **unidimensional**.

6. Why are interval scales better than ordinal scales?

Parametric statistics, such as the mean, standard deviation, analysis of variance, and associated statistics, make the assumption that the data are measured with an interval scale—i.e., the distances between the units are equal at all points along the scale. The simplest example is that 1° represents the same amount of thermal energy whether the temperature is 34° or 95°. Using parametric statistics on data measured on an ordinal scale, a scale where the differences between points of the scale do not represent equal amounts of the underlying variable, may result in mathematically correct answers that have no relation to the true state of affairs.

7. Is the lack of an origin or natural zero important?

The presence of an origin, or natural zero, is the characteristic that distinguishes interval scales from ratio scales. Both types of scales have equal units, but interval scale values cannot be expressed in ratios. It would make no sense to say that an object at 100° is twice as hot as an object at 50°.

In outcomes measurement, there are few, if any, ratio scales. All psychometric models suffer from the inability to produce ratio scales. The usual solution to the problem is to set the zero point arbitrarily on the logit scale at the average item difficulty, so that a person with a zero measure would have an average score on an item of average difficulty. As different scales measuring the same variable may have different zeros, equating the scales is necessary if measures on the different scales are to have the same meaning.

8. Why is unidimensionality important?

Well, you can't add apples and oranges. In order to add or subtract the numeric results of two items, those two items must be measuring the same thing, sharing a common line of inquiry. Combining two things that do not mean the same thing conveys little if any meaning and usually hides important differences between individuals. For instance, if the sum of a person's age and IQ was 150, it could equally describe a 75-year-old with a 75 IQ, a 40-year-old with a 110 IQ, and a 10-year-old with 140 IQ. Although these three people are characterized by the same number (150), they could hardly be thought of as interchangeable. In an unidimensional scale, persons with the same measure can be thought of as interchangeable, with regard to the trait measured by the scale.

9. Why is a common metric important?

In the true-score model, which is assumed when one simply sums across items measured in successive categories like a Likert scale, there are two metrics, one for the persons and one for the items. You can describe both the persons and items in terms of the mean or median score or the proportion of responses falling into each response category, but there is no way to relate the item scores to the person scores. That is, if a person who scored in the top category on half of the items was evaluated on an item where half of the persons evaluated were rated in the top category, what score would this person most likely receive? In the true-score model, there is no way to predict this outcome, because the items and persons are not measured on a common metric.

One of the distinct advantages of the Rasch family of psychometric models is that both the persons and items are measured on a common metric. Thus, the model specifies mathematically the probabilistic outcome of any interaction between persons and items. (In a deterministic model a person is in one category or another. In a probabilistic model, there is a probability that a person may be in any category.) That is to say, if a person with a measure of 0.0 logits (equal to the average difficulty of the items on a log-odds scale) is presented an item with a difficulty of 0.0, then it is possible to predict the person's most likely evaluation and the probability of the person receiving each of the possible scores.

10. How can a common metric help me to describe a patient's progress?

Typically, functional outcomes are norm-referenced—i.e., a person's measure is usually described by some population of interest, such as normal, admission and discharge status for a particular diagnosis, age group, gender, etc. This severely limits the interpretability of the scale because little is usually known about the relationship between competencies or skills of interest and measures on the outcome scales. What is important in being able to describe the patient's functional outcomes is how well the patient will be able to perform a variety of daily skills. It is possible to test the patient on all of the skills of interest, but this is time- and resource-consuming, and it is unnecessary if the items and persons can be calibrated (**calibration** is the process by which the raw scores resulting from observations are turned into measures for persons and items) on a common metric. The common metric and the probabilistic model which defines the relationship between person and item measures and expected scores allow for the construction of a domain-referenced scale that allows the patient's functional outcomes to be described in terms of the skills represented by the items, even if the patient was not evaluated on this skill.

The figure at the top of the facing page shows that a person with a score of 60 on a PECS© Motor Skills LifeScale™ would be independent on feeding (7), functional independent on position changes (6), limited independent on ambulation (5), and fair on endurance (4). Each of these ratings would have a specific descriptor that further defines the level of skills. In the case of endurance, fair would mean that the patient actively participates in 20 minutes of treatment before requiring a rest. The use of these descriptors allows the translation of a person's functional outcomes measure into the language of important skills that most persons think about, but at the same time maintaining the objectivity, replicability, and generalizability necessary in science.

Motor Skills Expected Scores

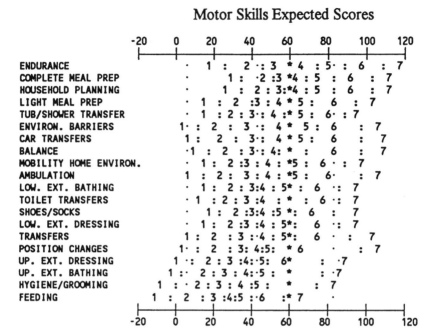

11. Aren't blanks the same as zero?

In most applications of Likert scales (where a person is rated on a numeric scale indicating intensity or severity), missing data (unadministered items) are problematic. Since the interpretability of the total score in the true-score model depends on every person being evaluated on the same set of items, the presence of unadministered (unanswered) items changes the meaning of the total score. A score of 7 on 10 items with no blanks does not mean the same thing as score of 7 on 8 items with 2 blanks.

12. How can you compensate for blank or missing data?

In the true-score model, there are two methods generally employed to solve the problem of blanks. The first, to delete any record with missing scores can result in the loss of significant amounts of data. The second involves assigning a value to the person based on some rule: One rule assigns the modal (most frequent) response for the item to the blank, and another assigns the modal response for the person to the blank. Sometimes the lowest response category is assigned for blanks. In the case of only two score categories (0 and 1), this may not be an inappropriate assumption, particularly if there is a reason to assume unattempted items were too hard for the person. But, as the number of score categories for each item increases (1 to 7 in the case of PECS), the use of the lowest (or highest) category as a replacement value becomes more problematic.

13. What is sample-freed measurement?

One of the properties of the family of Rasch psychometric models (models where the interaction between the person and the item is an exponential function of the difference between the person and item locations on the variable) is that the estimation of any parameter of interest is freed from the distributional properties of the remaining parameters. In other words, the estimate of the person measure does not depend on the difficulties of the specific items on which the person is being evaluated, and the estimate of the item measure (difficulty) does not depend on the ability of the persons to whom the items were administered.

In the true-score model, the estimates of both person and item locations are sample-dependent. If a functional assessment item is given to patients at the beginning of treatment, the average score on the item may be 2.4. The same item at the end of treatment might have an average score of 4.5. The change in the item score might be viewed as very positive, since the change in the score indicates that the patients responded to therapy. Unfortunately, this interpretation holds only if the item was administered to every patient on admission and discharge. Obviously, if the pre- and post-treatment scores for items are to have any scientific value, they must not be sample-dependent. That is to say, the estimates of item difficulty cannot depend on the distribution of the ability of the persons to whom the items are administered.

14. Give two reasons why sample-freed measurement is important.

1. Diversity of diagnostic populations served: With a wide variety of diagnostic categories representing many levels of severity, the need for a scale that maintains its structure (invariance of item difficulties) over different groups is essential if comparisons across different diagnostic categories are to be made. Even if two diagnostic groups use the same items, if the definition of the variable is different for the groups, then the results of the assessment for the two groups have a different meaning, even if the groups have the same average measures.

2. Increasing levels of care in the rehabilitation process need to have functional outcome measures at each level of care. As the patient's condition improves, the patient is assigned to the most cost-effective level of care. This implies that different patients in different levels of care will have different functional levels. For the measurement process to be as efficient and accurate as possible, the items used to assess the functional outcomes must match the level of care. Thus, persons in different levels of care will be assessed on different items. Having a functional assessment scale that will produce comparable assessments on a common scale for different levels of severity without exhibiting the floor and ceiling effects common to fixed scales is an important step in evaluating functional outcomes.

15. Why do we need to check the fit of the data?

The important psychometric properties—interval scales, a common metric for items and persons, and sample-freed estimation of item and person parameters—are consequences of the psychometric model if and only if the data "fit" the model. **Fit** in this sense means that the responses to the assessments can be described by the probabilistic expression for the appropriate Rasch model. In more simple terms, the outcome of any interaction between person and item can be determined by two things, the difficulty of the item and the status (ability) of the person. Anything else that influences this outcome in a systematic way is a threat to the use of the model, causes the data not to fit, and may invalidate the desirable properties. Fortunately, the fit of the data to the measurement model is easy to manage, and many of the computer programs designed to estimate the person and item parameters incorporate fit analysis into the calibration process.

16. How do we check the fit of the data?

The fit of the data can be assessed through the use of the simple difference between the observed response (X) and the expected response (E). The expected response is calculated from the probability expression for the model using the parameters that were estimated for the model. There is a residual (X–E) calculated for each item—person interaction in the data set. These residuals can be standardized to form approximate chi-squared statistics and combined in interesting ways to test specific threats to the measurement model. When the standardized residuals are summed across all of the items evaluated for a person, the sum becomes a person-fit statistic; when summed across all of the persons who were evaluated on a particular item, the sum becomes an item-fit statistic. There are a variety of ways these statistics are reported—mean squares, unweighted total (outfit), weighted total (infit)—but all of these fit statistics contain basically the same information, each having just been transformed in a different way to provide a different frame of reference against which to compare results. Since most of these statistics are sensitive to sample size, there is no simple rule indicating when the data should be considered too poor to be appropriately analyzed by the model, but there are several sources where general guidelines can be found.

17. Why do the scales need to replicate?

In functional outcome assessment, there is a need to be able to compare the results of the rehabilitation process across different diagnoses, treatment modalities, and institutions. To have a separate outcome measure for each combination of these three factors would lead to chaos. Outcome measures that replicate over institutions are necessary if there is to be any synthesis of the research findings from the many different research programs investigating similar problems. Outcome measures that replicate over different diagnoses are necessary if outcome data are to be used in program evaluation and quality management programs. Outcome measures that replicate over different treatment modalities are necessary to conduct treatment effectiveness or efficacy studies.

18. But what happens if the variables are not the same?

If the definition of the variable is not the same for two or more populations of interest, then the pretreatment and post-treatment raw scores or measures, either for individuals or groups, cannot be directly compared. Mathematical manipulations of the numbers is always possible, but since the definition of the two variables is not the same, there is no guarantee that the results of the mathematical or statistical analysis will represent a true picture of the relationship between the groups.

19. Is there some way to "correct" for this change in definition?

In many pre/post-assessment designs, there is an interaction between the variable and treatment. This interaction causes some of the items to become easier after treatment, while the difficulty of some other items is unaffected. Thus, the pretreatment assessment definition of the variable is not the same as the post-treatment assessment definition. In situations where there are pre/post-treatment differences in the definition of the variable, the t-test procedures for identifying items that have changed significantly can be used to identify the best set of items that maintain the difficulty order over treatment. This subset of items can then be used to determine changes in person measures due to treatment. Thus, the unidimensionality of the scale is maintained and differences between measures can be thought of as the distance along the variable that the treatment has moved the individual or group of individuals.

20. Why do we need all of the different scales?

There is nothing wrong with having different scales, as long as they share a common metric, i.e., the arbitrary origin imposed in the calibration process has been removed. A good example would be thermometers; despite all of the different types of thermometers and different scales, the whole system works because there is a single underlying interval metric. The different scales are simply linear transformations of that metric, and all thermometers, no matter what physical property they are based on, report temperature on that metric.

The situation with functional outcomes assessment is similar. There are a wide variety of circumstances that require different types of assessment instruments. In fact, the more focused the instrument is on the population being measured, the more accurate that measurement (the smaller the standard error of estimate) will be. So, we improve the utility of the measures by being able to focus the items on the population of interest.

21. Why do scales have to be equated?

Even if scales such as the FIM and PECS Motor Skills LifeScale are developed to assess similar outcomes and are separately determined to fit one of the Rasch family of psychometric models, the results of the two scales cannot be directly compared. Despite the similarity of the two scales, there is one important difference—the lack of a common origin. To translate from one scale to the other, one needs to know the difference between the two origins. The metrics of the two scales have equal units (logits).

22. How do you equate these two scales?

To remove the differences between the arbitrary origins of the FIM and PECS, the scales must be equated by either common item equating or common person equating. In **common person equating**, the entirety of both scales must be administered to a group of subjects (stable results are achievable with a sample size of 30–100). Simultaneously calibrating the total item set will result in a metric with a zero set to the average difficulty of the combined item set. In **common item equating**, a subset of items from one of the scales is administered with a subset of the second scale. The calibration of the second scale and the common items is then linked back to the original scale through a link constant that is based on the difference between the original item difficulty and the subsequent item difficulty for the subset of common items. The origin (zero) of either scale can then be transferred to the other. There are then three possible origins—the origin based on either of the original scales or the origin of the combined scale. The choice of the origin is unimportant, so long as the outcomes from both scales use the same origin.

23. Is it really worth all the effort?

Whether we like it or not, services rendered to persons with impairments and/or disabilities are being carefully scrutinized by managed-care programs to determine the value of the service. Value is a term which is based upon benefit per unit of cost. In the field of PM&R, the benefit gained by persons with impairments and/or disabilities is the outcome of change effected in their ability to perform daily activities. These outcomes still require "value"-based judgments to decide on the worth of the human investment.

BIBLIOGRAPHY

1. Fisher WP, Harvey RF, Taylor P, et al: Rehabits: A common language of functional assessment. Arch Phys Med Rehabil 76:113–122, 1995.
2. Harvey RF, Jellinek HM: Functional performance assessment: A program approach. Arch Phys Med Rehabil 62:456–461, 1981.
3. Harvey RF, Silverstein B, Kilgore KM, et al: Applying psychometric criteria to functional assessment in medical rehabilitation: III. Construct validity and predicting level of care. Arch Phys Med Rehabil 73:887–892, 1992.
4. Kilgore KM, Fisher WP, Harvey RF, Silverstein B: Diagnosis-based differences in Rasch calibrations of functional assessment scales. Arch Phys Med Rehabil 74:1254, 1993.
5. Kilgore KM, Fisher WP, Silverstein B, et al: Application of Rasch analysis to the Patient Evaluation and Conference System. Phys Med Rehabil Clin North Am 4:493–515, 1993.
6. Rasch G: Probabilistic models for some intelligence and attainment tests. Copenhagen Denmarks Paedogogski Institut, 1960. [Reprinted by University of Chicago Press, 1980.]
7. Silverstein B, Kilgore KM, Fisher WP, et al: Applying psychometric criteria to functional assessment: I. Exploring unidimensionality. Arch Phys Med Rehabil 72:631–637, 1991.
8. Silverstein B, Kilgore KM, Fisher WP, et al: Applying psychometric criteria to functional assessment in medical rehabilitation: II. Defining interval measures. Arch Phys Med Rehabil 73:507–518, 1992.
9. Smith RM: IPARM: Item and person analysis with the Rasch model. Chicago, MESA Press, 1991.
10. Smith RM: Applications of Rasch Measurement. Chicago, MESA Press, 1993.
11. Smith RM, Miao CV: Assessing unidimensionality for Rasch measurement. In Wilson Â (ed): Objective Measurement: Theory into Practice II. Norwood, NJ, Ablex Publishing, 1994.
12. Wright BD, Linacre JM: Observations are always ordinal; measurements, however, must be interval. Arch Phys Med Rehabil 70:857–860, 1989.
13. Wright BD, Masters GN: Rating Sale Analysis. Chicago, MESA Press, 1982.
14. Wright BD, Stone M: Best Test Design. Chicago, MESA Press, 1979.

4. PM&R EDUCATION

Joseph C. Honet, M.D., M.S.

1. AAMCACGMERRCPMRCMEAMAAHACMSSABMSABPMRSQSCIMACCME. What do all those initials have to do with PM&R education? Is this the genetic code for a physiatrist?

All future physiatrists go to medical schools that are accredited by the American Association of Medical Colleges (**AAMC**), although PM&R training is not a universal requirement in medical schools. The Accreditation Council for Graduate Medical Education (**ACGME**) is ultimately responsible for accrediting all residency programs throughout the United States. The Residency Review Committee (**RRC**) for PM&R actually accredits the PM&R residency committees, and this responsibility has been delegated by the ACGME. Accreditation is a voluntary process which, when successful, provides the residency program with a stamp of approval. The parents of the ACGME include the Council on Medical Education (**CME**) of the American Medical Association (**AMA**), the American Hospital Association (**AHA**), the Council of Medical Specialty Societies (**CMSS**), the AAMC, and the American Board of Medical Specialties (**ABMS**).

When the resident completes the graduate medical education program, he or she can be examined, which, if successfully completed, allows certification by the American Board of Physical Medicine and Rehabilitation (**ABPM&R**), which is a member society of the ABMS. Recently, the ABMS approved special qualifications (**SQ**) in Spinal Cord Injury Medicine (**SCIM**). During residency and certainly following residency, educational courses are used for continuing medical education, which is necessary for lifelong learning. These educational courses should be approved by the Accreditation Council on Continuing Medical Education (**ACCME**).

2. How do I get training in PM&R in my medical school?

Some medical schools require rotations in PM&R. However, if the school does not have required rotations or if more experience in physical medicine is desired, an elective rotation can be pursued at your own medical school. If the medical school, by some chance, does not have a Department of Physical Medicine, rotations can be arranged at other medical schools as an away elective.

3. Now that I have decided that I want to train in PM&R, how can I find out what steps I should take?

The *Graduate Medical Education Directory* of the American Medical Association (green book) is available at every medical school and lists the accredited programs in PM&R. The list is provided by state, city, name of the institution, program director (the person responsible for that residency program), address, length of program, number of positions, and ID number.

4. How can I tell whether the program provides the required education?

The green book also details the program requirements for PM&R, which is a listing of the requirements that the program must provide to be accredited by the RRC in PM&R. The programs provide either 3 years of PM&R with 1 extra year of clinical experience (internship), or a total of 4 years in the program which also includes 1 year of clinical experience.

5. What are some of the requirements, and why are they necessary?

The programs requires **4 years of training**, 1 of which is for obtaining clinical skills. This could be a year of internal medicine or family practice or some combination of these and other basic subjects that allow training in clinical care of patients ("primary care").

A minimum of 1 year must be spent caring for **inpatients** with rehabilitation problems, during which each resident must have at least 8 patients on a geographically located rehabilitation unit. This experience must be supervised, the patients must be seen on a regular basis, and the resident must participate in the interdisciplinary team process of rehabilitative care, which includes the patient and patient's significant others.

At least 1 year must be spent in the **outpatient** care of PM&R patients. This must include some time caring for patients with musculoskeletal and neuromuscular problems, which provides training in ambulatory care.

As of January 1, 1996, the newest requirements cover such things as the definition of PM&R, length of training, details of the clinical experience, requirements and responsibilities of the program director, requirements of the faculty and allied health staff, the subject matter that is required (including the clinical program, didactic program, journal clubs, and basic science requirements for the resident, faculty, and program evaluation), and the importance of Board results for the residents in the program.

6. Is there some trick to finding a good program?

You could ask for advice from the people in the PM&R department at your university or contact residents at your university or nearby institutions. They cannot tell you all the features of each program, but by way of the "grapevine," they can give you some directions and ideas. It would also be helpful to read the requirements and provide yourself with a list of questions that you would ask the program director when you visit the program. Information to ask the program director includes the results of previous residents on the certification examinations of the American Board of PM&R, the cycle of review and when the program will be reviewed again, and some of the concerns or lack of compliances in the program.

7. Is a small program or a large program better, or doesn't it make any difference?

Obviously, programs have different characteristics. Some programs spend more time on the care of rehabilitation patients (spinal-cord injury, closed-head injury, stroke, etc.) and others might spend more time on physical medicine patients (low-back pain, shoulder pain, sports injuries, occupational injuries, etc.). Obviously, every program must meet all of the requirements as part of the training, but certain programs may be heavier in one area than in another. Also, some programs are large, with 30 residents, and others may have as few as 2 residents per year (a total of 8). Some programs stress research more heavily.

You have to determine which of these characteristics best meet your needs. Are you more interested in rehab or the physical medicine aspects of the specialty, or are they equal in your mind? Do you want a more academic environment because you are interested in becoming a faculty member, and is research something that you want to pursue? Just as with everything else, you must make your choice based on your own personal characteristics and goals.

8. How can I get the most out of any program?

1. See as many patients as possible and be thorough in patient evaluations.
2. Ask questions of the faculty.
3. Make sure that all aspects of the specialty are covered (including the rehabilitation aspects, care of patients with musculoskeletal problems, experience in electromyographic exams, and other things such as pediatrics and geriatrics).
4. Constantly read the literature to be current, to have an idea of important principles, and to follow the constant updating of the specialty.
5. Understand how to evaluate and assess function of the CNS, other parts of the neuromuscular system, and the musculoskeletal system (e.g., gait evaluation).
6. Learn how to interact with the patient, the patient's significant others, the allied health team, other physicians, and, in this day and age, third-party payers.
7. Learn to lead the rehabilitation team.

9. Now I have had great training in PM&R, having completed the best residency program. Do I automatically become certified?

The goal of certification is to provide assurance to the public that a specialist in PM&R has successfully completed an approved educational program and has completed an evaluation process that includes an examination designed to assess the knowledge, skills, and experience of the candidate. Candidates must apply for examination to the American Board of PM&R (**ABPM&R**), and it must be done in a timely fashion, usually before November of the year prior to the exams. The ABPM&R provides a booklet of the information about applying for testing.

To become certified requires that you pass first a written exam (Part I) prepared by the ABPM&R and given in May of each year (can be taken during your senior year of residency). You are eligible to take Part II after 1 year of PM&R experience, if you pass Part I. This oral examination is also given in May. On successful completion of both parts of the examination, you are provided with a certificate from the ABPM&R. Currently, the certificate is time-limited and recertification is necessary within 10 years.

10. With all this certification, etc., is it really worth my time, effort, and anxiety to take the board examinations in PM&R?

Certification has always been important but has a new importance in this modern day of medicine. The public is more aware of the importance of certification in specialties and is asking it of individual doctors. In addition, many health maintenance organizations require certification to be accepted as a provider.

11. I am not ready to practice PM&R. Is there any subspecialty training that I can take for which I will be certified?

The ABPM&R has just recently been approved to provide special qualifications for spinal cord injury medicine (**SCIM**). Thus, successful completion of a 1-year SCIM training program allows the individual enrolled in the program to undergo an examination, again given by the ABPM&R.

BIBLIOGRAPHY

1. The Graduate Medical Education Directory. Chicago, American Medical Association, 1996. (Tel. 312-464-5000).
2. ABPM&R Booklet of Information. Rochester, MN, American Board of Physical Medicine and Rehabilitation, 1996. (Tel. 507-282-1776).
3. AAP Newsletter. Available from 7100 Lakewood Bldg, Suite 112, 5987 East 71st Street, Indianapolis, IN 46220. (Tel. 317-845-4200).
4. Directory of Physical Medicine and Rehabilitation Residency Training Programs. Available from 7100 Lakewood Building, Suite 112, 5987 East 71st Street, Indianapolis, IN 46220. (Tel. 317-845-4200).

5. RESEARCH CONCEPTS IN PM&R

John E. Hewett, Ph.D., David G. McDonald, Ph.D., and Jerry C. Parker, Ph.D.

"Many scientists owe their greatness not to their skill in solving problems but to their wisdom in choosing them."—E. Bright, 1952

1. What are the sources and characteristics of a good research hypothesis?

The sources of a hypothesis can be termed systematic and unsystematic.

There are at least three **systematic** sources: (1) from existing theory; (2) based on an integration of research literature; and (3) in applied research, out of need for a solution to a problem.

The **unsystematic** sources include, but are not limited to: (1) naturalistic observations; (2) listening to a colleague; and (3) the product of quiet reflection. A good idea is a good idea, regardless of its source.

What is a good **hypothesis**? It must be testable. The topic must be phrased in terms of variables that can be defined and measured, and it should be important rather than trivial or transient.

2. Why is the literature search important to the success of a research project?

The process of scientific discovery involves the combined efforts of many individual scientists. The hypotheses of a new investigator frequently were tested in the experiments of the past. Exploration of the experiments, data, and conclusions of the past provides a context for refinement of research questions.

3. What are the prerequisites for informed consent prior to conducting a research study?

Institutional Review Board regulations require four conditions for informed consent:

1. The participant must be **legally competent**; otherwise, consent from the guardian is required.

2. The consent must be **voluntary**; no pressures, even subtle, must be operating to sway a participant's choice.

3. Consent must be **truly informed**. The participant must receive and understand all necessary information prior to making a decision.

4. **Comprehension** of the consent information and awareness of the alternative choices must be assured. Complicated consent forms or technical jargon must be avoided.

4. How do basic and applied research differ?

Basic research is research in which the investigator seeks to discover fundamental laws of nature, without regard for their ultimate application in solving practical problems. It is also frequently described as **theory-driven**, since this form of research is generally based on hypotheses derived from existing theory.

Applied research is any investigation undertaken solely to solve some real-world problem, without regard for the theories or natural laws that may be relevant. The primary goal is to determine if a better solution can be found, and it is frequently described as **problem-solving** research. Examples of applied research would include a study of the relative comfort and maneuverability of several different wheelchair designs or a study of the relative effectiveness of two different methods of using a cane in patients with knee injury.

In the field of rehab medicine, many research projects are both basic and applied. For example, a study of the Functional Independence Measure (FIM) scores of AIDS patients is basic research in that it tells us something new about AIDS, but it is also applied research in that it gives us more information on management of AIDS patients as well as the usefulness of the FIM scale.

5. Why is theory important in science?

A theory is a relatively general statement of mechanisms or relationships derived from partially verified cause-and-effect relationships in nature. Theories are a motivating logical force in most basic research, which is often described as theory-driven research.

Good theories have the following characteristics:

1. They can account for existing data.
2. They have explanatory relevance (the explanation makes sense).
3. They can be tested.
4. They predict novel events or new phenomena.
5. They are parsimonious (make few assumptions).

Good theories also perform several functions:

1. They promote understanding.
2. They can be used to predict outcomes in systems processes.
3. They provide a framework for organizing and interpreting research results.
4. They generate research if they have heuristic or seminal value.

6. What is a variable? What types are there?

A variable is any phenomenon that varies. Variables can be sorted into various categories:

1. **Behavioral, stimulus, and organismic/subject variables.** A behavioral variable is any observable response of the patient or subject. Stimulus variables are quantifiable aspects of the experimental context that have potential effects on the response of subjects. Organismic/subject variables are any relevant characteristics of the subjects, such as age, gender, or diagnosis.

2. **Independent versus dependent variables.** The independent variable is the intervention or treatment administered by the investigator to the experimental group (example = an analgesic) and withheld from the control group (example = a placebo). The dependent variable is the outcome variable hypothesized to have a relationship to the independent variable in a study (example = measure of pain reduction produced by the analgesic).

3. **Extraneous variable or confound.** An extraneous variable is any variable (other than the independent variable) that can affect the dependent variable in a study. Extraneous variables can be especially troublesome if they mimic or cancel the effect of the independent variable. Examples include age, gender, drug effects, and diagnosis. Therefore, they must be controlled by holding them constant across groups in a study (example = using groups of equal age, gender mix, drug treatment, and diagnosis). An uncontrolled extraneous variable is called a confound.

4. **Latent versus manifest variables.** A latent variable is any theoretical concept or construct that is assumed to exist but cannot be measured directly, whereas a manifest variable is any measured variable that is used as an observed indicator of a latent variable.

7. What is the difference between categorical, ordinal, interval, and ratio measurements?

The concepts of categorical, ordinal, interval, and ratio measurement reflect increasing degrees of precision (reliability and consistency) in measurement with whatever methods are available.

Categorical measurement: naming or labeling only. Examples include studies in which subjects are grouped by category, such as gender, ethnic, or cultural background. The dependent variable (outcome variable) in a study can also be a categorical measure, such as "recovered" versus "not recovered."

Ordinal measurement: measurement by ranking in order or along a scale of mutually exclusive categories, meaning that measurement is precise enough to determine if one of two observations is greater or lesser than the second. Use of rating scales, such as the FIM, is an example of ordinal measurement.

Interval measurement: similar to ordinal measurement, except that, in addition, the units between successive steps on the scale are equal and constant. An example of interval measurement is temperature on the Fahrenheit scale: the difference between 30°F and 35°F is the same as the difference between 100°F and 105°F.

Ratio measurement: almost the same as interval measurement, except that in ratio measures, there is a known true zero point. Examples might be age or elapsed time in performance tasks.

8. What are the major types of research design? How do they differ?

In broad terms, there are four major types of research designs or strategies, plus an assortment of various specialized designs. The four major types are:

1. **True experiments** have four primary characteristics: (1) there is an independent and a dependent variable; (2) there is a high degree of control of extraneous variables; (3) they are repeatable (replication is feasible), which is a reason for publication of experiments in research journals; and (4) the experimental and control groups are formed by random assignment of subjects. This last characteristic is highly critical and unique to true experiments. True experiments are the leading scientific method for establishing cause-and-effect relationships, the primary long-range goal of most science.

2. **Quasi-experiments** are "almost" experiments, but not quite. The essential difference is that subjects are not allocated to groups by random assignment, but rather on the basis of some preexisting variable, which raises the question of some preexisting confound. Examples of quasi-experiments are common in medicine and include studies comparing almost any patient group with nonpatient controls, where a true experiment would not be ethical or legally permissible. Although quasi-experiments do not provide incontrovertible evidence of cause-and-effect relationships, the procedure still reveals relationships between variables.

3. In **correlational studies**, the investigator simply wishes to determine whether two variables are related, i.e., that they co-vary. The typical statistical procedure employed is the correlation coefficient. These studies do not establish causality, but the association demonstrated by this method can be further investigated.

4. **Descriptive studies** consist simply of collecting systematic observations and/or measurements of any real-world phenomenon, with no control of confounds or manipulation of independent variables. When conducted outside the laboratory, these studies are often called **naturalistic studies**. Surveys and clinical case studies are descriptive studies. Descriptive studies can be valuable in the early stages of any research area.

9. How do "between-subjects" and "within-subjects" designs differ?

In **between-subjects designs**, comparisons are made between groups of subjects, such as experimental and control groups. If there is more than one experimental group (common in drug studies), each group experiences only one level of the independent variable (e.g., high, medium, or low dose of the drug). In actual practice, most studies are, therefore, between-subject studies.

In **within-subjects designs**, there is only one group, but each subject experiences every value of the independent variable, usually in some counterbalanced order. The advantage of this procedure is that it may be preferable if there are small sample groups (subjects in short supply).

10. What do we need to know about statistics to be successful investigators in PM&R?

What is needed is a thorough understanding of the research question (significance, variables to validly answer, confounds). This type of information allows the investigator to interact successfully with a statistician. The statistician is then able to provide the statistical expertise to design the experiment and answer the question. A basic understanding of statistical techniques allows the investigator to effectively translate naturalistic observations and hypotheses into *answerable* questions.

11. What is meant by the term descriptive statistics?

Let $x_1,..., x_n$ denote a set of numbers. A descriptive statistic for this set of numbers is a number computed from the set that summarizes a particular type of information contained in the set. Examples of descriptive statistics are the mean ($\bar{x}$), median ($\tilde{x}$), standard deviation (SD), and percentiles (x_p). The median is the 50th percentile. The mean and median provide information about the middle of the set, and the standard deviation and various percentiles provide information about the spread of the data.

12. What is meant by inferential statistics?

Statistical inference is drawing conclusions about the population as a whole based on the information that is derived from a sample of that population. By population, we mean the totality of subjects who are of interest to us. By a sample, we simply mean a subset of all subjects of interest to us. There are three general types of statistical inference: point estimation, interval estimation, and hypothesis testing.

13. What is hypothesis testing?

A **statistical hypothesis** is a conjecture about a population. If the population is characterized in terms of parameters, then these hypotheses will be conjectures about the parameters of the population, such as the population mean and/or the population standard deviation (parametric statistical hypotheses). Suppose that we have a population of hemiplegic patients, and we would like to determine if the proportion of these patients who can complete a task differs from the proportion of control subjects who can complete the same task. Here, the **alternative hypothesis** is that the two proportions are not the same, and the **null hypothesis** is that the two proportions are the same.

If the population cannot be characterized relative to parameters, then our conjecture (hypothesis) will be about the population itself, and the procedures employed will be called nonparametric procedures. The most commonly used **nonparametric methods** are those based on ranks rather than on the raw data.

14. What are type I and type II errors?
The terms type I and type II errors are used in the context of hypothesis testing. A **type I error** is made when we conclude that a null hypothesis is false when, in fact, it is true. A **type II error** is made when the data lead us to conclude that the null is true when, in fact, it is not.

A test of a statistical hypothesis is a decision rule that tells us whether we should reject the null hypothesis in question. By the **alpha level** (α) of the test, we mean the probability of rejecting the null hypothesis when, in fact, it is true. By the **beta level** (β) of the test, we mean the probability of not rejecting the null hypothesis when it is false. This depends on the actual magnitude of difference that exists. The **power** of the test is $1 - \beta$.

15. Define probability.
The classical definition of the probability of an event is the number of times the event occurs, divided by the number of independent chances the event has to occur.

16. Define _p_-value.
Suppose we are testing a null hypothesis H_0 versus an alternative hypothesis H_A, and large values of the test statistic T support H_A. If H_0 is really true, we would not expect t, the value of T obtained from the observed data, to be large. If H_0 is really true, how likely is it that the sample should produce a value of $T \geq t$, the value actually produced? The _p_-value is a measure of this. Thus, a small _p_-value is an indication that the truth of the null hypothesis is unlikely.

17. What is meant by effect size?
The effect size is the average magnitude of change in the dependent variable (DV) produced by the independent variable (IV). It can be mathematically defined simply as the difference between group means (the experimental group mean minus the control group mean, which is the effect of the IV). This difference can be divided by the pooled standard deviation of the two groups combined or simply the control group to convert the effect size into standard deviation units, a form of standard score similar to another familiar standard score, the **z-score**. In this way, effect sizes obtained in different studies can be meaningfully compared. Cohen has provided a helpful definition of small, medium, and large standard effect sizes as those with values of about 0.20, 0.50, and 0.80, respectively. Effect size is an essential tool used in two important areas: statistical power analysis and meta-analysis.

18. How does one determine the optimal sample size in a study? How do you know if a given sample is large enough to answer the question?
The four variables, **sample size, statistical power, alpha,** and **effect size,** are interrelated in such a way that knowing any three allows one to estimate the fourth. Thus, for a given alpha, effect size, and power, the necessary sample size can be estimated.

Consider a hypothetical two-independent group study in which the experimenter sets the alpha at 0.05, the desired power at 0.80, and expects a relatively moderate effect size of 0.50. Then, using these values in appropriate tables, it can be determined that a sample size of 64 subjects in each group will be required with these specified parameters to reach a statistically valid conclusion. However, if one expects a relatively small effect (say 0.20, instead of 0.50), then the required sample size is almost 400 subjects/group in order to maintain a statistical power of 0.80.

One dismaying consequence of this fact is that an unknown number of published reports in the journal literature suffer from the common problem of relying on a sample size that is too small. This means that the resulting statistical power is considerably less than 0.80, often less than 0.50, in which case their odds of finding the effect are less than 50-50! When the experimenters also fail to reject the null hypothesis, then one must seriously consider that their report may represent a type II error, rather than a true finding of no effect of the independent variable.

19. What is the analysis of variance?

Analysis of variance (ANOVA) refers to a set of statistical methods associated with testing the equality of two or more means. For example, it could be used to determine if three different methods of teaching stroke patients how to do a task result in different mean times to complete the task.

20. What is meant by analysis of covariance?

Analysis of covariance combines regression and ANOVA methods for the purpose of forming ANOVA models with reduced error variance. It does this by making use of quantitative variables that are related to the independent variable. For example, in a study designed to determine if two populations have different numbers of foot abnormalities, there may be some possible additional variables that could affect the outcome variable of interest. One specific example would be the age of the subjects in the study. Age would be a variable that could affect whether an individual has a foot abnormality or not. Thus, age could be built into the statistical analysis as a covariate.

21. Define regression.

With regression, we are interested in building a model where one or more variables are used to predict another variable. In the **simple regression** model, we have a variable, called the independent variable, that is used to provide information about another variable, called the dependent variable. In **multiple regression**, rather than using just one variable to predict the dependent variable, two or more variables, called the independent variables, are used. As an example of a multiple regression model, the dependent variable might be the length of time that it takes to complete a task and the independent variables would be duration of disease, age, and weight.

22. How is meta-analysis done?

Meta-analysis is an objective (statistical) method of collectively analyzing the results of more than one study. The essential elements in conducting a meta-analysis are:

1. Identify the hypothesis or research question, conduct a literature search, and then determine the criteria for including and excluding existing studies.

2. Calculate the effect size (see Question 17) for each of the studies included. Studies with larger samples are weighted more heavily in the analysis.

3. Calculate whether the resulting overall effect size is or is not significantly greater than 0, a conclusion that is not always apparent to (subjective) narrative reviewers.

4. It can be determined at this point whether the overall effect of the independent variable was small, medium, or large, a finding that some would argue is even more important than knowing that the overall effect was significant or not.

The introduction of meta-analysis has provided exciting capabilities in synthesizing the results of diverse studies, and it promises to have an increasingly greater impact in the future.

BIBLIOGRAPHY

1. Campbell DT, Stanley JC: Experimental and Quasi-experimental Designs for Research. Chicago, Rand McNally, 1966.
2. Cohen J: Statistical Power Analysis for the Behavioral Sciences, 2nd ed. Hillsdale, NJ, Lawrence Erlbaum Assoc., 1988.
3. Colton T: Statistics in Medicine. Boston, Little, Brown & Co., 1974.
4. Cooper HM: Integrating Research: A Guide for Literature Reviews, 2nd ed. Beverly Hills, CA, Sage, 1989.
5. Hulley SB, Cummings SR: Designing Clinical Research: An Epidemiological Approach. Baltimore, Williams & Wilkins, 1988.
6. Shott S: Statistics for Health Professionals. Philadelphia, W.B. Saunders, 1990.
7. Smith ML, Glass GV: Meta-analysis of pyschotherapy outcome studies. Am Psychol 32:752–760, 1977.

6. MUSCULOSKELETAL ANATOMY AND KINESIOLOGY

Carson D. Schneck, M.D., Ph.D.

PRINCIPLES OF KINESIOLOGY

1. How do agonist, antagonist, and synergistic muscles operate to accomplish joint motion?

1. **Agonist**, or prime mover, is any muscle that can cause a specific joint motion. For example, the biceps brachii contracts to cause elbow flexion.

2. An **antagonist** is any muscle that can produce a motion opposite to the specific agonist motion. For example, triceps brachii is an antagonist to elbow flexion. Antagonists are normally completely relaxed during contraction of an agonist (except during a rapid ballistic motion).

3. **Synergistic** muscles normally contract to remove unwanted actions of agonists or to stabilize other (usually more proximal) joints. For example, during elbow flexion by the biceps brachii, the forearm pronators contract to remove the undesirable supination which the biceps would produce.

2. What forces normally produce motion at joints?

Muscle contraction and gravity, with each serving as the prime mover for about 50% of all joint movements.

3. Name the three types of muscle contraction.

1. **Shortening, concentric,** or **isotonic** contraction occurs when the muscle's force exceeds the load. Hence, the muscle shortens to produce joint motion while maintaining constant tension.

2. **Isometric** or **static** contraction occurs when the muscle force equals the load. The muscle maintains the same length, and the joint does not move.

3. **Lengthening** or **eccentric** contraction occurs when muscle force is less than the load. This normally occurs when gravity is the prime mover. To control the effect of gravity, eccentric contraction occurs in the muscle(s) that opposes the direction that gravity is tending to move the joint.

4. Two muscles together often perform the same function. How can you eliminate one of the muscles to evaluate the other muscle in relative isolation?

Three **muscle elimination procedures** are used commonly:

1. Placing a muscle at a **mechanical disadvantage** by positioning the part so that the muscle to be eliminated will have no substantial vector component in the direction of the function to be tested.

2. Placing a muscle at a **physiologic** or **length disadvantage** by positioning the part so that the muscle is slackened or has much of its shortening capability used up by performing a function other than the one being tested.

3. If the muscle to be eliminated has several functions, it can be **reciprocally inhibited** from participating in the tested function by forcibly performing a function antagonistic to one of its other functions.

5. How is muscle strength graded?

Manual muscle strength assessment is accomplished by proceeding cephalad down in the order of innervation from the brachial plexus, through the lumbosacral plexus. If specific nerves are in question, examine muscles in the proximal-to-distal order in which they receive their motor branches. Resistance is best assessed using the "make and break" technique, in which the examiner overpowers a patient's fixed mid-muscle-length contraction.

In clinical practice, the following hierarchy of ordinal ranked categories is used. For greater reproducibility, a continuous measure such as hand-held dynamometry is superior.

5 = normal power against gravity and the usual amount of resistance
4 = muscle contraction possible against gravity and less than the normal amount of resistance
3 = muscle contraction possible only against gravity, not with resistance
2 = joint movement possible only with gravity eliminated
1 = flicker of contraction with no movement
0 = no contraction detectable

SPINE

6. Name the major ligaments of the spine.
Anterior longitudinal ligament
Posterior longitudinal ligament
Ligamenta flava
Interspinous and supraspinous ligaments

7. What are the parts of the intervertebral disc?
A peripheral, laminated, fibrocartilaginous **anulus fibrosus** and a central, gel-like **nucleus pulposus**. The anulus fibrosus contains the fluid nucleus pulposus between the adjacent vertebral bodies. The nucleus pulposus serves as a hydraulic load-dispersing mechanism, so that as the spine bends in any direction, the compressive loads borne by that side of the disc are redistributed over a larger surface area, thereby reducing the pressure.

8. Why do most intervertebral disc protrusions occur posterolaterally?
1. The disc is reinforced anterolaterally by the anterior longitudinal ligament and posteromedially by the posterior longitudinal ligament. Posterolaterally, there are no extrinsic supporting ligaments.
2. The nucleus pulposus is eccentrically located closer to the posterior aspect of the disc, causing the posterior anulus to have the smallest radial dimension and offer the least support.
3. The posterior anulus is thinnest in the superior-inferior dimension at cervical and lumbar levels, causing it to suffer the greatest strain.
4. Since flexion is the most predominant spine motion, the posterior anulus receives the most repetitive tensile stresses.
5. The posterolateral anulus is subject to the highest intralaminar shear stresses, causing intralaminar separation.

9. Describe the course of the spinal nerves in the spine.
At most levels, **dorsal** and **ventral roots** joint to form **spinal nerves** as they enter the intervertebral foramen. The **dorsal root ganglia** are located on the spinal nerve at this point. As spinal nerves exit the intervertebral foramen, they terminate by dividing into **dorsal** and **ventral rami**. Cervical spinal nerves exit above the vertebra of the same number. The C8 spinal nerve emerges between the C7 and T1 vertebrae, which causes all thoracic, lumbar, and sacral nerves to exit below the vertebrae of the same number. Because lower spinal nerves must descend to their intervertebral foramina from their higher point of origin from the spinal cord, they typically occupy the upper portion of their intervertebral foramen.

10. Why do herniated lumbar intervertebral discs commonly miss the nerve that exits at that level and instead affect the next lower spinal nerve roots?
Lumbar intervertebral foramina are large, and because the nerves occupy the upper part of the foramen and the disc is related to the lower part of the foramen, posterolateral disc herniations

commonly miss the nerve in the foramen. Instead, they tend to affect the roots of the next lower spinal nerve, which occupy the most lateral part of the spinal canal before exiting from the next lower intervertebral foramen. For example, a herniated L4–5 disc will typically miss the L4 nerve and affect the L5 roots.

11. Where are the uncovertebral or Luschka's joints?

The lower five cervical vertebrae contain **uncinate processes** that protrude cranially from the lateral margins of the superior surface of their bodies. Luschka's joints begin to develop in the second decade of life as degenerative clefts in the lateral part of the intervertebral disc just medial to the uncinate processes. Degeneration begins at this point because it is where the cervical discs are narrowest in their superior-inferior dimension and hence subject to greatest tensile stresses during motion. Hypertrophic degenerative changes can involve Luschka's joints or the posterior portion of the cervical disc, which is the next thinnest part of the disc. Hypertrophic bars developing in the posterior disc can encroach both nerve roots and spinal cord.

12. What are lateral recesses? What is their significance?

Lateral recesses are a normal narrowing of the anteroposterior dimension of the lateral portion of the spinal canal at the L4, L5, and S1 levels. They occur because the pedicles become shorter in their AP dimension at these levels. This brings the superior articular processes and facet joints close to the posterior aspect of the lateral part of the vertebral bodies. The pedicle forms the lateral wall of the recess.

As the L4–S1 nerve roots descend the spinal canal, they each course through a lateral recess before exiting their intervertebral foramen. When hypertrophic degenerative changes involve the superior articular process, it can reduce the distance between this process and the vertebral body to < 3 mm, producing **lateral stenosis** with the potential for nerve root encroachment. Hypertrophic changes involving the more medially situated inferior articular process will more likely produce a **central stenosis** of the spinal canal. Facet joints also form the posterior boundary of the intervertebral foramen, where hypertrophic changes can produce **foraminal stenosis**.

13. What anatomic and mechanical features of the lumbosacral junction predispose L5 to spondylolysis and spondylolisthesis?

The steep inclined plane of the sacral angle (commonly 50° from horizontal) predisposes the L5 vertebra to slide forward on S1 under a gravitational load. This slippage is resisted by the impaction of the inferior articular processes of L5 against the superior articular processes of the sacrum. These forces and their reactions concentrate substantial shearing stresses on the **pars interarticularis** of the L5 lamina. Hence, **spondylolysis** is most commonly a stress fracture. Whether a **spondylolisthesis** develops depends on the ability of the anterior longitudinal ligament and iliolumbar ligaments to resist anterior displacement of the L5 vertebral body.

14. Are the deep back muscles contracted or relaxed in the upright position?

In the upright position, the spine is in relatively good equilibrium because the line of gravity falls through the points of inflection of each of the curves of the spine. As a result, activity in the major deep back muscles (erector spinae, semispinalis, multifidus and rotators) is negligible, and the ligaments of the spine resist any applied moments.

15. Which muscles are responsible for producing the major spine motions?

Flexion: The **anterior abdominal muscles** initiate flexion, but as soon as the spine is out of equilibrium, gravity becomes the prime mover under the control of an eccentric contraction of the **deep back muscles**. A concentric contraction of the deep back muscles returns the spine to an upright position.

Extension: Spinal extension is initiated by the **deep back muscles**, with gravity becoming the prime mover as soon as the spine is out of equilibrium. The **anterior abdominal muscles**

control gravity with an eccentric contraction and return the spine to an upright position with a concentric contraction.

Lateral bending: Lateral bending is initiated by the ipsilateral **deep back, abdominal, psoas major**, and **quadratus lumborum** muscles. Once started, gravity becomes the prime mover under the control of the same muscles on the contralateral side, which also contract concentrically to return the spine to the upright position.

Rotation: Rotation of the front of the trunk to one side is produced by the ipsilateral **erector spinae** and **internal abdominal oblique** muscles and the contralateral **deeper back** muscles and **external abdominal oblique**. Rotation of the face to one side is also produced by the ipsilateral **splenius**, contralateral **sternocleidomastoid** and other **cervical rotators**.

16. What do dorsal rami of spinal nerves innervate?

Dorsal rami innervate the skin of the medial two-thirds of the back from the interauricular line to the coccyx (top of the head to the tip of the tail), deep muscles of the back, posterior ligaments of the spine, and the facet joint capsules.

UPPER LIMB

17. What structure provides the strongest support for the acromioclavicular joint?

The **coracoclavicular ligament**, which descends from the distal clavicle to the coracoid process. This ligament must be torn to produce the major stepdown of the acromion below the clavicle in grade 3 acromioclavicular joint injuries.

18. What structural features cause the shoulder (glenohumeral) joint to be a highly mobile but relatively unstable joint?

The relatively poor bony congruence between the glenoid and humeral head and a slack capsule.

19. What dynamic features help maintain shoulder joint contact through the full range of abduction?

The **rotator cuff muscles** stabilize the shoulder by varying their medially directed vector forces. In early abduction, the **deltoid** tends to sublux the humeral head superiorly. This is offset by increased tension in the superior capsule by the simultaneous contraction of the **supraspinatus** and by the slightly downward vector pull of the **subscapularis, infraspinatus**, and **teres minor** muscles. In the middle range of abduction, the **subscapularis** turns off to allow the **infraspinatus** and **teres major** to externally rotate the humerus and bring the greater tubercle posteriorly under the acromion (which is the highest part of the coracoacromial arch). This prevents its impingement against the arch.

20. How does medial and lateral winging of the scapula occur?

The medial border of the scapula is normally kept closely applied to the thoracic wall by the resultant vector forces of its medially and laterally tethering muscles, the **trapezius** and **serratus anterior**. If the serratus anterior is paralyzed, the medial border will wing away from the chest wall and be displaced medially by the unopposed retraction of the trapezius (medial winging). If the trapezius is paralyzed, the medial border will also wing but be displaced laterally by the unopposed protraction of the serratus anterior (lateral winging).

21. What are the two major "crutch-walking" muscles of the shoulder?

The upward vector force of the crutches at the shoulder is primarily offset by the downward pull of the **pectoralis major** and **latissimus dorsi** muscles acting on the humerus.

22. Why is the elbow a relatively stable joint?

The trochlear notch of the ulna has a good grip on the humeral trochlea, and there are strong, relatively taut radial and ulnar collateral ligaments.

23. Where is the axis for pronation and supination of the forearm located?

Proximally, it passes through the center of the radial head; distally, it passes through the ulnar head. Hence, during pronation and supination, the radius scribes half a cone in space about the ulna.

24. How are major loads transferred from the radius at the wrist to the ulna at the elbow?

They are transferred across the **interosseous membrane**, whose fibers run primarily from the ulna upward to the radius. Hence, loads ascending the radius will tense this membrane and be transferred to the ulna.

WRIST AND HAND

25. Which carpal bones are most frequently injured?

The major weight-bearing carpal bones are most frequently injured: the **scaphoid** by a neck fracture, and the **lunate** with a palmar dislocation. In one-third of scaphoid fractures there is nonunion, since about one-third of scaphoids receive a blood supply only to their distal end. The lunate tends to dislocate palmarward during hyperextension injuries, because it is wedge-shaped with the apex of the wedge pointing dorsally.

26. Why does carpal tunnel syndrome cause no sensory abnormalities over the palm?

The palmar cutaneous branch of the median nerve passes superficial to the flexor retinaculum.

27. How can the flexor digitorum profundus be eliminated in order to test the flexor digitorum superficialis tendons in isolation?

To test the ability of the flexor digitorum superficialis to flex the proximal interphalangeal (PIP) joint of a finger, hold the rest of the fingers into forcible by hyperextension by resistance over the distal phalanges. This is effective because the individual tendons of the profundus generally arise from a common tendon that attaches to its muscle mass, while each of the tendons of the superficialis has its own separate muscle belly. Hence, placing the other fingers into extension puts all of the profundus under stretch and eliminates it as PIP joint flexor.

28. How can the extensor digitorum be eliminated to isolate and test the extensor indicis as the last muscle innervated by the radial nerve?

The extensor indicis is tested by metacarpophalangeal (MP) joint extension of the index finger with the other fingers held in flexion at their MP joints. This is effective because the tendons of the extensor digitorum are cross-linked over the dorsum of the hand by intertendinous connections. Therefore, if the rest of the tendons are pulled distally over their MP joints by forcible flexion, it tethers the tendon to the index finger distally and makes the extensor digitorum ineffective as an index finger MP joint extensor.

29. Why are the motions of the thumb at right angles to the similar motions of the fingers?

In the resting hand, the thumb is internally rotated 90° relative to the fingers. Hence, flexion and extension of the thumb occur in a plane parallel to the plane of the palm, and abduction and adduction of the thumb occur at right angles to the plane of the palm, with the thumb moving away from the palm in abduction and toward the palm in adduction. Opposition involves almost 90° of further internal rotation of the thumb at its carpometacarpal joint.

30. What is the normal digital balance mechanism of the fingers?

At the MP joint, there is one extensor, the extensor digitorum (though there is an additional extensor of the index and little fingers), balanced against four flexors—the interossei, lumbrical, and flexor digitorum profundus, and superficialis. At the PIP joint, there are three extensors—interossei and the lumbrical and extensor digitorum—balanced against two flexors—flexor digitorum profundus and superficialis. At the distal interphalangeal (DIP) joint, there are three extensors—interossei and the lumbrical and extensor digitorum—balanced against one flexor,

flexor digitorum profundus. The muscles contributing to the extensor balance form an extensor hood mechanism which splits into lateral and central bands over the PIP joint, with the central band inserting into the base of the middle phalanx and the lateral bands inserting into the base of the distal phalanx. Over the PIP joint, all three bands are connected by the **triangular membrane**, which holds the lateral bands in their normal dorsal position. An **oblique retinacular ligament of Landsmeer** splits off the lateral bands to tether them ventrally to the proximal phalanx.

LOWER LIMB

31. What structural features make the hip a relatively stable joint?

1. Good congruence between the femoral head and the deeply concave acetabulum, which with its labrum forms more than half a sphere.

2. Strong capsular ligaments, two of which—the iliofemoral and ischiofemoral ligaments—are maximally taut in the extended upright position (the usual weight-bearing position).

32. What are the unique features of the hip joint capsule and its blood supply? What is their clinical significance?

The anterior hip joint capsule attaches to the **intertrochanteric line of the femur**, thereby completely enclosing the anterior femoral neck. The posterior capsule encloses the proximal two-thirds of the femoral neck. Therefore, the femoral head and most of the femoral neck are intracapsular. This has two clinically important effects. First, it requires that most of the blood supply to the femoral head (mostly from the **medial femoral circumflex artery**) must ascend the femoral neck. Hence, except for the small branch of the obturator artery that enters the head with the ligament of the femoral head (ligamentum teres), most of the blood supply to the femoral head is compromised by femoral neck fractures. Second, because the capsule attaches to the femoral neck so low, the upper femoral metaphysis is intracapsular. Since the metaphysis is the most vascular part of a long bone, hematogenously spread infection to the upper femoral metaphysis can easily produce a septic arthritis. In most other joints, the metaphyses are extracapsular.

33. Even though the long, obliquely situated femoral neck predisposes the hip to high shearing forces and fracture, are there any physiologic advantages to this unique design?

The long, obliquely situated femoral neck has the salutary effect of displacing the greater trochanter farther from the abduction-adduction axis of the femoral head, thereby lengthening the moment arm of the gluteus medius-minimus muscles. In standing on one leg, the gravitational vector acting on the adduction side of the hip joint is on a moment arm approximately three times as long as the gluteus medius-minimus moment arm. Therefore, these muscles have to produce a force approximately three times as great as the gravitational vector to offset its hip adduction tendency. If the femoral neck were any shorter or more vertically oriented, as in a valgus hip, the gluteus medius-minimus moment arm would be shortened, requiring these muscles to apply more force to offset the gravitational vector. The long moment arm of the normal femoral neck thereby reduces the loads across the hip and helps protect the hip from degenerative arthritis.

34. What is the best way to test the right gluteus medius-minimus muscles?

Ask the patient to stand on the right leg. If these muscles are weak or paralyzed, the left side of the pelvis will sag under the influence of the gravitational adduction vector (Trendelenburg sign).

35. At what point in the gait cycle is the gluteus maximus most active? Why?

At heel strike of the ipsilateral limb. This offsets the effect of the ground reaction vector, which acts anterior to the hip at this point and therefore tends to cause the trunk to flex on the thigh.

36. When is the iliopsoas most active during the gait cycle? Why?

At toe-off the iliopsoas acts as a hip flexor to offset the ground reaction vector, which is then acting posterior to the hip to cause hip extension.

37. Why is the knee joint most stable in extension?
    1. Since the anterior portion of the femoral condyle is less curved than the posterior condyle, the congruence and area of contact between the **femoral** and **tibial condyles** are greatest in extension. Hence, the pressures acting across the knee are lowest in extension.
    2. The **tibial** and **fibular collateral ligaments** are maximally taut in extension.
    3. The **anterior cruciate ligament** is completely tense only in extension.

38. Why are the gastrocnemius and soleus muscles the most active lower limb muscles in standing?
    In quiet standing, the line of gravity falls slightly behind the hip joint, slightly anterior to the knee, and 2 inches anterior to the ankle joint axis. At the hip, the tendency of the line of gravity to hyperextend the hip is resisted by the tension in the iliofemoral (and ischiofemoral) ligaments. So hip flexor muscle activity is generally unnecessary. The line of gravity tends to hyperextend the knee, and tension in the posterior capsule probably helps resist this. However, the activity in the gastrocnemius muscle, which is primarily to stabilize the ankle, also helps prevent back-knee. At the ankle, the long moment arm of the line of gravity makes it a strong ankle dorsiflexor. The activity in the gastrocnemius and soleus muscles resists this ankle dorsiflexion tendency.

FOOT AND ANKLE

39. What is the most osteologically stable position of the ankle? Why?
    In dorsiflexion. Both the talar trochlea and tibiofibular mortise have wedge-shaped articular surfaces that are wide anteriorly and narrow posteriorly. In dorsiflexion, the wide anterior part of the talar trochlea is wedged back into the narrow posterior part of the tibiofibular mortise.

40. At what joint(s) does most of the pronation and supination of the foot occur?
    The subtalar joint permits most of the pronation (eversion) and supination (inversion) of the foot, but the transverse tarsal and tarsometatarsal joints also contribute.

41. When are the ankle dorsiflexor muscles active during gait?
    The ankle dorsiflexors are active isometrically during swing to prevent gravity from causing foot-drop, and eccentrically from heel strike to flat foot (the loading response) to control the plantar flexion vector exerted on the calcaneus by the ground reaction.

42. Which nerve of the foot is homologous to the median nerve in the hand?
    The medial plantar nerve. It generally supplies the plantar skin of the medial two-thirds of the foot and medial three and one-half digits, the intrinsic muscles of the great toe except for the adductor hallucis, the first lumbrical, and the flexor digitorum brevis (homologous to the flexor digitorum superficialis of the upper limb). The lateral plantar nerve is also homologous to the ulnar nerve.

BIBLIOGRAPHY

1. Bland JH, Boushey DR: Anatomy and physiology of the cervical spine. Semin Arthritis Rheum 20:1–20, 1990.
2. Cailliet R: Low Back Pain Syndrome. Philadelphia, F.A. Davis, 1995, pp 1–76.
3. Hayashi K, Yabuki T: Origin of the uncus and of Luschka's joint in the cervical spine. J Bone Joint Surg 67A:788–791, 1985.
4. Inman VT, Saunders JB, Abbott LC: Observations on the function of the shoulder joint. J Bone Joint Surg 26A:1–30, 1944.
5. Johnson RM, Crelin ES, White AA, et al: Some newer observations on the functional anatomy of the lower cervical spine. Clin Orthop 111:192–200, 1975.
6. Schneck CD: Clinical anatomy of the cervical spine. In White AH, Schofferman JA: Spine Care. St. Louis, Mosby, 1995, pp 1306–1334.
7. Schneck CD: Functional and clinical anatomy of the spine. Spine State Art Rev 9:1–37, 1995.
8. Turek SL: Orthopedics: Principles and Their Application. Philadelphia, J.B. Lippincott, 1984, pp 1123–1126.

7. NERVOUS SYSTEM ANATOMY

Stephen Goldberg, M.D.

1. What structures comprise the central nervous system (CNS)?
Spinal cord
Brainstem (medulla, pons, midbrain)
Cerebellum
Cerebrum
Diencephalon (everything that contains the name thalamus—thalamus, hypothalamus, epithalamus, subthalamus)
Basal ganglia (caudate nucleus, globus pallidus, putamen, claustrum, amygdala)

2. How many structures make up the peripheral nervous system?
31 pairs of spinal nerves
12 cranial nerves (although the optic nerve technically is an outgrowth of the CNS)

3. What is the autonomic nervous system?
The autonomic nervous system innervates smooth muscle, cardiac muscle, and glands. It includes the **sympathetic nerves**, which originate from spinal cord segments T1–L2, and the **parasympathetic nerves**, which originate from spinal cord segments S2–S4 as well as from four cranial nerves (CN): CN3 (oculomotor nerve fibers to pupil and ciliary body), CN7 (facial nerve fibers to sublingual, submaxillary, and lacrimal glands), CN9 (glossopharyngeal nerve fibers to parotid glands), and CN10 (vagus nerve fibers to heart, lungs, and GI tract to the splenic flexure).

SPINAL CORD

4. Name the five major divisions of the spinal cord.
Cervical, thoracic, lumbar, sacral, and coccygeal.

5. Where does the spinal cord end?
About the level of vertebrae L1–2.

6. How many nerves exit the spinal cord?
There are 31 pairs of spinal nerves: 8 cervical, 12 thoracic, 5 lumbar, 5 sacral, and 1 coccygeal. Each spinal nerve is the fusion of a dorsal and ventral nerve root.

7. What are the coverings (meninges) of the spinal cord?
The meninges surround the entire CNS and consist of the **pia**, which hugs the spinal cord and brain; the **arachnoid membrane**; and the **dura**, which is closely adherent to bone.

8. Where do you find the cauda equina?
The cauda equina ("horse's tail") is the downward extension of spinal cord roots at the inferior end of the spinal cord.

MOTOR AND SENSORY PATHWAYS

9. What are the major motor pathways to the extremities?
Corticospinal tract (pyramidal tract): extends from the motor area of the cerebral frontal cortex (Brodmann's areas 4, 6) through the internal capsule, brainstem, and spinal cord, crossing

over at the junction between the brainstem and spinal cord at the level of the foramen magnum. Therefore, lesions to the corticospinal tract above the level of the foramen magnum result in contralateral weakness, whereas lesions below the level of the foramen magnum result in ipsilateral weakness.

Rubrospinal tract: connects the red nucleus of the midbrain with the spinal cord
Tectospinal tract: connects the tectum of the midbrain with the spinal cord
Reticulospinal tract: connects the reticular formation of the brainstem with the spinal cord
Vestibulospinal tract: connects the vestibular nuclei of the brainstem with the spinal cord

10. What distinguishes an upper motor neuron lesion from a lower motor neuron lesion?
An upper motor neuron lesion generally refers to an injury to the corticospinal tract. The corticospinal pathway synapses in the anterior horn of the spinal cord just prior to leaving the cord. A lower motor neuron lesion is an injury to the peripheral motor nerves or their cell bodies in the gray matter of the anterior horn on which the corticospinal tract synapses.

Upper MN Defect	Lower MN Defect
Spastic paralysis	Flaccid paralysis
No significant muscle atrophy	Significant atrophy
No fasciculations or fibrillations	Fasciculations and fibrillations present
Hyperreflexia	Hyporeflexia
Babinski reflex may be present	Babinski reflex not present

11. How do the effects of corticospinal tract injuries differ from those of cerebellar and basal ganglia injuries?
All of the injuries produce motor problems. **Corticospinal tract** injuries cause paralysis.

Cerebellar injuries are characterized by awkwardness of movement (**ataxia**) rather than paralysis. The awkwardness is on intention—i.e., at rest, the patient shows no problem, but the ataxia becomes noticeable when the patient attempts a motor action. There may be awkwardness of posture and gait, poor coordination of movement, dysmetria, dysdiadochokinesia, scanning speech, decreased tendon reflexes on the affected side, asthenia, tremor, and nystagmus.

Basal ganglia disorders, like cerebellar disorders, are characterized by awkward movements rather than paralysis. The movement disorder, however, is generally present at rest, including such problems as parkinsonism, chorea, athetosis, and hemiballismus.

12. Name three major sensory pathways in the spinal cord.
   1. Pain-temperature—spinothalamic tract
   2. Proprioception-stereognosis—posterior columns (Proprioception is the ability to tell, with the eyes closed, if a joint is flexed or extended. Stereognosis is the ability to identify, with the eyes closed, an object placed in one's hand.)
   3. Light touch—spinothalamic tract and posterior columns

BRAINSTEM AND CRANIAL NERVES

13. Name the three parts of the brainstem.
The midbrain (most superior), pons, and medulla (most inferior).

14. What are the functions of the cranial nerves?
   CN1 (olfactory): smell
   CN2 (optic): sight
   CN3 (oculomotor): constricts pupils, accommodates, moves eyes
   CN4 (trochlear), CN6 (abducens): move eyes
   CN5 (trigeminal): chews, feels front of head
   CN7 (facial): moves face, taste, salivation, crying
   CN8 (vestibulocochlear): hearing, regulates balance

CN9 (glossopharyngeal): taste, salivation, swallowing, monitors carotid body and sinus

CN10 (vagus): taste, swallowing, lifts palate; communication to and from thoracoabdominal viscera to the splenic flexure of the colon

CN11 (accessory): turns head, lifts shoulders

CN12 (hypoglossal): moves tongue

15. What is Horner's syndrome?

Horner's syndrome is ptosis, miosis, and anhydrosis (lack of sweating) from a lesion of the sympathetic pathway to the face. The lesion may lie within the brainstem or within the superior cervical ganglion or its sympathetic extensions to the head.

16. Which cranial nerves exit from the three parts of the brainstem?

Midbrain—CN3, CN4

Pons—CN5, CN6, CN7, CN8

Medulla—(part of CN7 and CN8), CN9, CN10, CN12

CN11 exits from the upper cervical cord, goes through the foramen magnum, touches CNs 9 and 10, and then returns to the neck via the jugular foramen. The optic nerve lies superior to the brainstem. The olfactory nerve lies in the cribriform plate of the ethmoid bone.

17. What CNS areas connect with the brainstem?

The midbrain connects with the diencephalon above. The medulla connects with the spinal cord below. In addition, each section of the brainstem has two major connections (right and left) with the cerebellum. Two superior cerebellar peduncles connect with the midbrain; two middle cerebellar peduncles connect with the pons; and two inferior cerebellar peduncles connect with the medulla.

18. What are the two pigmented areas of the brainstem?

The substantia nigra, which lies in the midbrain, and the locus coeruleus, which lies in the pons.

19. What is the red nucleus?

The red nucleus lies in the midbrain. It receives major output from the cerebellum via the superior cerebellar peduncle. It has major connections to the cerebral cortex as well as to the spinal cord via the rubrospinal tract.

20. What is the medial longitudinal fasciculus (MLF)?

The MLF is a pathway that runs through the brainstem and interconnects the ocular nuclei of CNs 3, 4, 6, and the vestibular nuclei. It plays an important role in coordinating eye movements with head and truncal posture.

21. What is the Edinger-Westphal nucleus?

The Edinger-Westphal nucleus is the parasympathetic nucleus of the third cranial nerve in the midbrain. It supplies motor fibers responsible for pupillary constriction and lens accommodation.

22. What is an Argyll-Robertson pupil?

One of the classic signs of tertiary syphilis. The pupil constricts on accommodating but does not constrict to light. The lesion is believed to be in the midbrain.

23. What is the pathway for vision?

Optic nerve fibers extend from the retina to the optic nerve, to the optic chiasm, to the optic tract, to the lateral geniculate body, and to the visual area of the brain via the optic radiation. Optic radiation fibers that extend through the parietal lobe end up superior to the calcarine fissure in the occipital lobe. Optic radiation fibers that extend through the temporal lobe end up inferior to the calcarine fissure in the occipital lobe.

24. What causes a left homonymous hemianopsia? Bitemporal hemianopsia? Superior quadrantanopsia?

Left homonymous hemianopsia: a lesion to the right optic tract, right lateral geniculate body, right optic radiation, or right occipital lobe.

Bitemporal hemianopsia: a lesion to the optic chiasm, generally from a pituitary tumor.

Superior quadrantanopsia: a lesion in the inferior aspect of the optic radiation.

25. What is most peculiar about the exit point of CN4 from the brainstem?

CN4 is the only cranial nerve to exit on the posterior side of the brainstem. In addition, it crosses over the midline before continuing on its course.

26. If a child has a head tilt, how do you know if it is due to a CN4 palsy or to a stiff neck?

Cover one eye. If the head straightens out, the tilt is due to a CN4 palsy. The child tilts the head in a CN4 palsy to avoid double vision. Covering one eye eliminates double vision, so the head straightens out.

27. Which CNs exit at the pontomedullary junction?

CN6 exits by the midline; CNs 7 and 8 exit laterally.

28. Where do the motor and sensory branches of CN5 exit the brainstem?

Both exit the brainstem at the same point, in the lateral aspect of the pons.

29. What are the sensory branches of CN5?

V1—ophthalmic
V2—maxillary
V3—mandibular

30. Which cranial nerve nucleus extends through all sections of the brainstem?

The trigeminal sensory nucleus. Its mesencephalic nucleus (facial proprioception) lies in the midbrain. Its main nucleus (facial light touch) lies in the pons. Its spinal nucleus (facial pain/temperature) lies in the medulla and upper spinal cord.

31. What is the function of cranial nerve 7?

CN7 innervates the muscles of facial expression; supplies parasympathetic fibers to the lacrimal, submandibular, and sublingual glands; receives taste information from the anterior two-thirds of the tongue; and receives a minor sensory input from the skin of the external ear.

32. How does the facial weakness that results from a CN7 lesion differ from that due to a lesion of the facial motor area of the cerebral cortex?

A CN7 lesion (as in Bell's palsy of CN7, which occurs in the facial nerve canal) results in ipsilateral facial paralysis, which includes the upper and lower face. A cerebral lesion results in contralateral facial paralysis, confined to the lower face.

33. What is Mobius syndrome?

A congenital absence of both facial nerve nuclei, resulting in bilateral facial paralysis. The abducens nuclei may also be absent.

34. What are the nucleus ambiguus, nucleus solitarius, and salivatory nucleus?

The **nucleus ambiguus**, which lies in the medulla, is a motor nucleus (CNs 9 and 10) that innervates the deep throat, i.e., the muscles of swallowing (CNs 9, 10) and speech (CN10).

The **nucleus solitarius** is a visceral sensory nucleus (CNs 7, 9, 10) that lies in the medulla. It receives input from the viscera as well as taste information. It is a relay in the gag reflex.

The **salivatory nucleus**, which contains superior and inferior divisions, innervates the salivary glands (CNs 7 and 9) and lacrimal glands (CN7).

35. What does CN9 do?

CN9, the glossopharyngeal nerve, innervates the stylopharyngeus muscle of the pharynx and the parotid gland, and it receives taste information from the posterior one-third of the tongue. It receives sensory tactile input from the posterior one-third of the tongue as well as from the skin around the external ear canal. It also receives sensory input from the carotid body and sinus.

36. Which side does the tongue deviate to if cranial nerve 12 (hypoglossal nerve) is injured?

The tongue deviates to the side of the lesion. Imagine that you are riding a bicycle and your left hand becomes paralyzed. If you then try to push on the handle bars, the wheel will turn to the left. The genioglossus muscle, which is innervated by CN12 and pushes out the tongue, operates on a similar principle.

PERIPHERAL NERVES

37. What type of nerve fibers are found in anterior (ventral) nerve roots?
Mainly motor axons.

38. What type of nerve fibers are found in posterior (dorsal) nerve roots?
Mainly sensory axons.

39. What is found in posterior (dorsal) root ganglia?

Posterior root ganglia contain the cell bodies of sensory axons, but no synapses. This has important implications for electromyographers performing nerve conduction studies. If the lesion is proximal to the dorsal root ganglion, then sensory conduction will be normal in the peripheral nerve, since the cell bodies are intact.

40. What sensory features distinguish a peripheral nerve lesion from a CNS lesion?

Peripheral nerve lesions can be distinguished from CNS lesions by the different kinds of sensory and motor deficits that arise. Peripheral nerve lesions result in **dermatome**-type sensory deficits—i.e., there is a striplike loss of sensation along a particular area of the body, corresponding to the extension of individual peripheral nerves away from the spinal cord. L4–5 radiculopathies are particularly common, as are C6, C7, and C8 radiculopathies.

The CNS, however, is not organized by dermatomes. A CNS motor lesion will more likely result in a **general sensory loss** in an extremity rather than in the striplike dermatome deficit.

41. Which dermatomes are innervated by which nerves?
Some mnemonic aids for the dermatomes:
C1: no sensory distribution
C2: skull cap
C3: collar around the neck
C4: cape around the shoulders
T5: nipples
C6: "thumb suckers suck C6"
T10: belly button
L1 = IL (region of inguinal ligament)
L4: knee jerk
S1: ankle jerk

42. Can motor features distinguish a peripheral nerve lesion from a CNS lesion?

Peripheral nerve lesions produce lower motor neuron deficits. CNS lesions produce upper motor neuron deficits.

43. Which roots comprise the brachial plexus?

The brachial plexus contains the ventral rami of C5, 6, 7, 8 and T1.

44. Which nerves arise from the anterior (ventral) rami of the roots prior to the formation of the brachial plexus?

The **dorsal scapular nerve**, from C5 to the rhomboid and levator scapula muscles, is responsible for elevating and stabilizing the scapula. The **long thoracic nerve**, from C5, 6, and 7 to the serratus anterior muscle, is responsible for abduction of the scapula.

45. Which roots form the trunks of the brachial plexus?

The superior trunk arises from C5 and 6. The suprascapular nerve (C5) comes off the upper trunk and supplies the supraspinatus (abduction) and infraspinatus (external rotation) muscles of the shoulder. The middle trunk comes from C7. The lower trunk comes from C8 and T1.

46. What nerve is commonly affected in shoulder dislocations or fractures of the humerus?

The axillary nerve is commonly affected, resulting in weakness of abduction of the shoulder and anesthesia over the lateral proximal arm.

47. What is the thoracic outlet syndrome?

This syndrome, usually caused by an extra cervical rib that compresses the medial cord of the brachial plexus and the axillary artery, results in tingling and numbness in the medial aspect of the arm, along with decreased upper extremity pulses.

48. Describe the anatomy of the peripheral nerves to the upper extremity.

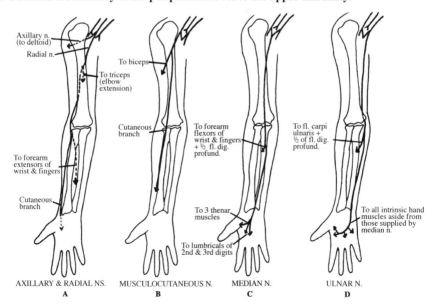

Anatomy of the nerves to the upper extremity. (From Goldberg S: Clinical Anatomy Made Ridiculously Simple. Miami, MedMaster, 1991; with permission.)

49. What motor functions are impaired by peripheral nerve injuries in the upper extremity?

Radial nerve (C5–8)—Elbow and wrist extension (patient has wrist drop); extension of fingers at MCP joints; triceps reflex

Median nerve (C8–T1)—Wrist, thumb, index, and middle finger flexion; thumb opposition, forearm pronation; ability of wrist to bend toward the radial (thumb) side; atrophy of thenar eminence (ball of thumb)

Ulnar nerve (C8–T1)—Flexion of wrist, ring and small finger (claw hand); opposition of little finger; ability of wrist to bend toward ulnar (small finger) side; adduction and abduction of fingers; atrophy of hypothenar eminence in palm (at base of ring and small fingers)

Musculocutaneous nerve (C5–6)—Elbow flexion (biceps); forearm supination; biceps reflex

Axillary nerve (C5–6)—Ability to move upper arm outward, forward, or backward (deltoid atrophy)

Long thoracic nerve (C5–7)—Ability to elevate arm above horizontal (winging of scapula)

50. Describe the anatomy of the lumbosacral plexus.

The roots of L1 through S4 contribute to the lumbosacral plexus. The lumbosacral plexus innervates the skin and skeletal muscles of the lower extremity and perineal area. As in the brachial plexus, its nerve fibers are extensions of anterior (ventral) rami.

Of the gluteal nerves, the inferior gluteal nerve supplies gluteus maximus, whereas the superior gluteal nerve supplies gluteus medius and minimus. Injury to the superior gluteal nerve (e.g., direct trauma, polio) results in the "gluteus medius limp": the abductor function of gluteus medius is lost, and the pelvis tilts to the unaffected side when the unaffected extremity is lifted on attempting to walk. To some, the gait resembles a sexy wiggle.

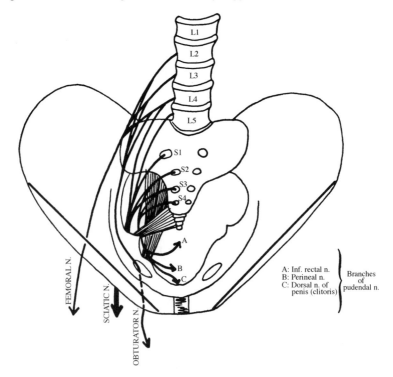

Overview of the lumbosacral plexus. (From Goldberg S: Clinical Anatomy Made Ridiculously Simple. Miami, MedMaster, 1991; with permission.)

51. Describe the route of the peripheral nerves to the lower extremity.

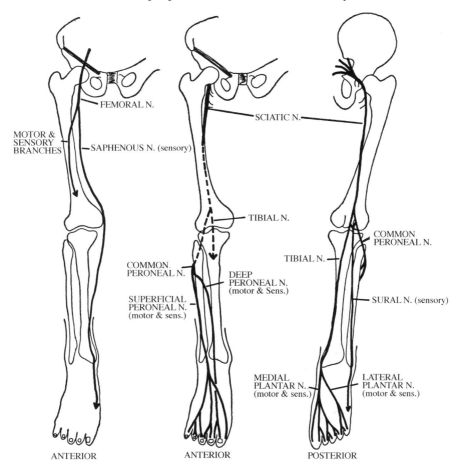

Anatomy of the nerves to the lower extremity. (From Goldberg S: Clinical Anatomy Made Ridiculously Simple. Miami, MedMaster, 1991; with permission.)

52. What motor functions are impaired by peripheral nerve injuries in the lower extremity?

Femoral nerve (L2–4)	Knee extension; hip flexion; knee jerk.
Obturator nerve (L2–4)	Hip adduction (patient's leg swings outward when walking)
Sciatic nerve (L4–S3)	Knee flexion plus other functions along its branches, the tibial and common peroneal nerves
Tibial nerve (L4–S3)	Foot inversion; ankle plantar flexion; ankle jerk
Common peroneal nerve (L4–S2)	Foot eversion; ankle and toes dorsiflexion (patient has high stepping gait owing to foot-drop)

53. Name the other branches of the lumbar plexus.

Iliohypogastric nerve (L1)—supplies abdominal muscles as well as skin over the hypogastric and gluteal areas

Ilioinguinal nerve (L1)—innervates skin over the groin and scrotum/labia

Genitofemoral nerve (L1, 2)—runs in the inguinal canal to reach the skin at the base of the penis and scrotum/clitoris and labia majora

54. What is meralgia paraesthetica?

Commonly found in obese individuals, it is a numbness over the lateral thigh that results from compression of the lateral femoral cutaneous nerve where it runs under the inguinal ligament.

55. Which nerve supplies the perineum?

The pudendal nerve (S2,3,4). Parasympathetic branches of S2,3,4 supply the bladder and are critical in bladder emptying. Sympathetic fibers to the bladder (from T11 to L2) promote retention of urine, but severing of sympathetic fibers to the bladder does not significantly affect bladder function.

CEREBRUM

56. What does the frontal lobe do?

Motor areas of the frontal lobe control **voluntary movement** on the opposite side of the body, including eye movement to the opposite side. The dominant hemisphere, usually the left, contains Broca's speech area, which when injured results in a motor aphasia (**language** deficit). Areas of the frontal lobe anterior to the motor areas are involved in complex **behavioral** and **executive** activities. Lesions here result in changes in judgment, abstract thinking, tactfulness, and foresight.

57. What does the parietal lobe do?

It receives contralateral light touch, proprioceptive, and pain sensory input. Lesions to the dominant hemisphere result in tactile and proprioceptive agnosia (complex receptive disabilities). There may also be confusion in left-right discrimination, disturbances of body image, and apraxia (complex cerebral motor disabilities, caused by cutting off impulses to and from association tracts that interconnect with nearby regions).

58. What effects do temporal lobe lesions have? Occipital lobe lesions?

Temporal lobe lesions in the dominant hemisphere result in auditory aphasia. The patient hears but does not understand. He speaks but makes mistakes unknowingly, owing to an inability to understand his own words. Lesions may result in alexia and agraphia (inability to read and write).

Destruction of an **occipital lobe** causes blindness in the contralateral visual field. Lesions that spare the most-posterior aspect of the occipital lobe do not cause blindness, but rather cause difficulty in recognizing and identifying objects (visual agnosia). A region of the occipital lobe also controls involuntary eye movements to the contralateral side of the body.

CEREBRAL CIRCULATION

59. What is meant by the terms anterior and posterior cerebral circulation?

The **anterior** circulation is the distribution of the internal carotid artery to the cerebrum via the anterior and middle cerebral arteries. The **posterior** circulation is the distribution of the vertebral arteries to the brainstem, cerebellum, and cerebrum via the basilar artery and posterior cerebral artery.

60. What brain region is supplied by the anterior cerebral artery?

The anterior cerebral artery supplies the midline of the cerebrum, specifically the frontal and parietal lobes and the superior portions of the temporal and occipital lobes.

61. Which brain region is supplied by the middle cerebral artery?

The lateral surface of the cerebrum. Specifically, as is the case for the anterior cerebral artery, the frontal and parietal lobes and the superior portions of the temporal and occipital lobe are supplied.

62. Which region is supplied by the posterior cerebral artery?

The medial and lateral surface of the cerebrum. Specifically, the inferior portions of the temporal and occipital lobes.

63. What is the first branch of the internal carotid artery?

The ophthalmic artery.

64. Where does the brainstem get its blood supply?

From the posterior circulation. Namely, branches from the vertebral arteries (to the medulla) and branches from the basilar artery (to the pons and midbrain).

65. What blood vessels supply the cerebellum?

The cerebellar blood supply comes from branches of the basilar artery: the superior cerebellar, the anterior inferior cerebellar, and the posterior inferior cerebellar arteries.

66. What is the blood supply of the thalamus and internal capsules?

From branches of the circle of Willis, including the lenticulostriate and choroidal arteries.

67. Which vessels comprise the circle of Willis?

The anterior communicating artery, the two anterior cerebral arteries, the two middle cerebral arteries, the two posterior communicating arteries, and the two posterior cerebral arteries.

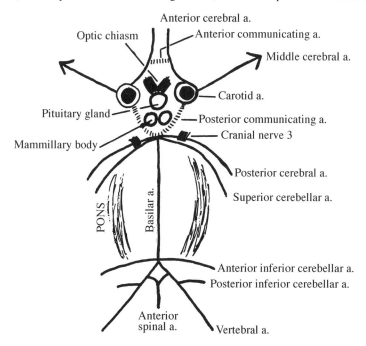

The circle of Willis. (From Goldberg S: Clinical Neuroanatomy Made Ridiculously Simple. Miami, MedMaster, 1995; with permission.)

68. Where does the spinal cord derive its blood supply?

The anterior spinal artery supplies the anterior two-thirds of the spinal cord. Two posterior spinal arteries supply the posterior third. Also, there are rich anastomoses from branches of the vertebral artery and aorta, so a stroke of the spinal cord is rare.

CEREBROSPINAL FLUID

69. Where is the CSF produced?
It is produced by the choroid plexus, which may be found in each of the four ventricles of the brain.

70. How much CSF is produced daily?
About 500 mL.

71. How does the CSF flow through the brain?
The CSF flows from the two lateral ventricles (in the cerebral hemispheres), to the single midline third ventricle (between the right and left thalamus and hypothalamus), to the single midline fourth ventricle (which overlies the pons and medulla), through the foramina of Magendie and Luschka (in the fourth ventricle), to the subarachnoid space (the space between the pia and arachnoid membranes), which lies outside the brain. CSF leaves the subarachnoid space by filtering through the arachnoid granulations of the superior sagittal sinus, where the CSF joins the venous circulation.

72. How do communicating and noncommunicating hydrocephalus differ?
In hydrocephalus, there is elevated CSF pressure and dilation of the ventricles secondary to obstruction to the flow of CSF. In **communicating** hydrocephalus, the obstruction lies outside the ventricular system, beyond the foramina of Magendie and Luschka. In **noncommunicating** hydrocephalus, obstruction occurs within the ventricular system before the foramina of Magendie and Luschka.

73. Where is spinal fluid extracted during a spinal tap?
Spinal fluid is extracted from the subarachnoid space between vertebrae L2 and S2. Normally, the fluid is extracted about vertebra level L4–5.

BIBLIOGRAPHY

1. Goldberg S: Clinical Anatomy Made Ridiculously Simple. Miami, MedMaster, 1991.
2. Goldberg S: Clinical Neuroanatomy Made Ridiculously Simple. Miami, MedMaster, 1995.
3. Goldberg S: Clinical Physiology Made Ridiculously Simple. Miami, MedMaster, 1995.
4. Kandel ER, Schwartz JH, Jessell TM: Essentials of Neural Science and Behavior. Norwalk, CT, Appleton & Lange, 1995.
5. Martin JH: Neuroanatomy: Text and Atlas. Norwalk, CT, Appleton & Lange, 1996.
6. Carpenter MB, Sutin J: Human Neuroanatomy. Baltimore, Williams & Wilkins, 1983.
7. Haines DE: Neuroanatomy: An Atlas of Structures, Sections and Systems. Baltimore, Urban & Schwarzenberg, 1991.

8. NEUROPHYSIOLOGY

Gary Goldberg, M.D.

1. As a rehabilitation clinician, why do I need to know about basic neurophysiology?
Rehabilitation assesses function and treats disability. Since many disabilities derive from lost function occurring as a result of structural or physiologic impairment, all rehabilitation clinicians must have a basic understanding of normal anatomy and physiology. The more one understands about normal physiology and the pathophysiology of the nervous system, the better one can appreciate the neurophysiologic mechanisms of disability and adaptation and the better one can begin to develop strategies for treating the disability. In Mountcastle's famous words: "Physiology is what transforms structure into action."

2. Name the basic elements of the neuron.

A typical vertebrate neuron gives rise to two types of processes: dendrites and axons. The axon is the transmission process that carries action potentials to points distant from the cell body. The action potential that travels down the axon is initiated at the axon hillock. Each neuron may communicate with up to 1000 other neurons through contact via synapses.

(Figure reproduced from Kandel ER, Schwartz JH, Jessel TM (eds): Principles of Neural Science, 3rd ed. New York, Elsevier, 1991, p 19, with permission.)

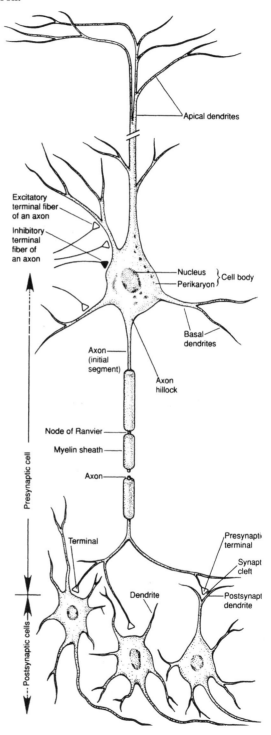

3. What is the basic function of the neuron?

Neurons come in many different shapes and configurations, but their basic function is to integrate activity impinging on the neuron and conduct this information from one place to another. Some neurons function primarily as processing elements in a network (e.g., the interneurons in the spinal cord gray matter), while others conduct information from one place to another along a long cylindrical cellular projection called the axon.

4. How do neurons integrate and transmit information?

Via chemicals that are released at the **synapses**. These chemicals, called **neurotransmitters**, either excite the neuron by depolarizing its membrane and thus creating an excitatory postsynaptic potential, or inhibit the neuron by hyperpolarizing the membrane and thus producing an inhibitory postsynaptic potential. Any particular neuron is constantly bombarded through the synaptic inputs to its dendritic tree by both excitatory and inhibitory influences, which are integrated and then control the overall state of excitation of the neuron, determining when and how frequently it will become excited enough to generate an **action potential**. That action potential can then be conducted along its axon to other neurons. This continual, dynamic process of integration of inputs by the neuron is the basis of computation within the nervous system. All the "action" that takes place in the neuron occurs at its membrane and involves transient local changes in the electrical properties of the nerve cell membrane, or **neurolemma**.

5. Explain what is meant by resting membrane potential.

All cellular membranes have ATP-dependent ion-exchange pumps that are used to control the movement of sodium and potassium ions between the intracellular and extracellular spaces. The electrical voltage in the intracellular space of all cells, by virtue of the high intracellular concentration of nondiffusable anions together with the action of the ion-exchange pump, is relatively negative (by just under 100 mV) compared to the extracellular space. The membrane is thus said to be "polarized," with its inside surface being relatively negative at rest compared to its outside surface. This is an important fact since all excitable tissue phenomena in muscle and nerve cells assume a **resting membrane potential** that keeps the excitable cell quiescent in the presence of a lack of excitation. However, this is not really a "resting" condition since it is *actively* maintained.

6. What is an ectopic membrane potential?

Any problem with the membrane-based ion-exchange pump or the relative permeability of the membrane to any of the major ionic species can result in a major fluctuation of the resting membrane potential in nerve and muscle fibers. This fluctuation can lead to unconstrained depolarization of the membrane to the threshold level, resulting in spontaneous excitation and discharge of the membrane with the production of an aberrant, or **ectopic**, action potential. This is one of the main physiologic ways that excitable cells respond to pathology and is the basis for ectopic discharge in excitable tissues, producing such phenomena as muscle fiber fibrillation and motor unit fasciculation.

7. How does the voltage-dependent ion channel work in this system?

In neuronal and muscle membrane (the neurolemma and sarcolemma, respectively), **voltage-dependent ion channels**, primarily for sodium and potassium, pop open transiently when the intracellular voltage drifts positive (i.e., the membrane depolarizes). At the threshold voltage, an explosive electrochemical process is initiated in which voltage-dependent **sodium channels** open in rapidly increasing numbers, and the transmembrane voltage rises sharply as sodium ions rush into the cell from higher concentration in the extracellular space to lower concentration in the intracellular space, producing a further rise in intracellular voltage and further depolarization of the cell membrane. This regenerative explosion is the basis of the sharp upswing of the nerve action potential. The voltage eventually levels off as the sodium channels become less sensitive (i.e., less likely to open) to the increased voltage and as voltage-dependent **potassium channels** open. The transmembrane voltage reverses, dropping toward the resting level. It actually overshoots the resting level, and the membrane becomes hyperpolarized for a short period called the **refractory period**, during which it is resistant to excitation.

8. Discuss the role of membrane refractoriness in conducting action potentials.

Postexcitatory refractoriness is a critical aspect of neural network dynamics that helps to constrain the excitatory phenomena in the nervous system. The duration of the refractory period determines how quickly a nerve can be repetitively excited and restricts the effective "bandwidth," or information-carrying capacity, of the neuron. This refractory mechanism produces an asymmetry of excitability around the area of depolarized membrane conducting the action potential. The membrane in front of the action potential remains excitable and ready to "fire up" while the membrane behind the action potential becomes transiently inexcitable and resistant to rebounding excitatory influence. This asymmetry prevents "backfiring" of the cell membrane and ensures that the action potential travels as a unidirectional wave of excitation down the length of the fiber.

9. Where do calcium ions operate in the action potential?

A transient "spike" of membrane depolarization is conducted from the cell body of the neuron down the axon as a wave of excitation. When it reaches the distal end of the axon at the presynaptic terminal, the depolarization spike initiates the flow of calcium ions into the presynaptic terminal through voltage-dependent calcium channels concentrated in the membrane of the presynaptic terminal, activating the cell that it contacts.

10. What are fibrillation and fasciculation?

In the mature neuromuscular system, a muscle fiber should normally generate an action potential and contract only when "it is told to" by a motor neuron. However, in muscle fibers with defective membranes that "leak" sodium ions from the extracellular to the intracellular space, spontaneous membrane depolarization leads to the spontaneous generation of a muscle fiber action potential and the autonomous contraction of the fiber. This autonomous contraction of a muscle fiber occurs in the presence of pathologic conditions that either remove the neural control over the muscle fiber or directly damage the muscle fiber membrane. This pathologic autonomous muscle fiber contraction is called a **fibrillation**, an invisible tiny twitch of an individual muscle fiber.

A similar type of electrical destabilization of the membrane of the motor neuron and motor axon leads to spontaneous generation of an ectopic action potential, which is conducted through the terminal branching of the fiber to all muscle fibers innervated by the motor neuron. This results in a synchronous autonomous contraction of all the fibers in the motor unit, producing a significant, visible twitch of the muscle called a **fasciculation**. Both phenomena are physiologic results of the loss of normal constraint over the excitation of nerve and muscle fibers in various neuromuscular disorders.

11. What is a neural network? What does it do?

A neural network is a set of neurons that are interconnected in a specified pattern. Through the conduction of activity from one place to another within the network and through the convergence and divergence of activity in different parts of the network as it is dynamically active, patterns of activation emerge. A network may be considered to have a set of inputs impinging on input neurons, a set of outputs generated by output neurons, as well as a set of neurons that mediate activity back and forth between input and output neurons. The general structure of a neural network includes input neurons that convey afferent information from the periphery and output neurons that convey efferent information to the periphery. These two general flows of information can interact at multiple levels, allowing an efferent flow to modulate an afferent flow and an afferent flow to modulate an efferent flow. These interactions help control what moves along the pathway from the periphery to more central structures to eventually enable perception to occur, and what moves along the pathway from central structures to the periphery to generate movement.

12. Give an example of a neural network.

The interaction of afferent and efferent flows helps the nervous system to differentiate when apparent movement of an external object is due to actual object movement in the external world versus self-generated movement that makes it seem as if the object is moving (e.g., eye movement). These two situations are distinguished by a so-called efference copy signal that is sent from the efferent system to the afferent system to inform perceptual areas that the apparent movement is due to self-generated movement. This mechanism can sometimes fail, leading to illusory perceptions of object movement, as when a patient has nystagmus and feels that the external world is actually jumping around with each eye movement, a symptom referred to as oscillopsia. This illusion can be produced by pushing with one's finger on the lateral aspect of the globe of the eye.

13. Outline the parts and functions of the peripheral nervous system.

Structure and Function of the Peripheral Nervous System

STRUCTURE	FUNCTION
Somatic	Controls voluntary movement
Afferent (sensory)	Transmits sensory information from periphery and surface (i.e., skin, muscles, joints) about the dynamic state of limbs, their articulation in space, and external environment
Efferent (motor)	Conducts voluntary motor control messages to skeletal muscle
Autonomic	Controls vegetative functions
Afferent	Receives sensory information about internal environment of body
Efferent	Sends control messages to smooth muscle of blood vessels, cardiac muscle, exocrine glands, and internal viscera
Parasympathetic	Maintains internal resources and internal homeostasis
Sympathetic	Involved in stress response

14. What comprises the motivational subsystem of the CNS?

The CNS has three major interacting functional subsystems: the sensory, motor, and motivational subsystems. The hypothalamus and the nuclei of the limbic system, such as the hippocampus and amygdala, are important parts of the motivational subsystem. This subsystem interconnects sensory and motor subsystems by making decisions about actions based on the detection of sensory context from both the internal and external environments. For example, the motivational subsystem activates the motor system to reach for an apple when the sensed internal nutritional state indicates a need for nourishment. The motivational subsystem must work in close conjunction with both the autonomic and somatic peripheral nervous systems by taking in information from both systems and coordinating activity in both systems.

15. How are the sensory systems of the nervous system organized?

There are several major sensory systems in the brain: somatosensory, special visceral afferent (taste), vestibular, auditory, visual, and olfactory systems. The somatosensory system is divided into the lemniscal system subserving epicritic sensations of light touch and vibration sense and the spinothalamic system subserving the protocritic sensations of pain and temperature. All systems except for the olfactory system transmit information to specialized regions of the thalamus. The interaction between the thalamus and cortex is a mutually excitatory interaction, and each sensation (except for olfaction) has a specific thalamic nucleus that is reciprocally connected to a well-circumscribed cortical area that functions as a primary receiving zone for that particular sensation. Other nonspecific thalamic nuclei are more diffusely connected to the cerebral cortex. The olfactory system connects directly into the amygdala, a critical nucleus of the limbic (motivational) system, as well as to olfactory regions of cerebral cortex. Unlike all other sensory systems, it does not connect through the thalamus to its cortical area.

16. How are the extrathalamic ascending neuromodulatory systems organized?

In addition to the sensory system projections to the cerebral cortex, a number of widely projecting systems connect to the cerebral cortex directly from nuclei in the reticular core of the brainstem and midbrain. These systems are characterized by the major neurotransmitter which each system utilizes to modulate cortical activity. These systems are extremely important in controlling the overall excitability and responsiveness, or tone, of different parts of the cerebral cortex and are especially important in regulating levels of consciousness and the sleep-wake cycle. Disruption of these systems is associated with the loss of consciousness that occurs with the diffuse axonal injury to the subcortical white matter in cranial trauma. Many neurotransmitter-based psychoactive medications function by influencing the operation of one or more of these major systems.

Major Extrathalamic Neurotransmitter Systems

NEUROTRANSMITTER	MAJOR SOURCE NUCLEUS	TYPICAL MEDICATION(S)
Acetylcholine	Nucleus basalis of Meynert	Benzotropine mesylate (antagonist)
Dopamine	Substantia nigra (pars compacta), ventral tegmental area	L-Dopa, bromocriptine (agonists)
Norepinephrine	Locus coeruleus	Methyphenidate, nortriptyline (agonists)
Serotonin	Raphe nuclei	Fluoxetine, sertraline (agonists)

17. What other substances function as neurotransmitters in the brain?

Additional neurotransmitter systems in the brain include those utilizing epinephrine and histamine, amino acids (e.g., GABA, glutamate, glycine), neuropeptides, hypothalamic and hypophyseal peptide hormones, and opioids (endorphins and enkephalins).

18. What is a motor unit?

The motor unit is the *functional element of voluntary movement*. It consists of the anterior horn cell, motor axon, nerve terminals, neuromuscular junctions, and all the muscle fibers innervated by the anterior horn cell. The CNS activates the anterior horn cell, which in turn activates the muscle fibers in the motor unit, to produce voluntary movement.

19. How does the motor unit work?

The anterior horn cell controls a significant number of muscle fibers, ranging up to several thousand muscle fibers in a single motor unit. Each time the anterior horn cell fires an action potential, the end result is a **synchronous** twitch of all the muscle fibers in the motor unit. Tension is graded in muscle by recruiting additional motor units and by increasing the firing rate of the motor units in the available pool that have been activated. A motor unit cannot be normally fired at a tonic rate less than about 6/second. The rate at which a motor unit starts firing when it is first recruited is called the **onset firing rate**. The rate at which a motor unit is firing when the next motor unit in sequence is recruited is called the **recruitment firing rate** or **recruitment frequency**.

The manner in which motor units in a muscle are recruited is generally very orderly and in a sequence from the population of smaller motor units innervated by motor neurons with smaller cell bodies, through to the population of larger motor units innervated by motor neurons with larger cell bodies. This process of recruitment from smaller to larger units is referred as the **size principle**. The size principle has a number of important functional implications. The units recruited initially in a contraction are generally slow-twitch oxidative units, while those recruited at higher tension levels are generally fast-twitch glycolytic units, ensuring that sustained low-level concentrations are performed by fatigue-resistant muscle fibers. Furthermore, the amount of incremental force (ΔF) added to a muscle contraction at any point during a graded activation is approximately proportional to the current force (F) being produced by the muscle. Therefore, the ratio of ΔF to F is a constant during the development of tension in a graded contraction of the muscle.

20. What is muscular co-contraction and what does it accomplish?

High-force output motor units cannot be immediately accessed but can only be recruited after low-force output motor units have first been activated. To obtain the rapid deployment of a large amount of force, the muscle may need to be "preloaded" so that it is already operating up in the range in which the high-force output units are starting to be recruited. Agonist-antagonist muscle groups will sometimes oppose each other in a **co-contraction** in order to "bias" a muscle into its higher output range, which enables more immediate access to the large-amplitude, fast-fatigable motor units and facilitates rapid production of large bursts of muscular force.

Muscle co-contraction is also important for the stabilization of proximal joints during more distal movement and also for situations in which forces across a joint must be absorbed through muscle contraction. Co-contraction is also used to stabilize a limb in anticipation of a dynamic load whose exact direction of force cannot be predicted.

On the other hand, in many gross motor activities, gravity acts as as sustained force that serves as the primary propulsive force, which is then controlled by low-grade, sustained eccentric muscle contractions. In this case, the muscles operate in their low range where the slow-oxidative low-amplitude units predominate and co-contraction just adds an unnecessary and wasteful burden. In such instances, agonist-antagonist interaction is controlled with patterns of **reciprocal inhibition** that produce a "push-pull" alternating interaction between muscles to produce opposing forces. Mechanisms for controlling the interaction of agonist-antagonist pairs of muscles in either co-contraction or reciprocal inhibition relationships are programmed to a great extent at the spinal segmental level.

21. How does a muscle fiber contract?

A twitch of mechanical energy is produced through the transient shortening of a muscle fiber whenever an action potential travels along the sarcolemma (i.e., muscle fiber cell membrane).

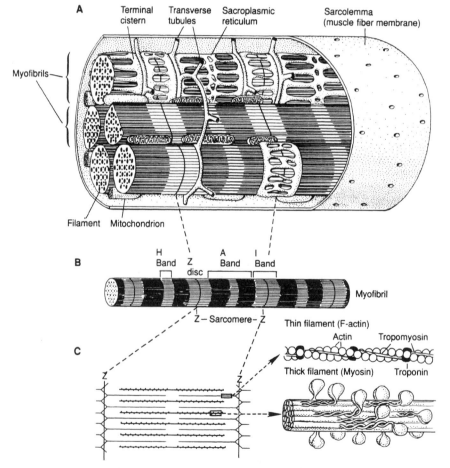

Muscle anatomy. (Figure reproduced from Kandel ER, Schwartz JH, Jessell TM (eds): Principles of Neural Science, 3rd ed. New York, Elsevier, 1991, p 549, with permission.)

The actual shortening of muscle is produced by the coordinated, relative movement of thin (**actin**) and thick (**myosin**) filaments within the **myofibrils** (see figure). Two factors are necessary for the contraction to develop: a supply of high-energy phosphate bonds for metabolic support of contraction (usually provided by ATP), and a supply of calcium ions. The movement is driven by cross-bridge molecules originating in the thick filaments and bridging across to the thin filaments. The binding of ATP to a cross-bridge causes it to release its contact with the actin-binding site on the thin filament. The ATP then splits, forming a high-energy state of the cross-bridge which extends and binds itself to another binding site on the thin filament. The cross-bridge moves from a high-energy state to a low-energy state in the process of bending and shortening, thus moving the thin filament in toward the center of the thick filament and drawing the Z lines on the sarcomeres closer together. A new ATP molecule then must bind to the cross-bridge in order to facilitate its dissociation from the binding site on the thin filament. The dissociated cross-bridge is then cocked and ready to attach to another binding site on the thin filament. This cycle repeats itself over and over as long as there is ATP present to drive the process.

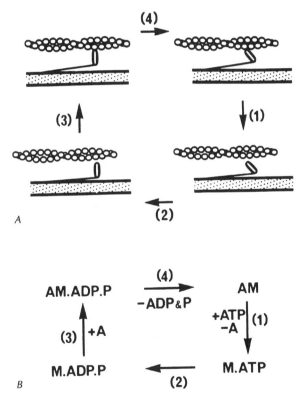

Steps in the contraction of a muscle fiber according to the sliding filament theory. Structural *(A)* and corresponding biochemical *(B)* changes. (Figure reproduced from Engel AG, Franzini-Armstrong C (eds): Myology: Basic and Clinical, 2nd ed. New York: McGraw-Hill, 1994, p 162, with permission.)

22. What role does calcium play in muscle contraction?

The forming of a cross-bridge can only occur when there are receptor-binding sites available on the thin filament for the cross-bridge to attach. In the presence of calcium ions, there is a conformational change in the thin filament that exposes the binding sites. When calcium is not present in the myofibril, contraction cannot occur because the binding sites are retracted. Thus, control of the contractile process reduces to controlling the concentration of calcium ions in the myofibril. The spreading excitation of the muscle fiber causes a release of calcium into the myofibril through voltage-dependent calcium channels that open in the membranes of the sarcoplasmic reticulum as the wave of depolarization spreads down the fiber. Calcium ions flow into the myofibril and activate the contractile process. Calcium ions are then rapidly and efficiently pumped out of the myofibril and back into the sarcoplasmic reticulum as the muscle fiber relaxes. This, then, is the basic process whereby the electrical phenomenon of transmitted membrane depolarization along the length of a muscle fiber is transformed into the mechanical phenomenon of muscle fiber shortening and muscle contraction.

23. Outline the sequence of events in muscular contraction.
Excitation-contraction coupling
1. Depolarization of sarcolemma with conduction of muscle fiber action potential
2. Internal fiber depolarization through transmission along T-tubule system
3. Release of Ca^{2+} from sarcoplasmic reticulum
4. Ca^{2+} diffuses into sarcomeres

Contraction
5. Ca^{2+} binds to troponin
6. Troponin–Ca^{2+} complex removes tropomyosin blockage of actin-binding sites
7. Myosin heads containing high-energy myosin–ADP–P_i complex attach to actin-binding sites and form cross-bridges between thick and thin filaments
8. Conformational energy-releasing changes occur in high-energy myosin heads that cause them to swivel, producing relative motion of the thick and thin filaments releasing ADP and P_i and returning the myosin head to its low-energy state
9. A new ATP molecule binds to the myosin head, allowing the release of the head from the actin-binding site
10. ATP splits to ADP and P_i, producing an high-energy myosin–ADP–P_i complex
11. Return to step 7 with repeating of cycle of steps 7–10 as long as actin-binding sites remain available for attachment

Relaxation
12. Ca^{2+} pumped back into sarcoplasmic reticulum
13. Ca^{2+} around thin filaments diffuses back toward the sarcoplasmic reticulum
14. Ca^{2+} released from troponin–Ca^{2+} complex
15. Troponin permits return of tropomyosin to blocking position
16. Myosin–actin cross-bridges break with addition of ATP to the myosin head, but new cross-bridges cannot form because the actin-binding sites are no longer available because of blocking action of tropomyosin

24. What is spasticity? Describe its neurophysiologic basis.
Spasticity is most often used to refer to abnormalities of movement in a limb in which there has been damage to centers that modulate the activity of the motor unit. A number of things go wrong with motor control and the process of voluntary activation of the motor units when centers above the level of the spinal segment are damaged. When motor control is dysfunctional, events can be viewed as "**negative**" phenomena, where activity that should normally be present is not or where normal activity patterns become abnormally attenuated, or "**positive**" phenomena, where activity patterns that are normally not present appear (e.g., pathologic reflex patterns) or where activity patterns that are normally present become abnormally exaggerated and distorted.

25. Name the six major descending tracts from the brain.
The circuits in the spinal cord at the segmental level are controlled by descending tracts from the brain.
1. Corticospinal tract (including lateral and ventral tracts) projecting from the cerebral cortex
2. Vestibulospinal tract projecting from the vestibular nuclei in the pons
3. Medial reticulospinal tract projecting from the pontine reticular formation

4. Lateral reticulospinal tract projecting from the medullary reticular formation
5. Rubrospinal tract projecting from the red nucleus in the midbrain
6. Tectospinal tract projecting from the superior colliculus in the tectum of the midbrain

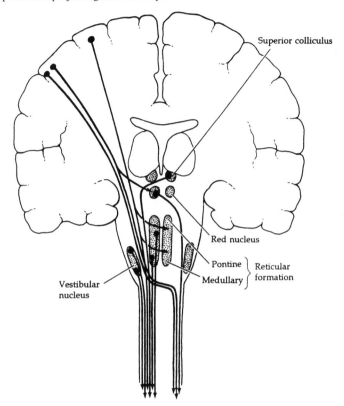

Descending fiber tracts from different parts of the brain to the spinal cord. (Figure reproduced from Nicholls JG, Martin AR, Wallace BG: From Neuron to Brain: A Cellular and Molecular Approach to the Function of the Nervous System, 3rd ed. Sunderland, MA: Sinauer Associates, Inc., 1992, p 534, with permission.)

26. How do each of the different descending tracts affect muscle tone?

Each of the descending pathways has a different influence on the background tone and dynamic activation of motor neuron pools and interneuronal circuits in the spinal cord.

The **vestibulospinal** and **reticulospinal** tracts are involved in the postural biasing of muscles and anticipatory postural adjustments that precede voluntary movements. The vestibulospinal and reticulospinal output neurons are generally excitatory to extensor motor neurons innervating extensor muscles in the arms and legs and are under inhibitory control from the cortical level. The loss of cortical inhibitory control over these pathways tends to facilitate extensor tone in the arms and legs, resulting in **decerebrate rigidity**.

The **rubrospinal** and **corticospinal** tracts both tend to balance the extensor drive by facilitating drive to flexor muscles. The rubrospinal tract in humans extends only into the cervical cord and thus can counteract extensor drive in the arms but not the legs. Thus, the **decorticate rigidity** in humans with large cerebral hemisphere lesions is primarily one of net facilitation of flexors in the arms and extensors in the legs. This is because loss of descending control from the cerebral cortex releases unopposed excitatory extensor drive from the vestibular and reticular formation areas to the lower limb extensor muscles, while flexor facilitation is released from the red nucleus to upper limb flexor muscles in projections in the rubrospinal tract.

27. What is the upper motor neuron syndrome?

When there is dysfunction of the descending inputs to the spinal cord, there is a degrading of the dynamic control of the motor neurons, and the patterns of activation of muscles in a limb that form the basis of normal limb function become disordered. This combination of findings—changes in response to passive sustained and dynamic stretch, disinhibition of antigravity postural subroutines, and disordering of voluntary patterns of muscle activation—depends on the exact way in which the descending pathways have been affected by the damage. This combination of changes can be thought of as a type of disordered motor control or as a syndrome, the **upper motor neuron syndrome** (UMNS), where the term "upper motor neuron" refers to any neuron in the central neuraxis which projects down to the spinal cord through one of the descending pathways.

The disorder of function associated with UMNS may be due to a wide variety of possible mechanisms, which could include altered response (usually exaggerated excitation) to passive stretch, an inability to generate voluntary activation of a muscle (i.e., decreased drive), or an inability to dynamically coordinate the activation of a set of different muscles in the limb. Additionally, over time in the paretic limb, there are changes in the fibrous architecture of the muscle that lead to changes in the passive visco-elastic properties of the muscle of an affected limb. Thus limitation of movement in chronic UMNS may be due to fixed contracture or may be exaggerated by a loss of distensibility of the fibrous matrix of the muscle.

28. What parts of the nervous system are involved in the control of voluntary movement?

The **motor cortex** is the cortical strip of the precentral gyrus. It is a somatotopically organized, electrically excitable region of the cerebral cortex that is involved in the execution of detailed aspects of voluntary fine movement, especially rapid, finely coordinated, "fractionated" movements of the fingers and toes.

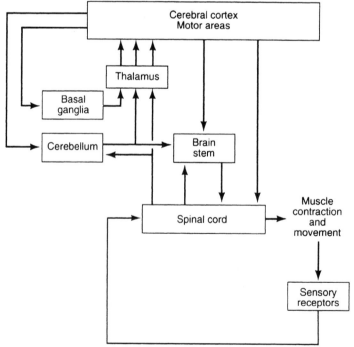

Levels of organization of the motor system. (Figure reproduced from Kandel ER, Schwartz JH, Jessell TM (eds): Principles of Neural Science, 3rd ed. New York, Elsevier, 1991, p 539, with permission.)

Areas in the **parietal cortex** and **frontal cortex** (in the "premotor" cortex) are involved in translating the intent to act into more global aspects of the task, such as its timing, sequential linkage of different subtasks, trajectory through extrapersonal space, and coordination of the postural stabilization and distal limb control in movement.

The **cerebellum** receives two inputs and has one output. This input, from the cerebral cortex and from the spinal cord, keeps the cerebellum informed about what is going on in the limbs, particularly with muscle and tendon stretch information. The cerebellum generates output back to the cerebral cortex that can then influence the ongoing outflow of activity from the cortex. There is thus a circular loop involved in cerebellar circuitry, called a re-entrant loop, since the output re-enters the general part of the nervous system (the cerebral cortex) from which input originated.

The **basal ganglia** consist of the striatum (the caudate and putamen nuclei), the pallidal nuclei (the external and internal segments of the globus pallidus), and a set of nuclei in the midbrain including the substantia nigra and subthalamic nucleus. The basal ganglia constitute a second, but differently connected, re-entrant loop with the cerebral cortex.

29. What is the role of the cerebellum in the control of voluntary movement?

The cerebellum is an important "meta-system" in voluntary motor control that enables the refinement and fine-tuning of motor performance through dynamic modulation of outflows from the motor cortex. This is done by correcting errors detected between the sampled outflow from the motor cortex, which conveys the details of the *intended* movement, and the sensory input from the periphery, which conveys the details of the *actual* movement.

The cerebellum can be viewed as being responsible for the discrete timing relationships within a pattern of muscle activations and may have some type of dynamic clocking function. The cerebellum rapidly performs precise adjustments of the dynamics of the sensorimotor linkage and muscle activation patterns to allow for progressively more rapid and accurate performance of a motor task as it is being practiced. As such, the cerebellum is an important site for motor learning and for the development of procedural memories (i.e., motor engrams). The automatization of motor skill performance frees up the cerebral cortex from the attentional load involved in taking care of all the details of execution.

30. What motor dysfunction is associated with cerebellar damage?

Deficient movement execution and coordination with the appearance of oscillations (**ataxic tremor**), inaccurate endpoint acquisition (**past-pointing**), and impairment of the timing of muscle activation in dynamic alternation and rhythmic movements (**dysdiadochokinesis**). There is a lack of precision in the timing of activation of bursts of EMG activity in agonist and antagonist muscle pairs, particularly for rapid "ballistic" movements which cannot be controlled with continuous feedback. A delay in the development of the braking effect of the antagonist burst that follows the acceleration produced by the initial agonist burst results in overshoot of the target, or past-pointing. This effect is exaggerated when movement speed increases, since the timing precision demands of the task become more severe. Errors are reduced by slowing down performance of the task and by focusing more attention on performance.

In the presence of cerebellar impairment, patients tend to try to simplify the problem of performing multijoint movements by focusing on the movement of one joint at a time in sequence, rather than attempting to move all joints simultaneously. The cerebellum adjusts stretch reflex gains to allow for appropriate dynamic load compensation necessary, for example, when an unexpected loading of the limb occurs. In the presence of cerebellar damage, load compensation responses are reduced or delayed, the gain of the stretch reflexes is reduced with resulting hypotonia, and the result is an underdamped limb that is prone to oscillation and overshoot.

31. What role does the basal ganglia play in voluntary movement?

Whereas the cerebellum is involved in the control and coordination of precise timing relationships between bursts of activity in different muscles firing within a pattern, the basal ganglia seem to be involved in the more global control of the timing of the pattern as a whole—i.e., its relative expansion or compression in time. This may be closely related to the clocking of internal ultradian rhythms. The striatum receive widespread input from all over the cerebral cortex, and the output of the globus pallidus goes to a limited area of the thalamus that interacts with a very limited region of the premotor and supplementary motor areas. The striatum appears to be subdivided into segregated modules, each of which receives inputs from different subregions of the cerebral cortex, suggesting a highly modularized system of re-entrant loops.

The basal ganglia may play a role in selecting specific motor patterns to be chosen from a vast repertoire of potential patterns based on current cortically processed sensory context. This probably occurs through a process of selective facilitation of a small subset of modular loops and massive inhibition of the remaining loops that allows only limited modules of the striatum to be allowed to inhibit regions of the globus pallidus, which then projects inhibitory output to the thalamus. Thus, the basal ganglia can be viewed as a selective filter of information flow converging on motor preparation regions of the cerebral cortex. They may therefore be involved in the process of selecting motor engrams to be activated in a certain context or setting up critical perceptuomotor linkages.

32. How does dopaminergic failure in the basal ganglia present clinically?

Dysfunction of the dopaminergic system within the basal ganglia results in problems with slowness of movement, impairment of initiation, and overall constriction of movement. Dopamine acts as a promoter and energizer of movement by playing a role in the selective facilitation of specific movements. It may also serve a role as a controlling influence on an internal sense of time. Thus, patients with dopaminergic insufficiency associated with parkinsonism have problems with estimating time intervals and accurately reproducing time intervals presented to them.

33. Explain the roles of different parts of the cerebral cortex in the planning and control of movement.

The cerebral cortex plays an important role in assuring that movements are integrated, coordinated, and contextually appropriate. Through emerging techniques, such as positron-emission tomography and functional MRI, that allow the activity of different parts of the brain to be imaged in the behaving human subject, we are able to learn more about the functional networks in the cerebral cortex that participate in conscious perception and volition.

One theory relates to how different parts of the cerebral cortex have evolved. The medial part of the cortex has evolved from the hippocampus, while the lateral part of the cortex has evolved from the primitive olfactory complex. This suggests that structures on the medial surface of the hemisphere, such as the **anterior cingulate cortex** and the **supplementary motor area**, are involved in the initiation and control of movements that are internally based, while the areas on the lateral surface of the brain, such as the **ventrolateral frontal lobe** and the **lateral parietal regions**, are involved in the detection and registration of external information and the integration of external cues into action control. In fact, the anterior cingulate cortex on the medial surface of the brain, just above the corpus callosum, appears to be part of an important **executive attention network** that is associated with conscious volition, while the lateral structures appear to be important elements of a perceptual orienting network and a **vigilance network** that focuses on external events. The cerebellum appears to be more closely associated with the lateral system, while the basal ganglia are most closely associated with the medial system. These different "premotor" systems, the medial and lateral, appear to relate to each other through reciprocal inhibition. Activation of the anterior circulate region and the executive attention network appears to be associated with the subjective experience of awareness or effort directed to performance—attention for action.

While we have much more to learn from this line of research in cognitive neuroscience, there are some emerging ideas that are of critical relevance to rehabilitation:

1. While elementary cognitive operations can be localized to different parts of the cortex, the performance of complex cognitive tasks is associated with activation of widely distributed neural systems. Different cortical regions work together to construct the necessary neural basis for the successful performance of the task.

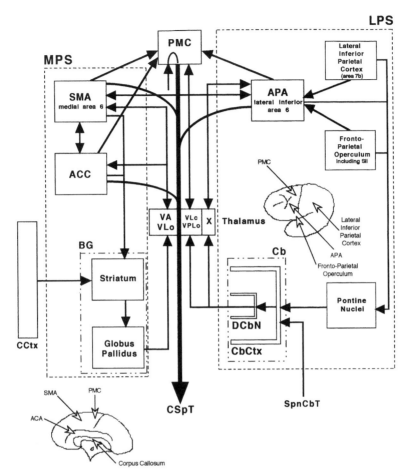

Structure and organization of the medial premotor system (MPS) on the medial surface of the hemisphere and the lateral premotor system (LPS) on the lateral surface of the hemisphere. In the MPS, the supplementary motor area (SMA) and the anterior cingulate cortex (ACC) project in topographically ordered fashion to the primary motor cortex (PMC). These areas are also in close relationship with the basal ganglia (BG). In the LPS, the arcuate premotor area (APA) on the lateral surface of the monkey brain projects similarly to PMC. The cerebellum (Cb) with the cerebellar cortex (CbCtx) and the deep cerebellar nuclei (DCbN) is part of the LPS and projects through the thalamus back to APA and PMC. The cerebellar cortex also receives direct afferents from the spinal cord by way of the spinocerebellar tract (SpnCbT). The BG receive input from broadly distributed regions of the cerebral cortex projecting to the striatum and project output back from the globus pallidus to the SMA and ACC via the VA and VLo nuclei of the thalamus. Outflow from the PMC, SMA, ACC, and APA projects to the spinal cord by way of the corticospinal tract (CSpT). Projections to the PMC influence the "gain" of sensorimotor "transcortical" loops that link sensory input to the PMC to the efferent projects from the PMC into the CSpT.

2. These distributed networks can reorganize to some degree following limited brain damage that interferes with function in some subset of the network (Frackowiak et al., 1991).

3. Less effort and attention are required to repeat a cognitive task recently performed, and when a skill is practiced, its learning and automatization is accompanied by a significant simplification of the neural network whose activation is associated with skill performance. While the executive attention network, including the anterior cingulate cortex, activates strongly while the task is novel and is first being performed, the activation of this network steadily drops down as

the subject becomes adept at performing the task with repeated occurrence. While the executive attention network quiets down, other areas pick up. For example, the insular regions of both hemispheres that show reduced activity during the activation of the executive attention system in the early stages of learning are reengaged (Raichle et al., 1994).

4. The topographic organization of maps in the brain (e.g., in somatosensory cortex) is dynamically maintained through experience and may undergo a process of limited reorganization in response to concentrated sensory experience in a motivated subject (Jenkins et al., 1990).

These principles document the adaptive capacity of the central nervous system, and particularly the cerebral cortex, and are beginning to provide a basis for a Rehabilitation Neuroscience that links fundamental advancements in our knowledge of the neurophysiologic basis of central nervous system functionality to innovations in rehabilitative care.

BIBLIOGRAPHY

 1. Deecke L, Eccles JC, Mountcastle VB (eds): From Neuron to Action: An Appraisal of Fundamental and Clinical Research. New York, Springer-Verlag, 1990.
 2. Dieber MP, Passingham RE, Colebatch JG, et al: Cortical areas and the selection of movement: A study with positron emission tomography. Exp Brain Res 84:393–402, 1991.
 3. Dumitru D: Electrodiagnostic Medicine. Philadelphia, Hanley & Belfus, 1995.
 4. Frackowiak RSJ, Weiller C, Chollet F: The functional anatomy of recovery from brain injury. In Chadwick DJ, Whelan J (eds): Exploring Brain Functional Anatomy with Positron Tomography (CIBA Foundation Symposium 163). New York, Wiley, 1991, pp 235–249.
 5. Glenn WB, Whyte J (eds): The Practical Management of Spasticity in Adults and Children. Philadelphia, Lea & Febiger, 1990.
 6. Goldberg G: From intent to action: Evolution and function of the premotor systems of the frontal lobe. In Perecman E (ed): The Frontal Lobes Revisited. New York, IRBN Press, 1987, pp 273–306.
 7. Goldberg G: Neurophysiologic models of recovery in stroke. Phys Med Rehabil Clin North Am 2:599–614, 1991.
 8. Goldberg G: Premotor systems, attention to action and behavioral choice. In Kien J, McCrohan CR, Winslow W (eds): Neurobiology of Motor Programme Selection. New York, Pergamon Press, 1992, pp 225–249.
 9. Jenkins WM, Merzenich MM, Ochs MT, et al: Functional reorganization of primary somatosensory cortex in adult owl monkeys after behaviorally controlled tactile stimulation. J Neurophysiol 63:82–104, 1990.
10. Kandel ER, Schwartz JH, Jessel TM (eds): Principles of Neural Science, 3rd ed. New York, Elsevier, 1991.
11. Latash ML: Control of Human Movement. Champaign, IL, Human Kinetics, 1993.
12. Pastor MA, Atreida J, Jahanshahi M, Obeso JA: Time estimation and reproduction is abnormal Parkinson's disease. Brain 115:211–225, 1992.
13. Patton HD, Fuchs AF, Hille B, et al (eds): Textbook of Physiology: Vol. 1. Excitable Cells and Neurophysiology, 21st ed. Philadelphia, W.B. Saunders, 1989.
14. Posner MI, Raichle ME: Images of Mind. New York, Scientific American Library, 1994.
15. Raichle ME, Fiez JA, Videen TO, et al: Practice-related changes in human brain functional anatomy during non-motor learning. Cerebral Cortex 4:8–26, 1994.

II. Caring for People with Disabilities

9. PRIMARY CARE ISSUES IN REHABILITATION

Richard S. Materson, M.D., and Susan M. Miller, M.D.

1. What sort of communication disorders should be watched for in a primary care practice?

Hearing impairments and other communication deficits resulting from cerebral palsy (CP) presumably are identified and evaluated in children while they participate in other educational services. Hearing loss is observed in approximately 15% of all children with CP. It is most closely associated with the athetoid form of this disease but can be seen in 7% of those with spasticity.

Unfortunately, once a person is out of their school system, access to hearing and communication services becomes limited. In one study, 22% of adults with CP were found to have mild to moderate hearing loss. Because it is easy to assume cognitive defects are the reason for lack of satisfactory communication, it is possible to overlook the need for audiologic evaluation. Many patients, however, would benefit from this service as well as augmentative communication systems prescribed by speech-language pathologists.

In addition, an estimated 8 million older Americans have a speech, language, or hearing problem. Again, assumptions about cognitive decline can cause treatable impairments to be missed.

2. What types of cardiac disease are seen in persons with neuromuscular diseases?

Duchenne's muscular dystrophy, Becker's muscular dystrophy, congenital myopathies, myotonic muscular dystrophy, limb girdle and fascioscapulohumeral muscular dystrophy, Friedreich's ataxia, and polymyositis are a few of the neuromuscular diseases that exhibit a high incidence of EKG and echocardiogram abnormalities.

In **Duchenne's muscular dystrophy**, healthy myocardium can be replaced by extensive fibrosis in the left ventricular (LV) wall and ventricular septum, and fatty infiltration can be noticed in the sinus and AV node. EKG abnormalities are therefore frequently noted in patients with this disorder. Echocardiography reveals a high incidence of mitral valve prolapse and LV contraction abnormalities. Usually, these myocardial impairments remain silent until late in the course of Duchenne's muscular dystrophy.

In **myotonic muscular dystrophy**, sudden death in these patients is frequently related to conduction disturbances, most commonly high-degree AV block or ventricular tachycardia. EKG abnormalities are evident in approximately 80% of all patients with this disease, but the incidence of sudden death and other cardiac conduction symptoms is low, from 4–12%. Complaints of palpitations, chest pain, and syncope that remain undiagnosed after a vascular or neurologic evaluation warrant advanced electrophysiologic studies. If His bundle studies are abnormal, placement of a pacemaker should be considered.

The cardiomyopathy of **Friedreich's ataxia** is demonstrated by cardiac muscle fiber hypertrophy, interstitial fibrosis, and active necrosis. These abnormalities manifest themselves in EKG changes seen in as many as 91% of patients, mostly in the form of repolarization abnormalities. Echocardiograms commonly reveal pathologies such as concentric LV hypertrophy and papillary muscle thickening in up to 86% of individuals. In one study of 82 people who died with Friedreich's ataxia, over one-half of them died with heart failure.

3. Is there any relationship between the development of stroke and future cardiac disease?

The major cause of death occurring 3 months or more after a stroke is myocardial infarction. Therefore, presentation of a cerebrovascular accident should suggest coexistent coronary artery disease in that same patient. This principle should be recognized also in the patient with a transient ischemic attack (TIA).

4. Can someone with a "stable" neuromusculoskeletal disease get worse over the years?

Yes. Many conditions can complicate a stable neuromuscular illness and even cause a decrease in function. Spasticity is one such condition. However, spasticity accompanies many diseases of the neuromuscular system, so it may be difficult to tell if the spasticity is of new onset or an exacerbation.

5. How can I tell if spasticity is a new condition or if it is detrimental to the patient's health?

While the primary cause of spasticity may be obvious (e.g., stroke or spinal cord injury), changes in the **pattern** of spasticity must be carefully examined for cause. Spasticity may be thought of as a clinical manifestation of pain in the insensate individual or in the individual unable to communicate due to coma or language dysfunction. Thus, the sudden onset of increased spasticity should not be treated with an automatic increase in therapy sessions and/or medications, as the condition cannot be assumed to be secondary to the nervous system disorder itself.

Factors such as fever and stress may influence the severity of frequency of the spasm. Common causes for an increase in spasticity also include bladder or renal infections, inadequate bowel evacuation, skin irritation from decubitus ulcers, ingrown toenails, hyperthermia and sunburn, abdominal emergencies, and occult fractures. Only treatment of the specific etiologic cause will reduce the patient's spasticity.

6. How do occult fractures occur?

In any condition that results in immobility, osteoporosis is a common phenomenon. Much effort has been devoted to the study of osteoporosis in the disabled and particularly in the spinal cord-injured population. Loss of bone begins early after a spinal cord injury. One study saw a 27% decrease in bone mineral density (BMD) only 4 months after injury, and by 16 months BMD has plateaued at 63% of normal.

In the osteoporotic individual, spontaneous fractures are frequently produced by minor trauma, such as a fall from a wheelchair. The incidence of fractures in spinal cord-injured individuals has been reported to be up to 6% at specialized treatment centers, and it is probably higher. Most fractures in persons with spinal cord injuries occur in the lower extremities, specifically the femur. Falls are the most common cause of trauma, but spastic movements also occasionally provoke fractures, as do motor vehicle accidents. Because pain is rarely a diagnostic clue in these cases, one must look carefully for signs of local swelling. Bruising and deformity may not necessarily appear in an individual with a spinal cord injury or any other lower extremity paralysis.

7. Can further spinal deformity occur in individuals who have chronic neuromuscular diseases?

Scoliosis secondary to neuromuscular disease is a common entity, particularly during the adolescent growth spurt. Whereas an idiopathic scoliosis produces recognizable curve patterns, neuromuscular disease generally causes a collapse in the spine, which gives rise to a characteristically long C-curve. Common causes of this process include muscular dystrophy, cerebral palsy, and early-age spinal cord trauma.

Most curves due to paralytic diseases extend to the pelvis, which provokes further problems than just the deformity itself. For example, a C-curve may cause an individual to bear weight more prominently on one ischium than the other, promoting the conditions necessary for decubitus formation. Concomitant pelvic obliquity can also result in a poor relationship between the femoral head and its acetabulum, leading to painful degenerative joint disease and the possibility of hip subluxation/dislocation.

8. Are there any spinal deformities besides scoliosis that are associated with chronic neuro-muscular diseases?

Disorders characterized by either choreoathetoid and/or spastic movements also have been associated with neurologic deterioration secondary to cervical spinal disease, probably because of the severe spondylosis that develops due to excessive movement. This degenerative joint disease eventually causes spinal stenosis, herniation, and other fixed deformities, resulting in radiculopathies and/or myelopathy that leads to a loss of functional skills. A full workup to evaluate spinal pathology should be initiated in adults with movement disorders who, after years of stable function, develop new neck pain, new incontinence, a decrease in their ambulatory status, or a change of hand dominance or hand skills.

9. Besides good diet and regular bowel program, how else can I monitor my patient's GI tract?

In all persons, the incidence of colorectal cancer increases with aging. Fecal occult blood testing is perhaps the most prevalent means of screening for this disease, but this method is ineffective in spinal cord-injured persons or other individuals who perform manual bowel programs. Rectal bleeding is reported in approximately 75% of these persons, due to hemorrhoids, mucosal prolapse, and other perianal pathologies seen in an aging population of persons who can require daily suppositories and manual stimulation to effect a bowel movement. Since testing for occult bleeding is not a reliable screening method, yearly rectal exams are necessary, and routine flexible sigmoidoscopy every 3–5 years in spinal cord-injured patients 40 years or older (even if asymptomatic) should be considered. A screening barium enema exam has also been suggested at age 50. Full colonoscopic examinations may be appropriate for those who report an increase in lower GI bleeding or a change in their usual bowel routine or who have a positive barium enema.

10. What sort of followup is required for the urinary tract of disabled individuals?

The incidence of death secondary to renal disease in those with neuromuscular bladder disorders has been significantly declining over the years, mainly due to the new management schemes for patients with this disorder. Maintenance of the catheter-free state and heightened knowledge regarding long-term renal follow-up, combined with improved technologic advances that allow satisfactory visualization and study of the upper and lower GU system, have probably accounted for most of the improvement in patient survival rates.

There is, however, no universally accepted program for urinary tract surveillance or evaluation. It is most important to systematically and periodically evaluate the upper tracts of the patient, whether or not symptoms are present. Asymptomatic patients, stabilized after the acute injury, should be evaluated annually for at least 5 years and then once every 1–2 years after. (Patients who develop symptoms are obviously evaluated as soon as possible.)

Controversy surrounds the specific of these yearly evaluations, but it seems traditionally expected to include a pertinent history and physical exam, urine culture, and visualization of kidney, ureter, and bladder anatomy.

11. Why are yearly serum creatinine measures not good enough for urinary tract followup?

Serum creatinine measures are similarly not subtle enough to assess renal function. The glomerular filtration rate must be decreased to approximately 30% of normal before the plasma creatinine level becomes abnormal. Loss of muscle mass, particularly in paraplegic and quadriplegic individuals, may allow the serum creatinine to remain normal even in the face of increasing renal dysfunction. Although creatinine clearance does measure kidney function, an adequately collected sample is frequently difficult to obtain.

12. How can I help my disabled female population receive the gynecologic care that they deserve?

The gynecologic care of women with disabilities is often lacking in a total program of primary health care. Besides issues of sexuality, the unmet needs of women with physical disabilities include lack of architectural accessibility to gynecologic care as well as little or no education in the options concerning birth control.

13. How does one make a GYN office accessible to a disabled female?

The physical space of the gynecologist's office must be well-designed to cater to the needs of women with both mobility and sensory limitations. Women with sight and hearing problems often need interpreters so as not to limit communication between patient and doctor. Because signed communication can be interpreted from across a room, attention must be paid to the design of the interview area to give the woman, her interpreter, and her physician absolute privacy as they discuss her medical needs.

For the women with mobility limitations, ramps, widened doorways and hallways, adequate bathroom space, and safety features (such as elevated toilet seats as well as hand rails) are all needed to provide accessibility to gynecologic care. Another especially important part of the gynecologic exam is an accessible table. To allow easy transfers from wheelchairs, the table should be able to be lowered to 19 inches. When a table with suitable height specifications is not present, adequate staff must be available to enable a safe and dignified transfer. Hand rails on exam tables promote a secure feeling among the individual who may experience sudden and unexpected spasticity. Leg supports and straps are also essential to allow for a more comfortable exam.

14. How can the patient be positioned for comfort as well as an adequate exam?

Changes in body position may be necessary for disabled females with mobility impairments. For example, patients with severe spasticity may be more comfortably examined in a knee-to-chest position with an assistant holding the legs away from the perineal area. Side-lying positions can also be attempted for these individuals, with the bottom leg flexed and upper leg placed on the examiner's shoulder. For patients with lower-extremity amputations, the woman may choose to hold the residual limb herself or have an assistant perform this task, rather than to attempt to place it into a stirrup. In those individuals with poor hip mobility, it may be necessary to flex one knee and gently abduct the other leg to provide for an adequate examination.

When patients must be examined in bed, a rolled blanket can be used to elevate the pelvis. This position, however, alters the usual angle of the pelvis in relation to the usual position of the speculum, so that the speculum may not always expose a cervix in mid-position or anteverted cervix. This problem can sometimes be avoided by reversing the position of the speculum so that the blade that usually pushes down will push up to expose the cervix.

In patients with spasticity, lidocaine gel applied to the perineal surface prior to the examination may decrease pain and thus spasms. Patients also should empty their bladders prior to examination, as pressure on a full bladder can induce spasms.

15. Are oral contraceptives appropriate for disabled patients?

Contraceptive information is frequently not discussed with disabled females but is an important part of their overall care. Choice of contraceptive device will depend on the patient's mobility as well as her fine finger movement and coordination. Some authors believe that decreased mobility, such as that seen in spinal cord injuries and other disabilities, is a strong contraindication to hormonal contraceptives (especially those containing estrogen) due to the increased risk of deep vein thrombosis. Others state that with careful monitoring of a patient's coagulation status, low-dose oral contraception may be used in those who are immobile, particularly in women with mild to severe leg spasticity. Other disabling conditions that do not lend themselves to the use of hormonal contraceptives include lupus erythematosus, high blood pressure requiring the use of antihypertensive medications, and known circulatory problems.

16. Is there anything specific that I need to know about the treatment of sexually transmitted diseases in disabled females?

In a female with sensory impairments of the pelvic region, sexually transmitted disease may go undetected. A high degree of suspicion based on such clues as an increase in spasticity and vague abdominal discomfort may be the physician's best diagnostic aid. Remember, when prescribing antibiotics (or any packaged mediations) for women with upper extremity limitations, the ease of package opening needs to be considered. Furthermore, patients with dysphagia may need to have "crushable" pills that can be placed in ground or pureed food or into thickened liquids or pudding.

17. How do I advise a disabled woman who wishes to become pregnant?

Because of wide ignorance, many people respond to a pregnant disabled female with surprise, rudeness, and even disgust. The decision to attempt a pregnancy is a private one for any female and loving partner, disabled or not.

Before a patient makes a final decision about child-bearing, possible medical complications of pregnancy to the mother and child need to be discussed. The mother also needs to plan for the care of the child if her own physical impairments are limited. However, there are many types of adaptive equipment and furniture that allow for both easier physical access to the child as well as his or her safety.

18. Besides decubitus ulcers, what else does a primary care physician need to know about the skin care of disabled individuals?

Though not frequently recognized, amputees have frequent skin abnormalities that can seriously affect their use of a prosthetic device and thus their ambulatory status. Regular attention to the skin of the residual limb of an amputee is important; a skin lesion considered a nuisance in anyone besides an amputee can lead to a disabling problem that prevents the wearing of the prosthesis.

Generally, keeping the residual limb and prosthetic socket clean with soap and water, and taking care to rinse and dry these areas well after washing, will go a long way toward preventing skin disorders. The socket may usually be cleaned with a dampened cloth. Both socket and limb should be allowed to air-dry overnight.

19. What other sort of skin problems can occur in the amputee?

If the surface layer of the skin, keratin, is not removed regularly by a friction-inducing activity (such as washing), it accumulates and grows thicker. The keratin will become drier and less flexible, eventually tearing, producing a rupture in the epidermis below that is a source of constant bleeding and oozing. The keratin itself collects into masses that appear wart-like (verrucous hyperplasia), which can become secondarily infected as well as painful and swollen. Antibiotics are required for treatment, as are the use of keratolytic agents. The primary cause of this disorder—failure to scrub the residual limb—must be eliminated so as it does not become a repetitive process. A lack of total socket contact can also cause this skin disease and should be sought if adequate hygiene has been documented.

Various abnormalities of the prosthetic device can strip excessive keratin off the surface of the skin and push it wavelike in the direction of the movement of the socket brim. This allows the keratin to accumulate in a small area; then pressure exerted upon it by the prosthetic brim drives it into the skin. A foreign body reaction is often induced, and the formation of abscesses, called epidermoid cysts, occurs. Treatment of this condition often requires incision and drainage. Individuals cannot wear their prosthetics during their recovery. This problem can be prevented by an adequately aligned prosthesis and a stump sock specifically designed to reduce friction.

Contact dermatitis can be seen in prosthesis wearers. It is easily diagnosed, as it is limited to the area of contact of the offending material against the residual limb. It is frequently caused by detergents used to wash stump socks or by inadequate rinsing of the soaps/detergents used for washing the sockets. Treatment is symptomatic as long as the offending material is identified and avoided. Occasionally, a prosthetic socket may contain chemicals that cause a contact dermatitis and therefore must be remade from nonallergic materials.

20. What kind of skin infections can affect the amputee?

Folliculitis	Hidradenitis (infection of sweat glands, usually in groin or axilla)
Furuncles	Fungal infections of groin and axilla

21. Is cancer a concern in the residual limb?

If the primary amputation was done because of a cancerous growth, malignant tumors of the residual limb can recur. Also, any lesion under the prosthesis suspicious for malignant melanoma should be biopsied immediately for definitive diagnosis.

22. When children are born with disabling illnesses, their parents often express that they feel alone. What do you tell them?

First of all, one of the best ways for parents to learn about raising children with disabling illnesses is by talking to other parents of children with similar conditions. The United Cerebral Palsy Associations (1-800-USA-5UCP) are terrific resources for parents of children with this disease and other illnesses. The National Information Center for Children and Youths with Disabilities (1-800-999-5599) can also help find support services for these parents.

23. Are the particular injuries that need to be considered when recommending recreational activities to wheelchair users and other disabled individuals?

All sports are associated with injury, whether the athlete is able-bodied or disabled. Several studies have attempted to classify the types of injuries that might be expected to be encountered by the physically challenged athlete. Not surprisingly, the available data seem to indicate that most injuries experienced are of a type similar to those seen in able-bodied athletes, i.e., soft tissue injuries such as sprains, strains, contusions, and abrasions.

24. What are the high-risk sports among the disabled population?

In order of injury frequency, track, basketball, road-racing, tennis, and field events. Injuries are most common in athletes between 21 and 30 years of age and in those training > 10 hr/wk.

25. What problems do disabled athletes have with temperature regulation?

Temperature regulation disorders may occur with athletes whose sweating response has been altered by their disease process, e.g., persons with spinal cord injuries. In the able-bodied athlete, evaporative heat loss occurs from all parts of the body. In the spinal cord-injured athlete, sweating below the level of lesion may be deficient. Depending on the location of the lesion, and particularly in extremes of weather, core temperatures during practice and competitions can soar to dangerous levels, leading to heat exhaustion and occasionally life-threatening heat stroke and autonomic dysreflexia. Dehydration from lack of adequate water intake and the absence of active musculature able to return lower-extremity venous blood and the heat it carries to the heart only serve to complicate this problem. Therefore heat loss in hot, humid conditions needs to be made more efficient in susceptible athletes (and competition observers) through the use of loose-fitting light clothing, adequate hydration, sufficient areas of shade, and the use of cool damp towels or water mist over the entire body's skin area to aid in heat loss through convection.

In cold, damp, or windy conditions, the problem is opposite. The disabled athlete, after competition, stops the excessive use of his muscles, the mainstay of heat production. The skin is damp with sweat, and the vasculature is as vasodilated as possible. Paralysis of affected muscles prevents shivering, the natural method whereby heat loss is controlled. The conditions then are ideal for hypothermia. Temperature loss is prevented by adequate hydration, this time with warm liquids, a change of dry clothing, and use of appropriate insulating blankets and other materials.

26. What unique problems does the insensate athlete encounter?

Insensate athletes are uniquely susceptible to decubitus ulcer formation and should carefully inspect their bodies after each workout and competition. Wheelchair athletes who strap their legs into chairs that produce the "knees-up forward-seated position" are especially at risk for increased pressure over the sacrum and ischial tuberosity. This increase in skin pressure, coupled with sweat causing tissue maceration and the shear forces created by the repetitive movement required for competition, sets up the conditions conducive to decubitus formation. Whereas the majority of ulcers occur over the sacrum and buttocks, improperly fitted footwear coupled with prolonged strapping into competitive wheelchairs can also produce decubiti over other bony prominences.

27. Are there other skin injuries that disabled athletes need to worry about?

Disabled athletes also exhibit a high percentage of skin injuries to the upper extremities. Blisters commonly develop on the hand and fingers of disabled athletes and on the inner arm due to friction from wheelchair tires. Irritation of the skin can occur at the area of the wheelchair seat-post and from rubbing against the back of the wheelchair. Blisters can be prevented by slow callus formation, taping the fingers and hands, padding the seat-post area of the wheelchair, and/or wearing a shirt or wrapping the upper arms to prevent repetitive friction from injuring the skin.

Abrasions, lacerations, and resultant skin infections occur commonly in wheelchair athletes, as fingers and thumbs catch on push rims, spokes, brakes, and the metal edge of an empty armrest socket. Preventive measures include removal of handbrakes, filing down of empty armrest sockets, and the use of plastic wheel guard covers. Again, protective hand padding is important. Areas of chronic irritation may need extra attention from friction-reducing materials, such as mole skin or a layer of petroleum jelly covered with adhesive tape.

28. What resources are available to disabled individuals interested in competitive and/or noncompetitive sports?

The authors recommend that the interested athlete review the listing of "Sports Associations" in *Sports 'N Spokes*, a magazine reporting on the issues and events in the area of disabled athletes. It is published bimonthly by the Paralyzed Veterans of America (2111 East Highland Avenue, Suite 180, Phoenix, AZ 85016-4702, 602-224-0500). In this resource athletic organizations are listed by sport and include associations of archery, basketball, billiards, bowling, aviation, golf, hockey, tennis, racquetball, road racing, motorcycling, quad rugby, outdoor sports, skiing, sailing, table tennis, swimming, softball, shooting, canoeing, rowing, scuba diving, and weightlifting, among others.

BIBLIOGRAPHY

1. Badell A, Welner S: The care of women with physical disabilities. In Seltzer VL, Pearse WH (eds): Women's Primary Health Care. New York, McGraw-Hill, 1995, pp 731–736.
2. Bloomquist LK: Injuries to athletes with physical disabilities: Prevention implications. Physician Sportsmedicine 14:97–105, 1986.
3. Booth DW: Athletes with disabilities. In Harries M, et al (eds): Oxford Textbook of Sports Medicine. Oxford Medical Publications, 1994, pp 634–646.
4. Cosman BC, Stone JM, Perkash I: The gastrointestinal system. In Whiteneck GG, et al (eds): Aging with Spinal Cord Injury. New York, Demos, 1993, pp 117–129.
5. Fisk JR, Bunch WH: Scoliosis in neuromuscular disease. Orthop Clin North Am 10:863–917, 1979.
6. Fowler WM, Johnson ER, Yong CC: Management of medical complications in neuromuscular disease. Phys Med Rehabil State Art Rev 2(4):597–615, 1988.
7. Fuji T, et al: Cervical radiculopathy and myelopathy secondary to athetoid cerebral palsy. J Bone Joint Surg 69A:815–821, 1987.
8. Glenn MB, Whyte J: The Practical Management of Spasticity in Children and Adults. Philadelphia, Lea & Febiger, 1990.
9. Levit F: Skin problems in amputees. In American Academy of Orthopaedic Surgeons: Atlas of Limb Prosthetics. St. Louis, Mosby, 1981, pp 443–447.
10. Lloyd LK: Long-term follow-up of neurogenic bladder. Phys Med Rehabil Clin North Am 4:391–409, 1993.
11. Lord J: Cerebral palsy: A clinical approach. Arch Phys Med Rehabil 65:542–548, 1984.
12. Nelson MR, Alexander MA: Pediatric-onset disabilities. In Felsenthal G (ed): Rehabilitation of the Aging and Elderly Patient. Baltimore, Williams & Wilkins, 1994, pp 407–413.
13. Price N, Schubert ML, Vijay MR: Gastrointestinal disease in the spinal cord injured patient. Phys Med Rehabil State Art Rev 1:475–488, 1987.
14. Reese ME, et al: Acquired cervical spine impairments in young adults with cerebral palsy. Dev Med Child Neurol 33:153–166, 1991.
15. Sawin KJ: Issues for women with physical disability and chronic illness. In Youngkin EQ, et al (eds): Women's Health: A Primary Care Clinical Guide. Norwalk, CT, Appleton & Lange, 1994, pp 697–719.
16. Shadden BB: Communication and aging: An overview. In Communication Behavior and Aging: A Sourcebook for Clinicians. Baltimore, William & Wilkins, 1988, p 4.
17. Stacy WK, Midha M: The kidney in the spinal cord injury patient. Phys Med Rehabil State Art Rev 1:415–423, 1987.

18. Waters RL, Sie LH, Adkins RH: The musculoskeletal system. In Whiteneck GG, et al (eds): Aging with Spinal Cord Injury. New York, Demos, 1993, pp 53–72.
19. Yatsu FM, DeGraba TJ, Harson S: Therapy of secondary medical complications of strokes. In Barnett HJM, et al (eds): Stroke, Pathophysiology, Diagnosis and Management. New York, Churchill Livingstone, 1992, pp 995–1004.

10. SATISFYING SEXUALITY DESPITE DISABILITY

Steven A. Stiens, M.D., Ruth K. Westheimer, Ed.D., and Mark A. Young, M.D.

1. What is sexuality?

Sexuality is the expression of a person's femaleness or maleness through personality, body, dress, and behavior; it is the personification of biologic gender, gender identity, and sexual orientation. It develops through physiologic cues from the body, experiences of self, maturation, socialization, societal reflection of the person, and intimate relationships. Sexuality, therefore, requires an evolving self-understanding, an ongoing opportunity for communication of self-perception, and responses from those around us. The context of sexual rehabilitation is the affirmation of the person's sexuality and enablement of sexual self-expression. The anticipation of patients' sexuality as a facet of their role in relationships is but one example of the power of therapeutic expectation.

2. What is sexual literacy?

Sexual literacy is the working knowledge of anatomy, physiology, and recent research pertaining to human sexuality theory and practice. The "sexually-literate" health professional must be comfortable with his or her own sexuality, suspend judgment, and express genuine willingness to pursue understanding and solutions with the patient and partner.

3. What are the subcomponents of personal sexual expression?

Sexual identity—phenotypic sex with objective expression and function of secondary sexual characteristics, anatomy, and physiology

Gender identity—the person's subjective sense of self as man or woman

Orientation—the focus of desire for sexual relationship

Intention—degree of aggression inherent in sexual fantasy and behavior

Sexual desire—interest in a variety of activity, frequency

4. How does disability affect body image and sexual self-concept?

The **body image** is the mind's picture of our own bodies, the perception we have of ourselves. It is closely associated with the awareness of our body (the afferent sensory barrage and central processing, "the experienced homunculus"). The expression and practice of sexuality are affected by self-esteem, body image, and interpersonal attachment. It is continually evaluated by the self. Despite adaptation to self, individuals often confront a society with a stigma and risk devaluation by others. Rehabilitation specialists must strive to help patients become fully self-aware, construct a body image, accept it, like it, and share it.

5. Isn't it important to have a relationship first?

Personal relationships begin with our attitudes about ourselves. Beyond self-perception is self-acceptance, self-esteem, and self-worth as a potential partner for another. The rehabilitation team must successfully reflect patients' personal values, reinforcing the value of their companionship to others. People who project self-respect and satisfaction are most fully capable of initiating relationships and graciously accepting others' attention. People who recognize their capabilities are most able to contribute them to a mutually complementary relationship. Consequently, rehabilitation must teach patients the necessity for taking risks of rejection in interactions with others.

6. What communications must there be with the patient's partner?

For patients who have a sexual partner, intervention is most effective if the partner is included in any communication between the rehabilitation professional and the patient on matters of sexual functioning. This is particularly true after a myocardial infarction, when the partner may be fearful about engaging in sexual activity that might produce another "attack" and perhaps even cause the patient's death.

Sexual issues must be integrated into the entire rehabilitation plan; partners in life need full inclusion in the rehab process. If possible, it is desirable to maintain a separation between roles of caretaker and sexual partner. This can be achieved with proactive planning for attendant care.

7. What are the physiologic changes associated with the four stages of the human sexual response as outlined by Masters and Johnson?

Excitement stage I: muscle tension, sympathetic activity, nipple erection
  Female: clitoris swelling, vaginal lubrication
  Male: penile erection, testes rise
Plateau stage II: heightened excitement, pulse 100–160 bpm, sex flush
  Female: clitoris withdrawals, vaginal vasocongestion
  Male: testes enlarge, Cowper's secretion
Orgasm stage III (seconds to minutes): rhythmic muscle contractions
  Female: uterus, vagina, and anus contract
  Male: ejaculation, bladder neck closes
Relaxation stage IV (minutes to hours): return to baseline, refractory period

8. Describe the physiology of the sexual response in women.

The uterus and ovaries receive only sympathetic innervation from the hypogastric nerve. Clitoral swelling and vaginal secretion are parasympathetically driven. At orgasm, the pelvic floor (pudendal nerve) contracts rhythmically.

9. How do neurologic injuries affect female sexual function?

Menstruation may not occur for 3 or more months after CNS trauma. Vaginal lubrication occurs with reflex stimulation as long as the conus and autonomic connections remain intact. After complete spinal cord injury at level T6 and above, psychogenic subjective arousal does not produce vaginal lubrication; manual clitoral stimulation produces reflex lubrication and increased vaginal pulse amplitude.

Fertility is generally not significantly affected by spinal cord injury. Pregnancy may be complicated by urinary tract infection, decubiti, constipation, and mobility limitations. Labor is initiated and driven hormonally. The delivery can be vaginal but should be anticipated and monitored, with autonomic hyperreflexia prevention and preparedness for forceps use or cesarean techniques.

10. How do erections occur?

Male erection is initiated by arterial vasodilatation and venous outlet constriction, which result in engorgement of the penile sinusoids. Autonomic penile innervation is via the pelvic plexus lateral to the rectum which carries the parasympathetic **nervi erigentes** (S2,3,4) and sympathetic **hypogastric nerve** (T12, L1) fibers to the penis. Somatic sensation and pelvic floor motor control are via the pudendal (S2,3,4) mixed nerve. Psychogenic erections are mediated via the lumbar sympathetics (T10–L2). Reflexogenic erection is primarily cholinergic (parasympathetic, S2,3,4) and the ejaculation detumescence process is primarily sympathetic, but a complex interplay of autonomic systems and other neurotransmitters also have roles in the process.

11. Describe the physiology of the sexual response in men.

Psychogenic stimuli can produce erection and emission containing spermatozoa via sympathetic facilitation. **Emission** is the sympathetically controlled process of deposition of seminal fluid in the posterior urethra. **Ejaculation** is the forceful delivery of the semen out of the urethra by the pudendal-innervated bulbocavernous and ischiocavernosus muscles. Ejaculation is typically ineffective after complete spinal cord injury (SCI) and can result in retrograde ejaculation (semen into the bladder). Ejaculation can be facilitated with a vibrator stimulus under the glans at the frenulum or inhibited by the squeeze technique (firm grasp of glans).

12. How do neurologic injuries affect the process of erection?

Past reviews have reported an overall 54–87% incidence of erection after SCI (60–90% upper motor neuron reflex, 10–30% lower motor neuron psychogenic or reflex). A recent study utilizing physiologic recordings defined erections as an increase in penile circumference of 3–6 mm and demonstrated 100% reflexogenic erection in upper SCI and in 80–90% of patients with lower motor neuron lesions. The capacity for tumescence with partial innervation is encouraging, but penile rigidity facilitates successful intromission (vaginal insertion of penis, not to be confused with "intermission").

13. What are the rehabilitation options for producing erections after neurologic injuries?

Without erection, satisfying intromission can be accomplished with the **stuffing technique** (pushing the penis into the vagina and stimulating the woman with friction and sustained pressure at the introitus). Erection can be produced noninvasively with **vacuum entrapment** and expansion of the penis, cavernosal engorgement can be maintained with a custom circular rubber-tension ring at the base of the penis.

Pharmacologic adjuncts have included **yohimbine** (not used in SCI) and **testosterone** (increases libido, minimal improvement of erections, use only if serum levels are low). Intracorporal injections with **papaverine** (a nonspecific smooth muscle relaxant) and/or **prostaglandin E1** produce erections if dosed properly, but such treatment requires written approval by the patient as these agents have not been approved by the FDA for this indication. These agents act by causing relaxation of smooth muscle and vasodilatation. Venous outflow is decreased through relaxation of corporal smooth muscle that occludes draining venues. Prevention and management of side effects such as priapism (cavernosal needle aspiration reduces pressure and removes medication) and corporal fibrosis with repeated injections require physician supervision and a 24-hour emergency plan.

Penile implants may be noninflatable (rigid or semirigid, not currently used in SCI) or inflatable and facilitate retention of condoms for urinary management. Rigid or malleable penile implants are not recommended for SCI or neurologic disorders because they can cause tissue erosion at insensate areas.

14. Does spinal cord injury affect male fertility?

Deficits in spermatogenesis documented by testicular biopsy have included tubular atrophy, spermatogenic arrest, and interstitial fibrosis. Seminal parameters show decreased sperm counts and motility as well as abnormal morphology. Repeated ejaculation reduces stasis and can improve sperm quality.

15. What is the PLISSIT model of sex therapy?

P = permission to be sexual
LI = limited information
SS = specific suggestions
IT = intensive therapy

This model presents a spectrum of interventional areas that can be addressed in part by each member of the interdisciplinary team.

16. Explain the components of the PLISSIT approach.

Permission—Sensitive questions regarding sexual function in history-taking are therapeutic affirmations of the patient's sexuality and role in the lives of others. Recognition and sensitive discussion of potentially embarrassing situations—bathing, bowel and bladder care—provide permission for the patient to discuss their emotional reactions and fears and to begin communications about adaptive solutions. Teaching the patient management techniques for angina, bronchospasm, autonomic dysreflexia, and prevention of incontinence prepares them for their own problem-solving in sexual exploration.

Limited Information—All rehabilitation programs should include lectures and discussion that educate the patient about the basic physiology and pathophysiology of the sexual response cycle and reproduction. One-to-one explanation of the unique effects of a patient's disease or injury should complement this review. This primary education should be the designated responsibility of one rehabilitation team member, with appropriate referral to another team member as needed for elaboration.

Specific Suggestions—Ideally, all team members contribute to successful sexual adjustment and function. For example, the training of the patient by the primary nurse for skin examination for sores can lead to reflections on body image. A *suggestion* might be an assignment for the patient or couple to *experiment with visual body exploration* and *survey patient sensation*. Such a couple can later be assigned *sensate focus exercises* and then advanced to a search for areas that might be new erogenous zones. Physical therapy education for a spouse on transfers and mat mobility might easily be generalized by couples for use in sexual positioning.

Intensive Therapy—The presence of impairments that contribute to role performance deficits demands formal attention and the response of a rehabilitation team member. On most teams, this is the psychologist.

17. How are sexual problems elicited?

A medical environment is an advantage that can achieve patient openness and honesty about sexual issues. Evaluations of sexual function start with the social history and move from the review of symptoms out through the physical examination to goal setting. This framework for questioning will make sexual questions "matter of fact" when you arrive at the urogenital system. Descriptions of sexual function will lead to opportunities to discuss situations and partners.

The mirror is the most important tool for the physical exam. The mirror allows the physician to visualize areas of the body with the patient and partners. An examination that includes the aid of a spouse for positioning lends itself to review of the patient's sensory, motor, and autonomic impairments. Potential for lubrication, reflexogenic erections, and positioning for intercourse can be sensitively addressed in such sessions.

18. Is there sex after stroke?

Sensory impairment, as opposed to mobility deficits, has been associated with decreased libido, decreased intercourse frequency, and erectile and perceptual disturbance. Issues related to aphasia, distortion of body image, and frontal limbic damage affect interest and performance. Women often experience difficulty with lubrication and require adjunctive creams to prevent dyspareunia.

19. Do people still want sex after going through a severe disability adjustment?

Depression, attitude, and self-perception all affect arousal. Use of explicit materials, memories, or conversations in person or by phone are often effective in reawakening desire. Self-exploration and stimulation reacquaint one with the recipe for satisfaction. Such self-knowledge provides a guide for pleasuring with partners.

20. When should a sex therapist be consulted?

Good sexual functioning depends not only on the physical health of the patients, but also on their libido. While the physical limitations caused by a disease or old age may require only some trial and error, the detrimental effects on the libido may be an issue that cannot be handled without guidance, particularly as the patient's sex partner may also be in need of assistance. Sex therapy need not be long-term, but even a few visits to a sex therapist should be recommended whenever issues involving difficulties of arousal are suspected by the primary physician.

21. Is there sex after a heart attack?

But of course! Myocardial infarction or heart disease in general need not preclude resumption of sexual activity. Contrary to popular myth, sexual activity is unassociated with the risk of sudden death in coronary patients. In fact, Ueno found that > 1% of sudden deaths in Japan happened during sex. The metabolic cost of sex in middle-aged married men is no more than 5 METS. Metabolic cost of intercourse in a familiar position is lower than in an unfamiliar position. For people resuming sexual activity after heart disease, foreplay may be a metabolically favorable "warm-up" (training) activity. Initial explorations can include masturbation to give the patient full control of the process. Thereafter, successive approximation of the previous routine can follow.

22. How important is it for the physician to give permission for sexual activity?

Change, especially a negative one occurring from an accident, disease, or aging, is often accompanied by fear. Patients frequently worry that they may aggravate their condition through sexual activity. This anxiety can affect sexual function as much as pathophysiology. Hearing the physician give permission to engage in sexual activity is a therapeutic step toward healthy sexual activity.

23. Can the location of erogenous zones really change after injury to the CNS?

Recent primate and human data demonstrate central sensory reorganization in response to injuries to the spinal cord or peripheral nerve. People with SCI have repeatedly reported areas in the zone of partial sensory preservation that are sexually exciting with stimulation. These areas can lead to the experience of orgasm with associated tachycardia and flushing above the lesion.

24. What is there to be afraid of?

Overcoming attitudinal and cultural taboos of intervention transcends barriers. Practices that bring together mutually sensate erogenous zones can become particularly satisfying parts of couples' repertoires: possibilities for **cunnilungus** (oral and lingual vulva stimulation) and **fellatio** (oral and lingual penile stimulation) should be explored. Unfortunately, a major barrier to sexual fulfillment after disability is our fears. This starts with fears of poor acceptance by a partner. Issues related to involuntary loss of urinary or bowel control are particularly ominous. Planning for sexual encounters reduces anxiety and makes them more conceivable.

25. How can humor help with sex after disability?

Humor puts people at ease. Disability often reduces physical control of situations. Humor offers a response to surprises and produces a playful atmosphere for persons to explore and bring pleasure to one another.

26. Do any organizations provide help for patients with sexuality issues?

Resources to Contact Regarding All Aspects of Sexuality of Disabled Individuals

ORGANIZATION	TELEPHONE	SERVICE
Through the Looking Glass 2198 6th Street Suite 100 Berkeley, CA 94710	510-848-1112	Focuses on services, research, and resource development for parents with disabilities; provides information about adaptive equipment and helps educate child protective services and parenting professionals.
Sex Information and Education Council of the United States 130 W. 42nd Street, Ste 350 New York, NY 10036	212-819-9770	Provides bibliographic information on topics of sexuality in disabled people, for consumers, parents, and professionals, includ-books, pamphlets, curriculum training manuals, journals, and newsletters.
United Cerebral Palsy Associates 1660 L Street, NW, #700 Washington, DC 20036-5682	800-USA-5UCP (V/TT)	Provides written information on sexuality issues and refers to appropriate local organizations (50% of persons receiving information from UCP have disabling conditions other than CP).

Courtesy of Richard S. Materson, M.D., and Susan M. Miller, M.D.

BIBLIOGRAPHY

1. Althof SE, Levine SB: Clinical approach to the sexuality of patients with spinal cord injury. Urol Clin North Am 20(3):527–533, 1993.
2. Annon J: The PLISSIT model: A proposed conceptual scheme for the behavioral treatment for sexual problems. J Sex Educ Ther 2:1, 1976.
3. Courtois FJ, Charvier KF, Leriche A, Raymond DP: Sexual function in spinal cord injury men: I. Assessing sexual capability. Paraplegia 31:771–784, 1993.
4. Donahue J, Gebbard P: The Kinsey Institute/Indiana University Report on Sexuality and Spinal Cord Injury. Sex Disabil 13:7–85, 1995.
5. Kreuter M, Sullivan M, Siostee A: Sexual adjustment after spinal cord injury—comparison of partner experiences in pre- and post-injury relationships. Paraplegia 32:759–770, 1994.
6. Lemon MA: Sexual counseling and spinal cord injury. Sex Disabil 11(1):73–97, 1993.
7. Monga T (ed): Sexuality and Disability. Phys Med Rehabil State Art Rev 9(2):299–420, 1995.
8. Sipski ML, Alexander CJ, Rosen RC: Physiological parameters associated with psychogenic sexual arousal in women complete spinal cord injuries. Arch Phys Rehabil 76:811–818, 1995.
9. Westheimer RK, Ruskin SA: Sex in Current Therapy in Physiatry: Physical Medicine and Rehabilitation. Philadelphia, W.B. Saunders, 1984, pp 530–535.
10. Westheimer RK: Sex for Dummies. Foster City, CA, IDG Books, 1995.

11. BEHAVIOR AND ADJUSTMENT IN THE REHABILITATION PATIENT

John Speed, M.B.B.S.

1. What role does the rehabilitation professional play in helping the patient adjust?

Rehabilitation practitioners must be prepared to guide newly disabled patients through the coping process, since "caring" for people with disability means far more than just ministering to their medical and functional needs. The clinician who has a solid understanding of the behavioral, emotional, and adjustment issues confronting the physically impaired population will be a more effective care-giver!

BEHAVIORAL COPING MECHANISMS

2. Name three important models of psychological adjustment to disability.
Behavioral model
Coping skills model
Stage theory model

3. Describe the behavioral model of psychological adjustment.

The behavioral model highlights the importance of external factors in establishing a person's adjustment. It emphasizes observable behaviors and deaccentuates internal factors and cognitive issues.

4. What are the seven adaptive tasks and coping skills included in the coping skills model?

The coping skills model emphasizes both behavioral and cognitive factors. Modeled after "crisis theory," this model encompasses seven important adaptive tasks and coping skills:

   1. Denying or minimizing the severity of a disability
   2. Seeking relevant information
   3. Requesting reassurance and emotional support

4. Learning illness-related skills
5. Establishing concrete goals
6. Rehearsing alternative outcomes
7. Identifying a general purpose or meaning for disability

5. Describe the stage theory model.

In the stage theory model, there is an orderly, predictable sequence of events or steps of emotional response for people facing disability. Analogous to Kubler-Ross' stages of grief and bereavement, stage theory typically begins with shock and ends in adaptation.

6. Do all people with disabilities of a particular type cope identically?

Although some general coping patterns may exist, there is little evidence that people react in specific and predictable ways to the onset of disability.

7. What are the common psychologic responses to spinal cord injury (SCI)?

Denial is a common response following SCI. Shortly after injury, many patients ask, "When am I going to walk again?" Pain and fear of dying may complicate one's ability to process information about prognosis. Many patients respond to the prognosis of paralysis with an assertion of will and strength—i.e., they will prove the physician wrong and walk out of the hospital. This may not be so much denial as evidence of the powerful resources a person draws upon in a time of adversity (i.e., hope).

8. Is a period of depression a precursor to healthy adjustment following SCI?

No, depression is not a requirement for successful adjustment. Stage theory of adjustment to disability suggests that denial is followed by depression, which is necessary for adjustment to occur. Depression, in turn, is replaced by feelings of dependency and hostility that must be worked through to reach the final stage of adjustment.

However, studies that looked for stages following SCI found more variability than similarity in the reactions of patients with SCI. It appears that depressive disorder affects a minority of patients in the first few months after injury. It does not appear to be a universal phenomenon, and when it does occur, it is not as severe or prolonged as expected. However, staff rating consistently overestimate the amount of depression actually present. This leads to the possibility of a Catch 22 situation; if the disabled person admits to depression, then that is a psychological problem; but, it the person denies depression, that constitutes denial, a psychological problem that needs treatment.

9. How do coping strategies differ in people with cancer compared to other disabilities?

Many strategies of cancer patients are similar to those seen in other persons with serious physical illness or disability. As with other conditions, psychosocial impairment may persist after the underlying physical problem has been resolved or improved. Pain, and the fear of pain, is a more frequent concern with cancer than with other disabling conditions. Due to the frequently progressive nature of cancer, the patient must be helped to adapt to multiple progressive losses and uncertainty regarding the future. Preparatory mourning can occur as family members begin to detach emotionally from the patient while he or she is still alive and functional. Empathetic confrontation of the family, including discussion of why such detachment is occurring, with assistance in planning supportive strategy, can help family members remain supportive while the patient remains alive.

10. What psychologic sequelae may be seen following severe burns?

Post-traumatic stress disorder is quite common among burn patients. Symptoms include re-experiencing the trauma through vivid, intrusive recollections or dreams, an exaggerated startle response, numbing of responsiveness to the outside world, difficulty with memory and concentration, avoidance of cues associated with the burn, and intensified distress when reminded of the burn.

CONVERSION DISORDER

11. What is a conversion disorder?

Conversion disorder is defined as a specific and enduring sensory or motor dysfunction, or symptom complex, involving the voluntary nervous system which **contradicts** known neurologic and musculoskeletal physiology and physical findings.

12. Where is conversion disorder most commonly seen?

Anyone working in the field of rehabilitation medicine will encounter patients with conversion disorder. It occurs in all settings—outpatient, consultation, or inpatient. If it is not appropriately diagnosed and managed, the symptoms and functional deficits will persist, leading to a great deal of frustration among patients, families, and the health care team. Conversion disorder is most common in adolescents and young adults. There is no gender preponderance.

13. What causes it?

1. Nonverbal communication theory—One expresses his or her wants and needs through physical symptoms.

2. Stress-diathesis model—Stress can present through the autonomic nervous system or, less commonly, the somatic nervous system.

3. Learned behavior—Symptoms are conditioned in an operant fashion. It the symptom elicits the patient's desired response from the environment, then the symptom will be maintained.

14. What factors are traditionally associated with conversion disorder?

Symptom symbolism (e.g., a professional marathon runner presenting to the emergency room with paraplegia the night before a race)

Secondary gain

Hysterical personality

La belle indifference

These conditions are common with conversion disorder but are not necessary for its diagnosis.

15. How is conversion disorder diagnosed?

Just like everything else in medicine, conversion disorder is best diagnosed by taking a careful history and, particularly, by performing a careful physical examination. The diagnosis of conversion disorder is *not* one of exclusion—there *must* be positive evidence demonstrating that the dysfunction is functional rather than organic. There can be variability from exam to exam, there can be failure of symptoms to conform to anatomic and physiologic patterns or innervation, or findings may vary with suggestion. Ratchety response on manual muscle testing, with giveway and inconsistency between different aspects of the examination, is suggestive of a nonorganic finding. Bizarre gait, slow motion movements, and "overflow" of movement are several findings on examination which should alert the examiner to the high probability of nonorganic weakness.

16. What types of treatment strategies are available?

Psychiatrically oriented (hypnosis, narcosuggestion, group therapy, or medication)

Modality oriented (functional electrical stimulation, electromyography, biofeedback)

Behaviorally oriented

17. What are the goals of behavioral management of conversion disorder?

1. To unlearn the maladaptive response.

2. To learn more appropriate means of interacting with the environment.

18. What do you tell the patient about the disorder?

Patients can be told that although the examination and diagnostic testing have definitively established that the brain, spinal cord, nerves, and muscles are intact, the messages that allow normal muscle function are somehow being blocked from getting through from the brain to the muscles. Preferably, the physician who has undertaken the diagnostic evaluation should counsel the patient as to the results of that workup and also mention that it is expected that function can be restored.

Typically, you should avoid discussing the diagnosis of conversion disorder with the patient; however, many patients are medically sophisticated and will want to know what the term is for this "blockage." In this case, the patient's physician and psychologist should confer. The best approach is simply to say, "It doesn't matter where the problem lies; the bottom line is that you have functional deficits, and this therapy approach can help you to improve your ability to function."

19. How do you do behavioral management of conversion disorder?

Treatment progresses along a sequence defined in advance, using a series of steps appropriate for the symptom complex; the patient is not allowed to progress to the next step in therapy until the previous one has been mastered.

- When not receiving therapy, the affected body part(s) is immobilized to prevent further incidental reinforcement of the abnormal motor function (e.g., when the lower extremities are involved, the patient is in a wheelchair, and when the upper extremities are involved, the patient has resting hand splints fitted).
- Copious praise is awarded the patient upon successful completion of a step in the training sequence. Where possible, there should be continuity of health care providers for the patient, and negative or "hopeless" statements (e.g., "I don't know what I can do for you") should be avoided. Patients are quick to pick up on any uncertainty or pessimism that a professional might demonstrate.
- Any type of out-of-hospital pass should be rarely offered and used very judiciously only for reinforcement of significant functional improvement late in the program, just prior to discharge.
- Adaptive equipment is to be actively avoided. At times, goal cards for each functional activity can help demonstrate to the patient that he or she is actually progressing.
- It should be explained that symptoms caused by "message blockage" can at times be made worse by stress, and this opens the door for psychological evaluation of the patient.

20. Where do you do behavioral management of conversion disorder?

Behavioral management is best achieved in an environment where significant control is attainable. Typically, inpatient rehabilitation units are preferred to an outpatient or psychiatric unit. Rehabilitation nurses and therapists are used to working with patients with significant functional deficits due to analogous organic conditions, but staff education as to the unconscious nature of conversion symptoms is critical to avoid their sense of being a victim of conscious manipulation.

BIBLIOGRAPHY

1. American Psychiatric Association: Diagnostic and Statistical Manual of Mental Disorders, 4th ed. Washington, D.C., American Psychiatric Association, 1995.
2. Delargy MA, Peatfield RC, Burt AA: Successful rehabilitation in conversion paralysis. BMJ 292:1730–1731, 1986.
3. Fishbain DA, Goldberg M, Khalil TM, et al: The utility of electromyographic feedback in the treatment of conversion paralysis. Am J Psychiatry 145:1572–1575, 1988.
4. Ford CV, Folks DG: Conversion disorders—An overview. Psychosomatics 26:371–383, 1985.
5. Gould R, Miller BI, Goldberg MA, Benson DF: The validity of hysterical signs and symptoms. J Nerv Mental Dis 174:593–597, 1986.
6. Helm PA, Fisher SV: Rehabilitation of the patient with burns. In DeLisa JA, Gans BM (eds): Rehabilitation Medicine: Principles and Practice, 2nd ed. Philadelphia, J.B. Lippincott, 1993, pp 1111–1130.
7. Klein MJ, Kewman DG, Sayama M: Behavior modification of abnormal gait and chronic pain secondary to somatization disorder. Arch Phys Med Rehabil 66:119–122, 1985.
8. Rohe DE: Psychological aspects of rehabilitation. In DeLisa JA, Gans BM (eds): Rehabilitation Medicine: Principles and Practice, 2nd ed. Philadelphia, J.B. Lippincott, 1993, pp 131–150.

9. Speed J: Behavioral management of conversion disorder: A literature review and retrospective study. Arch Phys Med Rehabil 77:147–154, 1996.
10. Teasell RW, Shapiro AP: Strategic-behavioral intervention in the treatment of chronic nonorganic motor disorders. Am J Phys Med Rehabil 73:44–50, 1994.
11. Trieschmann RB, Stolov WC, Montgomery ED: An approach to the treatment of abnormal ambulation resulting from conversion reaction. Arch Phys Med Rehabil 51:198–206, 1970.
12. Trieschmann RB: The psychosocial adjustment to spinal cord injury. In Bloch RF, Basbaum M (eds): Management of Spinal Cord Injury. Baltimore, Williams & Wilkins, 1986, pp 302–319.
13. Weintraub MI: Hysterical Conversion Reactions—A Clinical Guide to Diagnosis and Treatment. New York, SP Medical, 1983.

12. REHABILITATION OF PERSONS WITH SEVERE VISUAL IMPAIRMENT OR BLINDNESS

Stanley F. Wainapel, M.D., M.P.H.

1. Is vision rehabilitation relevant to physiatric practice?

Vision loss is one of the most common causes of functional disability among adults, and its impact on mobility, activities of daily living (ADL), or both is often profound. Moreover, severe vision impairment is likely to be a frequent concomitant of the conditions traditionally treated by physiatrists—i.e., stroke, amputation, hip fractures—and has been seen in 7% of patients admitted to an inpatient rehab unit. Maximizing visual perception is one component of a plan to maximize adaptive compensational outcome. Finally, in an environment where primary care is a favored model of medical management, it would be wise for physiatrists to have basic knowledge of the treatment of this highly prevalent sensory impairment.

2. What are common causes of visual impairment?

Among the elderly (those at highest risk for such problems), four conditions dominate all other etiologies of vision impairment:

Four Most Common Causes of Visual Impairment Among the Elderly

	AGE		
	< 65 YRS	65–75 YRS	75+ YRS
Senile cataracts	2.6%	9.6%	33.7%
Glaucoma	0.7	1.7	2.9
Diabetic retinopathy	1.1	1.7	3.0
Macular degeneration	0.6	4.1	15.4

Adapted from Morse A, Friedman D: Vision rehabilitation and aging. J Vis Impair Blind 80:803–804, 1986.

Among young and middle-aged adults diabetic retinopathy is the most frequent cause of vision loss, with diseases such as retinitis pigmentosa also beginning to assume greater importance. In children, congenital disorders (cataract) and disorders related to prematurity or neurologic disease (retinopathy of prematurity, cortical vision loss following anoxia or CNS infection) are among the more frequent etiologies.

3. How are visual impairments described and classified?

Visual impairment is usually described as **central** (visual acuity) or **peripheral** (visual field) deficits. Central deficits are either discrete (e.g,. scotomas) or diffuse (e.g,. lens opacity).

Peripheral deficits are described as concentric (loss of peripheral vision resulting in "tunnel vision," as in retinitis pigmentosa or glaucoma) or central (retention of peripheral fields only, as in age-related macular degeneration). Visual impairment can also be classified in terms of its severity, i.e., legal blindness or low vision.

4. What are legal blindness and low vision?

Legal blindness was defined by the Social Security Act of 1935 as:

1. Visual acuity of 20/200 or less in the better eye despite use of corrective lenses, or
2. Visual field of 20° or less in the better eye.

This arbitrary definition includes many people with some residual vision (only 15% of those who are legally blind are actually totally blind by virtue of having no light perception), and it unfortunately excludes many people with significant vision problems. These latter individuals are described as having **low vision**, which is usually defined as corrected visual acuity of less than 20/70 but better than 20/200, or visual field exceeding 20°. Those who are legally blind have greater access to state-funded vision rehabilitation services.

5. Does visual impairment affect physical function?

It most certainly does, which is a major reason for physiatrists to know about it. Several studies in the geriatric population have demonstrated that isolated visual impairment in older people produces significant deficits in basic ADLs as well as instrumental ADLs. Additional effects of visual impairment are social isolation and low employment rates.

It should also be noted that vision is one of the three major components of sensory feedback to maintain normal upright stance (proprioception and vestibular function are the other two), and its loss can be associated with increased risk of falling in the elderly, with a consequent rise in the risk of hip fractures.

6. How should the physiatrist screen patients for the presence of significant visual impairment?

A high index of suspicion, particularly in patients over age 65, is essential. Functionally based questions to ask could include:

1. Do you have any problems affecting your vision?
2. How do they affect your ability to get around or to do your daily activities?
3. Can you read newspaper print with (or without) your glasses?

The screening examination should include visual acuity using a portable Snellen eye chart or an ordinary newspaper (which documents acuity better or worse than 20/70) and visual fields using confrontation. If deficits are found or suspected, a full ophthalmologic evaluation should be obtained.

7. How can visually impaired patients gain access to vision rehabilitation services?

An ophthalmologic evaluation documenting the presence of "legal blindness" requires the submission of a form certifying the presence of this degree of visual impairment. The form goes to a state commission for the blind (this may vary from state to state), which then coordinates vision rehabilitation services to which such individuals are entitled. These may include social/vocational services, mobility and ADL training, low-vision equipment and other technology, and referral to the talking books library services. People with low vision may not be entitled to all these services, but they often can receive some of them through local facilities specializing in vision rehabilitation services.

8. What are the basic components of vision rehabilitation?

Vision rehabilitation techniques can be broadly grouped into two types, vision enhancement and vision substitution. These can be seen as analogous to orthotics and prosthetics, respectively. **Vision enhancement** uses devices or techniques that maximize the utility of any remaining visual function, while **vision substitution** utilizes technology or techniques that do not require any vision at all.

9. What are some vision enhancement techniques?
Vision enhancement techniques can be remembered with the mnemonic **IMAGE**:
 I = **I**llumination devices
 M = **M**agnification and large print
 A = **A**ltered contrast
 G = **G**lare reduction
 E = **E**xpanders of visual field

10. What are some vision substitution techniques?
Vision substitution techniques can be classified into:
Mobility: Cane, guide dog, sonic devices
Tactile: Braille books/devices, raised markings
Recorded: Talking books, radio reading services
Synthetic speech: Computers with verbal output, talking watches/calculators, etc.
Computer-generated vision systems
Special ADL techniques: Cooking techniques, money identification

11. Name some low-vision aids.
Vision enhancement
Magnifiers (hand-held, stand-alone, illuminated)
Telescopic lenses (monocular or binocular)
Closed-circuit television (CCTV) video magnifiers
Computer software providing magnification
Prisms for visual-field expansion
Nonoptical aids
Appropriate lighting (illumination)
Visors, tinted eye glasses (reduce glare)
Heightened color contrast (bold print pens, paper with extra-thick lines, white-on-black re-
 versal images for slides)

12. What kinds of mobility aids are used by blind or visually impaired patients?
Special mobility devices include the long white cane, laser cane, ultrasonic devices, and the guide dog. The guide dog is usually reserved for those with near-total blindness and is more likely to be used by younger adults. Finally, a friend or willing helper can offer his or her arm and walk alongside the person with a visual impairment (sighted guide technique).

13. How can computer technology contribute to the rehabilitation of visually impaired people?
On a basic level, simple "talking" devices, such as the talking watch, talking calculator, and talking glucometer (for blind diabetics), are obviously helpful ADL aids. At a more elaborate level, computers with synthetic speech output in combination with optical character recognition scanners, braille output, or voice-activated operation can open a world of informational and professional opportunities for people unable to read the computer screen or ordinary output from a printer.

14. What about some simple self-care devices that are low-tech?
Inexpensive ADL devices include the "talking" technology mentioned previously, raised-dot labeling of dials on kitchen equipment, high-contrast color surfaces in work areas, simple labeling systems for clothing (such as the use of variously shaped labels for each color), and the folding of dollar bills in particular ways to identify each denomination. The assessment of self-care needs of visually impaired persons and training in such strategies is customarily done by rehabilitation teachers, but in recent years occupational therapists have sometimes provided such services in selected settings.

15. What are the expected functional outcomes in patients with combined visual and neuromusculoskeletal disabilities (e.g., blind amputee)?

They are surprisingly good, particularly when vision loss preceded the more familiar physiatric diagnosis. In a study of 12 blind amputees, 75% became functional prosthetic users, and blind stroke patients have had similar results in inpatient settings.

16. Who pays for vision rehabilitation services?

Usually these services are covered through a state Commission for the Blind rather than by standard third-party payers such as Medicare and Medicaid. This funding (or lack of funding) is a reflection of the separate nature of the vision and medical rehab systems as they currently operate. A recent trend is the use of occupational or physical therapists as providers of vision rehab services. Under these circumstances, such services have been reimbursed by Medicare or Medicaid.

17. Where can my patients get more information on vision impairment and rehabilitation?

American Council of the Blind
1155 15th Street, NW, Suite 720
Washington, DC 20005
    202-467-5081
    800-424-8666
American Foundation for the Blind
11 Penn Plaza, Suite 300
New York, NY 10001
    800-232-5463
    212-502-7600
National Federation of the Blind
1800 Johnson Street
Baltimore, MD 21230
    410-659-9314
Council of Citizens with Low Vision
    International
5707 Brockton Drive, #302
Indianapolis, IN 46220
    800-733-2258
    317-254-1155
    317-252-1185

Jewish Guild for the Blind
15 West 65th Street
New York, NY 10023
    212-769-6200
The Lighthouse
111 East 59th Street
New York, NY 10022
    212-821-9200
    800-334-5497 (Information/referral)
    800-829-0500 (Mail order products)
National Library Service for the Blind
    and Physically Handicapped
1291 Taylor Street, NW
Washington, DC 20542
    800-424-8567
Resources for Rehabilitation
33 Bedford Street, Suite 19A
Lexington, MA 02173
    617-862-6455

BIBLIOGRAPHY

1. Altner PE, Rusin JJ, De Boer A: Rehabilitation of blind patients with lower extremity amputations. Arch Phys Med Rehabil 61:82–85, 1980.
2. Branch LG, Horowitz A, Carr C: The implications for everyday life of incident self-reported visual decline among people over age 65 living in the community. Gerontologist 29:359–365, 1989.
3. Carabellese C, Apollonio I, Rozzini R, et al: Sensory impairment and quality of life in a community elderly population. J Am Geriatr Soc 41:401–407, 1993.
4. DiStefano AF, Aston SJ: Rehabilitation of the blind and visually impaired elderly. In Brody SL, Ruff DL (eds): Aging and Rehabilitation Advances in the State of the Art. New York, Springer Publishing, 1986.
5. Faye EE: Clinical Low Vision. Boston, Little, Brown, & Co., 1984.
6. Felson DT, Anderson JJ, Hannah MT, et al: Impaired vision and hip fracture: The Framingham Eye Study. J Am Geriatr Soc 37:495–500, 1989.
7. Greenblatt SL: Providing services for people with vision loss. Lexington, MA, Resources for Rehabilitation, 1989.
8. Wainapel SF: Rehabilitation of the blind stroke patient. Arch Phys Med Rehabil 65:487–489, 1984.
9. Wainapel SF: Visual impairments. In Felsenthal G, Garrison SH, Steinberg FU (eds): Rehabilitation pf the Aging and Elderly Patient. Baltimore, Williams & Wilkins, 1993, pp 327–337.
10. Wainapel SF, Kwon YS, Fazzari PJ: Severe visual impairment on a rehabilitation unit: Incidence and implications. Arch Phys Med Rehabil 65:487–489, 1984.

13. REHABILITATIVE STRATEGIES IN THE HEARING IMPAIRED

J. Michael Anderson, M.D., Denise W. Thrope, M.S., CCC-A,
and Linda J. Anderson, O.T.R.

1. When is hearing loss a rehabilitation problem?

Difficulty hearing impairs many functional activities including communication, education, the exchange of ideas, the carrying out of orders, as well as the pure pleasure of listening and responding. A person begins to be socially incapacitated when hearing loss in both ears reaches 40 dB in the speech frequencies (500–3000 Hz). Only when the hearing loss is total or near-total (> 85–90 dB below normal) do we apply the term "deafness." Hearing loss implies a partial loss of function; only the profoundly damaged ear is unable to respond to amplified sound. When a physician learns that a patient's hearing cannot be corrected medically or surgically, suitable rehabilitation must be advised.

2. What can rehabilitation personnel do for hearing problems?

Evaluation for medical and/or surgical approaches to underlying problems should first be undertaken to identify correctable hearing problems. Hearing aids and augmentative hearing devices can be provided by an audiologist and are often used in conjunction with aural rehabilitation techniques. Other professionals who may help treat hearing impairment include educators of the deaf, speech therapists, and occupational therapists.

3. What are the signs and symptoms of hearing problems? How often do they occur?

Although persons with hearing impairment may report their difficulty in hearing, often they may be unaware of their problem. Others may first note a person's poor response to auditory stimuli. In the elderly patient, hearing loss may "masquerade" as dementia. The patient who is unable to hear speech or who has poor speech discrimination may not be able to respond to verbal or other aural stimuli and appear confused or demented. Other symptoms, such as tinnitus, sometimes may be the initial presentation of an underlying hearing problem.

Hearing problems that require some form of assistance affect over 20 million people in the United States, and a minimum of 12 million persons have a hearing loss great enough to handicap them. Over 2 million Americans are either totally deaf or lack sufficient hearing to understand speech.

4. What are the four types of hearing problems?

1. **Conductive hearing loss** occurs in patients with external or middle-ear disorders, such as otitis media, otosclerosis, and perforated eardrum. These patients have a normal inner ear and are hard of hearing because of a defect in the mechanism by which sound is transmitted to the inner ear. These persons can hear perfectly if the sound is amplified sufficiently and so are usually able to use hearing aids.

2. **Sensorineural hearing loss** is due to processes within the inner ear, cochlea, eighth cranial (cochlear) nerve, or brain and is associated with infection, trauma, toxic substance, degenerative disease, or congenital abnormality.

3. **Combined hearing loss** with both conductive and sensorineural components

4. **Central auditory loss** occurs when the brain's hearing center is not properly functioning. Sound of sufficient loudness may reach the center, but understanding is impaired, especially in a noisy environment. Such disorders are the most difficult to diagnose and treat and can be caused by various conditions, including tumors or head injury.

5. How are hearing problems clinically assessed on a rehabilitation service?

Easily administered hearing tests include use of whispered and spoken voice, watch tick, tuning forks, or similar devices. Audiometry screening with a portable pure-tone audiometry device (to test speech frequencies of 250–3,000 Hz) can be done by trained personnel (i.e., audiologist, speech therapist, nurse, occupational therapist, or physician). The 128-cycle tuning fork, commonly used to test vibration sensation, should not be used, as patients often have difficulty differentiating between feeling the vibrations and hearing them. The most useful tuning forks for testing hearing are those with frequencies of 256, 512, or 1,024 Hz. The tuning fork should be stroked between the thumb and index finger, gently tapped on the knuckle, or carefully activated with a rubber reflex hammer. Striking the fork too hard produces overtones as well as too intense a sound.

6. What are compensatory strategies and how are they used?

When a patient has a significant hearing problem, it impairs communication with every team member. The rehab team and hospital staff can "ignore" the hearing problem to minimize inconvenience or use compensatory strategies. Compensatory strategies include hand signs, gestures, written communication, speaking clearly and distinctly at a normal to slow speed in a well-lit environment (so the listener can observe facial expressions), and use of assistive listening devices, such as battery-powered voice amplifiers. A quiet area with a minimum of background noise is recommended. The family should be instructed in these techniques, and may be better able to interpret communicative gestures and non-verbal cues than will the rehabilitation staff.

7. How reliable is a hearing test in an aphasic or neurologically impaired patient?

Very often, an individual can be tested reliably even when neurologically impaired. The ability to detect tones does not require the higher centers of the brain. If the individual can be trained to respond to tones, a valid hearing test can be obtained. If such training cannot be completed, often speech threshold can be obtained with a little creativity, whether it be following instructions such as clapping hands or finishing the words to a familiar song. In a nonresponsive patient, physiologic tests can be utilized, such as brainstem evoked audiometry.

8. What the parts of an audiology evaluation?

Air conduction threshold testing obtains pure-tone thresholds at octaves from 250–8,000 Hz, as well as using speech stimuli in both ears under headphones. A **speech reception threshold** is obtained by presenting two-syllable words, called "spondee words," spoken down to a level where 50% of the words can be heard and repeated. **Speech recognition testing** is completed by presenting monosyllabic words at comfort levels. Generally, a list of 50 monosyllabic words is presented, and the percent correct is obtained for a speech recognition score. In **bone conduction threshold testing**, the bone oscillator is placed on the mastoid, and again pure-tone thresholds are obtained, from 250–4,000 Hz, to determine whether the hearing loss is conductive, sensorineural, or mixed. **Impedance audiometry** may also be performed to assess middle ear function and to check the acoustic reflex.

An audiologist who specializes in identifying, assessing, and providing nonmedical or surgical interventions, holds a masters degree, and is certified by the American Speech-Language-Hearing Association (ASHA), performs the evaluation.

9. Describe the treatment options for various hearing problems.

Treatment interventions for sensorineural and conductive loss may include hearing aids, assistive listening devices, and aural rehabilitation. For the profoundly deaf, cochlear implants are available. The cochlear implant is surgically implanted to stimulate the auditory nerve and provides awareness of sound, although not sound as a "normal" hearing person knows it. Some conductive losses can be helped through medical intervention, depending on the cause of the hearing loss.

A hearing aid generally does not help a purely central hearing loss, as the problem is not one of decreased volume. Aural rehabilitation, using speech-language pathology or audiology services, can be useful as a focusing technique. An assistive listening device can also be useful to improve the signal-to-noise ratio and to focus on the auditory information during therapy sessions.

10. How does a hearing aid work?

A hearing aid is a small electronic instrument that makes sound louder and thus easier to detect and understand. It does not correct a hearing loss, overcome reduced discrimination, or even provide normal hearing the way eyeglasses can provide normal vision, but it can make a tremendous improvement in quality of life. A hearing aid consists of a microphone to pick up the signal, an amplifier to make the sound louder, and a receiver which is a mini-loudspeaker to deliver the sound. It relies on a battery for power.

11. Describe the different types of hearing aids.

A number of different styles and types of hearing aids exist. The different styles vary in size from a **completely-in-the-canal** (CIC) hearing aid, which can barely be seen from the outside, to the **full-concha in-the-ear** hearing aid, probably the most prevalent, to a **behind-the-ear** hearing aid, which fits over the ear and relies on an attached ear mold to direct the sound into the ear. **Body-type** hearing aids also exist but are rarely used, in which the user wears a small box that serves as the hearing aid on the body with a cord or cords that snap into the ear molds.

Bone conduction aids often look like headbands and are used by individuals who cannot place the ear mold or hearing aid in the ear, possibly because of constant drainage or a malformation. Some newer types of hearing aids are programmed by a computer, and the user can select two or three different listening settings depending on the environment. Such **programmable hearing aids** are more expensive, and to achieve optimum success with such a device, an individual must be able to use it properly. It is not for everyone.

12. What is an assistive listening device?

An assistive listening device is any type of equipment or system that helps the hearing-impaired individual communicate more effectively, often in conjunction with or in place of a conventional hearing aid. These devices may be for personal use or part of a large room system. A **personal system** may use a hard wire from a speaker's microphone to the listener's headset or hearing aid or use FM radio waves or infrared light to transmit the sound information. The signal must be picked up by some type of receiver, which may be the telephone switch built into the hearing aid. **Room systems** usually rely on FM, infrared, or an audio loop system (which creates an electric current in a length of wire looped around the room). The signal can be picked up by a receiver obtained from the facility or through use of the telephone switch on the hearing aid, if it has one. Assistive listening devices, especially the personal type, are helpful to those who have difficulty in noisy situations, because only the message sent over the device is amplified and the background noise is not made louder.

More familiar assistive listening devices include closed captioning for television and telephone amplifiers. both of which can be purchased inexpensively. Other devices recommended for the severely or profoundly hearing impaired person include alerting devices such as a light connected to the telephone, doorbell, or fire alarms.

13. What is aural rehabilitation?

Aural rehabilitation is a process that addresses the effect of impaired hearing on the individual and attempts to provide strategies for coping with the communication deficit as well as psychosocial aspects of hearing loss. The most obvious form of aural rehabilitation is the fitting of a **hearing aid** and follow-up to teach the user realistic expectations and proper use of the device. **Auditory training** attempts to teach the hearing-impaired person to use residual hearing to its maximum. One goal is to relearn the sounds of both speech and the environment. Lessons in **speech reading** (lip reading) are another aspect of aural rehabilitation. **Counseling** the hearing-impaired individual, along with his or her family, to understand the degree that a communication deficit can impact upon life is also a part of aural rehabilitation. Thus, aural rehabilitation may involve a number of rehab professionals.

14. How can you tell which type of hearing aid is best for an individual patient?

The degree of hearing loss is important. A severe to profound hearing loss cannot be effectively corrected with a tiny, mini-canal hearing aid. The person's lifestyle, tolerance, and ability to manipulate the hearing aid are all important. A person with a significant hearing loss may be better off with an assistive listening device. Someone whose cognition is impaired would not be a candidate for a complex programmable hearing aid. The individual is being fit, not the hearing loss.

15. Why may some people dislike hearing aids? What barriers exist to use of the aids?

1. The primary reason people reject hearing aids is because they think it makes them seem old or disabled.

2. Hearing aids are *not* usually covered by insurance, and Medicare does not reimburse for the devices. Prices range from $500 to over $2,000 for a programmable instrument.

3. Some elderly patients have difficulty in manipulating the tiny controls and in inserting the aids into the ear canal.

16. When should I refer may patient for an ENT evaluation?

A patient complaining of a unilateral hearing loss, tinnitus, ear pain or drainage, and vertigo or dizziness not associated with other known factors should be referred. Any patient complaining of a hearing problem can be referred to rule out an underlying medical process. A patient with significant cerumen impaction may be an appropriate referral.

17. What types of hearing problems occur in children?

All types of hearing problems occur in children. Conductive hearing loss caused by **otitis media** is the single type seen more in children than in adults.

18. At what age can training begin in hearing-impaired children?

It is important to identify the presence of a hearing impairment in a child of < 2 years of age. If hearing loss is significant, a hearing aid may be prescribed. Additionally, it is necessary to begin sense training very early in life so that the child can learn lip-reading (speech reading) and the early simple vocal sounds. Most specialized schools for the hearing impaired accept children for training before 3 years in order to provide the extra training necessary. These children have educational delay, even with normal or superior intelligence.

19. How can hearing be assessed clinically in neonates and young children?

Clinical testing can be performed in infants, including preterm infants as young as 6 months' gestational age, if medically stable. Absence of a startle reflex can be a clue as to whether an infant hears. Attempts to localize a sound should occur between 8–12 months of gestational age in an infant with normal hearing.

Infants in the pediatric intensive care unit (PICU) or special care nursery (SCN) may have auditory suppression. The excessive noise levels in these areas may actually result in reduced responses to the auditory stimulation they receive. This type of auditory suppression is a normal adaptive response and is temporary. However, this auditory suppression may spuriously reduce the infant's response to behavioral hearing assessments, as the infant learns to "ignore" noise as a protection from overstimulation, and it must be considered with an infant whose response appears to be abnormal within the PICU or SCN settings.

The accuracy of **behavioral hearing assessments** varies in the preterm infant, who may have problems with motor control and weakness that preclude the consistency of the response to sound. It may be necessary to repeat this test on different days to verify the presence or absence of response.

Behavioral testing can be attempted in children as young as 6 months of age. It is performed in a sound-treated room and cannot rule out unilateral hearing loss. With small children, conditioning techniques, in which a sound is associated with a light or toy, have been successful. As the child reaches 2–3 years of age, he or she can frequently be taught "play audiometry"—for example, the child throws a block into a box when hearing a tone. Speech is an effective tool on a hard-to-test child, who at least may localize his or her own name, wave "bye-bye," or identify body parts down to very-low-intensity levels. Although not a complete frequency response, at least some hearing in the speech range can be implied from these responses.

20. How are physiologic hearing tests done?

The best known of the physiologic techniques is **brainstem auditory evoked response audiometry** (BAER), also known as auditory brainstem response or ABR, and brainstem evoked response audiometry (BSER). BAER involves placing an electrode on the child and presenting a stimulus, picked from the computerized system. A specific waveform response is recorded from the brainstem if the stimulus is heard. When the intensity of the stimulus is decreased, the response should show a decrease in amplitude and an increase in latency. A click stimulus or tone pips are utilized to assess higher frequencies. The test requires the infant to be quiet and preferably asleep.

21. What is otoacoustic emission testing?

An otoacoustic emission (OAE) test refers to a quick, noninvasive screening procedure that can identify a properly functioning cochlea if the sound can reach the inner ear. The otoacoustic emission refers to an "echo" from the hair cells of a normally functioning cochlea, which is reflected back through the middle ear where it is picked up by a microphone connected to a microcomputer. This procedure is used in a number of newborn screening programs to detect hearing loss of > 35 dB and holds promise for use in universal screening of newborns. The type of OAEs in such screening are transient evoked otoacoustic emissions.

22. How old should a child be before using a hearing aid or other device?

With accurate physiologic testing now available, infants can be fitted with hearing aids as soon as the hearing loss is verified. A child < 6 months of age can wear a hearing aid with the hopes that speech and language development can begin. A hearing loss of a moderate to severe degree or worse warrants intervention.

23. Besides hearing aids or other devices, what interventions are needed to ensure their safety and allow communication and education for infants or young children with hearing problems?

Early parental intervention and safety: Basic issues are addressed, such as being careful when opening doors which the child may not hear, replacing auditory fire alarms with intense visual alarms with flashing lights, and obtaining deaf signs to warn neighborhood motorists.

Enrichment of visual and tactile sensory environment: Normal toys can be purchased to provide a variety of visual, tactile, and auditory stimulation. Hammers, drums, rattles, and other "musical" toys can encourage participation in an experience of rhythm, vibration, and auditory stimulation for musical enjoyment. Use of talking books, audio tapes, and spoken language are to be encouraged. Toys using sound frequencies that are within the child's unimpaired range should be encouraged.

Basic sign: Parents should learn basic sign and use it with the child from the time the hearing loss is detected.

Protection of the child's remaining hearing: Use of ear plugs for swimming or bathing may be advised. Seeking early medical care for suspected ear infections or "allergies" will help prevent further damage. Physicians should be told of the child's hearing loss before prescription medications are given, so as to avoid inadvertent toxic injury associated with medications.

24. What resources are available for hearing-impaired children and their parents?

As soon as a child or infant is identified with a hearing loss, the best referral is to an audiologist or a school for the deaf. If neither of these is available, the child's school system, local United Way agencies, and social workers may offer further advice. Very often, a school system will have a child-find or parent-infant program that can be helpful.

Parental support groups may educate the parents in the various school options available within a community and about their rights and responsibilities. Parental support groups are also important for preventing child abuse, which occurs more commonly to the handicapped child.

The American Speech-Language-Hearing Association (ASHA) and Self-Help for Hard of Hearing People, Inc. (SHHH) provide information, offer support groups, and serve as advocates on issues of concern for the hearing-impaired.

BIBLIOGRAPHY

1. American Speech-Language-Hearing Association, Ad Hoc Committee on Screening for Impairment, handicap, and Middle Ear Disorders: Audiologic screening. ASHA 36(6–7):53–54, 1994.
2. American Speech-Language-Hearing Association, Committee on Infant Hearing: Guidelines for the audiologic assessment of children from birth through 36 months of age. ASHA 32(50):37–41, 1991.
3. Byrne D: Key issues in hearing aid selection and evaluation. J Am Acad Audiol 3(2):67–80, 1992.
4. Curnock DA: Identifying hearing impairment in infants and young children [editorial]. BMJ 307(6914): 1225–1226, 1993.
5. Ebert DA, Heckerling PS: Communication with deaf patients. JAMA 273:227–229, 1995.
6. National Institutes of Health Consensus Development Conference Statement: Early identification of hearing impairment in infants and young children. Int J Pediatr Ororhinolaryngol 27:215–217, 1993.
7. Popelka GR, Gates GA: Hearing aid evaluation and fitting. Otolaryngol Clin North Am 24:315–428, 1991.
8. Tyler RS, Tye-Murray N, Gantz BJ: Aural rehabilitation. Otolaryngol Clin North Am 24:429–445, 1991.

14. THE AMERICANS WITH DISABILITIES ACT AND OTHER FEDERAL LEGISLATION ON DISABILITIES

Leighton Chan, M.D., *and Mary Richardson*, Ph.D., M.H.A.

1. What legislation has addressed the civil rights of individuals with disabilities?

Unsuccessful attempts were made to include disabled individuals in the Civil Rights Act of 1964, and it was not until the Rehabilitation Act of 1973 that the federal government began to address the issue of discrimination against those with disabilities. More recently, the Americans with Disabilities Act has further expanded the rights of individuals with disabilities.

2. What is the American with Disabilities Act?

The Americans with Disabilities Act (ADA) was signed into law by President George Bush in 1990. Most people are aware that the ADA requires removal of architectural barriers in some facilities; however, the ADA is much more than just building codes and regulations. The ADA takes aim at discrimination and articulates goals for equal opportunity, full participation, independent living, and economic self-sufficiency. It documents that people with disabilities, as a group, occupy an inferior status in our society and are severely disadvantaged socially, vocationally, economically, and educationally. It calls for a "clear and comprehensive national mandate for the elimination of discrimination against individuals with disabilities" and provides enforceable standards for doing so.

Specifically, the ADA is designed to prevent discrimination against those with disabilities in several settings: employment, public services, public accommodations, and telecommunications.

These rights had been partially protected by the Rehabilitation Act of 1973, which prohibited discrimination in programs receiving federal assistance. The ADA extends these rights to cover entities not receiving such funds, so that private concerns, such as businesses and restaurants, must abide by the ADA.

3. How does the ADA define disability?

The ADA defines **disability** as:

(A) a physical or mental impairment that substantially limits one or more of the major life activities of such individual,

(B) a record of such impairment,

(C) being regarded as having such an impairment.

4. Are individuals suffering from drug and alcohol addiction considered disabled by the ADA?

The drug and alcohol provisions of the ADA protects those who are **recovering** alcoholics and **former** drug abusers. The ADA will not protect an alcoholic who is unable to perform his or her job due to alcoholism, nor will it protect current drug abusers.

5. How does the ADA affect the employer and workers with a disability?

The ADA defines an **employer** as anyone engaged in an industry effecting commerce who has 15 or more employees. The ADA prohibits discrimination by the employer against any **qualified individual** with a disability in regard to hiring, promotions, discharge, compensation, training, or other privileges of employment. Qualified individuals are those who, "with or without **reasonable accommodation**, can perform the **essential functions** of the employment position that such persons holds or desires." Reasonable accommodations must be made by the employer unless it poses **undue hardship** on the operation of the business.

The ADA specifically prohibits an employer from using screening methods and selection criteria that do not pertain to the requirements of the job and/or are meant to deny opportunity to the candidate because of his or her disability. The employer must clearly articulate the skill demands of the position and the performance expectations. If a person can meet those demands and expectations with reasonable accommodation by the employer, then he or she must be considered equally with other candidates, regardless of disability.

6. What government agency is charged with administering the ADA?

The **Equal Opportunities Employment Commission** (EOEC) is one of several federal agencies with regulatory responsibility for the ADA. They are in charge of issuing regulations concerning employment and the ADA, and many of these rules are published in the Code of Federal Regulations. In general, however, the Commission has opted for a case-by-case approach to resolving important issues, such as defining what constitutes reasonable accommodation, undue hardship, and the essential functions of employment. Luckily, many of these definitions were resolved during the legal challenges to section 504 of the Rehabilitation Act of 1973, which contained similar wording.

7. What are the Public Service Provisions of the ADA? Must all public transit be accessible?

Title II of the ADA states that "no qualified individual with a disability shall be excluded from participation in, or be denied the benefits of, the services, programs, or activities of a public entity or subjected to discrimination by such entity." **Public entities** are defined as state and local governments and the National Railroad Passenger Corporation.

The title goes on to describe specific requirements for **public transportation**. In general, all public rail systems must have an accessible car within 5 years. Retrofitting existing public buses is not required, but all new vehicles purchased or leased must be accessible, and good faith efforts must be made to acquire accessible used vehicles.

8. What are the Public Accommodations Provisions of the ADA?

Title III of the ADA specifies that "no individual shall be discriminated against on the basis of disability in the full and equal enjoyment of the goods, services, facilities, privileges, or accommodations of any place of public accommodation by any person who owns, leases (or leases to), or operates a place of public accommodation." Places of public accommodation include health care facilities, hotels, restaurants, professional offices, museums, and others. Religious organizations are exempted.

9. Must all private businesses be made accessible to individuals with disabilities?

Title III of the ADA requires that preexisting places of public accommodation remove architectural barriers only if this is readily achievable—i.e., "if this is easily accomplished and able to be carried out without difficulty or expense." Specific accessibility guidelines to be applied during new construction or remodeling are published by the Architectural and Transportation Barriers Compliance Board. Among the basic changes that may be needed for compliance include:

1. Installing ramps
2. Making curb cuts
3. Widening doorways
4. Removing high pile carpets to allow wheelchair accessibility
5. Installing accessible toilets
6. Providing interpreters
7. Installing Braille and large-print signs

Not all accommodations need be elaborate. Many changes, such as adding visual aids for those with hearing disabilities and installing paper cup dispensers at water fountains, are easily achievable and inexpensive.

Compliance with this title of the ADA has been an ongoing issue, particularly in regard to retrofitting existing facilities. In general, large institutions such as universities and corporations, have opted for a collaborative rather than confrontational relationship with local compliance boards. However, compliance by smaller institutions has been hampered by limited avenues of enforcement.

10. Describe the Telecommunications Provisions of the ADA.

Title IV of the ADA encourages the Federal Communications Commission to make telecommunications facilities available for hearing-impaired and speech-impaired individuals. It requires that all federally funded public service announcements on television include closed captioning (subtitles). Title IV also requires that the telecommunications industry create the infrastructure necessary to utilize closed captioning.

11. How is the physiatrist affected by ADA?

The ADA changes the relationship between the government and persons with disabilities. Prior to ADA, many felt the government's role was to fund entitlement payments to those who were unable to work. The ADA, on the other hand, places strong emphasis on what people can do and protecting equal rights. This emphasis dovetails nicely with the primary goals of rehabilitation medicine: using the team approach to maximize function and preserve independence. A physiatrist, then, must know the rights afforded to persons with disabilities by the ADA and make sure the individual and rehabilitation team are well versed in them so that these goals can be achieved.

In regard to the employment provisions of the ADA, a physiatrist and the rehabilitation team may be called upon to help define the strengths and limitations of an individual and to specify any modifications that might be necessary to allow that individual to meet the requirements of a job. Therefore, a physiatrist must be aware of what questions to ask an employer and have a good grasp of assistive technology that might help a patient perform specific job-related tasks. (See also chapters 16 and 84).

12. How do persons with disabilities fund their medical care?

For those who do not have an individual private insurance policy or a group policy through work, the most common way for persons with disabilities to acquire medical insurance is through Medicare and Medicaid. Those injured while working may have their medical bills covered through workers' compensation.

13. What is Medicare?

Medicare was created under the Social Security Act of 1956. It is a federally run program that provides health care coverage to those who have paid a Medicare payroll tax during their working years. In addition, family members of those who qualify may also be covered. In 1994, Medicare provided health care coverage for 36.7 million people.

In general, Medicare benefits begin when one retires and applies for Social Security benefits, but no earlier than age 65. An eligible individual can apply for benefits earlier in life if he or she is disabled or has renal disease.

14. How is Medicare organized?

Medicare coverage is divided into two parts. **Part A** covers the cost of inpatient hospitalization and home health services, as well as stays in skilled nursing facilities and hospices. **Part B** is a voluntary program and requires additional payments by the beneficiary. It covers the services of physicians, outpatient clinic visits, and many ancillary services, such as x-rays and lab tests. Many private insurance companies offer Medicare supplemental coverage for those items not covered in Part A or B.

15. How does Medicare pay for inpatient rehabilitation?

For acute care hospital stays, Medicare pays hospitals under a prospective payment system outlined in the Social Security Amendments of 1983. This system is based on **diagnosis-related groups** (DRGs), in which the hospital gets a fixed amount of money for each patient based on the diagnosis, regardless of how long the patient stays.

Inpatient rehabilitation, on the other hand, is currently exempt from this prospective payment system and is paid under the **Tax Equity and Fiscal Responsibility Act of 1982** (TEFRA). Under this Act, rehabilitation facilities are reimbursed in a fee-for-service manner up to a certain limit for each patient discharged.

16. What is Medicaid?

Authorized under Title XIX of the Social Security Act, Medicaid provides health insurance to many low-income patients as well as some persons who are disabled and medically needy. The Medicaid program is funded jointly by federal and state dollars. The federal government issues broad guidelines to the states, who administer the programs. Regulations concerning eligibility, coverage, and reimbursement vary from state to state. In 1995, Medicaid provided medical assistance to 36 million people.

17. How does a person with a disability qualify for Medicaid?

In general, Medicaid is a **means-tested** program—i.e., if a qualified individual has an income and resources below a certain level, then he or she is eligible for coverage. However, not all poor individuals qualify. For instance, healthy adults without children cannot be covered by Medicaid regardless of their income and resources. Individuals who might qualify include pregnant women, families with children, as well as the aged, blind, medically needy, institutionalized, and disabled. Often these individuals have to "spend down" their resources until they qualify.

To qualify for Medicaid on the basis of **disability**, an individual needs to be receiving **Social Security Insurance** (SSI) payments for that disability. The SSI program requires that the individual must be "unable to engage in any substantial gainful activity by reason of a medically determined physical or mental impairment expected to result in death or that has lasted or can be expected to last for a continuous period of at least 12 months." In addition, these recipients may have to pass a means test.

18. What services are covered under Medicaid?

Medicaid coverage varies widely from state to state. In general, Medicaid requires that states cover the cost of medically oriented services delivered primarily in institutional settings, such as hospitals and nursing homes. Several states, such as Oregon, have Medicaid waivers to design their own package of benefits. Coverage of many items, such as prescription drugs and dental care, is optional, and states are not required to include them in their Medicaid package.

19. If I have a disability, how can I receive income assistance?

Poverty is commonly associated with disability. With costly medical bills and poor earning potential, those with disabilities are economically disadvantaged and can come to rely on public assistance. There are two major federal programs to provide income assistance to individuals with disabilities: Social Security Insurance (SSI) and Social Security Disability Insurance (SSDI).

SSI is linked to the Medicaid system and provides financial assistance to low-income individuals who are aged, blind, or disabled. To qualify on the basis of disability, a person must be "unable to engage in any substantial gainful activity by reason of a medically determined physical or mental impairment expected to result in death or that has lasted or can be expected to last for a continuous period of at least 12 months." (SSI determination for children is different and based on a categorical definition of disability.) In 1987, an estimated 4.4 million individuals received SSI payments, including 1.5 million older Americans and 2.9 million persons who were blind or disabled.

SSDI is similar to SSI but is linked to the Medicare system. Therefore, to get SSDI benefits, one has to have worked and paid into the Social Security System. Applicants for SSDI must meet a definition of disability similar to that for SSI. Physicians assess when a person cannot work or is ready to return to work. Eligibility is reevaluated approximately every 3 years. In 1988, 3 million individuals received $15.9 billion in SSDI payments.

20. If I have a disability, will the state or federal government help me get back to work?

Federal involvement in vocational rehabilitation for persons with disabilities was greatly expanded by the Rehabilitation Act of 1983. Title I of the Act provided federal grants to state vocational rehabilitation agencies and outlined guidelines under which these agencies operate. Currently, Congress is considering numerous changes to the Rehabilitation Act, so consult your local vocational rehabilitation office for up-to-date regulations.

In general, to be eligible for vocational rehabilitation, a person must have a physical or mental impairment that results in a substantial impediment to employment. In addition, it must be determined that they can benefit from vocational rehabilitation services. Since vocational rehabilitation is not an entitlement program, states are not mandated to provide services to all who qualify. In fact, states are required to prioritize services to those with the most severe disabilities including amputees and individuals with paraplegia, quadriplegia, stroke, and other neurologic disorders. Title I requires that each person receiving vocational rehabilitation have an **Individualized Written Rehabilitation Program** (IWRP) to outline the goals and specific services required. The client or his or her representative must review the IWRP and comment on it.

21. If I have a child with a disability, what will the federal and state governments do to protect his or her education?

Federally mandated education for children with disabilities began in the mid 1970s, when several studies revealed only a few states attempted to educate more than half their children with disabilities. In 1975, Congress passed the **Education for All Handicapped Children Act** (EHA). This Act was later incorporated into **Individuals with Disabilities Education Act** (IDEA), and together they have served to define state obligations in regard to education of children with disabilities.

22. Which children are covered under IDEA?

By law, any state that accepts federal funds under IDEA must have a "zero reject" policy and provide assistance to **all who qualify**. In general, all children aged 3–21 years are eligible for educational assistance under IDEA if they meet eligibility criteria. A child must have one of several specific conditions listed in the Act, including mental retardation, deafness, orthopedic impairments, traumatic brain injury, and others. In addition, this health conditions must "adversely affect educational performance" and require special education.

It is important to note that not all children with disabilities require special education. For instance, a child with paraplegia may need some physical accommodations to attend school but will probably do regular course work.

23. What type of education is the state required to provide?

Under IDEA, all qualified children must be provided with a **free appropriate public education** (FAPE), including special education and related services in the **least restrictive setting**. The Act further mandates that "to the maximum extent appropriate, children with disabilities . . . are educated with children who are not disabled." States are obligated to provide the necessary assistive technology and other personnel to achieve these goals.

The intent of IDEA is to promote the mainstreaming of children with disabilities into regular classrooms with the rest of their peers. It is felt that this improves the education of all students, including those without disabilities. Clearly, however, mainstreaming is not appropriate for all individuals, and for some children, a more controlled environment may represent the "least restrictive setting."

The educational goals for children with disabilities, including the educational setting, are set out in an **Individual Education Plan** (IEP), produced by the school district for each qualified child. Educational goals vary depending on the student's capabilities. The goals may be similar to those for nondisabled students, or they may be focused on achieving "self-care skills." In addition, the IEP must have a **"transition services statement"** that helps coordinate the movement of the student from school into the next step, such as independent living or vocational rehabilitation.

24. What is the physiatrist's role in the education of children with disabilities?

While the physiatrist is not directly involved with creating the IEP, they are important in identifying children who might be candidates for educational assistance. In addition, they provide written guidance to the school concerning the educational impact of the disability. Physiatrists are also responsible for coordinating the interdisciplinary team's efforts to outline a student's plan for school health maintenance activities and therapies. Physiatrists can also inform caregivers about the crucial need for the prevention of secondary disabilities, such as joint contractures.

25. How has the federal government helped promote assistive technology?

The Technology-Related Assistance for Individuals with Disabilities Act (Tech Act) was signed into law in 1988 in response to the growing awareness of the role of technology in the field of rehabilitation.

The Act defines assistive technology as a combination of both devices and services. The term **assistive technology device** means "any item, piece of equipment, or product system whether acquired commercially off the shelf, modified, or customized that is used to increase, maintain, or improve the functional capabilities of individuals with disabilities." **Assistive technology services** means "any service that directly assists an individual with a disability in the selection, acquisition, or use of an assistive technology device." These definitions were later amended into the Individuals with Disabilities Education Act in 1990. In addition to providing definitions, The Tech Act also provides funding to the states for research efforts, demonstration projects, educational programs, as well as direct provision of assistive technology to patients.

BIBLIOGRAPHY

1. Julnes R, Brown S: Assistive technology and special education programs: Legal mandates and practice implications. Law Educ Desk Notes 3(4):54, 1993.
2. Melvin D: The desegregation of children with disabilities. DePaul Law Rev 44:603, 1995.
3. Perlman L, Kirk F: Key disability and rehabilitation legislation. J Appl Rehabil Counsel 22(3):25, 1991.
4. Pope A, Tarlov A: Disability in America. Washington, DC, National Academy Press, 1991.
5. Richardson M: The impact of the Americans with Disabilities Act on employment opportunity for people with disabilities. Annu Rev Public Health 15:96, 1994.
6. Rothstein L: Disabilities and the Law. New York, McGraw-Hill, 1992, p 55.

15. PERSONAL ENABLEMENT THROUGH ENVIRONMENTAL MODIFICATIONS

Shoshana Shamberg, O.T.R./L, Steven A. Stiens, M.D., and Aaron Shamberg, M.L.A.

"Rehabilitation is often like surgery from the skin out."

– Stiens, 1994

1. What is the relationship between the physical environment and personhood?

Essentially, behavior is carried out/played out against or through the medium of the physical environment. The human maturation process requires physical interaction with the environment to develop functional mobility and to facilitate physical adaptation. The variety of physical capabilities acquired in this interaction defines our freedom to move about and modify the environment to our personal specifications. These experiences of "mastery" are internalized as self-discovery and development. Our mastery becomes a behavioral pattern that is successful and is acted out in our relationship to the world that surrounds us. It is uniquely human to adapt to the environment and to adapt the environment to our specifications.

2. How does a new injury or illness affect this relationship?

Immediately after a catastrophic illness or injury, the experience of the lived body is radically distorted. The **body image** is altered due to new deficits in perception, sensation, motor performance, and loss of body parts. Environmental perception may be altered due to sensory deficit or neglect. This situation is compounded by the **depersonalization** of hospitalization. The person is separated from the familiar immediate environment of their clothes and personal objects (keys, watch, jewelry) and is confined to a bed, horizontal. The patient's relationship to the environment is determined in the interaction of patient pathophysiology with the institution. Communication as a means to share personal identity and to alter the physical environment frequently dominates the interaction. Patients may be labeled as "problems" due to repeated requests for assistance.

This situation of **person in a new body in the environment** can be compared to that of an infant in a crib testing the environment. This testing and modifying the environment through verbal and physical interaction are crucial for beginning the problem-solving process and eliminating potential barriers to independence. The new relationship must be redeveloped through physical interaction "anew" in the changed body. The patient carries memories, impressions, attitudes, and fantasies about their new physical state into this reality. Early "experiments" of environment interaction in the new state confirm or refute such impressions and color the person's future expectations. The ongoing process of adaptation is an **operant process** that is facilitated by multiple repetitions, spontaneous activities, and a variety of perceptual and physical interactions.

3. What is the role of the rehabilitation team in this process?

The rehabilitation professionals should facilitate the patient's articulation of feelings and memories of satisfaction with past physical "prowess" and experiences with the physical world in the new relationship. Alterations in the patient's immediate and intermediate environment reachieve an ongoing expression of personhood and enable the person to successfully interact with the physical environment. The patient moves toward reachievement of self-feeding, dressing, and use and manipulation of environmental controls (bed, call light, TV, phone). Independent transfers and mobility to and from the bed are achieved as soon as possible.

The goal is for the patient to rediscover a healthy interaction with the environment, which the patient can generalize to the achievement of his or her personal goals for the future. This may require the demonstration of "solutions" offered through technology or environmental design early in the rehabilitation process.

4. What assessment techniques can be used by the interdisciplinary team to target environmental barriers and formulate solutions to maximize functional independence?

The full capabilities of the patient are difficult to predict early in the rehabilitation process. Initial emphasis must be placed on the team's knowledge of the patient's activity before the injury. Such knowledge can be elicited through **retrospective sociobehavioral mapping** (review a typical 1-week period for patient location, activity, and companionship).

The chronology of the rehabilitation process can be understood as a continuum that starts with the design of the person's immediate environment (braces, wheelchair, etc.) and progresses to the intermediate environment (their home). The community and natural environments are emphasized during the latter phases of the process.

Assessment of the home environment can include floor plans, photographic/video depictions, or home visits. The progression to home must include experimentation and interaction with the environment after physically entering it (therapeutic leave of absence, pass, predischarge home visits, community outings). In essence, the goal is to progressively design an environment that enhances personhood and reflects the characteristics and goals of the patient in concert with others living in the home.

5. Describe two transitional environments in current use as part of community rehabilitation units today.

Independent living trial apartment. An environment designed to simulate a patient's home, where he or she may reside for a brief period before actual discharge. The patient's family or other social support may choose to visit or live in this simulated home environment to receive comprehensive training and to practice assistive care. Problem-solving and generalization of skills attained during the inpatient rehabilitation process slow adaptation to the traditional home environment and identification of new foci for rehabilitation intervention.

Simulated community environments provide safe challenges to the patient, while he or she works on refining maximum functional skills. For example, functional skills must be combined in real-world challenges requiring memory and problem-solving as well as mobility.

6. How are the intermediate (residential) environmental needs of a person assessed and met before discharge home?

The rehabilitation team and the patient collaborate to determine present and to anticipate evolving patient capabilities and demands imposed by the change in environment. These solutions for the removal of barriers in the home include environmental modifications, assistive devices, and ADL training in the home environment.

A building contractor and/or designer knowledgeable in accessibility issues, in consultation with the patient and interdisciplinary team, can then determine the structural feasibility of the suggestions, the cost of each recommended modification, and equipment and installation costs. To determine which modifications will be implemented initially and in the future, the patient must prioritize them in terms of immediate requirements to maximize safety, independence, and use of the environment for daily activities, as well as in terms of financial constraints.

Before discharge, the modifications should be phased in to ensure safe and direct access to at least one exterior entrance, a bathroom, and the bedroom. If the patient is able to move and function in the environment, renovations can be phased in until full access is achieved to the areas used by the patient.

Evaluation and documentation should include the following:

1. **Tasks** that the patient must perform for daily activities must be determined and the task requirements defined.

2. Through observation of the patient performing daily activities and moving through the environment, a task analysis of each activity is documented. Focus is on the patient's physical, cognitive, and sensory strengths and deficits affecting functional performance and on any environmental barriers that are creating obstacles or problems.

3. Determine interventions that can easily and immediately be provided, such as ADL training, rearrangement of the environment, and assistive devices.

4. A **home visit** by members of the rehabilitation team, before discharge of the patient, is ideal. Photographic and/or video documentation of this visit is helpful to formulate a solution. Determine which environmental modifications can be implemented immediately and provide information to the patient and the family so that they can find the appropriate professionals to begin construction of accessible features before the patient's discharge to the home environment. A rehabilitation professional who is specially trained as an accessibility and assistive technology consultant can provide comprehensive solutions to create a barrier-free environment. Phasing in construction may be necessary. Assistive devices and environmental modifications must be compatible with the patient's daily functioning in a variety of situations. The need for adaptability, portability, and ease of use must be carefully considered.

5. If necessary and appropriate, caregivers should be provided ADL training to assist the patient in performing daily activities and self-care with the greatest level of independence and safety. The training may be videoed so that this information can be carried over in the home environment.

7. After the patient is relocated at home outside the hospital, what other assessments are needed to help change the immediate environment to meet personal needs?

Once the patient is home and using the environment, further biosocial and functional assessment by an occupational or physical therapist accessibility consultant may be necessary to continue to maximize functional independence in self-care and make caregiving as easy as possible. **Role changes** may result from a disability that prevents the patient from returning to a previous job or to duties in the home. Transitions to this new status can be less stressful if adequate preparation is accomplished through **family scenario mapping** (verbal review of family activities to define tasks by interest and aptitude) and by practice in such areas as kitchen activities, housekeeping, childcare, martial relations, accessing tools and equipment needed for self-care, etc.

8. What are some resources available to plan home modifications?

American Association of Retired Persons, Fulfillment, K St. NW, Washington, DC 20049

Abilities OT Services, Inc—comprehensive functional and environmental assessments, accessibility consultations, and educational programming. 1-410-358-7269

Abledata—database of free information, listing over 17,000 adaptive devices. 1-800-346-2742, 1-301-588-9284 (MD)

Access Board-ATBCB—technical assistance and resource manuals on accessibility guidelines and compliance issues. ADA resources. 1-202-272-5434 (voice), 1-202-272-5449 (TT), 1-800-872-2253

American Occupational Therapy Association (AOTA)—information for employers and consumers concerning ADA and accessibility and the OT ADA Consultant Network. 1-800-SAY-AOTA (members), 1-800-755-8550 (consumers and employers)

Center for Universal Design, North Carolina State University—research publications, seminars, newsletter on accessible design and legislation, and the Housing Design Advisors Network. 1-919-515-3082, 1-919-737-3032 (TDD), 1-800-647-6777

Easter Seals Society. 202-232-2342, 202-462-7379 (Fax)

Housing and Urban Development (HUD). 1-800-795-7915

Institute for Technology Development, Advanced Living Systems Division—research and information on accessible design and products. 1-601-634-0158.

National Association of Home Builders, Research Center—publications on senior housing and accessible products. 1-301-249-0305, 1-800-368-5242

National Easter Seal Society—videos, publications, resource information, and sensitivity training on a variety of disability issues. 1-312-726-6200, 1-312-726-4258 (TDD)

National Organization on Disability (NOD)—publications and newsletter concerning ADA, disability rights, and accessibility; also specializing in accessibility for places of worship. 1-202-732-1139, 1-202-732-5316 (TDD)

Paralyzed Veterans Administration (PVA), Access Information Bulletin—discusses issues in accessible design, construction, and retrofitting. 1-800-424-8200

Trace Research and Development Center, University of Wisconsin—database of products and organizations on computer access for persons with disabilities. 1-608-262-6966

Volunteers for Medical Engineering (VME)—future home resource center for assistive technology and adaptive design. 1-410-666-0086, 1-410-666-9023 (Fax)

9. What areas of the home are considered in a functional home assessment?

In a **functional home assessment**, an occupational therapist follows the sequence of movements the patient would take through the home. The therapist considers such environmental elements as parking, exterior walkways and driveway, steps, exterior lighting, lawn maintenance, security, entrances, doorways, interior hallways, living/dining room layout and type furniture, floor surfaces, switches and environmental controls (heating, lighting, air conditioning, etc.), interior lighting, doorway width, location of telephones, interior stairs and handrails, accessing and use of bathroom (especially toilet and tub/shower), kitchen layout and appliances, storage, laundry facilities, basement access, location of breaker/fuse boxes, need for ECUs (environmental control units) and personal emergency response systems, locations and use of fire extinguisher and smoke alarms, need for intercom system, safety, and security. Accessing closets and dressers is also important.

10. How is accessibility defined in the community environment?

Government legislation has established accessibility guidelines at the federal, state, and local levels. These regulate the type, location, design, and layout of both public and, in some cases, private spaces. Most building design is based on the use of space by an average person and may not meet the needs of individuals with disabilities, tall or short stature, or any other physical or cognitive characteristics that do not fall into society's norm. The **Access Board**, a federal agency responsible for developing these guidelines, has organized numerous task forces, comprised of disability advocates and national experts in the design and construction industry, to develop accessibility guidelines that address construction of all types of environments. The goal is eventually to develop a single set of design and construction guidelines that can be adopted by any state to comply with all previous federal legislation dealing with accessibility of environments for children as well as adults with a variety of abilities and disabilities. Due to separation of church and state, religious organizations are exempt from complying with federal accessibility guidelines.

11. What rights does a tenant with a disability have?

The **Fair Housing Act of 1988** mandates accessibility compliance and civil rights protection in private housing. Persons with disabilities, are provided equal access to housing and a mechanism for filing complaints if their civil rights are violated. According to this law, the resident cannot be denied the opportunity to modify the rented home to meet individual needs for accessibility. However, the cost of the modification is the responsibility of the renter. The landlord may require that the work be done by a professional approved by him, and an escrow account may be established in which the tenant must place funds of the cost of returning the residence to its original state. Modifications that may be easily used by other tenants and do not change the nature of the residence would not be required to be remodified, such as widening doorways, levered handles, grab bar solid blocking, etc. A physician's order stating that these modifications are a medical necessity would enable the tenant to deduct the cost as a medical expense.

Section 504 of the **Rehabilitation Act of 1973** mandates that public housing and housing subsidized with federal funds be accessible and adaptable to meet the needs of tenants with disabilities.

12. What elements should be considered when making an apartment accessible?

Exterior features: Parking spaces should be level and located near an accessible entrance. Each space should be at least 96 inches wide and have an adjacent access aisle at least 60 inches wide. Two accessible parking spaces may share a common access aisle. One no-step entrance may be created by grading the entrance at a height level to the ground level or garage entrance; by constructing a porch lift, outdoor chair lift, or stair glide; or by constructing a ramp. The **ideal grade** on an exterior uncovered ramp is 1:20 (20 inches of ramp length for every inch of height). The **maximum grade** should not exceed 1:12 or 4. If an entrance is 2 feet from ground level, the ideal ramp length is 40 feet. A level platform at the top of the ramp should provide adequate turning radius for a wheelchair to maneuver and turn, and a 24-inch area on the latch side of the door to allow approach.

All door thresholds should be ¼-inch high or less, removed, or beveled. All doorways should be 36 inches wide with at least a 32-inch clearance when the door is open. An alternative to widening existing doorways is to install **swing clear hinges**, which allow the door to open clear of the door frame, thereby increasing the door clearance by approximately 2 inches. Door-closing pressure should be 5 lbs or less. **Automatic door openers** and **keyless locks** create easy access for any resident of the apartment building with limited upper body strength and hand function. Levered door handles or door knob adapters may make it easier to use door hardware.

Interior features: Motion sensitive, photosensitive, or automatically timed lighting along walkways and entrances provides security and visual cueing for safety and direction. Walkways and hallways should be 48 inches wide. Elevator controls must be located at an accessible height from a wheelchair and should have tactile and auditory indicators for each floor. Outlets and switches should be located approximately 18 inches from the floor.

The turn radius in each room of the apartment should allow enough space for a wheelchair to turn and maneuver, usually a minimum of 60 inches in diameter. In tight spaces, such as in a kitchen and bathroom, open areas underneath counter tops and sinks and open shower stalls can be utilized for this turning area.

Multilevel or adjustable sink heights and counter tops provide accessibility from standing and seated positions. Plumbing should be installed toward the back wall with **hot water pipes insulated** to prevent burns. Single-levered faucet handles are most universal. Automatic faucets, hand dryers, wall-mounted electric toothbrushes, and soap/shampoo dispensers may be installed for a person with limited hand function and upper body strength. Toilet height of 17–19 inches allows horizontal transfers from the wheelchair and limits the degree that an adult must bend when getting up and down. However, for a child or short adult this may be too high.

An adequate **grab bar system** provides support throughout the tub and toilet areas and must be located at the height that promotes safe movement and good body mechanics. A **hand-held shower head** on an adjustable-height track can be used for bathing from a seated and standing position. Tub lifts, which lower a person into a tub, can be controlled by hydraulic, battery, or manual mechanisms. A rubberized mat and tub strips provide a non-slip surface. An angled mirror and a side-mounted medicine cabinet can be used from a standing or seated position. Adequate lighting is of the non-glare type, preferably with sconces and multiple bulbs or adjustable intensity. A **ground fault intercept outlet (GFI)** prevents electrocution form the use of electrical appliances near a sink or other source of water. **Contrasting the color of surfaces**, especially background and foreground, enables people with visual or cognitive impairments to see and define surfaces.

In the kitchen, cabinets should allow enough toe space for wheelchair clearance. A U-shaped or L-shaped kitchen design provides efficiency of movement and work. Use a side-by-side refrigerator with adjustable shelves and drawers. A side-swing wall oven installed in an accessible counter top or one with adjustable height should have staggered burners and side- or front-mounted controls to prevent accidental burns when reaching. An angled mirror installed on the back wall allows a seated person to view the contents of pots. A **pull-out shelf** or cutting board installed beneath the oven or near the stove and sink areas provides a stable surface for transferring hot items from the oven as well as a working surface usable from a seated position. All appliances and sinks should have counter space on both sides so that heavy items can be slid from one place to another without excessive lifting. The sink should have a maximum depth of 6 inches. A **long, retractable water hose** on the sink makes cleanup and filling pots on the burners easy if installed nearby. **Task lighting** over work areas affords extra lighting. **Lazy Susans** in the cabinets and the refrigerator allow access to items toward the back of shelves, and easy glide, pull-out shelving creates accessible storage in cabinets while decreasing the need for reaching and bending.

A **fire extinguisher** located at an accessible height and location is very important. A message board or tape recorder can be used for notes and directions on the use of small appliances. Large knobs or buttons on the stove, dishwasher, and microwave controls are helpful, but existing ones often can be adapted. A strip outlet with a single on/off switch for small appliances can be installed toward the front of a lower cabinet under the countertop work surface.

In the living room, seating should be firm and high enough for smooth transfers and movement from sitting to standing. Sturdy arm rests with a good grasping surface provide stability for good body mechanics. An electric-powered, lounge lift chair or a spring-loaded seat lifter can also promote safety and increase independence. Tight, short-loop carpeting, preferably glued to the floor or with a dense, firm, thin pad, allows easier and safer movement. **Environmental control units (ECUs)** enable regulation of thermostats, lighting, stereos, and television from a single location or portable control unit. Intercoms to entrances and other rooms and remote door openers decrease the need to move quickly.

13. What is visitability? Why is this movement important?

Visitability is a design concept for residential households that promotes the creation of communities in which people of all abilities and disabilities especially mobility impairments, can get into the door and use at least one bathroom when visiting neighbors. Key features of visitability include at least one no-step entrance, at least 32-inch clearances on all doorways with $1/2$ inch or less thresholds, and a bathroom door and interior space that is large enough for wheelchair access, especially to the toilet and sink areas. This concept provides a bridge from the intermediate to the surrounding community environment and fosters social interdependence (neighbor role) and relationships that can offer natural supports for persons with disabilities. This concept is being promoted by **Concrete Change**, an organization based in Atlanta and created by Eleanor Smith, a wheelchair user.

14. Give some examples of accessible features for visually impaired persons.

1. **Increased lighting with reduced glare:** Situate lighting to reduce shadows; use shades, sconces, or recessed lighting to diffuse direct lighting; etc.

2. **Contrasting solid color of surfaces:** Defines objects and spaces, especially background and foreground (e.g., contrasting the color between the floor and wall and/or door, toilet seat and floor, etc.).

3. **Tactile indicators:** Raised letters or voice output on controls and signage. Use of large print with high contrast.

4. **Vary textures:** Provide cues for direction, dangerous situations, and boundaries (e.g., different floor textures, simple patterns, etc.)

5. **Illuminated switches** for appliances, lights, etc.

6. **Nonskid, matte-finish floor surfaces:** decrease glare and perceptual distortions.

15. Give some examples of accessible features for hearing impaired persons.

1. Use of **TDDs** for telephone communication, fax machine, and telephone relay systems.

2. Handy access to **paper and writing implement** for communication.

3. **Vibrating devices** such as alarms on clock, smoke alarms, telephone, door bell, baby monitor.

4. **Smoke alarms** and other signals (door bells, telephone, etc.) with visual alerting devices. Access to oral and sign language interpreters when needed.

5. **Amplification devices** to eliminate background noises and increase volume of desired noise.

6. **Furniture arrangement** so that seating is facing and adequate lighting so that the person can use visual cues when speaking.

16. A single woman with mild dementia had to be discharged home. Suggest possible environmental solutions for challenges she may face.

1. Provide environmental cues to address safety, memory, and communication deficits.

2. Personal emergency response system with medication management. Training in the use of the devices and monitor ability to learn.

3. Automatic medication management system that is set up weekly by a homecare nurse.

4. Burglar alarm and posted fire escape plan that has been learned, practiced, and monitored regularly.

5. Smoke alarms that are hot-wired with battery back-up.

6. Emergency lighting in case of power failure.

7. Daily call to monitor ability to care for herself.

8. Meals on wheels and use of microwave with electric hot water pot.

9. Electric range or microwave oven. Avoid use of a gas stove. Automatic turn-off controls to address memory deficits.

10. Post instructions on the step-by-step use of all appliances and their safety issues.

11. Preprogram telephone numbers used most for one-button speed calling.

12. Use of a tape recorder to record daily instructions or for message taking.

13. Provide opportunities for the patient to access as many community resources as needed to maintain her independence, health, and safety and promote socialization—e.g., support groups, religious associations, social service agencies, transportation.

17. Which is the most dangerous room in the house?

The bathroom. Bathroom accidents are one of the leading causes of death and disability in the older population. Shower and tub falls rank as the third leading cause of accidental death in the 50-plus age group. More than half of all accidents could be prevented with some sort of environmental modification.

18. What is aging in place?

According to a 1990 study conducted by the American Association of Retired Persons, 86% of seniors (65 years and older) want to "age in place," i.e., remain in their present homes as long as possible. In 1986, the figure was 78%. This shows an increasing desire for older adults to do whatever is possible to obtain the resources and means to make their homes fit their changing needs as they age or become disabled. One in 10 elderly move against their wishes due to the environmental limitations of their present homes. Most of these people are homeowners who have occupied the home for 20+ years, and 86% of these homes are mortgage-free. Many spouses or family members provide partial or full-time caregiving when needed, rather than choosing a nursing home or specialized senior housing. Environmental modifications, adaptability of the environment, specialized equipment, services, and ADL training can assist in providing seniors and people with disabilities with this goal, maximizing quality of life, autonomy, and health.

BIBLIOGRAPHY

1. EOEC and Department of Justice: Americans with Disabilities Act Handbook. Washington, DC, Government Printing Office, 1991.
2. Freiden L, Cole JA: Independence: The ultimate goal of rehabilitation for spinal cord-injured persons. Am J Occup Ther 39:734–739, 1985.
3. Grandjean E: Fitting the Task to Man: An Ergonomic Approach. London, Taylor & Francis, 1986, pp 263–357.

4. Pedretti LW: Occupational Therapy: Practical Skills for Physical Dysfunction. St. Louis, Mosby, 1985, pp 436–461.
5. Shamberg S: The accessibility consultant: A new role for occupational therapist under the ADA. Occup Ther Pract 4(4):14–23, 1993.
6. Shamberg A, Shamberg S: Re-entry begins at home: Maximizing independence through environmental modifications. Nat Head Inj Found TBI Challenge 2(1):4–8, 1994.
7. Stiens DW, Stiens SA: Environmental modifications and role functions: Redesign of a house for a family with a paraplegic father. J Am Parapleg Soc 16(4):278–279, 1994.
8. Wylde M, Baron-Robbins A, Clark S: Building for a Lifetime: The Design and Construction of Fully Accessible Homes. Newtown, CT, Taunton, 1994.

16. ASSISTIVE TECHNOLOGY

Michael L. Boninger, M.D.

1. Why read this chapter on assistive technology (AT)?

In addition to your insatiable thirst for knowledge, reasons for learning about AT include:

1. You have to sign the AT prescription and want to make sure that the AT service provider follows it.

2. It may help provide better patient care.

3. There were a lot of AT questions on boards last year.

2. What is assistive technology?

The U.S. government defines AT in Public Law 100-407 as: "Any item, piece of equipment or product system whether commercially off the shelf, modified, or customized that is used to increase or improve functional capabilities of individuals with disabilities."

This definition highlights a most important point—that AT is used to improve function. When thinking of examples of AT, images of chrome moly mag wheelchairs with onboard computers and guidance systems may come to mind. A more useful example, however, is eyeglasses. This low-cost, easy-to-use, effective, widely available device increases functional capabilities in individuals with visual impairment.

3. What legislation has impacted the provision of AT?

AT is more widely used, at least in part, because of legislative efforts on behalf of individuals with disabilities. This legislation has specified that **reasonable accommodations** in a **least restrictive environment** be made for all people with disabilities. The following list is a summary of legislation that affects delivery of AT services:

1. *Rehabilitation Act of 1973*: mandated reasonable accommodations in a least restrictive fashion for federally funded employment and higher education.

2. *Education for All Handicapped Children Act of 1975* (PL 94-142): extended the Rehabilitation Act of 1973 to include children aged 5–21.

3. *Handicapped Infants and Toddlers Act* (PL 99-457): extended PL 94-142 to include infants and aged 3–5.

4. *1986 Amendments to Rehabilitation Act of 1973* (PL 99-506): required states to include provisions for AT in vocational rehabilitation, including equal access to electronic office equipment.

5. *Technology-Related Assistance for Individuals with Disabilities Act* (PL 100-407): first legislation specifically related to AT; provided planning and funding for equipment and research to states.

6. *Americans with Disabilities Act (ADA) of 1990* (PL 101-336): civil rights act for disabled, included all citizens, not just federal and state employees, in all of the above acts.

Two additional acts passed since the ADA of 1990 have updated early laws to comply with ADA wording. The end result is legislation that prohibits discrimination based on a loose definition of disability. In order to not discriminate, businesses, schools, and government are required to make reasonable accommodations, such as providing AT (i.e., a standing wheelchair to get into files) or making modifications to structures (curb cuts, entrance ramps).

4. What functions can AT devices replace?

Human function can be broken down into the broad categories of sensing, processing and effecting. Each of these functions can either be augmented by, or substituted for, using AT. Examples of these functions are straightforward, with the exception of processing. If an individual has difficulty remembering to take medication, he or she may be able to augment his or her memory by recording a reminder to take the pill at 12:00 noon in a memory book. If he or she is unable to remember to check the memory book, then an electronic alarm can be programmed to chime with a reminder to take the pill at noon each day. This alarm would replace the function of memory.

5. How are AT devices controlled?

The human operator controls the AT through movement or muscle activation. If a person can move it, AT can use it. The figure shows the points on the body that can be used to control AT. These points range from the ankle to diaphragm to eyes. The effectiveness of each control point is related not only to gross and fine motor control, but also to a person's cognitive and sensory ability.

Movements interact with the AT device by way of switches. These switches or control interfaces can take numerous forms. Simple switches may vary dramatically in size to allow for problems with motor control. Each switch can have multiple positions or can be placed in series with another device, such as a scanner. As other industries drive the technology of control interfaces, individuals with disability will benefit. One prime example of this is voice recognition, which has improved by leaps and bounds due to the demands of industry.

6. Can one controller be used to control a number of devices?

Picture an individual with a C5 spinal cord injury: She controls her wheelchair with a joystick, her computer with a tongue keyboard, and her environmental control unit with a pointer. Having a separate control for each device not only does not make sense, but it is also costly and inefficient. Some integrated controllers are available now, and in working toward the ideal situation of a single control running a number of devices, the International Standards Organization is using a specified M3S port to control all types of AT devices. Additional work is being done on smart controllers that enable a user to drive a wheelchair and use an augmentative communication device at the same time (walking and talking together).

7. Define augmentative and alternative communication (AAC).

AAC is communication that *requires something other than a person's own body*. A ready example is the pencil; a more rehabilitation-relevant example is a communication board. A communication board contains either letters or pictures that can be pointed at in order to communicate. These simple devices should be suggested immediately when an individual is unable to communicate. The literature is replete with cases of individuals who were thought to have very low intelligence until they were provided with a means to communicate.

8. What types of AAC devices are out there?

Basic AAC takes an input from a control interface and, through processing, produces written and/or auditory (spoken) output. Systems differ by the type of interface and amount of processing. Communication boards involve no processing and therefore are very slow. They do, however, have the benefit of being portable, never breaking down, and working in any environment.

If an individual is able to type, communication will be much faster. Methods have been developed to increase the rate of word production, including numeric codes and abbreviations that represent words, word-prediction based on the first letters selected, and symbolic representation of words. These rate-enhancing systems can require considerable cognitive ability, which may be a limiting factor.

9. What is the problem with these AAC devices?

They are slow. Most speech occurs at rates of 150–175 words/minute. Even with rate enhancement, word output with single finger control can be as slow as 3–5 words/minute. This disparity results in speaking individuals dominating conversations and can inhibit full participation by an individual with communication problems. New rules of communication must be learned by everyone.

10. What is an environmental control unit (ECU)?

Many of the objects in an individual's environment are electronically controlled and operated. An ECU is a device that allows an individual with disability to control these items. The most widely used ECU is the TV remote control, although for this to be considered in AT, it must be used by an individual with a disability. ECUs require a control interface (see question 5) which, through house wiring, infrared, ultrasound, or other method, transmits signals that control lights, appliances, phone, and other electrical devices.

11. When should an ECU be "prescribed"?

Simply put—as soon as possible. Early use (in the acute care hospital) of an ECU by a patient with a high spinal cord injury can reduce anxiety, increase motivation for rehabilitation, and free up nursing time. In addition, early use of an ECU may increase the chances of its use at discharge from rehabilitation. In the acute care setting the ECU can control the nurse call, TV, and lights and allows the patient a feeling of control.

Another population to whom the ASAP motto applies is children. Allowing a child with a disability control over his or her environment may help prevent behavioral problems in the future. Geriatric patients at nursing homes have also been shown to benefit from access to an ECU.

12. Can we get a robot to feed her lunch? (Or, what is available to manipulate the environment?)

No, R2D2 has not arrived. However, many of the best aids for manipulating the environment are low-tech, such as reachers and mouth-sticks. Two specific electromechanical devices that are commercially available are feeders and page-turners. Feeders consist of a control switch, a turntable to position foods, and a spoon or scooper. The feeders require the food to be prepared and set-up in a specific way. Page turners allow an individual to read without assistance or a mouth-stick to turn pages. Alternatives such as talking books are another option.

13. What about robots?

Although robotics holds promise for the future, there are very few robots currently in use by individuals with disability. Robotics developed for industry have little application in AT in that they usually do one task repeatedly and are used for their strength, precision, and speed. Also, control systems for robotics are difficult to design because robots often have a number of degrees of freedom, all of which require independent control. To solve this problem, researchers have developed workstations that place all the items to be manipulated (food, phone, toothbrush) in specified locations with respect to the robot arm. Unfortunately, this requires the user to perform all the associated tasks in a restricted environment and may prevent social interaction. Current research is focusing on wheelchair-mounted robot arms and robots that can sense the position of the object to be manipulated.

14. Besides glasses and hearing aids, what other sensory aids are available?

A considerable number of devices are available that provide alternative sensation through technology. One such device takes visual information detected by a camera and translates this spatial data into vibrating pins. As the scanner sees an "E," an array of vibrating pins provides tactile stimulation in the shape of an "E." The user must recognize the shape as an "E" and incorporate this information into a word as it is scanned. Pictures can also be scanned with this device.

An alternative device uses a video camera to scan a typed page and then, through optical character recognition, translates this material into either braille or auditory output. This translation can generally be done with a standard personal computer.

Electronic travel aids act as an alternative to vision by sensing, through lasers or ultrasound, any obstructions in a path. They have advantages over a cane in that they can detect objects that are farther away, but, unlike a cane, they do not provide proprioceptive feedback through tactile input. These devices can be mounted to wheelchairs.

Each of the devices listed has a number of different forms with advantages and disadvantages. The physician, who may not be knowledgeable about the technical aspects of these devices, works as part of a multidisciplinary team to prescribe and deliver the best AT available.

15. Discuss the elements of the "letter of medical necessity."

An unfortunate fact of life in medicine is financing. This issue is even more troublesome when dealing with ATs, especially in individuals with limited insurance. The letter of medical necessity should include:

Diagnoses—ICD-9-CM code(s) (you should have these memorized by your PGY-2 year)

Functional limitation—balance disorder, hemiparesis, weakness, pain

Patient status—"Due to the patient's functional limitation, he or she is unable to . . . [perform activities of daily living, communicate verbally, perform work activities, etc.].''

Use of equipment—"The use of equipment will . . . [allow the patient to function independently, return home, give independent wheelchair mobility in the home and community, etc.].''

Description of equipment
   Wheelchair—electric, manual, one-arm drive
   Wheelchair frame—lightweight, reclining
   Wheelchair accessories—armrest, casters, axle
   Other—bathing aids, communication aids, back support

Rationale—goal and benefits to patient
   Safety, safe positioning for activity
   Cost-effectiveness in prevention of secondary complications
   Access to workplace or school
   Past experience, interventions, and results

Duration–of expected use

16. Is a prescription and letter of medical necessity the only way a patient can get an AT device?

Fortunately, no. There are other funding sources that do not require a prescription, such as vocational rehabilitation offices. In addition, many individuals purchase their ATs independently, either because insurance will not help or because they would rather have final control of their purchase.

BIBLIOGRAPHY

 1. Cook AM, Hussey SM: Assistive Technologies: Principles and Practice. St. Louis, Mosby-Year Book, 1995.
 2. Cooper RA: Intelligent control of power wheelchairs. IEEE Eng Med Biol 14:423–431, 1995.
 3. Cooper RA: Rehabilitation Engineering Applied to Mobility and Manipulation. London, Institute of Physics Publishing, 1995.
 4. Efthimiou J, Gordon WA, Sell GH, et al: Electronic assistive devices: Their impact on the quality of life of high level quadriplegic persons. Arch Phys Med Rehabil 62:131–134, 1981.
 5. Foulds R: Rehabilitation Robotics. In Proceedings of the Innovations in Rehabilitation Engineering Workshop. Baltimore, MD, 1994, p 40.
 6. Hobson D, Trefler E: Fundamentals of rehabilitation engineering [course notes]. Pittsburgh, School of Health and Rehabilitation Sciences, University of Pittsburgh 1994 [Unpublished].
 7. Jones RD, Hooper RH, Armstrong DI, et al: Microprocessor-based multi-patient environmental-control system for a spinal injuries unit. Med Biol Eng Comput 18:607–616, 1980.
 8. Mann WC: Use of environmental control devices by elderly nursing home patients. Assist Technol 4:60–65, 1992.
 9. Miller GA: Language and Speech. San Francisco, W. H. Freeman, 1981.
10. Schwartzberg JG, Kakavas VK: Guidelines for the Use of Assistive Technology: Evaluation, Referral, Prescription. Chicago, American Medical Association, Department of Geriatric Health, 1994.
11. Van Woerden JA: M3S: A general purpose interface for the rehabilitation environment. In Proceedings of the Second European Conference for the Advancement of Rehabilitation Technology. Stockholm, Sweden, 1993, p 22.1.

III. Rehabilitation Assessments

17. THE PHYSIATRIC ASSESSMENT

Marvin M. Brooke, M.D.

1. Who consults the physiatrist to issue an assessment? What drives the decision?

Requests for consultation are worded differently by referring physicians, social workers, or therapists, depending on their experience: "Please, transfer to rehab," "Mobilize and move out!," "I can't do anything else for her," "Is he disabled?," "I've tried X, Y, or Z, what next?"

It is more helpful if the request includes the originating service's assessment of the problem and a specific question. Consults often recognize only a fraction of the patient's impairment, disability, and handicap spectrum, and they often occur late in the treatment course.

2. What are the objectives for a comprehensive physiatric consultation?

1. Establish the diagnosis and relate it to functional performance.
2. Provide a functional prognosis.
3. Quantify a functional level.
4. Develop a rehabilitation problem list.
5. Formulate a short, intermediate, and long-term rehabilitation plan.
6. Orchestrate the consultations and interventions through the interdisciplinary process to achieve scheduled goals.
7. Translate the plan and intervention for the originators of the physiatric consultation.
8. Answer the question of the initial consultation and then inform of the proposal for comprehensive rehabilitation intervention.
9. With the approval of the attending physician, explain the intervention plan to the patient and family (interdisciplinary family conference), emphasizing their participation in the process.

3. Does the way the physiatrist carries out the history, physical, and assessment impact the rehabilitation patient's emotional adjustment and participation in the rehabilitation plan?

Individuals with the new onset of a significant disability usually are, consciously or subconsciously, facing immediate profound threats to their definition of self and personal goals. The fears may include death, pain, loss of power and control over the simplest mobility, self-care, and independence, and embarrassment due to skin, bladder, and sexual changes. Severe disability, without effective adaptation, may increase the risk for loss of marriage, family, friends, home, social organizations, job, and economic control. They may fear the recurrence of previous psychological problems, an inability to cope with stress, or an inability to make the behavioral and "motivational" changes necessary for rehabilitation.

The individual's relationship with his or her physician can be very constructive and supportive if it communicates a solution based on thorough, honest, and clearly organized information gathering. Individuals in crisis need accurate, honest, understandable, and prioritized information. They also need clear agreement on the goals, obstacles, and resources available as they work through the crisis. This makes it much more likely that the individual will agree with the team on a plan of action and work toward the goals. The value of accurate information and leadership in a crisis is often underestimated in rehabilitation as in other areas.

4. How do the differences between PM&R and the other traditional medical specialties impact the physiatric evaluation and examination?

PM&R utilizes an educational model that teaches the patient about his or her illness and how to remain independent. It goes beyond the traditional medical model in which the physician prescribes treatment to be done for, or to, the patient.

The physiatrist needs to carry out the evaluation in a manner that gathers the information necessary to teach a patient about his or her illness and rehabilitation, and with a method that demonstrates an organized and effective response based on accurate information. PM&R is focused more than any other specialty on the function of the individual in all roles in society, so the physiatric history and physical will include specific questions about, and often demonstration by the patient of, functional abilities. Certain aspects of the history, physical, and functional evaluation are emphasized because of their importance to function and the rehabilitation process. These usually include functions of mobility, self-care, bladder, skin care, sexual impairment, social function including architectural accessibility, educational and vocational areas, and cognitive and psychological function.

5. How is a physiatric history organized to produce a rehabilitation database?

The general outline of the history should be modified depending on the setting and purpose. The goals of the history are to derive pertinent medical information (risk factors, rate of progression, symptoms of other illness and complications), to assess the patient's personal response to illness (experience or anticipation of limitation) and to begin an open dialogue that engages the patient in goal-setting with the rehabilitation team.

1. Patient profile: age, social role, occupation, future plans
2. Chief complaint: functional effects perceived as most significant barriers
3. History of present illness
4. Functional history: previous activity, functional capacity, current function
5. Past medical history: past and current diagnoses, future risks
6. Review of systems
7. Family history: medical and functional capacity for patient assistance
8. Architectural setting, accessibility of home, work, and community

6. What are the objectives of the physiatric physical examination?

- Screen for new illnesses that could affect functional performance or rehabilitation participation
- Identify "regions of risk" for deterioration (skin, bladder, bowel, contractures)
- Identify and quantify secondary impairments (provides a baseline)
- Identify limitation in task performance (disability) specifically pertinent to short-term goals (i.e., transfers, gait)
- Demonstrate the patient's capabilities to him or herself and family

7. How is range of motion measured?

The anatomic position of all joints is defined with 0° as the starting point. Passive range of motion (PROM) is passive movement done by the examiner. If the patient performs it actively without assistance, it is called active range of motion (AROM). If the patient actively moves and the examiner assists to gain more range of motion, it is called active assistive range of motion (AAROM).

A goniometer is used with a hinge at the functional center of joint motion, one arm pointed at 0° in normal anatomic position and the other arm aligned along the bone of the extremity moving. Usually, the measurement of range of motion is recorded with the distal extremity being measured starting from the anatomic position as 0° and the end point of the range being the degrees moved away from zero. Raising one's arm straight overhead toward the sky would be 180° of shoulder abduction, and lifting your forefoot off the floor while your heal stays on the floor gives 20° of ankle dorsiflexion from the neutral, anatomic position.

8. How is hip range of motion measured?

Flexion contractures are common and can be hidden by lumbar lordosis. The **Thomas test** requires the patient to lie supine on a flat firm surface. The hip opposite the side to be measured is flexed maximally to the chest which flattens the lumbar lordosis. The **Kottke method** of measurement puts the hinge of the goniometer just superior to the trochanter, with one arm parallel to the maximally extended femur and the other aligned perpendicular to a line drawn from the anterior iliac spine to the posterior iliac spine.

9. Which common contractures occur and why?

Contractures commonly occur because patients are positioned in positions of comfort, decreasing stress on painful joints, with muscles that cross multiple joints shortened, and without stretching powerful muscle groups. The muscles that cross multiple joints include the hamstrings, rectus femoris, and finger flexors. The common bed position of comfort, which is unfortunately bad for range of motion, includes hips flexed and externally rotated, knees flexed, ankles plantarflexed, and upper extremities flexed and internally rotated.

10. How is muscle strength graded on the manual muscle test?

The patient's strength is tested manually. Values are compared to those of the opposite side, the examiner's strength, and the examiner's impression of normal strength for age and sex. The common grading scale of the manual muscle test is as follows:

0   No palpable or visible movement
1   Trace movement
2   Full ROM with gravity eliminated
3   Full ROM against gravity
4   Full ROM taking some resistance but not normal strength
5   Full ROM and normal strength for age and sex

Manual muscle testing was originally designed to follow patients with lower motor neuron and muscle diseases and represents an ordinal scale. Grades 4 and 5 are subjectively differentiated. Muscles that are able to take substantial resistance should be tested in mid-length using the "make and break" technique. In inter-rater reliability studies, physicians agreed to exact grades in 60% and to within one grade in 91% of muscles tested. Currently, the **handheld myometer** offers a portable continuous measure of torque generation by various groups that has high reliability.

BIBLIOGRAPHY

1. Guides to the Evaluation of Permanent Impairment, 4th ed. Chicago, American Medical Association, 1993.

18. NEUROLOGIC EVALUATION OF THE REHABILITATION PATIENT

Rajiv R. Ratan, M.D., Ph.D.

1. Summarize the major parts of the neurologic examination.

Mental status
Cranial nerves
Motor function—tone, power, adventitial movements, reflexes
Sensory function—pain, temperature, vibration, proprioception, stereognosis, two-point discrimination
Cerebellar function
Gait

MENTAL STATUS AND COGNITIVE FUNCTION

2. What should bedside cognitive or mental status testing include?

Standard mental status testing is extensive, making it difficult for physicians to remember. In an attempt to encourage easier use of the examination, the mnemonic **COMO ESTAS**, the Spanish phrase for "How are you?," can be used to denote the components of the examination:

C = Cognitive functions; i.e., calculation, concentration, insight, judgment
O = Overview; i.e., appearance, attitude, level of consciousness, movements
M = Memory; i.e., recent and remote
O = Orientation; i.e., to person, place, and time

E = Emotion; i.e., affect and mood
S = Speech; i.e., fluency, form, comprehension
T = Thought; i.e., process, content, perceptual disturbances
A = Attention; i.e., abstract thinking, recall, intelligence
S = Something else that the practitioner has forgotten that might be important for the patient

3. What are often the earliest unequivocal symptoms of metabolic or toxic encephalopathy?

Metabolic encephalopathies are among the most common causes of changes in mental status. Etiologies include recreational or prescribed drug intoxication, electrolyte imbalance, hypoxia, and liver disease. **Attention** and **cognition** are the most sensitive indicators of metabolic encephalopathy but are difficult to evaluate if the examiner does not know the premorbid personality or intellect. Under such circumstances, defects in **orientation** and **grasp of test situation** are the most sensitive indicators of brain dysfunction.

Specific questions to be asked include: What time is it? What day is it? How long does it take to reach home from the grocery store (or other well-defined place familiar to the patient)? Disorientation to person and place but not time is rarely observed in structural disease and can be a sign of nonorganic illness or hysteria.

4. Define dementia. What is required for its diagnosis?

Dementia is a clinical state characterized by a significant loss of function in multiple cognitive domains that is not due to an impaired level of arousal. Dementia does not necessarily indicate any specific etiology. Thus, its diagnosis is not synonymous with a progressive course, and it does not imply irreversibility.

The diagnosis requires serial examinations over time that document a decline in intellectual function or a single evaluation of cognitive function with evidence of a higher level of intellectual function in the past. Delirium, psychiatric problems, and focal CNS abnormalities such as stroke must be excluded. An altered level of consciousness is incompatible with an initial diagnosis of dementia. Once dementia is clinically suspected, a work-up must be done to ascertain its etiology.

5. How can aphasia be distinguished from dysarthria?

Aphasia is a disorder of language; dysarthria is a disorder of articulation. In dysarthria, naming, fluency, repetition, and comprehension are normal. Additionally, the patient can read and write with no errors.

6. What should a bedside evaluation for aphasia include? What abnormalities are seen in the major syndromes of aphasia?

1. **Anomia**—A cardinal feature of many aphasic syndromes. Naming of common objects, such as a pen or watch, is a good initial test of aphasia.

2. **Fluent or nonfluent**—Fluency refers to normal speech rhythm and output. Circumlocutions, use of empty word and incorrect words (e.g., "coon" for car), and syntactical errors can be associated with fluent speech. In nonfluent aphasias, speech is constipated and generated

only with a great deal of effort. Nonfluent aphasias are generally associated with cerebral damage anterior to the Rolandic fissure (motor cortex), while fluent aphasias are believed to be posterior to this anatomic structure (sensory cortex).

   3. **Comprehension**—Ask the patient to point at the door, window, or electric light. Ask two- or three-step commands, such as: "Take your right hand, touch your nose, and stick out your tongue."

   4. **Repetition**—Ask the patient to say: "No ifs, no ands, no buts" or "Around the rugged rock, the rugged rascal ran."

7. Name some types of aphasias.

Broca's—abnormal naming, nonfluent, normal comprehension, abnormal repetition
Wernicke's—abnormal naming, fluent, abnormal comprehension, abnormal repetition
Global—abnormal naming, nonfluent, abnormal comprehension, abnormal repetition
Conduction—abnormal or normal naming, fluent, normal comprehension, abnormal repetition
Anomic—abnormal naming, fluent, normal comprehension, normal repetition

8. Does severity of aphasia correlate with efficiency of communication?

   While the severity of aphasia correlates significantly with communication difficulty, other factors need to be considered in maximizing communication skills of the aphasic patient. Information about impairment and training in compensation should be given to the spouse and family as well as the patient. Evaluation of aphasic patients should include a neuropsychological assessment to differentiate aphasia from apraxia, visuoconstructive difficulties, and neglect.

9. Define unilateral neglect.

   Unilateral neglect is defined as *a lack of orienting responses to stimuli presented unilaterally*. Neglect cannot be diagnosed unless the primary sensory or motor modalities required to sense or orient the particular stimulus are intact. Neglect can be unimodal (i.e., visual neglect) or multimodal (i.e., performing complex tasks, such as dressing, when the patient fails to cover the neglected side). Hemineglect is most commonly associated with right hemisphere strokes but can be seen with strokes or with tumors affecting either hemisphere. Neglect is prognostic of poor functional recovery.

10. After excluding visual field defects and disorders of eye movements, how does one evaluate neglect at the bedside?

   1. Line bisection—Have the patient mark the center of 5 horizontal lines, each presented separately on a sheet of paper.

   2. Line cancellation—Present the patient with a single sheet of paper on which 20 lines in varying orientation are drawn on each half of the page.

   3. Letter cancellation—Instruct the patient to mark all the *A*'s on a sheet of paper. There should be 8 *A*'s on the sheet, 4 on each side, with 70 distractor letters (e.g., D, L, F, R).

   4. Clock construction—Have the patient place numbers as they would appear on a clockface within an outline circle on a piece of paper.

   With the above tests, performance on the left side can be compared with performance on the right side.

CRANIAL NERVE EVALUATION

11. How should one evaluate the integrity of a patient's visual fields?

   Stand about 3 feet in front of the patient, and ask him or her to view your nose. Hold your hands to either side of your face, midway between your eyes and the patient's. Briefly present 1 or 2 fingers from each hand, and ask the patient to indicate the number of fingers on each hand. Give the patient one or two trials the make sure the nature of the trial is understood. The hands should be moved so that all four quadrants of the visual field are tested. These tests will enable detection of a field defect or neglect.

During testing, encourage the patient to maintain fixation of your nose. If the patient is cooperative, bedside confrontation of the visual fields can provide diagnostic information. In the uncooperative, dysphasic, or lethargic patient, visual threat may cause an asymmetric blink response if there is a field deficit or neglect.

12. What do defects in the separate visual fields indicate?

Deficits confined to one eye are usually caused by disease of the globe, retina, or optic nerve. Deficits in both eyes (binocular) can be nasal (the half of the visual field of each eye toward the nose) or temporal (the half of the visual field of each eye toward the temple). Bitemporal deficits imply impairment of fibers crossing the optic chiasm (e.g., from pituitary tumor) or homonymous (i.e., the same field of vision for both eyes), indicating disease of the optic tract, radiation, or cortex. Temporal lobe (inferior) lesions usually result in superior homonymous field defects, whereas parietal lobe (superior) lesions usually produce lower homonymous field defects.

13. How do you distinguish a field defect due to malingering or hysteria from an organic field defect?

In nonorganic field loss, the most frequently encountered defect remains the same size regardless of distance from the eye and is often described as tunnel vision. In organic field loss, the size of the intact field increases as the distance from the eye increases.

14. What is the first question to ask a patient who complains of diplopia (double vision)?

"Does the diplopia go away when you cover one eye?" Monocular diplopia (double vision that persists with only one eye viewing) is usually due to a problem of the lens or cornea. Binocular diplopia (double vision that disappears with only one eye viewing) is usually due to a paralysis of extraocular muscles.

15. How does one evaluate the seventh cranial nerve?

Paying particular attention to the nasolabial folds and palpebral fissures, look for facial asymmetry at rest and during spontaneous facial movements. Then systematically test the frontalis muscle ("raise your eyebrows"), orbicularis oculi ("Close your eyelids and don't let me open them"), buccinator ("Blow out your cheeks"), elevators of the lips ("Show me your teeth, smile"), orbicularis oris ("Purse your lips and don't let me open them").

Upper motor lesions generally cause lower facial weakness, with slight asymmetry of the palpebral fissures and little or no weakness of the orbicularis oculi. Lower motor neuron lesions result in weakness of the upper and lower parts of the face and can involve taste (chorda tympani) and tearing (greater superficial petrosal nerve).

16. Define the different types of dysphagia.

Dysphagia can be due to mechanical factors or neurologic dysfunction. Each of these types of dysphagia can be oropharyngeal or esophageal.

17. Name some common neurologic causes of oropharyngeal dysphagia.

Stroke	Syringobulbia
Brainstem tumor	Myasthenia gravis
Motor neuron disease	Myopathies
Demyelinating disease (multiple sclerosis)	Parkinson's disease

MOTOR FUNCTION

18. Define spasticity and rigidity.

Spasticity is the increased resistance appreciated by the examiner when he or she moves a joint briskly. This hypertonicity is sometimes called **clasp-knife** spasticity because, like a pocket knife blade, the initial resistance fades away as the joint is flexed.

Rigidity is defined as increased resistance appreciated by the examiner throughout the range of joint movement. It is like bending a lead pipe and thus is referred to as **lead pipe** rigidity.

19. Name some diseases commonly associated with spasticity.

Diseases that involve damage to the corticospinal tracts (upper motor neurons), such as stroke, brain tumors, multiple sclerosis, traumatic brain and spinal cord injury, cerebral palsy, and cervical spondylosis.

20. What diseases are commonly associated with rigidity?

Diseases that involve damage or dysfunction of the extrapyramidal system (basal ganglia), such as idiopathic Parkinson's disease or drug-induced parkinsonism (e.g., metoclopramide, haloperidol, reserpine).

21. What historical features suggest proximal muscle weakness?

Legs
  Inability to get up from a chair or toilet without using one's hands
  Inability to get out of a car
Arms
  Inability to comb's one hair or brush one's teeth
  Inability to carry grocery bags or young children

22. What are the clinical features of a myopathy?

Nearly symmetric proximal muscle weakness without muscle wasting, with normal sensory examination, and with intact or slightly decreased reflexes.

23. List some of the common causes of myopathy in the rehabilitation setting.

Steroids	Duchenne's muscular dystrophy
Alcohol	Polymyositis
Zidovudine (AZT)	AIDS
Hypothyroidism	Mitochondrial diseases

24. What is the critical clinical difference between myopathies and disorders of the neuromuscular junction (e.g., myasthenia gravis)?

While the distribution of weakness is similar in these disorders, neuromuscular junction diseases are characterized by **fatigability**. They worsen with use and recover with rest.

25. What historical features suggest distal weakness?

Arms—Inability to button, open jars, or hold onto things
Legs—Frequent tripping or unusual wear on the toes of the shoes

26. What are the clinical features of peripheral neuropathies?

Distal weakness which may be asymmetric or symmetric, with atrophy, possible fasciculations, sensory loss, and absent reflexes.

27. Name some of the common causes of peripheral neuropathy.

The causes can be classified by mnemonic **DANG THE RAPIST**:

D = **D**iabetes	**R** = **R**heumatic (collagen vascular)
A = **A**lcohol	**A** = **A**myloid
N = **N**utritional	**P** = **P**araneoplastic
G = **G**uillain-Barré	**I** = **I**nfections
T = **T**rauma	**S** = **S**ystemic diseases
H = **H**ereditary	**T** = **T**umors
E = **E**nvironmental toxins	

28. How can peripheral neuropathies be distinguished from spinal cord lesions?

Spinal cord lesions usually cause weakness that is distal more than proximal. They are characterized by a sensory level below which there is a decrease in sensation, distal symmetric weakness, hyperreflexia, and bowel and bladder problems. Peripheral neuropathies can have glove-and-stocking sensory loss, dermatomal sensory loss, or sensory loss in the distribution of a single nerve. They are also characterized by loss of reflexes rather than hyperreflexia. Finally, some types of neuropathies involve the bladder or bowel. However, peripheral neuropathies cause bladder disorders of emptying, while spinal cord lesions usually cause bladder disorders of storage.

29. What pattern of weakness is commonly seen after a hemispheric stroke?

Hemispheric strokes involving the internal capsule (subcortical) or cortical motor strip result in hemiparesis of the contralateral limb. The pattern of weakness is typically extensors greater than flexors in both the upper and lower extremity. In subcortical strokes, the face, arm, and leg are affected equally, whereas in cortical strokes, the face, arm, and leg are affected unequally.

30. Describe one grading system for reflexes.

0   Absent reflex
1   Hypoactive reflex, or normal reflex that can only be elicited with reinforcement
2   Normal reflex
3   Hyperactive reflex. A clear indicator is elicitation of other reflex responses when testing one reflex. For example, if testing the biceps, and the brachioradialis and finger flexors are also elicited, this suggests hyperreflexia.
4   Clonus

31. What can you do if you get no response when eliciting a reflex?

Make sure to strike the blow crisply, change the tension on the muscle, vary compression of the tendon with your finger, or try reinforcement. Reinforcement can be done by having the patient perform a strong voluntary contraction of a muscle you are not testing. For example, have the patient bite down to facilitate elicitation of the biceps reflex.

32. How is clonus at the ankle elicited?

Quick dorsiflexion of the foot followed by continuous light pressure against the ball of the foot. The continuous light pressure opposes the reflex plantar flexion elicited by quick dorsiflexion.

33. What does the presence of clonus indicate?

Hyperreflexia due to an upper motor neuron lesion. Nonsustained clonus can also be elicited in patients who are anxious.

34. What happens to the abdominal and cremasteric reflexes in a cervical spinal cord lesion?

They are usually absent. When testing this reflex, remember that the abdomen should be relaxed. The abdominal reflex response is difficult to obtain if the muscles are too tense.

35. What is the Babinski sign?

The Babinski sign is dorsiflexion of the great toe in response to a plantar stimulus. It indicates an interruption of upper motor neuron tracts to the lumbosacral reflex centers as seen in diseases such as spinal cord injury, stroke, and multiple sclerosis.

SENSORY EXAMINATION

36. Define the primary and secondary sensory modalities.

Primary sensory modalities include pain sensation, temperature sensation, light touch, proprioception, and vibration sense. Primary sensory loss can be due to a lesion in the periphery, spinal cord, brainstem, or thalamus. Stereognosia (form sense, as in identifying a nickel or penny placed in the hand) and topognosia (ability to localize skin stimuli) are **secondary sensory** or cortical sensory modalities. Cortical sensory abnormalities can be diagnosed only when primary modalities are intact and are referable to lesions in the contralateral parietal cortex.

37. What is the proper way to test pain sensation?
With a clean safety pin. The advantage of the safety pin is that it has a blunt and a sharp end, thus allowing the reliability of the patient to be tested. The pin should be disposed of after the examination.

38. What is the proper way to test position sense?
Position sense should be tested in the hands or feet. The distal end of the third or fourth digit or toe should be used, as these have the least cortical innervation and are thus most sensitive to a loss in position sense. The digit should be grasped laterally and moved up or down or maintained in the neutral position. It is helpful to perform the test a few times with the patient's eyes open to be sure communication is established. With the eyes closed, the patient should make no mistakes on five trials. If abnormalities are found in one digit or two, other digits or toes should be tested.

39. What frequency tuning fork should be used for vibration testing?
256 cps

40. How is the Romberg test performed? What does a positive Romberg signify?
The Romberg test examines the integrity of the dorsal columns. It is *not* a test of cerebellar function. The proper procedure for the Romberg test is to ask the patient to stand with his or her heels together. With the patient's *eyes open*, note whether he or she sways. Then have the patient close his or her eyes. If the swaying is dramatically worse and the patient almost falls, the Romberg is considered "positive," and a dorsal column or proprioceptive defect is suggested. Patients normally sway slightly with the eyes closed, but never fall. Patients with cerebellar disease usually sway more with the eyes open as well as closed. In the Romberg test, the visual information for balance is being removed (by having the patient close his/her eyes), thus placing the responsibility for balance solely on the proprioceptive system.

41. Name the anatomic landmarks that mark different dermatomes.

C2—angle of the jaw	T10—umbilicus
C6—thumb	L4—knee cap
C7—middle finger (third digit)	L5—big toe
C8—little finger (fifth digit)	S1—lateral foot
T4—Nipple	S4, 5—perianal area

CEREBELLAR TESTING

42. What are the clinical features of cerebellar disease?
The main features of cerebellar dysfunction can be remembered by the mnemonic **HANDS Tremor**:

H = **H**ypotonia
A = **A**synergy (lack of coordination)
N = **N**ystagmus (ocular oscillation)
D = **D**ysarthria (speech abnormalities)
S = **S**tation and gait (ataxia)

Tremor = Coarse intention tremor

43. How can cerebellar ataxia be distinguished from a sensory ataxia?

Cerebellar Ataxia	Sensory Ataxia
Nystagmus	Loss of vibration and position sense
Hypotonia	Hypotonia
Coarse intention tremor	Loss of reflexes
Dysarthria	Ataxia worse with eyes closed (positive Romberg)

44. What is the best way to describe someone with cerebellar dysfunction?
They look drunk.

45. What is the typical stance of someone with cerebellar dysfunction?
A broad-based gait.

46. How can gait coordination be tested?
Have the patient tandem walk. Ask him or her to step along a straight line, placing the heel of one foot directly in front of the toe of the other foot.

47. How can coordination of the arms be tested?
Have the patient perform a finger-to-chin test. The patient is instructed to touch the examiner's finger, then touch his or her own chin. This sequence is repeated several times with the examiner altering the position of his or her finger with each trial. The chin is used instead of the nose because many patients with cerebellar dysfunction have such poor coordination that they are in danger of poking their own eye. If the patient undershoots or overshoots the examiner's fingers, the test is considered indicative of cerebellar dysfunction.

48. What is the heel-to-shin test?
This is another test of leg ataxia. With the patient lying down or sitting, he or she is instructed to place the heel of one leg on the opposing knee and to run the heel down to the shin.

49. Name some common causes of cerebellar dysfunction seen in the rehab setting.
Strokes
Multiple sclerosis
Anticonvulsants (phenytoin, phenobarbital, carbamazepine)

BIBLIOGRAPHY

1. Astrachan JM: Como estas, a mnemonic for the mental status examination [letter]. N Engl J Med 324:636, 1991.
2. Butter CM, Kirsch N: Combined and separate effects of eye patching and visual stimulation on unilateral neglect following stroke. Arch Phys Med Rehabil 73:1133–1139, 1992.
3. Caplan L: The Effective Clinical Neurologist. Oxford, Blackwell, 1990.
4. DeMeyer W: Technique of the Neurologic Examination: A Programmed Text, 3rd ed. New York, McGraw Hill, 1980.
5. Johnson RT, Griffin J: Current Therapy in Neurologic Diseases, 4th ed. Philadelphia, B.C. Decker, 1994.
6. Sundet K: Assessment of aphasia in relation to communication and cognitive impairments among stroke patients. Scand J Rehabil Med Suppl 26:60–69, 1992.

19. GAIT ANALYSIS

D. Casey Kerrigan, M.D., and Susan R. Ehrenthal, M.D.

"A journey of a thousand miles begins with a single step."—Lao Tzu

1. Why is gait more costly in energy terms than wheelchair ambulation?

The body's center of gravity must rise and fall with each step during gait, while in wheelchair ambulation, the center of gravity does not rise and fall. There is much work associated with this rise and fall. To calculate an estimate of the work done to walk a certain distance, multiply the vertical displacement of the center of gravity by the body weight and the number of steps.

2. What is a gait cycle?

A gait cycle can be considered the functional unit of gait. It is also referred to as a stride. **Stride length** is the distance between sequential corresponding points of contact by the same foot. **Step length** is the distance between sequential corresponding points of contact by opposite feet. Each stride or gait cycle comprises two steps.

3. What is cadence?

The number of steps per unit time. The average adult cadence is 90–120 steps/minute, with an energy cost of approximately 100 cal/mile.

4. What is a normal adult step length and step width?

Normal step length is about 38 cm. A normal base, or the distance between the center of the heels, is 6–10 cm.

5. Describe the terminology of gait analysis.

The classic terminology of gait such as heel strike, heel-off, and toe-off is "outgaited," since these terms are often not applicable in certain disabilities. The "hip" lingo divides gait into three functional tasks: **weight acceptance, single limb support,** and **limb advancement.** These first two terms comprise the stance period, while the latter comprises the swing period. Stance can be further subdivided into the following phases: **initial contact, loading response, midstance, terminal stance,** and **preswing.** Swing consists of three phrases: **initial swing, mid-swing,** and **terminal swing.**

6. How much of a typical walking cycle is spent in the stance phase? How much in the swing phase?

At normal walking speed, approximately 60% of a gait cycle is spent in stance and 40% in swing. The relative amount of time in stance decreases as the speed of walking increases.

7. What is the difference between walking and running?

Double support usually comprises 20% of a normal walking gait cycle. The relative amount of time spent in double support decreases as the speed of walking increases. *Walking turns to running when there is no longer a period of double support.*

8. What does it mean to walk like an Egyptian?

It is just a song.

9. Name the six determinants of gait.

1. Pelvic rotation
2. Pelvic tilt
3. Knee flexion
4. Foot motion
5. Knee motion
6. Pelvic lateral displacement

10. What is the deal with the six determinants of gait?

These six factors are utilized in normal human gait to minimize the movement of the center of gravity as predicted by the simple compass model of gait described by Saunders, Inman, and Eberhart. The center of gravity normally travels along a sinusoidal up-and-down and side-to-side formal path with each step. If instead of having a mobile pelvis, knees, and ankles, we had inflexible lower limbs, we would walk much like a compass. With such a compass gait, the center of gravity would go up and down much more, resulting in a much more inefficient gait. These determinants are mechanisms or events we utilize to reduce and smooth out the path of the center of gravity.

11. How do these six determinants of gait work?

The first five determinants primarily deal with raising the center of gravity's would-be lowest point at double support or lowering its would-be highest point at midstance. The sixth determinant has to do with reducing the center of gravity's horizontal displacement.

Pelvic rotation: With 4° of pelvic rotation in either direction during double support, the limbs are essentially lengthened. This effectively raises the center of gravity's would-be lowest point.

Pelvic tilt: Occurs in midstance. The pelvis normally dips 4° on the swing side and carries the center of gravity along with it. This lowers the center of gravity's would-be highest point.

Knee flexion: This determinant, which occurs in midstance, also effectively lowers the center of gravity's would-be highest point.

Foot and knee motion: The ankle pivots on the posterior heel at initial contact. The pivot point progresses to the forefoot by terminal stance. These combined actions act to heighten the center of gravity's would-be lowest point. The knee and foot motions also act to smooth the motion into a sinusoidal curve.

Lateral displacement of the pelvis: The hip joints are separated in the horizontal plane by the pelvic width. Valgus alignment at the knees combined with hip adduction places the feet closer together. This allows less excursion of the center of gravity in the horizontal plane.

12. Where is the normal center of gravity? How much does it move during ambulation?

It is approximately 5 cm anterior to the second sacral vertebra. The average total displacement of the center of gravity is about 5 cm in the vertical axis and 5 cm in the horizontal axis for an average adult male step. If it were not for the determinants of gait, the displacement would be about 10 cm. The actual displacement of the center of gravity varies depending on a person's height and step length, but it is always approximately one-half of what it would be if it were not for the determinants of gait.

13. When is the center of gravity at its highest and lowest points in walking? In running?

In walking, it is highest in midstance during single limb support and lowest at initial contact during the double support. Interestingly, in running it is at its highest point in the "flight" phase and at its lowest point in midstance of single limb support.

14. If I walked through a tunnel that was exactly my height, would I bump my head?

No, your height in midstance of gait is less than your standing height due to knee flexion and pelvic tilt. But don't run!

15. What is considered a comfortable walking speed?

A comfortable walking speed is one in which the energy cost per unit distance is at a minimum (i.e., comfort equates with efficiency). This is about **80 meters/min** or **3 mph**, with an energy cost of 4.3 kcal/min. Abnormal biomechanics result in an increased energy cost, which is usually compensated for by a slow walking speed.

16. Can a plastic or metal ankle-foot orthosis (AFO) reduce the energy cost of hemiparetic ambulation?

Both types of braces can significantly increase walking speed and reduce energy expenditure. An AFO reduces energy cost by simulating pushoff and raising the center of gravity in terminal stance (most important). Also, foot-drop is prevented in swing phase. In hemiplegic subjects, energy expenditure per unit distance was 74% above normal using an AFO but 88% without one. There was no significant difference between energy expenditure based on which type of AFO was used. Interestingly, it was easier to negotiate stairs when no AFO was used.

17. How do different assistive devices affect energy expenditure?

In healthy subjects, the use of either a cane or crutches with a partial weight-bearing gait required approximately 18–36% more energy per unit distance. Non-weight-bearing gaits using forearm crutches required 41–61% more energy per unit distance. There are no differences in energy expenditure when comparing the use of axillary or forearm crutches with one another.

18. What is the difference between kinematics and kinetics?

Kinematics is the study of the motions of joint and limb segments. **Kinetics** is the study of forces or torques that cause joint and limb motion.

19. When is a gait laboratory analysis indicated?

It is particularly useful in cases of upper motor neuron pathology. In many cases, the static evaluation of strength and tone may be deceptive. For instance, spasticity evident on static examination may not be apparent during ambulation. Gait analysis provides a respectable quantifiable measure of the requirement and result of a therapeutic intervention. It can be useful to assist in selecting the correct orthosis, therapy program, or surgical procedure. It may suggest a different treatment plan for a patient whose performance has plateaued.

20. What is an antalgic gait?

In an ambulator in pain, gait is modified to reduce weight-bearing on the involved side. The uninvolved limb is rapidly advanced to shorten stance on the affected side. Gait is often slow and steps are short to limit the weight-bearing period. Initial contact is avoided to decrease jarring.

21. What is steppage gait?

It is a compensatory gait using excessive hip and knee flexion to assist a "functionally long" lower leg and foot to clear the ground. For instance, it may be seen with an equinus (plantarflexion) deformity, gastrocsoleus spasticity, or with weak dorsiflexors.

22. Which gait disorder can be detected *before* the patient enters the room?

The foot-slap of a patient with a partial foot-drop can be heard as the foot rapidly moves from initial contact to loading response. Moderately weak (grade 4 or 3) dorsiflexors are the cause; during the period from initial contact to loading response, they must eccentrically contract to slow the forward fall of the body. If dorsiflexors are very weak (grade 2 or worse), a steppage gait is used, as there is not enough strength to lift the forefoot off the ground; this gait is silent.

23. What are the possible causes of equinus in swing?

Excessive plantarflexion in swing may be caused by:
1. Heel cord contracture
2. Spasticity of the soleus, gastrocnemius, or posterior tibialis muscles
3. Weak dorsiflexors

24. What are possible causes of genu recurvatum during the stance period of gait?

Knee hyperextension may be caused by:
1. Plantarflexion contracture (causing a knee extension moment through the closed kinetic chain)
2. Quadriceps weakness
3. Plantarflexor spasticity
4. Quadriceps spasticity

25. What is a Trendelenburg gait?

A Trendelenburg gait is characterized by **lateral trunk-bending toward** the supporting limb during the stance phase. The trunk will bend toward the affected side to keep the center of gravity directly above the hip joint. This maneuver eliminates the need for hip abductors and decreases the forces across the hip joint. A useful intervention is the introduction of a cane to be used contralaterally during the stance period of the affected side.

26. What are the two causes of a Trendelenburg gait?

The most common cause is **hip pain**, usually from osteoarthritis. Lateral trunk-bending serves to reduce the forces across the hip joint. The second cause is **weak hip abductors**. If hip abductors are weak bilaterally, the trunk will sway side to side, causing a "waddling" gait.

27. What is the gait pattern in a person with weak hip extensors?

A person with weak hip extensors walks with an **extensor lurch**. The trunk is hyperextended at the hip to prevent rapid forward fall at initial contact (jack-knifing).

28. When does an infant acquire the ability to walk supported? To walk unsupported? To run?

An infant generally walks with support by 1 year, walks unsupported by 15 months, and runs by approximately 18 months. By 3 years old, a mature gait pattern is established.

29. How does a toddler's gait differ from that of an adult?

Toddlers walk with:
1. A wider base of support
2. A reduced stride length with a higher cadence
3. No heelstrike
4. Little knee flexion during stance
5. Absence of reciprocal arm swing
6. External rotation of the entire leg during the swing phase

30. What alterations in gait parameters may be seen in the older adult?

A safer, more stable gait is obtained by shorter step lengths, an increased double-support stance period, and decreased pushoff power.

31. In the erect body position, where is the line of gravity relative to the hip, knee, and ankle joints?

The line of gravity passes behind the hip and in front of the knee and ankle. This allows the hip to be supported by the iliofemoral ligament and the knee to be supported by the posterior popliteal capsule with no muscular effort. Ankle stability is maintained by continuous contraction of the gastrocsoleus.

32. When walking with a heavy load, what features of the gait cycle are altered?

The step length is decreased. The period of double support is prolonged.

33. During which activity is leg-length discrepancy most apparent?

Running

34. At how many degrees does a knee flexion contracture significantly interfere with gait?

At 30°, all phases of the gait cycle will be abnormal. Contractures of this severity or greater essentially produce a leg-length discrepancy.

BIBLIOGRAPHY

1. Berger N, Edelstein J: Lower limb prosthetics [dissertation]. New York, New York University Post-Graduate Medical School, 1990.

2. Fisher S, Gullickson G Jr: Energy cost of ambulation in health and disability. Arch Phys Med Rehabil 59:124–133, 1978.
3. Gonzalez E, Corcoran PJ: Energy expenditure during ambulation. In Downey JA (ed): Physiological Basis of Rehabilitation Medicine, 2nd ed. Boston, Butterworth-Heinemann, 1994.
4. Harris GF, Wertsch JJ: Procedures for gait analysis. Arch Phys Med Rehabil 75:216–225, 1994.
5. Hoppenfield S: Physical Examination of the Spine and Extremities. Norwalk, CT, Appleton-Century-Crofts, 1976.
6. Kerrigan DC, Glenn MB: An illustration of clinical gait laboratory use to improve rehabilitation management. Am J Phys Med Rehabil 73:421–427, 1994.
7. Lehmkuhl LD, Smith LK (eds): Brunnstrom's Clinical Kinesiology, 4th ed. Philadelphia, F.A. Davis, 1987.
8. Perry J: Gait Analysis: Normal and Pathological Function. Thorofare, NJ, Slack, 1992.
9. Rose J, Gamble JG (eds): Human Walking, 2nd ed. Baltimore, Williams & Wilkins, 1993.
10. Saunders JBCM, Inman VT, Eberhardt HD: The major determinants in normal and pathological gait. J Bone Joint Surg 35A:543–548, 1953.

20. NEUROPSYCHIATRIC ASSESSMENT AFTER BRAIN INJURY

Marilyn F. Kraus, M.D., and Constantine Lyketsos, M.D.

1. How does neuropsychiatry differ from traditional psychiatry?

Neuropsychiatry is applied neuroscience. Whereas in traditional psychiatry, the diagnosis is based on a description of symptoms and not necessarily an etiology, in neuropsychiatry, the brain and its function are the primary concern and symptoms are derivative. The focus is on the evaluation and treatment of cognitive, mood, and behavioral sequelae in patients with neurologic disease or injury. This includes disorders such as stroke, dementias, traumatic brain injury (TBI), developmental disorders, and other neurologic disorders.

2. What possible neuropsychiatric sequelae are seen in early stages of coma recovery?

Patients may have any constellation of cognitive deficits, mood disturbances, personality changes, or behavioral problems. The nature and severity of these disorders depend on a number of factors, such as location and size of lesion, duration of coma and posttraumatic amnesia, premorbid level of function, history of substance abuse or previous brain injury, psychosocial factors (the patient's support system and other resources), age and medical health, and stage of recovery.

In patients who are in the early stages of coma recovery, there may be symptoms similar to a **delirium**. They may be confused, disoriented, or combative. Significant deficits in arousal, attention, and concentration may be evident. **Sleep disturbances** are common, and the patient may show psychotic features, such as **delusions** (false beliefs) or **hallucinations**.

3. What neuropsychiatric disorders are seen after coma or head injury?

Some disorders may be chronic and may even arise after a period of time. These include disorders of **mood** and mood regulation, **cognitive disturbances** such as memory deficits, and **behavioral dyscontrol** such as in frontal lobe syndromes. Disorders of **language**, such as Broca's and Wernicke's aphasias, occur more commonly following stroke than TBI, due to the common involvement of the middle cerebral artery territory in stroke.

4. Outline the basic mechanisms of injury in TBI.

A **penetrating injury** occurs when the skull is fractured and a foreign object enters the brain tissue.

Contusions are best described as superficial damage to the cortical convolutions of the inferior surfaces on the frontal and temporal lobes, which occur when the brain is forced against the inside surfaces of the skull. This can occur with blunt trauma or in acceleration-deceleration type injuries. If the injury is proximal to the site of the blow, it is a **coup** injury. Often the force of the blow causes the brain to be forced against the opposite surface of the skull, resulting in damage distal to the site of the blow, or **contrecoup** injury. The most common sites of contusions are the orbital frontal and anterior and lateral temporal lobes.

Diffuse axonal injury is almost inevitably a result of acceleration-deceleration injuries. When the brain is subject to rotational and acceleration-deceleration forces, individual axons can be stretched or sheared. Because this is usually a diffuse process, it may not be visible on CT or MRI scans.

Hematomas and **hypoxia** can be secondary mechanisms of injury in the acute period following injury and can result in broader areas of damage.

Free radicals and **excitotoxic neurotransmitters** are released following trauma or stroke and can also result in secondary damage. Examples are glutamate, aspartate, and nitric oxide.

5. How is the severity of the head injury determined?
Duration of loss of consciousness, initial score on the Glasgow Coma Scale (a 15-point scale that determines depth of coma), and length of post-traumatic amnesia (PTA) are generally the measures used to determine severity.

Measures Used to Determine Severity of Injury

	SEVERITY OF INJURY		
	MILD	MODERATE	SEVERE
Glasgow Coma Scale	13–15	9–15	≤ 8
Loss of consciousness	< 30 min	≤ 24 hrs	> 24 hrs
Length of PTA	0–24 hrs	1–7 days	> 7 days

6. What is posttraumatic amnesia (PTA)?
PTA is the period of time after a patient emerges from coma during which he or she has no continuous memory for day-to-day events—i.e., there is impaired memory for new information. The end of PTA is defined as the return of continuous memory.

A standard measure used to assess PTA is the **Galveston Orientation and Amnesia Test**. In moderate and severe injuries, this test appears to correlate fairly well with outcome. The relationship is not so clear in milder head injuries, which historically have been more difficult to define in terms of prognostic indicators.

7. How does the neuropsychiatrist approach the evaluation of the brain-injured patient?
In TBI, several things are important. First of all, a good **history** of the injury includes the type of trauma, duration of coma, duration of PTA, as well as associated injuries. History of previous brain injury and substance use must also be considered.

The evaluation of the patient's **current clinical status** includes an assessment of cognition, mood, or behavioral disturbances. Family and staff interviews help establish diagnosis.

In most cases, **neuropsychological testing** will be requested. This battery of tests is designed to define deficits in areas such as memory, language, and problem-solving. A description of the patient's premorbid functioning and personality is an essential factor in determining prognosis and in guiding a realistic rehabilitation program, including vocational and community re-entry.

8. What types of cognitive deficits are encountered in stroke patients?
Any variety and combination of deficits are possible. The resulting deficits depend primarily on the **type** and **location** of the lesion. Attention and concentration deficits are common, although

stroke can also result in a mood disturbance. In fact, cognition in general can be worsened when a mood disturbance is present. Neuropsychological testing remains the best way to define deficits and plan interventions accordingly.

9. What cognitive deficits occur after traumatic injury?

The different mechanisms of injury in TBI result in a wider range of possible effects. Acceleration-deceleration injuries, as in a car accident, can result in more diffuse injury, referred to as diffuse axonal injury. As with stroke, any combination and severity of cognitive deficits can be seen following trauma. But, there is the added difficulty of more diffuse injury which may not be readily apparent on CT or MRI scans.

10. Discuss the principles of using pharmacologic agents to treat neuropsychiatric symptoms following brain injury.

Treatment may be aimed at specific symptoms or proposed underlying pathology. For example, clinical symptoms such as depression or attention deficits can be identified and treated based on existing pharmacologic regimens. The primary difference between brain-injured and non-brain-injured patients is the enhanced sensitivity to side effects, as well as potential effects of medications on recovery, seen with brain injury. So a critical role of the physician is to avoid drugs that could worsen the recovering patient's condition and outcome. A consultation will often be required to choose appropriate pharmacologic intervention.

11. Can cognitive deficits be treated?

In general, the common nonspecific symptoms such as arousal, attention, and concentration can often be improved with certain medications. The drugs often used include those used to treat attention deficit disorder, such as the psychostimulants **methylphenidate** and **D-amphetamine**. They are usually well-tolerated in brain-injured patients and may also be effective for other disturbances, such as depressed mood or behavioral problems. Memory may improve with these treatments, although it is not clear if this is only secondary to improving attention and concentration.

Dopaminergic agents such as amantadine can be useful, particularly when symptoms are part of a frontal lobe syndrome.

Cognitive rehabilitation is gaining increased acceptance as an important component in the rehab of brain-injured patients. It may be particularly critical in the acute stage of recovery (up to 6 months postinjury) and could complement pharmacotherapy. It often involves techniques to retrain the patient in specific domains such as memory and attention. Different theoretical frameworks have been proposed to guide remediation strategies, and recent assessments support their effectiveness.

12. How is mood assessed in the brain-injured patient?

Primarily by examination of the patient and interviewing family and staff. **Depression** can be common following brain injury, but it does not always present in a typical manner. In general, a mood disturbance should be suspected when the patient's degree of disability is greater than would be expected given the severity of injury, or when the patient fails to meet rehab goals or cooperate with treatment. It is not unusual for some mood-disturbed patients to deny a depressed mood on questioning. Other disturbances of mood, such as **mania**, can result but are not as common. Treatment is similar to that used for patients with a primary diagnosis of mania, except that the anticonvulsants may be a more effective and safer choice than lithium, which may cause more side effects in a brain-injured patient.

13. How common is depression following stroke?

Depression can be a significant complicating factor in stroke, affecting about 30–60% of patients in the first year. Three types of mood disorders are seen in these patients. The first type resembles the **major depressive disorder** described in the DSM-IV. The symptoms are those classically associated with depression, such as sadness, anxiety, loss of energy, sleep and appetite problems, and thoughts of death or suicide.

Minor depression can also occur, with similar symptoms but of lesser intensity. This syndrome can often be missed. It is very similar to the **dysthymic disorder** described in DSM-IV.

The third disorder can present as an **indifferent, apathetic state** or with **inappropriate cheerfulness**. There can be slowness, agitation, and loss of interest.

There is also evidence that patients with **left-sided lesions** are more vulnerable to develop a depression. Also, the closer the lesion to the frontal pole, the greater the risk.

14. Is there a similar risk for mood disturbance following TBI?

Yes. Clinically, the magnitude of risk appears to be similar to that for stroke, although lesion location does not appear to be as important. Mood disturbances can present in a variety of ways. It is not unusual for the affective symptoms to be subtle, but for behavioral manifestations to predominate, such as irritability, uncooperativeness, apathy, and poor progression or effort in rehab. The mood disturbances may not necessarily meet traditional psychiatric criteria, but may present more as **mood lability** or **dysregulation**. Often, these can be treated successfully with a combination of pharmacologic and behavioral intervention.

15. What pharmacologic interventions are appropriate for patients with depression after brain injury?

In many ways, it is similar to the treatment of nonimpaired depressed patients, but there are significant considerations. The major concern involves the uncertain effects of chemicals on a damaged brain. These patients tend to be more sensitive to side effects, such as from anticholinergic agents. Also, because they often have impairment of cognition, it is better to avoid agents that could further aggravate these, such as the tertiary tricyclics (imipramine, amytriptyline).

Often, the newer serotonergic agents, such as sertraline and fluoxetine, can be very effective and well tolerated. Fluoxetine can be more beneficial if low arousal or fatigue is a problem, as well as attention and concentration problems. The psychostimulants (methylphenidate or dextroamphetamine) can be excellent choices, as they have a very good risk-benefit ratio. They have the added advantage of potentially improving attention, concentration, and memory. Also, animal studies have suggested that these agents may have a positive effect on cortical recovery.

16. What changes in personality can occur following brain injury?

Personality changes result from two factors. First, damage to structures directly responsible for behavior and emotion. Second, cognitive deficits can change perception, which in turn affects the patient's response to his or her environment. It is important to educate the families concerning these possible changes, as they will tend to interpret the patient as purposefully aggravating them or being mean or difficult.

Personality changes exist on a spectrum with other behavioral problems. On the milder end, there is an exaggeration of the patient's premorbid negative personality traits. Families may complain that the patient has become a "different person," and children can appear hyperactive or develop symptoms consistent with attention deficit disorder. Closed head injuries often result in injury to the frontal and temporal lobes, areas that regulate behavior and emotional response.

17. List the possible behavioral disturbances that can follow brain injury.

Depending on the location and severity of the injury, different types of behavioral disturbances can occur:

Irritability	Poor self-regulation of behavior
Lability	Poor judgment and insight
Impulsivity	Risk-taking
Aggression	Sexual disturbances
Poor ability to plan	Disturbances of regular sleep/wake cycles
Poor motivation	Mood dysregulation

18. What behavior problems are common following frontal lobe injury?

In TBI, the frontal lobes are a very common site of injury. Depending on the severity and location of the injury, these patients can show personality disturbances such as irritability, impulsivity, mood disturbances, aggressive behavior, as well as specific cognitive disturbances. They can show poor insight and judgment, particularly in regard to their own disability. In general, when there is significant injury to the frontal lobes, the ability to monitor and control behavior is impaired.

19. How can these behavioral problems be managed?

Treatment consists of several components: pharmacologic agents, behavioral strategies, and education and support of the family. In a rehab setting, it is important to assess the problem adequately and to work with the staff to set up a structured **behavioral program**. Frontal lobe patients often lose the ability to control or monitor their own behavior, but respond well when consistent external structure is set up.

Pharmacologic intervention may be helpful, depending on the exact nature of the problem. In some cases, **dopaminergic agents**, such as amantadine or L-dopa/carbidopa, improve impulsivity and aggression. Other agents can be useful, such as the anticonvulsants **carbamazepine** or **valproate**. Often, a combination of agents may be necessary.

20. What problems can follow injury to the temporal lobes?

The temporal lobes are another common site of injury in head trauma. The clinical syndromes that can result are even more variable than for frontal lobes injury. Different regions of the temporal lobes are responsible for receptive language (**aphasias**), high-level integration of sensory input, memory (**amnesia**), and emotional expression.

21. What types of aggressive behavior can follow brain injury?

Aggressive behavior following brain injury can range from mild verbal abusiveness to physical assaultiveness. It is important to characterize the aggressive behavior. Is the patient labile? Is there strong affect associated with the behavior? There are scales designed to quantify and characterize the aggression, such as the **Overt Aggression Scale**.

Aggression is a symptom that can have a variety of underlying causes. If it is part of a frontal lobe syndrome, then the treatment may differ from that for aggression resulting from psychosis, mood lability, or a seizure disorder. Dysregulated, aggressive behavior is a complex area that can have a significant impact on the patient's ability to return home and to the community.

22. How can aggression be managed in the rehab setting?

It can be managed behaviorally, pharmacologically, or by a combination of both methods. A variety of pharmacologic agents can be used, depending on the particular case. The anticonvulsants, dopaminergic agents, beta-blockers, antidepressants, or opioid antagonists may be helpful. The aggression must be carefully characterized to choose an appropriate treatment. If the aggression results from a mood disturbance, an antidepressant may be helpful. In some cases, there may be clinical or EEG evidence of temporal lobe epilepsy. In cases of severe brain injury, the aggression can be more of a reflexive or predatorial type, e.g., the patient who does not appear to get upset but strikes out at anyone who enters his visual field. Remember that aggression is a symptom, not a diagnosis. Treatment may often be trial and error.

23. How common are seizures following brain injury? Can they affect the patient's mental status?

The incidence of epilepsy developing within 5 years of a closed head injury is about 2–5%. The incidence following penetrating injuries is much higher. The frequency following stroke ranges from 6–13%.

Because the type of seizure can often be **complex partial**, this contributes to the risk of developing psychiatric symptoms. If an underlying dysrhythmia or epileptiform disorder is suspected as the cause of symptoms such as aggression or mood disturbances, a trial of an anticonvulsant may be warranted.

24. Discuss the postconcussive syndrome.

Postconcussive syndrome is a term usually reserved for a collection of symptoms that can follow relatively mild head injury. A number of somatic, cognitive, mood, or behavior changes can occur: headache, dizziness, tinnitus, hearing loss, blurred vision, light and noise sensitivity, altered taste and smell, irritability, lability, depression, anxiety, memory problems, attention and concentration problems, fatigue, sleep disturbances, slowed reaction time, slowed information processing time.

Although most patients who develop these symptoms show resolution over time, a significant minority show persistent difficulties. When indicated, pharmacologic treatment is aimed at target symptoms and may involve the use of antidepressants or psychostimulants.

25. How are sleep disturbances following brain injury managed?

Sleep disturbances can be a significant problem following brain injury and are often overlooked. Lack of sleep can worsen cognition, behavior, and mood and undermine treatment attempts. Disturbed sleep is very common in the first few months following TBI and may or may not resolve. Daytime sleepiness can also be a problem.

Treatment consists of medication and behavioral management. Often, the serotonin agents (fluoxetine, sertraline) can be helpful in regulating the sleep/wake cycles. Nortriptyline can be helpful if the patient has trouble remaining asleep. Pyschostimulants (methylphenidate, *d*-amphetamine) can be used for daytime sleepiness and consequently help normalize sleep at night. Trazodone is another choice.

Behaviorally, standard sleep hygiene should be used. The patient should keep regular hours, avoid caffeine, alcohol, and tobacco, and activities that are too stimulating before bedtime. If a sleep disorder is persistent and treatment refractory, a sleep study is warranted.

ACKNOWLEDGMENT

Supported in part by NIH grant no. T32-AG 00149.

BIBLIOGRAPHY

1. Duke LW, Weathers SL, Caldwell SG, Novack TA: Cognitive rehabilitation after head trauma: Toward an integrated cognitive/behavioral perspective on intervention. In Long CJ, Ross LK (eds): Handbook of Head Trauma. New York, Plenum Press, 1992, pp 165–187,
2. Evans RW: The postconcussion syndrome and the sequelae of mild head injury. Neurol Clin 10:815–847, 1992.
3. Faught E, Peters D, Bartolucci A, et al: Seizures after primary intracerebral hemorrhage. Neurology 39:1089–1093, 1989.
4. Fedoroff J, Starkstein S, Forrester A, et al: Depression in patients with acute traumatic brain injury. Am J Psychiatry 149:918–923, 1992.
5. Gualtieri CT: Neuropsychiatry and Behavioral Pharmacology. New York, Springer-Verlag, 1991.
6. Kraus MF: Neuropsychiatric sequelae of stroke and traumatic brain injury: The role of the psychostimulants. Int J Psychiatry Med 25:39–51, 1995.
7. Levin H, Kraus MF: The frontal lobes and traumatic brain injury. J Neuropsychiatry Clin Neurosci 6:443–454, 1994.
8. Silver JM, Yodofsky SC: Aggressive disorders. In Silver JM, Yodofsky SC, Hales RE (eds): Neuropsychiatry of Traumatic Brain Injury. Washington, DC, American Psychiatric Press, 1994, pp 313–353.
9. Starkstein SE, Robinson RG: Neuropsychiatric aspects of cerebral vascular disorders. In Yudofsky SC, Hales RE (eds): The American Psychiatric Press Textbook of Neuropsychiatry. Washington, DC, American Psychiatric Press, 1992, pp 449–472.
10. Yudofsky SC, Silver JM, Jackson W, et al: The overt aggression scale for the objective rating of verbal and physical aggression. Am J Psychiatry 143:35–39, 1986.

21. MANUAL WHEELCHAIRS

R. *Lee Kirby*. M.D., F.R.C.P.C.

1. Discuss briefly the importance and prevalence of wheelchair use.

The wheelchair is arguably the most important therapeutic tool in rehabilitation, equivalent in importance to vaccination in preventive medicine or antibiotics in curative medicine. In 1992, there were 1,072,000 wheelchair users in the U.S. (4.2 per 1000 population); about 75% of the wheelchairs were manually propelled. The prevalence is much greater among the elderly.

2. How safe are wheelchairs?

The long-term use of wheelchairs can result in chronic or repetitive stresses—for instance, on shoulders, peripheral nerves, and skin. Each year in the U.S. there are about 50 wheelchair-related deaths and over 36,000 wheelchair-related injuries that lead to an emergency department visit. About 75% of deaths and injuries occur because the users tip over or fall from their chairs.

3. Compare the ride of folding- and rigid-frame wheelchairs.

The flexibility of the folding frame leads to a more comfortable ride and makes it more likely that all four wheels will remain in contact with uneven terrain. Rigidity provides a responsive feel to wheelchair propulsion and turning because the applied forces are not damped by flexion of the chair. A rigid frame also allows more precise wheel alignment.

4. Why is seat depth important?

If the seat is too short and the thighs are unsupported, the area over which the forces are distributed is reduced, thus increasing pressure. A seat that is too long can cause pressure sores in the popliteal space or may force the user to scoot forward into a slumped (lumbar-kyphotic) position.

5. How is the seat height lowered?
- Use drop hooks to lower a rigid seat surface below the level of the side rails.
- Select a higher axle position for the rear wheel.
- Use a rear wheel with a smaller diameter.
- Steps 2 and 3 will tilt the seat backward unless the casters are also modified.

6. What are the pros and cons of increasing the seat-plane angle?

Pros: the seat-plane angle (the angle of the seat plane relative to the horizontal, usually 1–4° higher in front) may be accentuated to reduce (1) spasticity, (2) tendency for the user to slide forward on the seat, or (3) lumbar lordosis.

Cons: the accentuated angle makes transfers more difficult and puts more weight on the ischial tuberosities.

7. What are the considerations in choosing a wheelchair cushion?
- Virtually all personal wheelchairs should be fitted with a removable cushion for pressure distribution, shock absorption, and/or positioning.
- Very flexible cushions should be supported fully by the seat surface (preferably rigid) so that they do not fold over the seat margins.
- In choosing the cushion materials (e.g., foam, air, gel) and their distribution and shape, consider such issues as sensibility, pressure distribution, presence of spasticity or flaccidity, and incontinence. For instance, a user with spasticity may benefit from an anterior wedge and a slight pommel between the thighs. A user with flaccidity, who rests with the knees apart, may benefit from more lateral support.
- Decisions about the cushion should be made early, because the dimensions of the compressed cushion affect various wheelchair dimensions (e.g,. backrest, armrest, seat height).

8. How high should the backrest be?

- The upper border of the backrest should be 1–2" lower than the scapulae for users who propel their own wheelchairs, to minimize irritation from rubbing during propulsion.
- Higher backrests (sometimes with headrests) provide more support and more area for pressure distribution for users who do not propel the wheelchair independently or use a recliner.
- Backrests that do not extend above the lumbar region are increasingly common and are surprisingly well tolerated if the lumbosacral area is supported. Such low backrests have the advantage of permitting great freedom of upper body and trunk movement.

9. What should the backrest angle be?

- The angle of the backrest is commonly tilted back about 8° from vertical (i.e., ~95° from the seat plane).
- Users of lightweight wheelchairs may prefer to increase the seatplane angle and reduce the backrest-to-seatplane angle. Such a relatively forward inclination of the backrest assists the user in applying force to the wheels by preventing the trunk from being pushed backward with each arm thrust.
- For users with weak trunk muscles, increasing the backrest-to-seatplane angle ("recline") decreases the likelihood of falling forward onto the lap, obviating the need for a chest strap in some cases. Recline reduces the pressure on the ischial tuberosities in proprotion to the extent of the recline. However, because the mechanical axis of a backrest with variable recline is usually below and behind the anatomic axis of the user's hip joint, shear forces are produced by the relative movement of the back of the chair and the back of the user.

10. What about tilt?

- Tilt is a change in the position or attitude of the seat rather than a change in the posture of the user (relative position of body parts).
- Tilt obviates the shear problem of recliners and is less likely to induce spasticity.
- Tilt reduces the pressure on the ischial tuberosities in proportion to the extent of the tilt.

11. What are the pros and cons of desk-length armrests?

- Desk-length armrests (without the forward one-third) allow a closer approach to a desk or table but may not provide enough length to be useful for sit-to-stand transfers. This limitation can be circumvented if the armrests are reversible.
- In the reversed position, the notch allows better access of the arms to the wheels for propulsion but eliminates lateral support of the trunk through the armrests.

12. What is a wrap-around armrest? What is its principal advantage?

The rear attachment of the wrap-around armrest is behind the frame rather than beside it. This allows the rear wheels to be placed closer to the frame, narrowing the outside width of the wheelchair without narrowing the seat width.

13. What are the considerations in choosing the footrest height?

- The lowest point on the footrests should be at least 2" above the floor to avoid being caught on obstacles and incline transitions.
- If the footrests are too high, the thighs are lifted from the seat, increasing the presssure on the ischial tuberosities.
- If the footrests are too low (or removed), the front edge of the seat will bear more weight than appropriate, with the potential for pressure ulceration under the distal thighs. Also, there will be less support for forward leans.

14. What should the knee-flexion angle be?

The usual "hanger angle" is 60–70°. Elevating the footrests (extending the knees) reduces edema and knee-flexion contractures but decreases forward stability, both because the center of gravity is altered and because footrests serve as forward antitippers. Elevation of a single footrest may lead to a violent, yawing tip. Also, there can be relative movement between the elevating footrest and the user if the axes of the mechanical and anatomic joints are not colinear. Some elevating footrests accommodate for shear by either a gooseneck attachment that raises the mechanical axis or a telescoping mechanism that lengthens the footrest as it is elevated. Some wheelchairs set the knees in flexion of > 90°. Potential benefits include tighter turns, closer access to objects, protection of the feet, ease of transport of the wheelchair, and inhibition of spasticity. By bringing limb segments closer to the yaw axis, hyperflexion also allows faster turns (as a spinning skater gains speed by bringing the arms closer to the body). Disadvantags include: (1) users with long legs may be difficult to accommodate; (2) a small caster diameter and caster trail may be needed to avoid swiveling of the caster into footrests or heels during changes in direction; (3) the footrests are less effective as forward antitip devices; and (4) the hyperflexed position may occlude circulation and cause pressure lesions under the points where pressure is applied to achieve hyperflexion.

15. What are the pros and cons of front-rigging taper?

Some manufacturers provide models that are narrower in front, creating a tapered (or wedge) configuration that permits tighter cornering and holds the legs together. Potential disadvantages include aggravation of hip deformities (e.g., chronic or recurrent dislocation), pressure lesions on the lateral aspects of the lower legs, and interference with side transfers if the legs are tightly jammed in place, or interference with floor-to-seat transfers if the pelvis is too wide for the user to sit on the footrests.

16. How does rear-axle position affect the wheelchair?

Raising the axle lowers seat height and rear stability, raises forward stability, tilts the wheelchair backward, and causes a cambered wheel to toe out. **Moving the axle back** raises rear stability, decreases the ease of doing wheelies, limits the ability to lift the front wheels, reduces traction, lengthens wheelbase, and increases rolling resistance and downhill-turning tendency.

17. How do the wheel locks affect the likelihood and violence of a rear tipping accident?

The static rear stability of a wheelchair is decreased when the wheels are locked, because the axis of rotation is at the wheel-ground interface with the locks on and at the level of the rear-wheel axle with the locks off. However, once beyond the stability limits, a rear tip is slower and less violent if the wheels are locked (or equivalently grasped).

18. Define camber. How does it affect the wheelchair?

Camber is the angle, usually 3–9°, that results when the distance between the tops of the rear wheels is less than the distance between the bottoms. Camber provides a natural angle for the arms to address the wheels during propulsion, protects the user's hands from doorways or other players in sports, reduces downhill-turning tendency on side slopes, and increases ease of turning and lateral stability. Changing the camber produces many mechanical effects that may require compensation, such as lengthening the wheelbase, tilting the wheelchair backward, toe-out, and altering the caster-stem angle and caster-trail distance. Camber increases wear on wheel bearings and rolling resistance and creates a wider track that causes more difficulty in tight spaces. Furthermore, a cambered wheel, even if perfectly aligned when all four wheels are on the ground, will toe out during a wheelie in proportion to the wheelie angle. Unless compensations are made, camber increases forward stability and reduces rear stability because of some of the above effects.

19. What is toeing error? How can it be corrected?

The rear wheels are "toed in" when the fronts of the rear wheels are closer to each other than the backs; the opposite configuration is "toe out." Symmetric toeing error with a malalignment of as little as 2° increases rolling resistance quite dramatically. Asymmetric toeing may cause the wheelchair to deviate persistently to one side. If the wheelchair has an axle-adjustment plate, toeing error can be eliminated by adding washers under the front or back bolts. If the axle is housed in a tube of fixed alignment, the tube can be rotated.

20. Define caster trail and flutter.

Caster trail is the distance on the ground between two points: one obtained by dropping a vertical from the caster axle, the other by projecting the caster-swivel axis to the ground. The greater the trail, the greater the diamater that must be kept free of the rear wheels, footrests, and heels if the caster is to swivel freely.

Caster flutter (or shimmy) is the tendency for the casters to oscillate from side to side at a certain speed. Flutter can be annoying, increases rolling resistance, and may cause an unintentional change in direction. To decrease shimmy at normal rolling speeds, one can reduce the size and weight of the caster, increase the caster trail, or increase the proportion of the weight on the casters.

21. Why should the caster stems be vertical?

If the caster stems (and hence the axes around which the swivel occurs) are not vertical, the caster axle is lower at one swivel extreme than the other. Thus the wheelchair may "settle" after it comes to a halt. In starting up, the user may have to overcome some resistance to get the caster "uphill."

22. Why do many wheelchair users remove the rear antitippers or adjust them into ineffective positions?

Most antitippers have a limited range of adjustability. When adjusted to prevent full rear tips, they interfere with maneuverability (e.g., by "grounding out" during incline transitions or by preventing the wheelchair from being tipped back sufficiently to get the casters up a curb).

23. Where should a wheelchair user carry a load to maximize or minimize the effect on stability?

- To raise rear stability, the footrest position is the first choice; to lower rear stability, use the high-rear position.
- To raise forward stability, use the low-rear position; to lower forward stabilty, use the footrest position.
- To minimize the effect of added loads on stability, use the lap or under-the-seat position.

24. How much input should the wheelchair user have in the prescription process?

The prescription process should involve the user fully (and, if appropriate, the family or other caregivers). For the first wheelchair, the user's limited experience necessitates heavy reliance on the clincal team. As users gain more experience, they are able to participate more fully.

25. What are the steps in the prescription process?

1. The clinical team needs to assess the user, particularly his or her impairments, diagnoses, prognosis, residual abilities, extent of social participation, goals of wheelchair use, priorities (because tradeoffs are invariably necessary), and bodily dimensions.

2. The clinical team develops a list of the ideal wheelchair and seating features for the user.

3. The list of ideal features is compared with what is available from a reputable manufacturer in the user's price range and from a local dealer.

4. The user test-drives the chairs under consideration with a member of the clinical team.

5. Once the appropriate wheelchair is purchased, the user is trained in its use and maintenance.

6. After a few months of wheelchair use (and periodically thereafter), the situation should be reviewed and adjustments made.

BIBLIOGRAPHY

1. Axelson P, Minkel J, Chesney D: A Guide to Wheelchair Selection: How to Use the ANSI/RESNA Wheelchair Standards to Buy a Wheelchair. Washington, DC, Paralyzed Veterans of America, 1994.
2. Bergen AF, Presperin J, Tallman T: Positioning for function: Wheelchairs and other assistive technologies. Valhalla, NY, Valhalla Rehabilitation Publications, 1990.
3. Brubaker C: Ergonometric considerations: Choosing a wheelchair system. J Rehabil Res Dev Clin Suppl 2:37–48, 1990.
4. Cooper R: Rehabilitation Engineering Applied to Mobility and Manipulation. Philadelphia, Institute of Physics, 1995.
5. Denison I, Shaw J, Zuyderhoff R: Wheelchair Selection Manual: The Effect of Components on Manual Wheelchair Performance. Vancouver, British Columbia Rehabilitation Society.
6. Kirby RL: Wheelchairs. In Lazar R (ed): Neurorehabilitation. New York, McGraw-Hill, 1996.
7. Kirby RL: Wheelchair stability: Important, measurable and modifiable. Technol Disabil 5:75–80, 1996.
8. Wilson AB Jr: How to Select and Use Manual Wheelchairs. Topping, VA, Rehabilitation Press, 1992.

22. SWALLOWING AND DYSPHAGIA

Arthur A. Siebens, M.D., and Bryan O'Young, M.D.

1. Describe the three stages of swallowing.

It is customary to divide the passage of food and drink from mouth to stomach into oral, pharyngeal, and esophageal stages. These subdivisions are somewhat arbitrary because the structures that correspond to these three stages are continuous, and the coordination of these structures such as the tensions, motions, and nervous system events are not necessarily isolated by stage. In general, during the **oral stage** the swallowing entity (the bolus) is created. In the **pharyngeal stage**, the bolus is propelled from the mouth into the esophagus without contamination of the airways (nasopharynx or larynx). In the **esophageal stage**, the bolus is conducted from the pharynx into the cervical esophagus, through the thorax, and into the stomach. Flow of the bolus is away from the mouth and retrograde flow is abnormal. Clearance of the passageway is complete and prompt. Prolonged residual collections in the mouth, pharynx, or the esophagus are considered abnormal.

2. In the foodway from mouth to stomach, the oral, pharyngeal, and esophageal muscles act like a pump that is valved for unidirectional flow. Identify seven of these functional valves.

Valves relevant to unidirectional flow during swallowing. (a) Lips. Sealing of the lips prevents the bolus from retrograde flow outside of the mouth during the oral stage. (b) Tongue. Posterior thrust of the tongue against the wall of the pharynx prevents reflux from pharynx to mouth during the pharyngeal stage. (c) Velum. Elevation of the velum prevents oronasal reflux. (d and e) Epiglottis and vocal folds. Downward tilting of the epiglottis, the elevation of the larynx, the contraction of the laryngeal intrinsic muscles (not shown in figure), and the apposition of the vocal folds complete the sealing of the larynx. (f) Cricopharyngeus. Contraction of the cricopharyngeus prevents reflux from the upper esophagus to the pharynx. (g) Gastroesophageal sphincter. Its contraction prevents retrograde flow from the stomach into the esophagus. *(Continued below.)*

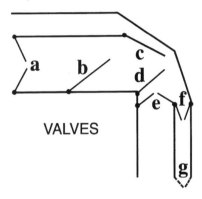

VALVES

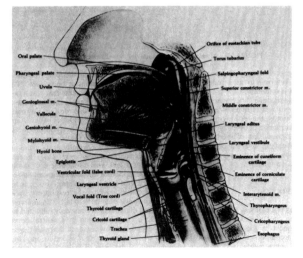

Sagittal schematic of the pharynx, larynx and mouth. (From Siebens AA: Rehabilitation for swallowing impairment. In Kottke FJ, Lehman JF (eds): Krusen's Handbook of Physical Medicine and Rehabilitation. Philadelphia, W.B. Saunders, 1990, pp 765–777, with permission.)

3. What role does the tongue play in swallowing?

In the **oral stage** of swallowing, the tongue assists in mixing and transport functions. Its action prepares foods by directing their course for mastication and wetting them with saliva. It also controls the transport of the prepared bolus from front to back of the oral cavity.

During the **pharyngeal stage**, it propels the bolus into the pharynx and seals the bolus within the pharynx by forceful apposition to the soft palate (velum) and posterior pharyngeal wall. Its piston or plunger action contributes to raising pharyngeal chamber pressure.

4. Describe the function of the cricopharyngeus muscle.

The cricopharyngeus controls flow between the pharynx and cervical esophagus. Its continuous contraction between swallows prevents air from entering and esophageal contents from refluxing. Its relaxation during the pharyngeal stage allows low-resistance passage of food into the esophagus. It functions, therefore, as a foodway gatekeeper.

5. Name three factors that promote passage of liquid from the pharynx into the cervical esophagus.

1. Gravity, if the pharynx is vertical
2. Increased pressure within the pharynx attributable to lingual thrust and shortening of the pharyngeal constrictors
3. Timely relaxation of the cricopharyngeus

6. Where is the "swallowing center"?

The "swallowing center" is a conceptual entity rather than a precise neuroanatomic site. Inasmuch as the afferent and efferent fibers of the glossopharyngeal and vagus nerves have their nuclei and multiple connections primarily in the dorsal medulla, this area, the **reticular formation**, is a critical one for swallowing. It is critical also for other vital functions relevant to the cardiovascular and respiratory systems.

7. Where is the glottis?

The glottis is the space between the vocal folds, also known as the "true cords" (in contrast to the "false cords" or ventricular folds). The space expands and decreases with inspiration and expiration, respectively, and is obliterated tightly during swallowing as the vocal folds snap together. Failure of timely glottic closure is one predisposition to airway penetration.

8. What is the principal motor nerve innervating the intrinsic muscles of the larynx?

All muscles intrinsic to the larynx are innervated by the inferior or recurrent laryngeal nerve except one, the cricothyroid muscle, which is innervated by the superior laryngeal nerve. Both nerves are special efferent fibers of the nucleus ambiguous (cranial nerve X) to these striated muscles.

9. What is the primary sensory nerve of the pharynx? The larynx?

For the pharynx it is the glossopharyngeal (IX), and for the larynx, the vagus (X), via the superior and inferior (recurrent) branches.

10. Define "silent" aspiration.

Contamination of the larynx or upper trachea with foodway contents without the elicitation of cough. The discovery of coughless aspiration is a result of fluoroscopic examination (modified barium swallow). Regrettably, detection readily escapes the bedside evaluation.

11. Describe the Heimlich maneuver.

The Heimlich maneuver is used to dislodge food that is stuck in the airway and that the patient cannot cough out. The maneuver consists of wrapping one's arms around the upper abdomen of the victim and squeezing mightily and quickly in a brief but fervent hug from the back. The intent is to force the victim's abdominal contents against the diaphragm, thereby increasing the air pressure in the lungs sufficiently to blow out the food plug. Dr. Heimlich described this maneuver in *JAMA* in 1975.

12. How useful is a bedside swallowing study?

For many patients, the bedside swallowing assessment is not a reliable basis for determining whether feeding by mouth is safe, because airway contamination during swallowing can occur independently of any outward sign such as coughing or a "moist voice." The patient with a tracheostomy is an exception, in that suctioning foodway contents from the trachea is clear evidence of airway contamination. Regrettably, there is no simple way to detect airway contamination at the bedside in many patients, and VFSS remains the gold standard for swallowing assessment.

13. What is "quad coughing"?

Quad coughing is a technique that aids expiratory airflow for maintaining patency of the airway. *Quad* indicates *quadriplegia*, which is commonly associated with paralysis or weakness of the muscles of forceful expiration, primarily the abdominals and intercostals. Cough assistance is given to the supine "quad" patient by pushing with one's outstretched hands on the abdomen and lower ribs synchronously with the patient's cough effort after deep inspiration. Normal cough airflow velocity is achieved despite the paralysis. Clearing of tracheobronchial secretions as well as aspirated material can be achieved.

14. How does the volume of saliva produced in 24 hours compare with the volume of urine produced in this period?

Surprisingly, normal output of saliva is similar to the normal output of urine—approximately 1.5 liters/24 hrs.

15. What drugs can be used to increase or decrease the flow of saliva?

The salivary glands are innervated by branches of the cranial division of the parasympathetic system coursing initially in the VIth (submandibular and sublingual glands) and IXth (parotid gland) cranial nerves. The terminal transmission is cholinergic, a muscarinic (glands and smooth muscles) as opposed to a nicotinic (skeletal muscle) effect of acetylcholine. **Propantheline** (Pro-Banthine) is among the blocking agents that decrease salivation. **Pilocarpine** is among the agents increasing salivary flow. Drying of the mouth is a common side effect of some antidepressants and of irradiation to the head and neck for the treatment of cancer.

16. What is a videofluoroscopic swallowing study? How is it different from an esophogram?

A videofluoroscopic swallowing study (VFSS) is a fluoroscopic procedure that visualizes what happens within the head and neck when food or liquid is placed in the mouth and swallowed. The bolus is made visible usually by adding barium. Both passage of the bolus and motions of structures are visualized and recorded on videotape, including whether the airway is protected from contamination by foodway contents. Playing the videotape at slow speed facilitates a precise understanding of swallowing dynamics.

Because the study is intended to reflect normal eating and drinking, VFSS is conducted with the subject standing or sitting. Gravity plays an important role in this position, interfering with the analysis of muscle contraction for bolus propulsion, particularly with respect to the esophagus. An esophogram, or contrast study of esophageal function, is conducted in the horizontal position for this reason.

17. Who should be referred for a VFSS?

Patients who complain of difficulty in swallowing (dysphagia) or who are thought to have an abnormality of swallowing. A swallowing assessment is commonly performed by a speech-language pathologist with specialized knowledge in swallowing. VFSS will likely be done in collaboration with a radiologist or another physician with privileges to perform fluoroscopy.

18. How much aspiration is too much?

No one knows. It is safe to assume that much is worse than a little and that solids are worse than liquids. However, acidity is an important variable, as pH 2.4 destroys lung.

19. What are the key prognostic factors to consider in recovery of swallowing function?

1. An **etiology compatible with physiologic change**. For example, inability to swallow safely commonly follows stroke. If there is general improvement neurologically, swallowing function is likely to change as well. However, if the neurologic and cognitive impairments remain unaltered, swallowing impairment is likely to remain. The length of time required for physiologic change varies greatly, extending to years in neurogenic dysphagia particularly.

2. The **capacity to incorporate compensations**. Overcoming resistance to modifying behavior is a necessity for much of rehabilitation. The resistance may be cognitive, as in the multiply disabled child who aspirates; emotional or psychophysiologic, as in hysterical dysphagia; or physical and physiologic, as in dysphagia associated with head and neck surgery for cancer.

3. The **acceptance of empiricism and imagination** as a useful strategy for problem-solving. A positive and creative attitude by both staff and patient is a part of a "let's try this" approach.

20. What are some common compensations for dysphagia?

Compensations for dysphagia are mostly measures to protect the airway. There are many. Dysphagia may be bolus-specific, with airway contamination being more likely with thin liquids than with thick ones, for example. Thickening liquids would be one compensation. Flexing the neck or **"chin tuck"** may prevent entry of liquid into the larynx, probably by facilitating forward motion of the larynx. Turning the head during swallowing may compensate for weakness of one side of the pharynx with pooling of retained fluid. Exercises to strengthen the muscles that elevate the larynx and teaching the patient to exhale immediately after swallowing may be helpful for obvious reasons. Teaching the effectiveness of compensations is best documented by VFSS. Teaching compensations is a bulwark of "swallowing rehabilitation."

21. Can patients with tracheostomy or ventilator dependency swallow?

The presence of a tracheostomy and its cannula is compatible with normal swallowing. However, it is commonly believed that the cannula may interfere with rise of the larynx and so inhibit the normal motions of swallowing. Also, with the absence of expiratory airflow through the glottis, the sweeping of the larynx and pharynx by the flow of expired air does not occur. Finally, the presence of a foreign object, the cannula, in the trachea may desensitize the airway, thereby raising the threshold for coughing and throat-clearing activity normally incident to airway contamination.

22. How is the modified Evans blue dye test used?

The **Evans blue test** of swallowing function is used in patients with tracheostomy. A diazo dye is applied to the tongue, and tracheal suctioning is used to detect the dye's presence in the trachea (positive test if dye is present). No dye should appear (negative test). A **modified Evans dye test** consists of feeding the patient boluses or foods colored by the dye. There is a good correlation between the Evans blue and modified Evans blue tests in that patients who test negative with the dye also test negative when given dyed food. A negative dye test is a reasonable basis for beginning oral feeding.

23. What factors should you consider when determining NPO versus PO status?

Pulmonary pathology due to aspiration in the presence of documented airway contamination during swallowing is a specific contraindication for oral alimentation and hydration. In the absence of pulmonary pathology ascribable to aspiration, PO ingestion despite aspiration is a judgment call. Among the variables are the patient's cognitive state and zeal for eating, the magnitude of airway contamination during swallowing, the characteristics of what is unsafely swallowed, the effectiveness of compensatory strategies, and the assumed capacity of the individual to withstand chronic aspiration. Because swallowing itself is the best exercise for its recovery, NPO is disadvantageous to treating dysphagia, even if indicated for protecting the respiratory system.

24. Will a gastrostomy prevent aspiration?

No. A gastrostomy provides an alternative to swallowing for nourishing the patient. It does not protect against aspiration of saliva or of gastric contents which reach the pharynx by reflux.

25. Why do stroke patients have the most difficulty swallowing thin liquids?

Thin liquids freely disperse into all the nooks and crannies of the pharynx and larynx. They also leak through compromised valves, such as the appositions of the vocal folds or the velum against the posterior wall of the pharynx. Thicker liquids, on the other hand, disperse less freely. The dysphagic patient often has greater difficulty protecting the airway against penetration by thin than by thick liquids.

26. How are ultrasound and manography used to evaluate swallowing?

Ultrasound has proved useful primarily in studying the oral stage of swallowing, in particular the motions of lingual muscles. It has not found use in studying pharyngeal or laryngeal events, where imaging involves contrast.

Manography, or the study of pressures, has been applied to esophageal dynamics for years. Transducers which can be placed within the foodway and the simultaneous recording or presentation of pressure and fluoroscopic image on a single video monitor (videofluoromanometry) are recent technologic advances which hold promise.

27. How does a unidirectional valve facilitate safe swallowing in a patient with a tracheostomy?

A unidirectional valve added to the tracheal cannula allows inspiration through the cannula into the airway but blocks expiration through the cannula, forcing expired air through the glottis and upper airway. Restoring phonation and throat-clearing capability are among the advantages. The preservation of expiration through the larynx helps blow out foodway contaminants which might otherwise penetrate more deeply into the airway. A number of valves have been made over the years, including ball valves and membrane valves, such as the popular Passy-Muir valve.

BIBLIOGRAPHY

1. Bartlett JG: Aspiration pneumonia. In Baum GL, Wolinsky E (eds): Textbook of Pulmonary Disease. Boston, Little, Brown, 1983, pp 583–593.
2. Cogen R, Weinryb J: Aspiration pneumonia in nursing home patients fed via gastrostomy tubes. Am Gastroenterol 84:1509–1512, 1989.
3. Hassett JM, Sunby C, Flint LM: No elimination of aspiration pneumonia in neurologically disabled patients with feeding gastrostomy. Surg Gynecol Obstet 167:383–388, 1988.
4. Heimlich JH: A life-saving maneuver to prevent food choking. JAMA 234:398–401, 1975.
5. Kirby N, Barnerias MJ, Siebens AA: An evaluation of assisted coughing in quadriparetic patients. Arch Phys Med Rehabil 47:705–710, 1966.
6. Linden P, Kuhlmeier KV, Patterson C: The probability of correctly predicting subglottic penetration from clinical observations. Dysphagia 8:170–179, 1993.
7. Linden P, Siebens AA: Dysphagia: Predicting laryngeal penetration. Arch Phys Med Rehabil 64:281–284, 1983.
8. Siebens AA: Rehabilitation for swallowing impairment. In Kottke FJ, Lehman JF (eds): Krusen's Handbook of Physical Medicine and Rehabilitation. Philadelphia, W.B. Saunders, 1990, pp 765–777.
9. Siebens AA, Tippett DC, Kirby N, French J: Dysphagia and expiratory air flow. Dysphagia 8:266–269, 1993.
10. Tippett DC, Siebens AA: Using ventilators for speaking and swallowing. Dysphagia 6:94–99, 1991.

23. NUTRITIONAL ASSESSMENT AND MANAGEMENT

Eli D. Ehrenpreis, M.D., and Tim L. Popovitch, M.S., R.D., L.D.

1. What is meant by malnutrition?
An imbalance between nutrient intake and bodily requirements. It is due to faulty or inadequate nourishment from malassimilation, insufficient food intake, or dietary indiscretion.

2. Name some common methods to assess the nutritional status of a patient.
Nutritional history
    Changes in body weight, food diaries, GI symptoms, ability to obtain food, general mental status, and swallowing ability
Clinical evaluation
    Physical examination
        Muscle strength
        Skin evaluation
        Neurologic exam
    Anthropometric measurements
        Height and weight
    Biochemical studies
Medical record review
    Prior history of nutritional deficiency or intestinal diseases
    Documented weights from previous clinical visits

3. How does kwashiorkor differ from marasmus?
Kwashiorkor is a form of malnutrition in which protein deficiency predominates. It is characterized by peripheral edema, skin changes, and abdominal distension. **Marasmus**, another form of malnutrition, results in profound muscle wasting with dry skin and loss of subcutaneous fat. Overlap between these two syndromes may be seen in some malnourished patients.

4. What does the term wasting syndrome mean?
Wasting syndrome is rapid loss of weight, often accompanied by loss of lean body mass. It may occur in patients with chronic renal failure. The HIV wasting syndrome, an AIDS-defining illness, is the involuntary loss of > 10% of baseline body weight accompanied by chronic diarrhea or weakness and documented fever. It carries a poor prognosis.

5. How common is malnutrition in hospitalized patients?
The incidence of malnutrition in hospitalized medical patients in the United States is between 30 and 50%.

6. How does one assess a patient's energy requirement?
Energy requirements for individuals are estimated by determining the basal metabolic rate (BMR). Requirements vary in individuals according to their level of activity. A variety of methods are used to estimate the BMR:
  1. Harris-Benedict equation
     Male kcal: $66 + (13.7 \times \text{weight in kg}) + (5 \times \text{height in cm}) - (6.8 \times \text{age})$
     Female kcal: $655 + (9.6 \times \text{weight in kg}) + (1.8 \times \text{height in cm}) - (4.7 \times \text{age})$
  2. Simple estimation
     30 kcal/kg – 25%

   3. Hamwai formula
      Desirable body weight (lb) × 10 = basal kcal required
   4. Kilocalories per kilogram method
      Sedentary activity: Ideal body weight (IBW) × 20–30
      Light activity: IBW × 25–35
      Moderate activity: IBW × 30–40
      Marked activity: IBW × 45–50
   5. WHO method
      Uses a table to predict BMR based on body weight
   6. Indirect calorimetry
   7. Direct calorimetry

7. How is ideal body weight calculated?

Ideal body weight is a person's weight that is considered "normal" for a particular age, sex, and body frame. It is estimated from comparison tables, the most common of these being the Metropolitan Life Insurance Tables.

8. How does distribution of body fat differ between men and women?

Men generally have distribution of excess body fat higher (abdominal) than women (thighs and buttocks). The old adage for this is apples (men) and pears (women). The percentage of fat in the body is higher in women than men in all age groups.

Percentage of Body Fat by Age

	M (%)	F (%)
Newborn	14	14
10 yr	13	19
15 yr	13	25
25 yr	21	28
65 yr	28	34

9. What serum markers are diminished in patients who are malnourished?

Cholesterol	Total protein
Triglycerides	Albumin
Creatinine	Prealbumin
Blood urea nitrogen	β-carotene
Total lymphocyte count	

10. What is meant by nutritional support? How is it administered?

Nutritional support is the provision of necessary nutrients (calories, protein, water, vitamins, and minerals) to patients who are unable to take in these nutrients on their own by eating. Nutritional support is administered in two primary ways: enteral and parenteral.

11. What are common indications for total parenteral nutrition (TPN) in hospitalized patients?

Careful assessment of patients for malnutrition and inability to achieve adequate nutrition should be made prior to initiation of TPN in hospitalized patients. Indications for TPN include:
Inability to eat
Nonfunctioning or poorly functioning GI tract
Hypermetabolic conditions with decreased ability to take in nutrients
Protracted nutrient losses with severe malnutrition
Pre- and post-surgery with expected prolonged course prior to return to normal bowel function
Preop patients who are malnourished
Adjunctive therapy in patients with inflammatory bowel disease

12. What are common complications of total parenteral nutrition?

TPN requires the placement of a catheter into a central vein for administration to prevent phlebitis from high nutrient concentration of administered solutions.

Catheter-related complications	Specific nutrient deficiencies
Pneumothorax	Fatty acids
Thrombophlebitis	Trace elements (e.g., Se, Zn)
Carotid artery laceration	Vitamins
Mediastinal hematoma	**Septic complications**
Hydrothorax	Line sepsis
Brachial plexus injury	Septic shock
Metabolic complications	Local wound infection
Hypoglycemia	
Hyperglycemia	
Abnormal serum levels of other electrolytes	

13. What role does glutamine serve in metabolism?

Glutamine has received attention in nutrition-related research because of its presumed role in maintaining mucosal integrity in the small intestine. Addition of glutamine to parenteral and enteral nutritional formulas normalizes intestinal morphometry in patients receiving chemotherapy and radiation. Glutamine has also been shown to result in improvement in metabolic parameters (such as fluid and nitrogen balance) in animal models of hypermetabolism and in the clinical setting.

14. How does weight loss affect prognosis in malnourished patients?

Weight loss of > 20% is associated with significant deficits in organ function, resulting in increased morbidity and mortality. Weight of < 48% of IBW is considered to be incompatible with survival. This information is based on data from concentration camps in World War II and political prisoners voluntarily fasting in Northern Ireland.

15. How is enteral nutrition support administered?

Oral intake of liquid supplements
Nasogastric feeding tubes
Gastrostomy or jejunostomy tubes
    Endoscopically placed
    Surgically placed

16. What common complications are seen with enteral nutrition support?

Mechanical	Gastrointestinal	Metabolic
Tube displacement	Diarrhea	Hypoglycemia
Aspiration	Constipation	Hyperglycemia
Nasopharyngeal irritation	Nausea/vomiting	Other electrolyte disturbances
Skin irritation		Individual nutrient deficiencies
Wound infection		
Fasciitis		
Tube occlusion		

17. What is the difference between a PEG and a PEJ?

The introduction of techniques for endoscopic placement of percutaneous feeding tubes has allowed for administration of nutrients to a large number of patients who cannot eat but are poor surgical candidates. **Percutaneous endoscopic gastrostomy** (PEG) tubes are placed directly from the exterior of the abdominal wall into the stomach. **Percutaneous endoscopic jejunostomy** (PEJ) tubes, which may reduce the risk of aspiration, require a mature PEG tract. A thin tube is placed into a preexisting PEG. The tip of this tube is then dragged with an endoscope and deposited in the distal duodenum or proximal jejunum.

18. How does one choose the appropriate form of enteral nutritional support?

Initially, the length of time enteral support will be required is determined. Short-term naso-gastric feedings or long-term PEG or PEJ feedings may be needed. Secondly, a formula based on the patient's capacity to absorb and digest nutrients is selected. There are a number of formulas available are specifically tailored to clinical conditions (e.g., malabsorption, diabetes, renal and hepatic diseases).

19. What methods are available for assessing the adequacy of administered nutritional support?

Clinical

Daily weights	Temperature
Vital signs	Motor strength
Fluid balance	Calorie counts

Laboratory

Electrolyte panel	Transferrin levels
Glucose dipsticks	Prealbumin levels
Triglyceride levels	Retinol-binding protein to assess visceral
Transferrin	protein status
Completed blood counts	Acid-base balance
Nitrogen balance	Vitamin and mineral status

20. How does fiber affect bowel function?

Delays emptying of food from the stomach
Decreases intestinal transit time (soluble fiber)
Increases intestinal transit time (insoluble fiber)
Increases fecal volume
Increases gas production (H_2, CO_2, methane) in the colon from fermentation

21. What is the difference between soluble and nonsoluble fibers?

Soluble fibers (gums, pectin, and mucilages) form gels which decrease intestinal transit time. Insoluble fibers binds with water to form a sponge-like consistency that increases transit time. Soluble fibers also lower serum cholesterol levels, which insoluble fibers do not.

Soluble dietary fibers	Insoluble dietary fibers
Pectin	Lignin
Gum	Cellulose
Mucilages	Some hemicellulose
Some hemicellulose	

22. What is the average daily fiber intake in the United States?

1.5 gm/1000 kcal (or 3–5 gm/day). The American Dietetic Society recommends 20–35 gm/day (10–13 gm/1000 kcal).

23. Which vitamins are antioxidants?

Vitamins C, E, and A.

24. What are the fat-soluble vitamins? What conditions cause deficiencies in these?

Vitamins A, E, D, and K. Intestinal disorders causing fat malabsorption, such as celiac sprue, scleroderma, and small bowel resection, cause deficiencies of these vitamins. Vitamin D deficiency also occurs in renal failure and with decreased sunlight exposure.

25. What vitamin deficiencies are commonly seen in the United States?

None. Nutritional deficiencies are seen in individual patient groups, however.

Patient Group	Deficiency	Etiology
Alcoholic	Thiamine, folate	Poor intake
AIDS	B_{12}, zinc, β-carotene	Malabsorption
		Hypermetabolism?
Elderly	B_{12}	Lack of intrinsic factor
		Achlorhydria
Small bowel resection	B_{12}, fat-soluble vitamins	Malabsorption
Pancreatic disorders	B_{12}, fat-soluble vitamins	Malabsorption
Celiac sprue	Fe, folate, fat-soluble vitamins	Malabsorption
Gastric resection	Fe, B_{12}	Malabsorption
Pregnancy	Fe, folate, Ca	Increased requirement

BIBLIOGRAPHY

1. Burkitt DP, Walker ARP, Painter NS: Effect of dietary fiber on stools and transit times, and its role in the causation of disease. Lancet 2:1408–1414, 1972.
2. Fischer JE: Total Parenteral Nutrition, 2nd ed. Boston, Little, Brown & Company, 1991.
3. Florida Dietetic Association: Handbook of Medical Nutrition Therapy: The Florida Diet Manula, 1995 ed. Tallahassee, Florida Dietetic Association, 1995.
4. Groff JL, Gropper SS, Hunt SM: Advanced Nutrition and Human Metabolism, 2nd ed. St. Paul, West Publishing, 1995.
5. Guenter P, Muurahainen N, Simons G, et al: Relationships among nutrition status, disease progression, and survival in HIV infection. J Acquir Immune Def Syndr 6:1130–1138, 1993.
6. International Life Sciences Institute Nutrition Foundation: Present Knowledge in Nutrition, 6th ed. Washington, DC, International Life Sciences Institute, 1990.
7. Krotkiewski M, Bjorntrop P, Sjostrom L, et al: Impact of obesity on metabolism in men and women: Importance of regional adipose distribution. J Clin Invest 72:1150–1154, 1983.
8. National Research Council: Recommended Dietary Allowances, 10th ed. Washington, DC, National Academy Press, 1989.
9. Page CP, Hardin TC, Melnik G: Nutritional Assessment and Support: A Primer, 2nd ed. Baltimore, Williams & Wilkins, 1994.
10. Shils ME, Olson JA, Shike M: Modern Nutrition in Health and Disease, 8th ed. Malvern, PA, Lea & Febiger, 1994.

24. SPEECH-LANGUAGE PATHOLOGY EVALUATION AND TREATMENT

Donna C. Tippett, M.P.H., M.A., CCC-SLP

1. Explain the difference between speech and language.

The term **speech** refers to motor acts that result in the production of sounds through the co-ordination of muscles involved in respiration, phonation, resonance, and articulation. The term **language** refers to symbolic organization of sounds into meaningful and purposeful words and sentences to represent thought.

2. Who should be referred for a speech-language pathology evaluation?

The short answer is that you can refer anyone for a speech-language evaluation who has a communication or swallowing impairment. The etiologies of these disorders may be **developmental** (e.g., developmental language delay secondary to mental retardation, dysarthria secondary to cerebral palsy) or **acquired** (e.g., aphasia following left hemisphere stroke, dysarthria associated with multiple sclerosis, alaryngeal speech following laryngectomy, dysphagia secondary to brainstem stroke). If there is a question regarding the appropriateness of the referral, the speech-language pathologist can perform a screening evaluation before giving a lengthy assessment.

3. What are some examples of problem areas that speech-language pathologists treat?

Speech-language pathologists screen, identify, assess and interpret, diagnose, rehabilitate, and sometimes prevent disorders of:

Speech: articulation (dysarthria), fluency (stuttering), voice (dysphonia)

Language: aphasia

Oral-pharyngeal function: dysphagia

Cognition: disorders of attention, orientation, and memory following closed head injury

4. Are some individuals poor candidates for speech-language therapy?

It is difficult to make a definitive statement regarding candidacy for speech-language therapy given the diversity of patient populations and disorders seen by speech-language pathologists. However, it is usually true that treatment should be deferred for patients who are obtunded, sedated, or very ill. Variables which may be of prognostic value include:

Age at onset of disorder: the older the patient, the poorer the prognosis

General health: the healthier the patient, the better the prognosis

Motivation and cooperation: high degrees of motivation and cooperation are favorable prognostic signs

Environmental factors: family support can facilitate carryover of treatment objectives

Etiology: progressive diseases are associated with poorer outcomes, but therapy still may include compensatory strategies to facilitate communication and swallowing

Initial speech-language pathology evaluation results: responsiveness to diagnostic therapy is a favorable outcome variable

5. How are the aphasias classified?

There is no universally accepted nomenclature, and several schemes use different names for the same combinations of symptoms (e.g., Wernicke's aphasia = receptive aphasia = syntactic aphasia). One commonly used classification system, associated with the **Boston school of aphasia,** relies on an examination on fluency, comprehension, repetition, and word finding to make the diagnosis.

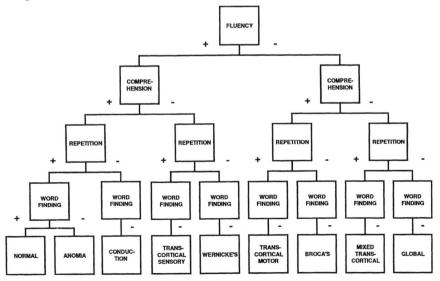

Classification of aphasias.

Aphasias are often difficult to classify in practice. It is important to distinguish fluent aphasias from language of confusion or psychotic speech. Fluent aphasias localize to the temporal area of the brain and may not be associated with a hemiparesis, making some people think the patient is just nuts. (Hint: these aphasic patients often have a hemianopsia or other subtle neurologic deficit). Dysfluent aphasias are more anterior, near the motor strip, and usually associated with a right hemiparesis, so the diagnosis of a stroke is readily apparent.

6. Name some common evaluation tools used to assess aphasia.

Comprehensive Tests of Aphasia

TESTS	PURPOSES	AREAS ASSESSED
Boston Diagnostic Aphasia Examination	Generates test scores for diagnosis of classic anatomically based aphasias	Conversational and expository speech Auditory comprehension Oral expression Understanding written language Writing Supplementary language and nonlanguage tests
Porch Index of Communicative Ability	Measures overall communicative ability and tracks recovery of language ability over time	Pantomine Reading Auditory Verbal Visual Writing Copying
Western Aphasia Battery	Classifies various aphasic syndromes and evaluates severity of impairment	Spontaneous speech Comprehension Repetition Naming Reading Writing Praxis Construction

7. Explain some of the terminology associated with aphasia.

Neologisms: substitutions of entirely invented words for correct ones

Semantic paraphasias: word substitutions belonging to the same semantic class (e.g., *chair* for *table*)

Phonemic paraphasias: substitutions of one sound for another (e.g., *fable* for *table*)

Jargon: fluent but incomprehensible speech due to severity of paraphasias

Telegraphic speech: speech output which includes substantive words (e.g., nouns, verbs) but omits grammatical modifiers (e.g., articles, conjunctions, pronouns)

Agrammatism: sparse, hesitant, groping speech limited to the most essential content words

Logorrhea: "press of speech"; fluent speech with unnecessary words and neologisms; speech is more abundant than normal speech

Echolalia: meaningless repetition of other's utterances, meaningless repetition of other's utterances

Palilalia: pathologic repetition of syllables or sounds; associated with degenerative brain diseases

8. What is VAT, VIC, MIT, and PACE therapy?

These represent treatments designed to address specific problems.

VAT—Using Visual Action Therapy, global aphasic patients learn to associate objects and their functions with action pictures and drawings of objects and later to produce gestures to indicate objects.

VIC—Using Visual Communication Therapy, global aphasic patients learn to use a system of arbitrary symbols to respond to commands, answer yes/no questions, and express needs and feelings.

MIT—Melodic Intonation Therapy, used with Broca's aphasics, capitalizes on preserved melodic production in the right hemisphere to facilitate speech production. Patients are taught to intone phrases, initially in unison with the speech-language pathologist and later independently.

PACE—Promoting Aphasics' Communicative Competence emphasizes a functional rather than a question-answer approach. The patient and clinician convey information in conversation using whatever means is necessary—speech, gesture, drawing, writing, mime.

9. What are language of confusion and language of generalized intellectual impairment: How are these differentiated from aphasia?

Neuropathologies of Language	Etiologies	Features	Distinguishing Characteristics
Language of confusion	Diffuse, bilateral cerebral hemisphere damage, often traumatic	Reduced recognition and understanding of environment, faulty memory, unclear thinking, disorientation, irrelevance, confabulation, confusion on open-ended tasks	Intact vocabulary and syntax; performance can improve if structure is provided
Language of generalized intellectual impairment	Diffuse, bilateral cerebral hemisphere damage (e.g., dementia)	Deterioration of performance in more difficult language tasks; reduced efficiency in all modes; greater difficulty on tasks requiring better retention, closer attention, powers of abstraction and generalization	Language impairment roughly proportional to impairment in other mental functions; evidence a lack of information rather than irrelevance
Aphasia	Commonly left unilateral cerebral hemisphere damage	Impaired ability to understand and/or express language (i.e., listening, speaking, reading, writing)	Language impairments disproportionate to impairment of other intellectual functions

10. What is crossed aphasia?

An aphasia following a lesion in the hemisphere ipsilateral to the preferred hand (i.e., a right-handed person becoming aphasic following a right hemisphere lesion, a left-handed person becoming aphasic following a left hemisphere lesion). Even though this phenomenon is quite unusual (occurring in < 2% of right-handed aphasics and 30% of left-handed aphasics), the Wada test is often performed prior to temporal lobotomies to confirm language dominance. This test involves injecting a barbiturate into a carotid artery, anesthetizing one hemisphere, and causing loss of language if that hemisphere is dominant.

11. Can an adult become a stutterer following a stroke?

Cortical dysfluency is described primarily in association with left hemisphere cerebrovascular accidents (CVA), but also following right CVAs, bilateral CVAs, closed head injuries, and penetrating head injuries. Dysfluency can also be psychogenic. Distinguishing neurogenic from psychogenic dsyfluency can be complicated and require a therapeutic trial to determine the diagnosis. Neurogenic dysfluency can persist for several weeks to several years. Psychogenic dysfluency is characterized by rapid responsiveness to treatment.

12. Define apraxia.

Apraxia is a disorder of the execution of learned movement that cannot be explained by weakness, incoordination, sensory loss, or lack of attention to commands. Cortical lesions are considered the neuroanatomic basis for apraxia in general. Apraxias include those of construction, dressing, gait, and speech.

Two anatomic explanations for apraxias have been advanced. In the **disconnection theory**, apraxia results because motor areas are isolated from cortical areas subserving language comprehension and visual abilities. For example, the motor ability to whistle may be intact, and an individual may whistle spontaneously, but when asked to whistle, the individual cannot perform this action on command. In the second theory, apraxia is thought to result from lesions occurring in cortical centers that store movement patterns. This theory does not explain why these movements can be performed adequately at times.

13. What is apraxia of speech?

It is one of many types of apraxia and is characterized by highly variable and unpredictable substitutions of sounds, often unrelated to intended sounds, blockages and repetitions similar to stuttering, and slow effortful output secondary to reduced capacity to program the positioning of speech muscles and the sequencing of muscle movements for the volitional production of sounds. There is no significant weakness, slowness, or incoordination of speech muscles in reflexive or automatic acts.

14. What is agnosia?

Agnosia is a disorder of recognition that may occur in any of the major sense modalities despite adequate perception in these modalities (e.g., audition, vision, tactile sensation). An **auditory agnosia** is an inability to match an environmental noise with its sound source. For example, a patient may not be able to recognize a watch from its ticking but can identify a watch placed in his hand. A **visual agnosia** is an inability to identify an object on visual confrontation. For example, a patient may not be able to identify his wife when shown a picture but can describe her appearance (e.g,. blonde hair, brown eyes).

15. What is alexia with agraphia? Without agraphia?

Alexia with agraphia is a defect in reading and writing. Speaking and listening may be completely spared. The lesion is in the left angular gyrus, which bridges the posterior temporal and parietal regions. In severe cases, patients may be unable to match upper and lower case letters, write letters from dictation, or transcribe from print into cursive. Milder forms are characterized by slow reading and errors in spelling and syntax.

In **alexia without agraphia**, or pure word blindness, the ability to recognize words is lost, although auditory comprehension, oral language, and writing are unaffected. These patients can write but cannot read their own handwriting! They may "read" laboriously via letter-by-letter spelling. The lesion is in the splenium of the corpus callosum, left visual cortex, and lingual gyrus. The language area of the left hemisphere is deprived of all visual input from both the left and right hemispheres.

16. What is pure word deafness?

In pure word deafness, auditory comprehension of language is profoundly impaired without affecting speaking, reading, and writing. These patients can hear and react to sounds (e.g,. car horn, glass breaking), but they generally cannot repeat what is said to them. If they can repeat, their productions are phonemic approximations. The lesion destroys both the major primary auditory cortex (Heschl's gyrus) and the subcortical fibers; therefore, information cannot reach Wernicke's area. The adjacent auditory center is destroyed, and the contralateral one is isolated by interruption of transcallosal fibers.

17. What is Gerstmann's syndrome?

This syndrome includes acalculia, finger agnosia, right/left confusion, and agraphia. Patients cannot add or subtract simple numbers, identify fingers on their hands, tell left from right, or write, even though upper extremity function is intact. The lesion is in the parieto-occipital region of the left hemisphere.

18. Describe the typical communication deficits seen in patients with right cerebral hemisphere damage.

These patients demonstrate relatively intact language but impaired communication abilities. Key features are insensitivity to context (i.e., missing nuances and subtleties), difficulty organizing information in a meaningful way (e.g., answering questions with tangential, unnecessary information), difficulty "reading" facial expressions and gestures, inability to understand figurative language, lack of affect, caustic sense of humor, neglect or denial of their deficits, better performance on structured than open-ended tasks, and writing errors (e.g., omission of strokes, letters or words; perseveration of strokes, letters, words; failure to dot *i*'s and cross *t*'s; extra capitalization).

19. How are dysarthria classified?

As with the aphasias, dysarthrias can be classified in a variety of ways—by age at onset, etiology, cranial nerve involvement, or speech component involvement. A well-known classification system is the Mayo Clinic approach, which reflects neuroanatomic and neurophysiologic bases for dysarthrias. Six types of dysarthria were delineated:

Flaccid dysarthria (in bulbar palsy)
Spastic dysarthria (in pseudobulbar palsy)
Ataxic dysarthria (in cerebellar disorders)
Hypokinetic dysarthria (in parkinsonism)
Hyperkinetic dysarthria (in dystonia and chorea)
Mixed dysarthria (in disorders of multiple motor systems, such as multiple sclerosis)

20. What are the components of speech production?

Speech production can be divided into the processes of **respiration, phonation, resonance, and articulation**. The respiratory mechanism provides the driving force for speech production. The larynx is the primary determinant of voice quality. The movement of the soft palate (velum) determines resonance quality. Lingual, labial, and mandibular function affect articulation.

21. How is speech production assessed?

The speech-language pathologist assesses speech production by examining nonspeech and speech aspects of each component of oral motor function. Perceptual deviations are analyzed to classify the type of dysarthria. Speech intelligibility is rated at a single word level and in conversation. An overall level of severity is assigned depending on the degree of impairment in speech and nonspeech tasks and unintelligibility.

Nonspeech and Speech Tests of Oral-Motor Function

COMPONENTS	EXAMPLES OF NONSPEECH TESTS	EXAMPLES OF SPEECH TESTS
Respiratory mechanism	Breathing rate at rest	Maximum sustained phonation
Larynx	Elevation with swallow	Ability to change loudness
Velum	Velar position at rest	Maintenance of oral/nasal contrasts
Tongue	Lingual range of movement	Lingual articulation
Lips/face	Facial symmetry	Labial articulation
Jaw	Mandibular strength against resistance	Mandibular assist for articulation

22. What is diadochokinesis?

The capacity for rapid, repetitive, alternate movement of a part of the body from one position to another (e.g., pronation, supination) as well as repetitive articulatory movements. Speech-language pathologists test this by requiring patients to repeat several nonsense syllables—*puh, tuh, kuh*—and the multisyllabic combination *puh-tuh-kuh*. Normative data are available for the number of repetitions over time: for example, norms for a 6-year-old are 20 repetitions of *puh* in 4.8 sec, 20 repetitions of *tuh* in 4.9 sec, 20 repetitions of *kuh* in 5.5 sec, and 10 repetitions of *puh-tuh-kuh* in 10.3 sec. Both slow and excessively fast diadochokinetic rates suggest neuromuscular abnormalities.

23. How does a speech-language pathologist improve a patient's speech intelligibility?

Dysarthria therapy is two-fold—one aspect is increasing patients' physiologic support for speech (e.g., range and speed of movement of articulators, respiratory support for speech, laryngeal coordination), and the other part is teaching them to make the best use of their residual physiologic support. Physiologic support can be improved by modifying posture, increasing strength, improving tone, and/or enhancing coordination. For example, a speech-language pathologist and physical therapist may collaborate to improve respiratory support for speech through the use of an abdominal binder or use isometric exercises to increase strength of articulators. Speech-language pathologists also design drills that patients practice to address specific problems, such as clearly articulating lingual consonants. Compensatory techniques can be taught, such as decreasing rate of speech and "over-articulating" to facilitate precise consonant production, minimizing background noise to compensate for reduced vocal intensity, or planning phrasing of words to avoid speaking on residual air.

24. What are some communication alternatives to natural speech?

Alternatives can be divided into oral and nonoral options. A familiar oral option is the use of an electrolarynx by a laryngectomee. Nonoral options include handwriting, gestures, and augmentative communication systems which range from simple alphabet and picture boards to sophisticated computer systems.

25. Explain how patients with tracheostomy can speak.

If a patient has a tracheostomy cannula with a deflated cuff or a cuffless cannula, the patient can speak by plugging the tracheostomy cannula if that is medically appropriate, occluding the tube intermittently with a finger (the hygiene of this practice is questionable at times) or applying a unidirectional valve to the hub of the cannula. A unidirectional speaking valve remains open during inspiration, allowing the patient to inhale at the level of the cannula, but closes during expiration, forcing airflow through the larynx and allowing phonation to occur.

BIBLIOGRAPHY

1. Darley FL, Aronson AE, Brown JR: Motor Speech Disorders. Philadelphia, W.B. Saunders, 1975.
2. Fletcher SG: Time-by-count measurement of diadochokinetic syllable rate. J Speech Hear Res 15:763–770, 1972.
3. Geschwind N: The apraxias: Neural mechanisms of disorders of learned movement. Am Sci 63:188–195, 1975.
4. Goodglass H, Kaplan E: Assessment of Aphasia and Related Disorders. Philadelphia, Lea & Febiger, 1972.
5. Heilman KM, Rothi LJG: Apraxia. In Heilman KM, Valenstein E (eds): Clinical Neuropsychology. New York, Oxford University Press, 1985.
6. Myers PS: Profiles of communication deficits in patients with right cerebral hemisphere damage. In Brookshire RH (ed): Clinical Aphasiology: Proceedings of the Conference. Minneapolis, BRK Publishers, 1979.
7. Netsell R, Daniel B: Dysarthria in adults: Physiologic approach to rehabilitation. Arch Phys Med Rehabil 60:502–508, 1979.
8. Siebens AA, Tippett DC, Kirby N, French J: Dysphagia and expiratory air flow. Dysphagia 8:266–269, 1993.
9. Tippett DC, Siebens AA: Distinguishing psychogenic from neurogenic dysfluency when neurologic and physiologic factors coexist. J Fluency Dis 16:3–12, 1991.
10. Tippett DC, Siebens AA: Using ventilators for speaking and swallowing. Dysphagia 6:94–99, 1991.
11. Tippett DC, Siebens AA: Preserving oral communication in individuals with tracheostomy and ventilator dependency. Am J Speech-Lang Pathol 4:55–61, 1995.
12. Wertz RT: Neuropathologies of speech and language: An introduction to patient management. In Johns DF (ed): Clinical Management of Neurogenic Communicative Disorders. Boston, Little, Brown, 1985.

25. INTERDISCIPLINARY ROLE OF THE PHYSICAL THERAPIST

Elizabeth Augustine, P.T., M.S.

1. What is physical therapy (PT)?

The American Physical Therapy Association defines PT as a health profession whose primary purpose is the promotion of optimal human health and function through the application of scientific principles to prevent, identify, assess, correct, or alleviate acute or prolonged movement dysfunction.

PT derives from the ancient art of medicine that the Greeks and Romans employed (i.e., massage, water, etc.). The practice of PT today is more comprehensive and complex and falls within four categories: **therapeutic exercises, electrotherapy, hydrotherapy,** and **massage.** By using a combination of techniques within these categories, physical therapists are able to rehabilitate patients to their highest level of function.

2. When did the profession of PT begin in the United States?

Modern PT began in the U.S. during World War I. At that time, physical therapists were called **reconstruction aides**, and their purpose was to rehabilitate wounded soldiers. **Mary McMillan** has been recognized as the first physical therapist in the United States. She received her training in England and worked there before returning to the U.S. in 1915. During the 1940s with World War II and the 1950s with the national polio epidemic, the demand for physical therapists grew. The practice of PT has expanded from the traditional hospital setting to outpatient clinics, home health agencies, private practice, schools, rehabilitation centers, skilled nursing facilities, and other.

3. How are goals formulated in PT?

Before the physical therapist assesses the patient, he or she will review the patient's medical chart and then talk with the physician and, when possible, members of the patient's family to determine the patient's prior level of function, diagnosis, current functional status, and precautions. The therapist then interviews the patient and assesses vital signs, cognition, range of motion, strength, deep tendon reflexes, sensation, skin integrity, balance, coordination, mobility status (bed mobility, transfers, wheelchair mobility, and gait), safety, endurance, and rehabilitation potential.

The therapist integrates this information and establishes short-term and long-term goals based on the discrepancies between the patient's prior level of function and current status. In general, the goals are organized hierarchically to enhance recovery and promote independence as soon as possible. The physical assessment determines the techniques, equipment, frequency and duration of treatment required to achieve the goals.

After a catastrophic injury, mobility limitations often determine the level of care a patient will require and the respective rehabilitation intervention. As such, a focus of therapy that emphasizes safe personal mobility with modified techniques (equipment) or natural support (family, hired attendant) is critical to an overall program that transitions a patient from institution to home.

4. How can PT goals be best defined to express the expected outcomes?

Goals are positive measurable statements documenting physical capabilities and functional activity. They are established to provide a focus for therapeutic intervention, as well as the participation of the interdisciplinary team and the patient's social support system. They must relate directly to the personal goals of the patient and the overall objectives of the long-term rehabilitation plan.

5. What is the role of the physical therapist within the interdisciplinary team?

After the therapist has made an initial evaluation of the patient's current status, this information is presented at the patient's care conference. Together, the different members of the rehab team establish an integrated treatment plan and goals for the patient. The therapist's responsibilities during the patient care conferences are:

1. To communicate the patient's mobility capabilities and restrictions
2. To update the team on the patient's progress and/or regression
3. To be attentive to the goals of the other team members and facilitate their achievement through patient interaction during PT sessions.

6. A 74-year-old man with Parkinson's disease fell at home and was unresponsive. At the hospital, the patient has dehydration, and his wife relates that her husband has lost weight and has been eating poorly lately. The wife's own health problems prevent her from caring for her husband at home. After hospitalization, he is transferred to a skilled nursing facility for rehabilitation. What should be his integrated treatment plan and goal?

Different rehabilitation professionals make their initial assessments and meet with the director of nurses during the patient's care conference to establish an integrated treatment plan and rehab goals plus discharge planning. The patient's number-one problem is identified as his poor nutritional status. On their initial evaluations, Nursing noted that the patient does not eat all of his meals (< 50%), Speech noted he has poor swallowing skills due to poor head position, Occupational Therapy reported that he requires moderate assistance for self-feeding skills, and Physical Therapy noted his poor sitting posture.

Goal (functional outcome): The patient will be able to sit independently with good posture for 30–60 minutes during 3 meals/day and feed self independently, consuming 75–100% of the meal within 3 weeks.

Treatment plan: During lunch, the patient will have good sitting posture (with 50–75% verbal and tactile cueing to maintain midline position for 20 minutes before fatiguing) to facilitate swallowing while the patient feeds self with appropriate foods (with 25–50% verbal and tactile cueing) and consumes 50–75% of the meal under the direction of the occupational therapist.

The patient's poor swallowing skills are secondary to poor sitting posture. The physical therapist will instruct the occupational therapist in the appropriate verbal and tactile cueing for the patient to maintain midline with good sitting posture during a meal. For continuity of the treatment plan, the occupational therapist will instruct the patient's nurse and/or family member of the specific intervention and expected outcomes, so that they can reinforce these skills with the patient when the occupational therapist is not present. As the patient continues to improve during his PT sessions (which focus on sitting balance and truncal muscular strengthening) and requires less cueing, the physical therapist will relay this new information to the occupational therapist so that adjustments can be made in the lunchtime treatment plan.

BIBLIOGRAPHY

1. American Physical Therapy Association: Physical Therapy Education and Societal Needs: Guidelines for Physical Therapy Education. Alexandria, VA, APTA, 1984.
2. Fletcher GF, Banja JD, Jann BB, Wolf SL: Rehabilitation Medicine: Contemporary Clinical Perspectives. Philadelphia, Lea & Febiger, 1992.
3. Scully RM, Barnes MR: Physical Therapy. Philadelphia, J.B. Lippincott, 1989.

26. OCCUPATIONAL THERAPY

Nancy Carlson, M.S., O.T.R./L

"Man through the use of his hands as energized by mind and will can influence the state of his own health."

—M. Reilly, occupational therapy's hypothesis

1. What information does the OT evaluation provide?

Occupational therapists implement individual person-centered treatment to achieve constructive patient performance in self-care, work, and leisure. The OT evaluation explains how the patient's physical, psychological, and cognitive limitations interfere with performance of self-care, work, and leisure tasks. Intact and impaired motor, sensory, cognitive, and perceptual skills are assessed. Functional abilities in self-care and occupational role-related tasks are addressed.

2. What type of questions is the OT evaluation likely to answer?

1. Is the patient capable of dressing independently?
2. Is the patient safe when preparing meals?
3. Is the patient able to perform duties as a parent or employee?

3. Explain the differences between performance areas and performance components.

In Uniform Terminology, occupational **performance areas** are self-care, work, and leisure. **Performance components** are the specific skills or abilities of the patient. Performance components contribute to the patient's ability to function in specific performance areas.

Occupational Performance Areas

Activities of daily living
1. Grooming
2. Oral hygiene
3. Bathing
4. Toilet hygiene
5. Dressing
6. Feeding and eating
7. Medication routine
8. Socialization
9. Functional communication
10. Functional mobility
11. Sexual expression

Work activities
1. Home management
2. Care of others
3. Educational activities
4. Vocational activities

Play or leisure activities
1. Exploration
2. Performance

Performance Components

Sensory motor components
1. Sensory integration
   Sensory awareness
   Sensory processing (tactile, visual, etc.)
   Perceptual skills
2. Neuromuscular
   Reflex
   Range of motion
   Muscle tone
   Strength
   Endurance
   Postural control
   Soft-tissue integrity

Cognitive integration and components
1. Level of arousal
2. Orientation
3. Recognition
4. Attention span
5. Memory (short-term, long-term, etc.)
6. Sequencing
7. Categorization
8. Concept formation
9. Intellectual operations in space
10. Problem-solving
11. Generalization of learning
12. Synthesis of learning

3. Motor
    Activity tolerance
    Gross motor coordination
    Crossing the midline
    Laterality
    Bilateral integration
    Praxis
    Fine motor coordination/dexterity
    Visual motor integration
    Oral motor control

Psychosocial skills and psychological
    components
    1. Psychological
    2. Social
    3. Self-management

4. What is SOAP? How is it reflected in the typical OT evaluation?

The OT evaluation includes various components known as **SOAP:**

S = **Subjective** information on patient's alertness, motivation, preferences, concerns

O = **Objective** information on current level of functioning in ADLs, IADLs, upper-extremity function, endurance level, skin condition, cognitive abilities, perceptual skills

A = **Assessment** of performance levels and their relation to occupational performance

P = **Plan** of intervention strategies, goals, and recommended timetable

5. What are long-term goals and short-term goals?

Long-term goals (LTGs) and **short-term goals** (STGs) are short quantifiable statements that focus the efforts of the therapy process. They are developed from the patient's current level of functioning and the self-care, work, and leisure tasks that the patient is expected to perform. Both STGs and LTGs are derived in collaboration with the patient and prioritized to meet unique and immediate needs. STGs are usually set to be accomplished within a week or a few weeks; LTGs describe an expected level of functioning in a performance area. For a patient with cardiopulmonary disease, an LTG may be "patient will complete morning self-care without rest periods." An STG contributing to this LTG may be "patient will bathe in the shower for 5 minutes without shortness of breath 3 of 5 days."

6. Define ADLs.

Activities of daily living (ADLs) are activities that each person must do on a daily basis for self-care. Eating, dressing, bathing, and grooming are examples of the ADL tasks. The ability to complete these tasks without assistance is valued highly by the North American culture and is considered paramount to rehabilitation. Most people wish to attain independence with these tasks following injury or a disease process. Since independence in ADL tasks represents a cultural bias, however, it is important to determine each patient's perspective before initiating intervention.

7. How do instrumental ADLs differ?

Instrumental ADLs, or IADLs, are similar to ADLs in that they are necessary for living independently. IADLs involve the patient's work and leisure tasks and are strongly related to patient roles. Meal planning, preparation, service and clean-up, marketing, care of home and clothing, and yard work are examples of IADLs. The table illustrates a common method of scoring ADL and IADL abilities.

ADL and IADL Scoring

SCORE	QUALITATIVE TERM	DESCRIPTION
1	Total assistance	Patient is unable to do any part of the task.
2	Maximum assistance	Patient requires maximum physical assistance or verbal cues to complete the task, assistance with 75% of the task.
3	Moderate assistance	Patient requires moderate physical assistance or verbal cues to complete the task; assistance with 50% of the task.

(Table continued on following page.)

ADL and IADL Scoring (Continued)

SCORE	QUALITATIVE TERM	DESCRIPTION
4	Minimal assistance	Patients requires minimal physical assistance or verbal cues to complete the task; assistance with 25% of the task.
5	Supervision	Patient is able to perform the task without physical contact but needs cuing or coaxing and/or cannot be left alone because of cognitive deficits, poor balance, or other safety issues.
6	Modified independent or independent with setup	Patient is able to complete the task once someone sets it up for him (e.g., dresses self once the clothing has been selected and obtained, or feeding self once adaptive equipment has been set up).
7	Independent	Patient is able to complete the task, including setup, with or without adaptive equipment; note should be made of adaptive equipment used.

8. What is the tradition of the occupational therapy process and outcome?

OT as a profession is deeply rooted in the philosophy that people are self-directed, adaptive beings who engage in purposeful activity. This purposeful activity comprises human **occupation**. OTs promote health through increased skill, competency, or efficacy. The OT profession emerged from a mental health tradition: precursors were WWI reconstruction aides who helped soldiers with wartime neuroses. The field was further advanced by Adolph Meyer, M.D., the first chairman of psychiatry at Johns Hopkins, who introduced the idea that humans need and are nurtured by activity. Throughout the years, occupational therapy has retained its psychiatric roots. It seeks to establish and restore both physical and psychosocial well-being in everyday living.

9. How does manual muscle strength relate to ADLs?

Muscle strength is measured by a specific procedure called a manual muscle test (MMT). MMT scores the maximum contraction of a muscle or muscle group. Good to normal muscle strength is necessary to complete ADLs with good endurance.

Muscle Strength Scoring

SCORE	GRADE	DESCRIPTOR	DESCRIPTION
0	0	None	No muscle contraction can be seen or felt
1	T	Trace	Contraction can be felt, but there is no motion
–2	P–	Poor minus	Part moves through incomplete ROM with gravity decreased
2	P	Poor	Part moves through complete ROM with gravity decreased
2+	P+	Poor plus	Part moves through incomplete ROM (< 50%) against gravity or complete ROM with gravity decreased against slight resistance
–3	F–	Fair minus	Part moves through incomplete ROM (> 50%) against gravity
3	F	Fair	Part moves through complete ROM against gravity
3+	F+	Fair plus	Part moves through complete ROM against gravity and slight resistance
4	G	Good	Part moves through complete ROM against gravity and moderate resistance
5	N	Normal	Part moves through complete ROM against gravity and full resistance

10. How do OT evaluations differ for the various diagnoses?

All OT evaluations address similar occupational performance areas—self-care, work, and leisure—but all OT evaluations are not identical. They differ based on the type of health care facility and the patient diagnosis. Since different diagnoses manifest differences in performance components, assessment varies with specific deficit areas.

Impaired Performance Components Related to Common Diagnoses

IMPAIRED PERFORMANCE COMPONENT	COMMON DIAGNOSIS
ROM, muscle strength	Neurologic and neuromuscular conditions, including CVA, head injury, multiple sclerosis, ALS, cerebral palsy
UE AROM/PROM	Quadriplegia, burns, UE amputation, arthritis, multiple sclerosis, ALS, orthopedic, and other traumatic injuries
UE coordination	Head injury, cerebral palsy, CVA, multiple sclerosis, tumors, and other neurologic conditions
Mobility without UE involvement/LE dressing	Paraplegia, osteoarthritis, LE amputations, burns, hip/knee fractures and replacements
Cognitive, perceptual, and sensory	Head injury, CVA, multiple sclerosis, Parkinson and Alzheimer diseases, mental retardation, spinal cord injury, head injury

UE, upper extremity; LE, lower extremity; CVA, cerebrovascular accident; ALS, amyotrophic lateral sclerosis.

11. Which evaluation tools are used most frequently?

Occupational Performance	*Performance Components*	*Environment Assessment*
ADL	**Upper-Extremity Functioning**	**Traditional**
Canadian Occupational Performance Measure	Manual Muscle Test dynometer	Postoccupancy Evaluation
Katz Index	Pinch gauge	Person-Environment Fit Scale
Barthel Index	Goniometer (ROM)	The Enabler
Kenny Self-Care Examination	Semmes-Weinstein monofilaments	The Source Book
Functional Independence Measure	Weinstein Enhanced Sensory Test	Accessibility checklist
Klein-Bell ADL Scale	Purdue Pegboard	Multiphasic Environmental Assessment Procedure
Work	Jebsen-Taylor Test of Hand Function	Comprehensive Occupational Assessment and Training System (COATS)
Loma Linda Univ. Activity Sort	Nine-Hole Peg Test	
WEST Tool Sort	Moberg Pick-Up Test	**Computerized**
Social and Prevocation Information Battery-Revised	Minnesota Rate of Manipulation Test	Assessment Tool
Occupational Skills Assessment Instrument	Crawford Small Parts Dexterity Test	Home Modification Workbook
Vocation Adaptation Rating Scales	Box and Block Test	The Source Book
Vocational Behavior Checklist	Bennett Hand Tool	LIFEASE
Functional Capacity Evaluation	WEST	
Leisure	O'Connor Finger Dexterity Test	
Activity Index (revised)	**Cognitive-Perceptual Tools**	
Meaningfulness of Activity Scale	Lowenstein OT Cognitive Assessment	
Leisure Diagnostic Battery	Test for Orientation for Rehabilitation Patients	
Leisure Satisfaction Questionnaire	Galveston Orientation and Amnesia Test	
Minnesota Leisure Time Physical Activity Questionnaire	Motor Free Visual Perception Test	
	Allan Cognitive Level Test	
	Mini-Mental Status Examination	
	Motor Free Visual Perception Test	
	Test of Visual Perceptual Skills	
	MEAMS (Middlesex Elderly Assessment of Mental Status)	
	Psychosocial Tools	
	Comprehensive OT Evaluation	
	Social Interaction Scale	
	Task Checklist	

12. Why is evaluation of the patient's home environment, workplace, and community crucial to the assessment process?

Occupation—participation in self-care, work, and leisure activities—occurs in the context of specific environmental settings: e.g., bathing in the bathroom, cooking in the kitchen, word-processing at a desk, and shopping at the mall. The environment influences these functions, and environmental adaptations and modifications permit individuals with disabilities to function with maximum independence in their homes and communities: e.g., ramps for increased access to a wheelchair-bound patient, removal of small throw rugs for an elderly person with poor visual acuity, etc.

In the environment, social and psychological barriers are often as detrimental as physical barriers and must be evaluated in the assessment process. Patients with AIDS, for instance, may be unable to participate in work and leisure activities because of society's misperceptions of the disease. It is important to begin assessment of the environment—home, work, and community— early in the rehab process. Equipment requires time for funding approval and delivery, and people require time for emotional and attitudinal adjustment.

BIBLIOGRAPHY

1. American Occupational Therapy Association—Representative Assembly: Uniform terminology for occupational therapy, 2nd ed. Am J Occup Ther 43(12):808–814, 1989.
2. Bowker AM: Assessment: The keystone of treatment planning. Occup Ther Health Care 1(2):25–32, 1993.
3. Christiansen C, Baum C: Occupational Therapy: Overcoming Human Performance Deficits. Thorofare, NJ, Slack, 1991.
4. Daniel MS, Strickland LR: Occupational Therapy Protocol Management in Adult Physical Dysfunction. Gaithersburg, MD, Aspen, 1992.
5. Hopkins HL, Smith HD: Willard and Spackman's Occupational Therapy. Philadelphia, Lippincott, 1993.
6. Granger CV, Hamilton BB, Linacre JM, et al: Performance profiles of the functional independence measure. Am J Phys Med Rehab 71(2):84–89, 1993.
7. Pedretti LW, Zoltan B: Occupational Therapy: Practice Skills for Physical Dysfunction. Baltimore, Mosby, 1990.
8. Reed KL: Quick Reference to Occupational Therapy. Gaithersburg, MD, Aspen, 1991.
9. Reilly M: The 1961 Eleanor Clark Slagle Lecture—Occupational therapy can be one of the great ideas of 20th century medicine. Am J Occup Ther 16:1–19, 1962.
10. Trombly CA: Occupational Therapy for Physical Dysfunction. Baltimore, Williams & Wilkins, 1995.

27. PSYCHOSOCIAL ASSESSMENT

Jacquelyn Dayton, M.S.W., C.S.W.

1. How does the social worker contribute to the psychosocial well-being of the patient?

By trying to understand what happened to the person and what effect this has on his or her psychologic or social functioning. Through interview the social worker elicits the patient's personal perception of disablement and the impact on his or her life. These open encounters are therapeutic in themselves. The social worker then reflects patient perceptions and goal priorities during interdisciplinary team meetings. Through counseling and therapy, the social worker enhances the patient's personal role performance, coping skills, and family function.

2. Do all patients have to see a social worker?

On a rehab unit, it is expected that the social worker assess and provide services to *every* patient. This differs from the situation on an acute care medical unit, where many patients have illnesses that resolve quickly so that they may only be hospitalized for 24 hours. Most rehab patients stay on the unit for at least 10 days and experience some residual effects of their illnesses. Adjustment, both physical and emotional, may be necessary for a safe community discharge. Therefore, the doctor should strongly encourage people to work with the social worker and should alert the social worker about any patient who seems to be especially in need.

3. What exactly is the role of the social worker?

A social worker's purpose in the rehab process is twofold. First, she or he helps the person to plan for his or discharge home in a timely manner so that the plans are in place by the time the person is ready to go. Second, the social worker helps patients deal with the stress caused by the sudden and drastic changes in physical, social, and emotional functioning. The social worker coordinates the interdisciplinary plan to minimize the biopsychosocial impact on the life of the person and the family.

4. What areas are addressed by the social worker in preparing the patient for discharge?

The first areas of focus are on the physical and social aspects of the person's situation. The social worker must understand what happened to the person and what his or her level of disability will be. Obviously, the level of function will differ for a person who has had a hip replacement and a person who has had a stroke. Bearing this in mind, the worker assesses the person's needs in relation to the home environment:

Does he or she live in a house or an apartment?

Are there stairs to climb?

Does the person live alone?

Does he or she have friends or family nearby to assist with care?

Are there financial resources available to hire help if necessary?

What type of assistance can be provided by the health insurance (assuming that the person has health insurance)?

If there is no insurance, is he or she eligible to apply for Medicaid?

The social worker must find the answers to these questions quickly, given increasingly shortened hospital stays. Then she or he must act as the patient's advocate and help arrange the necessary supports to effect a safe and timely discharge.

5. What are the common stresses that the social worker can help the patient face?

Rehabilitation social work deals with the stress caused by the sudden and drastic changes in the patient's physical, social, and emotional functioning. In addition, the family may feel anger and reluctance to care for the patient at home or overwhelmed with the decisions and responsibilities of discharge planning. As long-term therapy is not possible, the social worker's role is to provide supportive short-term counseling to help the patient and family deal with the imminent crisis of the impending discharge.

Naomi Golan has written of the material-arrangemental axis and the psychosocial axis. Along the first axis, the social worker helps the patient and family carry out the concrete tasks of arranging for community care. Having the family apply for Medicaid or work with the physical and occupational therapists to learn the patient's care are two examples of this. Simply taking some action helps the person to feel more in control of the problem and thus promotes a sense of competency. Along the second axis, the person continues to grapple with the stress of the change. This stress does not go away immediately and sometimes not at all. However, the person and family can get a sense of pride from adapting to the illness.

6. What are the usual discharge options?

When a persons comes to a rehabilitation unit, the expectation is that he or she will return to his or her previous living situation. In the ideal situation, the patient will be able to take care of his or her own personal needs with little or no assistance. In most cases, though, the patient needs some help with personal and household chores. Usually, these needs can be met with a combination of informal supports (i.e., family or friends) and homecare services, such as a visiting nurse, physical therapist, or home health aide. Such services may be reimbursed by the health insurance company. For patients with greater needs or with little support at home, other options for care must be considered:

Long-term care facility: When the person is extremely dependent on others for care, the need is greater than community resources can meet, and a long-term care facility must be considered. Such a facility, also called a skilled nursing facility or subacute rehabilitation facility, exists to provide care for patients who are chronically ill. Physical, occupational, and speech therapy are provided, but only to maintain the person's current level of functioning.

Subacute facility: This facility exists to provide therapy to people who are progressing but at a slower rate, too slow to justify care on an intensive rehab unit. For example, a person with a broken hip may not be allowed to put full weight on the affected limb for a few months. A subacute facility can help the person to continue to regain strength until the weight-bearing status is increased.

Again, planning for such a transfer can be very distressing. The social worker must guide the family through this process and act as advocate for them.

BIBLIOGRAPHY

1. Alter M, Roth EJ, Stiens SA, Young MA: How to choose an appropriate rehab program. Patient Care (Oct 30), 1995.
2. Hanks M, Poplin DE: The sociology of physical disability: A review of the literature and some conceptual perspectives. Deviant Behavior: An Interdisciplinary Journal 2:309–328, 1981.
3. Meyerson L: The social psychology of physical disability: 1948 and 1988. J Soc Issues 44:173–188, 1988.
4. Nagler M: Perspectives on Disability: Text and Readings on Disability. Palo Alto, CA, Health Markets Research, 1993.

28. VOCATIONAL REHABILITATION COUNSELING

Rochelle Habeck, Ph.D., and Ruth Torkelson Lynch, Ph.D.

"The two essential tasks in life are to love and to work."

—Sigmund Freud

1. What is a vocation? How does it relate to personhood and disability?

A vocation is a person's life work. In our dominant culture, one's occupation plays a central role in personal and social identity and is viewed as a potential source of meaning and life satisfaction. From a psychological perspective, one's vocation is often an important medium for developing self-concept and self-esteem. From the social perspective, work determines much of one's social situation in the community, such as place of residence, social network, family well-being, income, insurance and benefits. When disability interferes with one's vocational role, and that role has played a significant part in the person's identity and socioeconomic well-being, then the impact of disability has a far greater effect than on function alone.

2. What is vocational rehabilitation?

Vocational rehabilitation (VR) is the coordinated and systematic process of professional service devoted to an individual with disability to enable and sustain employment. The basic components of VR services are vocational assessment, counseling, goal-setting and service planning, case management, intervention with service delivery, job placement, and follow-up. The **outcomes** of the VR process for people with disabilities are participation in competitive employment, personal job satisfaction, and satisfactory job performance.

3. Who are qualified providers of VR and what do they do?

Rehabilitation counselors (RCs) provide VR services to persons with disabilities. Qualified professionals possess the master's degree in rehabilitation counseling and are certified rehabilitation counselors (CRC). They are vocational experts who operate from a counseling base and an ecological perspective to provide a broad range of services for individuals with disabilities related to vocational goals and independent living. RCs function as problem-solvers with clients to determine barriers to vocational adjustment within specific environments and to plan and implement interventional strategies. RCs assess psychosocial and vocational impacts of disability and orchestrate a wide array of environmental resources to effect appropriate employment outcomes. This includes interventions directed toward the individual to develop individual capacities as well as interventions directed toward the (work) environment to remove barriers and accommodate the needs of individuals with disabilities.

4. What role does VR play in a comprehensive rehabilitation program?

The vocational services component plays several essential roles:

1. Expresses the program's belief and commitment that patients can become and will be assisted in becoming full participants in society despite disablement.

2. Establishes vocational goals that provide a focus and incentive for other treatment goals and interventions within the rehab setting (e.g., effort at maintaining skin integrity and enhancing range of motion and ADL skills is reinforced for the person who sees how these goals relate to being able to engage in rewarding life activities and relationships).

3. Specifies the tasks, skill requirements, and environmental factors of the target outcome setting.

4. Provides direct intervention to reduce the effect of handicapping factors and disability on the person.

5. Directs the process from the inception toward economic productivity and self-satisfaction, which are values in the cost-benefit analysis of comprehensive rehabilitation.

5. Which patients should be referred for vocational rehabilitation counseling?

Persons with either short-term or long-term career disruption due to injury or illness can potentially benefit from VR counseling. In addition to assisting individuals whose career paths have been altered by disability, RCs can help individuals with disabilities save their jobs and/or careers through accommodations, such as job modification or redesign. Also, persons of school or working age who have not established a vocation or work history prior to disability are likely to require comprehensive VR services.

6. At what point in the rehabilitation process should VR begin?

For individuals who were employed at the time of injury, the team should establish communication immediately about vocational concerns with the individual, family, and employer. Expectancies seem to form soon after a disability occurs, on the part of the workplace (supervisor, coworkers, employer, etc.) as well as the individual and family. Once the period of crisis has stabilized and the bond with the employer and work role is less robust, it is more difficult to engender vocational expectations and negotiate options. Furthermore, the eligibility requirements for disability benefit programs create unintended disincentives that can discourage return to work by the individual and family. The probability of reemployment drops dramatically when a person is away from work for more than 30–60 days, and the probability decreases to 10–20% by 2 years.

Early and effective contact with the workplace, including plans for resumption of employment, reaffirms the bond between the employer and employee and develops awareness of alternatives for effectively using the patient's future capacities. Early intervention and counseling increase the probability of return to work by assisting the person, family, and employer to develop effective coping strategies for the short-term and desirable expectations for the future. Early vocational interventions directed toward the person focus on counseling to develop motivation, personal control, goal-setting, and problem-solving capabilities.

7. How are goals and outcomes determined in VR?

The major goal of VR is paid employment in the competitive labor market as a means to full participation in society. In the past, this goal was not deemed feasible for many clients because of the severity of their disabilities. With increasing options for support resources (e.g., personal care assistants, job coaches, health insurance continuation in trial work periods) and environmental accommodation (e.g., accessible buildings, job modifications, assistive technology), type and severity of disability are less significant determinants of vocational outcomes. Rather, vocational goals are formulated from a combination of:

- Individual factors—e.g., interests, values, mental and physical abilities, education, work experience, age
- Environmental factors—e.g., desired place of residence, community resources
- Policy factors—e.g., legal and benefit requirements
- Labor market opportunities
- Program funding

In our post-ADA society competitive employment and independent living are now presumed as potential goals for all individuals.

8. Is a full-time job the only goal of VR services?

Full-time, competitive employment is not the universal goal of all individuals, with or without a disability. Part-time employment, employment with temporary or permanent supports in the community, self-employment, and home-based programs are also viable outcomes of the VR process. In some cases, temporary or transitional objectives, such as independent living in the community, enhanced education, or skill training, may need to be pursued first to improve the chances of achieving and retaining competitive employment as an eventual goal. However, VR services that result in outcomes other than paid employment may be less desirable or not reimbursable in some policy systems.

9. How are specific VR services determined in each case?

Many of the services and interventions provided in the VR process depend on the needs and goals of the client, which are determined in the assessment process. However, the particular public and/or private policies and programs applicable to the individual's disability and employment circumstances (e.g., compensable work injury, automobile accident, military-related condition, long-term illness, or disability) will determine (a) eligibility for services, (b) priority for services, (c) nature and extent of services, (d) acceptable outcomes, (e) provider of services, and (f) concurrent policy initiatives (e.g., ADA, Social Security, personal care funding). Each program and policy has its own definition of disability and benefit provisions and therefore differs in eligibility criteria and service options.

In the case of a work-related injury covered under **workers' compensation**, the goal of VR is to return the injured worker to the preinjury job (or an alternative position) as quickly and efficiently as it is feasible and safe to do. Therefore, services are focused on rapid job placement using transferable skills and accommodations, with limited support for preparation for a new career.

Within **pediatric rehabilitation**, where the client is school-aged and has no prior work experience, VR services may focus on career development and career exploration through vocational education and temporary employment or internships in the community, in conjunction with the school program and rehabilitation facilities. Plan development and advocacy for future educational and vocational services from the appropriate resources (e.g., special education, state vocational rehab agency, automobile insurance carrier) are other major aspects of service.

10. How do environmental influences impact VR planning and service delivery?

An individual's characteristics and the person's functional limitations are certainly not the only determinants of independent living and employment outcomes. Discriminatory policy and practices as well as environmental barriers are also major handicapping factors. VR services must address modifications in both the physical and interpersonal aspects of the worksite:

Physical structures (e.g., equipment or architectural features)
- Modify the physical environment of the workplace
- Restructure job duties or process so that essential functions can be performed
- Provide augmentative or assistive devices, equipment, qualified readers, or interpreters
- Coordinate accessible transportation

Interpersonal elements (e.g., coworkers and supervisors)
- Teach direct supervisors how to facilitate accommodation needs with production and performance requirements
- Solicit supportive coworkers (**natural supports**) to provide accommodations or assistance
- Develop endorsement by management of the accommodation plan

Interventions will be most effective when the client, VR counselor, and individuals from the targeted environment are in close collaboration.

11. What types of interventions are used to help people return to employment?

Return-to-work services for individuals employed at the time of disability onset include:
- **Early vocational intervention**—supportive counseling; planning and coordination with the individual, representatives of the workplace, and medical providers
- **Worker–environment assessment**—work capacity evaluation, functional job analysis, worksite demands
- **Vocational counseling** and **case management**—analysis of work history, values, and interests; goal-setting; problem-solving; coordination of resources/services
- **Worker-environment interventions**—individual adaptations, job accommodations, worksite modifications
- **Reassessment and problem-solving**—follow-up services upon return to work

12. What interventions are used to help people who *don't* have jobs to return to?

Placement services are available for individuals who have a vocational goal and are ready for employment but do not have a job or employer to return to:
- **Job-search skills training**
- **Direct placement assistance and job development**
- **Supported employment** (for individuals with severe disabilities)
- **Other approaches** (e.g., work hardening, on-the-job evaluation, volunteer work, work-adjustment training)

13. Describe a possible VR plan for an individual with chronic low back pain who is returning to a preinjury job.

Vocational intervention at the **person** level:
- Analysis of the person's functional capacities in relation to the demands of preinjury work
- Counseling regarding the impact of the injury on the individual's career
- Coordination of rehab efforts to maximize that individual's confidence, strength, endurance, and flexibility to perform the demands of the job

Vocational intervention at the **environmental** level:
- Detailed analysis of the work environment and job demands
- Determine if aspects of the job, or the worker's method of performing the job tasks, can be modified to accommodate current functioning and reduce chances of further aggravation of the condition

Vocational plan—develop and negotiate gradual return to work or temporary modified duty plan with all parties to assist the individual in an early transition back to work.

14. Describe the VR plan for an individual with traumatic brain injury who was unemployed at the time of injury.

Vocational intervention at the **person** level:
- Assess residual skills, determine interests and aptitudes, develop a career plan

Vocational intervention at the **environmental** level:
- Consider requirements of suitable occupations and work environments and potential accommodation strategies (i.e., rely on residual functioning, avoid areas of disability)

Vocational plan—provide social skills training for use at the work environment; provide occupational retraining through continuing education or on-the-job training; use volunteer placement to develop general work behaviors or supported employment with a job coach to teach work skills at the job site; provide placement assistance or continued supported employment services depending on severity and capacities.

15. An individual with a spinal cord injury wishes to return to the former job. However, the person has substantial limitations in performing essential duties of the preinjury job, even with accommodations. What are the VR options?

1. **Same employer, same job:** If the person can return to the prior job, then the counselor can prepare a list of proposed solutions to maximize access and job performance (e.g., modifications to enhance building access, streamline the work station, accommodations for performance of job functions)

2. **Same employer, different job:** If return to the prior job is not feasible, even with accommodations, alternative employment within the company would be pursued, including retraining for the new job duties.

3. **New employer, different job:** A comprehensive plan to develop a new occupation with a new employer would be the third course of action.

16. Who pays for VR services?

The costs of **inpatient** VR services are usually bundled as an essential service through the per-diem rate of the rehab center or hospital or billed directly on a fee-for-service basis to the identified payer. Payment may be denied if these services are not covered within the policy. Typically, if the cost of services is billed to a third party, prior approval of the VR plan and the estimated services and costs are negotiated with the payer's claim representative. For individuals who lack insurance, coverage for early vocational services may be sought from the state VR agency through advocacy by the rehabilitation team.

The costs of **outpatient** VR services may be paid by a variety of sources. Typical private payers include workers' compensation insurance, long-term disability insurance, and auto insurance. Individuals who have no insurance or applicable coverage, who are unemployed, or who qualify for Medicare or Medicaid should apply for services from the state VR program, which are paid for through tax dollars.

17. Where can VR services be obtained in the community?

There are three major external sources for obtaining VR services:

1. **State division of vocational rehabilitation.** Each state has a public VR program that is funded through state and federal appropriations to provide services to individuals with mental or physical impairments. Referrals can be made directly to the local officer of the state VR agency.

2. **Private sector providers.** This is the fastest-growing segment of VR service providers, due in part to privatization of service delivery. These providers may be found in a variety of settings including independent practice, rehabilitation facilities, community agencies, linked regional networks, interstate corporations, and insurance companies. To make a referral to a private provider, the team should contact the payer to discuss the need for VR services and help determine who the appropriate provider will be.

3. **Employer-based programs.** Many employers, particularly large organizations which are self-insured, have some type of internal process for disability management and return to work, especially since the advent of the ADA.

BIBLIOGRAPHY

1. Boschen KA: Early intervention in vocational rehabilitation. Rehabil Counsel Bull 32:254–265, 1987.
2. Brodwin MG, Tellez F, Brodwin SK (eds): Medical, Psychosocial, and Vocational Aspects of Disability. Athens, GA, Elliott & Fitzpatrick, 1993.
3. Maki DR, Riggar TF (eds): Rehabilitation Counseling: Profession and Practice. New York, Springer, 1996.
4. Parker RM, Szymanski EM (eds): Rehabilitation Counseling: Basics and Beyond, 2nd ed. Austin, TX, Pro-Ed, 1992.

5. Roessler RT: A conceptual basis for return to work. Rehabil Counsel Bull 32:98–107, 1988.
6. Rubin SE, Roessler RT: Foundations of the Vocational Rehabilitation Process, 4th ed. Austin, TX, Pro-Ed, 1995.
7. Scheer SJ (ed): Medical Perspectives in Vocational Assessment of Impaired Workers. Gaithersburg, MD, Aspen, 1991.

29. RECREATIONAL THERAPY

David Tostenrude, C.T.R.S.

1. What is a recreation therapy (RT)?

Therapeutic recreation is defined by the National Therapeutic Recreation Society as services "to facilitate leisure, recreation, and play for persons with physical, mental, emotional, or social limitations in order to promote their health and well-being." RT is further defined by the American Therapeutic Recreation Association "as treatment services which restore, remediate, or rehabilitate in order to improve functioning and independence."

RT was incorporated into the medical model in the veterans and military hospitals during World War II. Sports and recreation programs were included in the rehabilitation process to address the needs of the "whole" person. Since then, RT has developed national professional organizations and therapists have been incorporated in many other settings.

2. Define leisure.

Leisure is defined differently by each of us. No matter how active or inactive an individual is, leisure has a part in that person's life. Leisure is activity, apart from the obligations of work, family, and society, to which the individual turns at will, for either relaxation, diversion, broadening his or her knowledge, or spontaneous social participation. Some people spend time outdoors hiking, boating, or mountain climbing, while others prefer working in the garden. In rehabilitation, it is critical to assess "what" leisure is to a person in order to identify the needs of the individual.

3. What is a recreation therapist?

A **Certified Therapeutic Recreation Specialist** (CTRS) is an individual who has fulfilled certification requirements through the National Council for Therapeutic Recreation Certification. To be awarded the CTRS certificate, an individual must meet eligibility requirements which include a professional internship and then pass the national exam. An RT is skilled professional, with a baccalaureate, masters, or doctorate degree in Therapeutic Recreation or in Recreation, with a specialization in Therapeutic Recreation from an accredited college or university.

4. How does the recreation therapist interact with the interdisciplinary rehab team?

The RT assesses the impact of the injury, disease, or disability on the patient's leisure lifestyle. Then, the RT presents his or her assessment to the team which then becomes part of the overall interdisciplinary plan. In addition, the role of the RT is to develop an individualized RT program that reflects not only the expressed needs of the patient but the treatment philosophy and the immediate goals of the other disciplines. The RT communicates with the other team members through documentation and charting, involvement in weakly team meetings, and coordination of interdisciplinary goals and interventions.

5. What programs does a recreation therapist involve the patient in?

RTs design leisure activities to obtain functional outcomes. Patients are involved in activities depending on the benefits associated with the specific activity, level of supervision targeted by the team or goals, and assessed capabilities of the patient.

1. **Treatment services**—The provision of prescribed leisure activities that directly promote functional improvement of skills and independence.

2. **Leisure education**—Programs designed for the acquisition and enhancement of diverse leisure-related knowledge, skills, and attitudes.

3. **Recreation participation**—Activities allow for self-motivated leisure activities that provide the opportunity for leisure skill development, self-expression, creativity, and enjoyment.

In all of these programs, the social environment, supervision, and locus of control are dependent on the RT's assessment of the patient needs and the nature of the activity. The RT must be flexible and attentive to the needs of the patient population, while having competency at evaluating leisure activities for their participation requirements and potential benefits.

For example, **aquatic therapy** is a popular modality for treatment to address spasticity, tone reduction, increase endurance, and cardiovascular fitness. Additional benefits include relaxation, swimming stroke development, improved self-image, and socialization. The RT assists the patient in locating community resources at home to continue after discharge. Aquatics may be part of the initial therapy program, but as the patient progresses, swimming may become an optional activity. In this aspect of the program, goals for aquatics then become self-directed rather than rehab-discipline-supported.

6. What outcomes does a recreation therapist attempt to achieve?

The outcomes targeted by the RT are a reflection of those specific needs of the individual. RT outcomes reflect improved adjustment to disability/illness, successful independence in the community, increased awareness of community resources, or the obtainment of leisure skills. Outcomes are measured through demonstration of knowledge or skill, reports of satisfaction, or behavioral observation. The RT is challenged to develop behavioral outcomes that identify the abstract nature of competence, independence, self-determination, and quality of life.

7. Describe community reintegration.

Community reintegration is facilitated by the RT, who assists the patient in transition from the hospital to living in the community. This experience is essential in the process of rehabilitation in order to develop confidence and to improve coping with often long-term hospitalizations associated with rehabilitation. As part of this program, natural supports are identified and included in this training to support independence and opportunities outside the home. Natural supports are family members, peers, and community programs. **Community outings** allow the patient to practice skills in the "real world." Outings are often accomplished either alone or in group settings depending on the patient goals. Community outings are an invaluable tool that involve the patient in experiences demanding interaction with peers and the public. These experiences challenge the patient's perception of disability and thereby improve adjustment, leading to a greater self-concept.

8. What is "play" therapy?

In addition to the many goals addressed in leisure, an important aspect of "play" is **coping**. Play is effective therapy because patients perceive involvement as nonthreatening. They do not have to make decisions during the activity that may affect their life, address possible dependency, or disability. The requirement is that they focus on the activity, and the result is skill acquisition, enjoyment, social stimulation, and stress reduction.

9. Is it just fun for the patients?

RT programs are fun. Additionally, they are designed not only to reflect the outcomes targeted for the patients, but also the interests of the patients. If you are working with an individual who used to paint for self-expression and relaxation, then an effective approach may be to get them involved in painting during rehabilitation. This work could reflect then the state of coping, self-concept, as well as relationships to society.

Individuals demonstrate natural behaviors and skills when they are acting without prompting. A key aspect of RT is the ability to involve patients in situations where they look past the long- or short-range goals associated with the activity, and thus the individual learns more and demonstrates the actual obtainment of a skill. An example is wheelchair mobility. The clinic provides an environment full of cues, scrutiny, and modification for accessibility. However, put that patient outdoors, and they suddenly have to contend with natural distractions, traffic, other people, weather, and terrain. This unique equation forces problem-solving from the patient and draws on their creativity, judgment, and skill. During this experience, the RT will see whether a patient has learned the skill adequately or needs further attention.

10. Why do RT programs differ so much from facility to facility?
RT programs differ widely among facilities because in addition to their CTRS training, many RTs have expertise and certifications in crafts, music, aquatics, downhill skiing, wilderness education, or sports, to name a few. An RT will use these skills to develop creative opportunities for goal achievement and skill acquisition. An RT program will develop a character that better addresses the diverse interests and backgrounds of the patients. Other influences include the resources of the RT department and the local community and the mission and vision of the medical center, rehabilitation section, and staff.

11. Why should you get the patient involved in the RT program?
The interdisciplinary team is made up of many professionals who interact with patients from different angles. The result is a holistic method of caring for the individual. As Abraham Maslow demonstrated in his theory of Self-Actualization, a "healthy person" is one who is able to satisfy both basic needs and higher metaneeds. These **metaneeds** include self-esteem, belongingness and love, safety, the ability to direct one's own life, and a sense of meaning to one's life. RT addresses these priorities in each patient and targets the outcomes to obtain independence and awareness beyond disability. An individual who is involved in meaningful activity and focus on wellness spends less on medical care in the long run.

BIBLIOGRAPHY

1. Dumazedier J: Toward a Society of Leisure. New York, Free Press, 1967, pp 16–17.
2. National Therapeutic Recreation Society: Code of Ethics. Arlington, VA, National Recreation and Park Association, 1990.
3. Peterson C, Gunn S: Therapeutic Recreation Program Design: Principles and Procedures. Englewood Cliffs, NJ, Prentice Hall, 1984, p 12.
4. Weiten W: Psychology Applied to Modern Life, 2nd ed. Monterey, CA, Brooks/Cole, 1986, pp 61–63.

30. REHABILITATION NURSING

Cynthia Zejdlik, R.N.

1. What is rehabilitation nursing?
The scope of rehabilitation nursing practice extends from primary preventive care through acute episodes of illness or injury, rehabilitation periods, community reintegration and beyond, to address health throughout the lifespan, including aging issues. The nursing process involves competencies in the interrelated steps of assessment, diagnosis, outcome identification, implementation, and evaluation, and includes an understanding of the following core concepts: communication, family and crisis theory, the change process, adjustment, adaptation, and coping, cultural diversity, group process and dynamics, functional status, growth and development, learning process, sexuality, socialization, role theory, safety, prevention, optimum wellness, quality of life, and advocacy.

2. How did the specialty practice of rehabilitation nursing evolve?

The foundation of rehabilitation nursing was laid during the mid-1800s when Florence Nightingale developed her first treatment plans that provided physical and psychological support while encouraging independence. By the turn of the century, rehabilitation references began to appear in nursing curricula and early journals. During World War I, the Red Cross recruited nurses to employ remedial exercises to returning soldiers, which laid the roots for medical social services and, eventually, the disciplines of occupational and physical therapy. By the 1950s, specialized education for rehab nurses started to appear, as the concept of custodial care began to crumble and the movement toward community reintegration for people with disabilities grew. The concept of specialized training and continuity of assignments has developed over the decades and reinforced the need for nurses with an in-depth understanding of rehabilitation and all of its complexities.

3. Which specialty nurses' associations are directly concerned with the rehabilitation field?

American Association of Neuroscience Nurses (founded in 1968)

Association of Rehabilitation Nurses (ARN, founded in 1974)

American Association of Spinal Cord Injury Nurses (founded in 1983)

The ARN offers Certification in Rehabilitation Nursing (the Certified Rehabilitation Registered Nurse, CRRN) based on a core curriculum and examination process with continuing educational requirements.

4. What are some rehabilitation nursing roles?

Primary care nurse. A designated registered nurse is accountable for the design and implementation of all aspects of nursing care for a patient in any given period of time.

Clinical nurse specialist. An expanded role implemented to advance clinical practice, education, consultation, and research, the clinical nurse specialist provides expertise in complex rehabilitation situations; guides the educational process for patients, families, and staff; and may provide consultation activities such as case-finding and management, marketing and community relations, or liaisons with payers.

Rehabilitation nurse case manager. According to the ARN, case management is defined as the process of planning, organizing, coordinating, and monitoring the services and resources needed to respond to an individual's health care needs, and it describes the various roles as facility- or agency-based, insurance-based or independent case manager.

Generalist practice. The professional nurse practicing as a generalist functions in a variety of capacities depending on basic education, specialized education including certification in rehab nursing, and clinical experience.

Advanced practice nurses. These nurses possess a graduate degree in nursing with a specialized focus, including interdisciplinary collaboration essential to comprehensive rehabilitation.

5. How do nurses implement rehabilitation?

Based on research to determine how to create a therapeutic milieu on a spinal cord injury unit, Nelson described optimal implementation of rehabilitation as four phases of community integration. These transitional phases, in one form or another, are adapted to multiple settings and specific disability populations.

1. **Buffering** is the nurturing and protective process of lessening, absorbing, or protecting individuals with a newly acquired disability against the shock of multiple ramifications and the indignities of being a patient.

2. **Transcending** helps people recognize and rise above culturally imposed limitations and negative beliefs about people with disabilities.

3. **Toughening** focuses on compensating for physical limitations, gaining independence, and maintaining social interactions without "using" the disability.

4. **Launching** exposes the disabled individual to the real world, explores the range of options for living in the community, promotes autonomy and decision-making, and enables the

person to leave the rehab program. Very often problems that people with disabilities face in community reintegration are social ones. Therefore, the more realistic links that can be made to the world "outside," the better.

6. How do rehabilitation nurses approach goal-setting in the rehab environment?

People often speak of rehabilitation as a journey without a map, where nurses are seen as guides or bridges. Expertise developed by rehab nurses has made it possible to predict functional expectations and help establish realistic goals for groups of individuals with similar disabilities. In the beginning, goals may be typically described as nursing goals, because individuals have little knowledge of what their potentials may be. As the rehabilitation process evolves, nurses seek active partnerships with individuals, and goals are modified to become more specific.

There is also a natural progression from simple to more complex tasks over the course rehabilitation. Continuous problem-solving is essential. In addition to psychosocial adaptation, maintaining optimal physiologic functions are of paramount concern, such as respiratory, cardiovascular, nutritional, urinary, bowel, and skin management. Re-establishing mobility and independence is as integral to nursing as it is to therapists and physicians. Nurses follow through and integrate what is learned in therapeutic sessions into daily activities, such as eating, bathing, dressing, transferring, and so on. Nurses also enhance the value of therapeutic sessions, treatments, and exercises by promoting general health measures, particularly to promote good nutrition, manage basic bodily functions reliably, and minimize pain and fatigue.

7. How do rehabilitation nurses know how hard to push?

Knowing when and how hard to push is critical. Most people who are newly disabled want staff to do a lot of things for them, which fosters unnecessary dependency. There is a balance between knowing when to assist and when the person needs to help himself or herself.

There is a big difference between getting tough and getting angry. Inexperienced staff do not always see the difference. When they watch an experienced staff member get tough with a patient, they interpret that it is acceptable to get angry, talk back, or freely ventilate their own feelings. Patients are able to discern the nurse's underlying motivation: whether it is to help become more independent, as in the case of toughening up, or that the nurse is frustrated, angry, or too busy.

BIBLIOGRAPHY

1. Association of Rehabilitation Nurses: Standards and Scope of Rehabilitation Nursing Practice, 3rd ed. Skokie, IL, ARN, 1994.
2. Hoeman S: Conceptual bases for rehabilitation nursing. In Hoeman S (ed): Rehabilitation Nursing: Process and Application. St. Louis, Mosby, 1996, pp 3–20.
3. Morrisey A: Rehabilitation Nursing. New York, G.P. Putnam's Sons, 1951.
4. Morrison M: On the threshold of outcomes management. Rehab Manag (Oct/Nov):105–107, 1992.
5. Mumma C, Nelson A: Models for theory-based practice of rehabilitation nursing. In Hoeman S (ed): Rehabilitation Nursing: Process and Application. St. Louis, Mosby, 1996, pp 21–23.
6. Nelson A: Developing a therapeutic milieu on a spinal cord injury unit. In Zejdlik C (ed): Management of Spinal Cord Injury. Boston, Jones & Bartlett Publ., 1992, pp 212–213.
7. Rehabilitation Nursing Foundation: The Specialty Practice of Rehabilitation: A Core Curriculum, 3rd ed. Skokie, IL, RFN, 1993.
8. Zejdlik C: Management of Spinal Cord Injury, 2nd ed. Boston, Jones & Bartlett Publ., 1992.

IV. Electrodiagnostic Assessment

31. GENERAL PRINCIPLES OF ELECTRODIAGNOSIS

Dennis D. J. Kim, M.D.

1. What is electrodiagnosis?

Electrodiagnosis is the process of taking a guided history and physical examination and recording spontaneous and evoked electromagnetic signals from a patient's nerves and muscles to clarify the etiology of symptoms and findings. The activity is recorded with a needle electrode and transmitted, via an amplifier, to an oscilloscope or digital visual display and a loudspeaker.

A physician called an **electromyographer**, who is usually a physiatrist or neurologist, carries out this process in three steps: examination, integrative interpretation, and reporting. The results indicate whether or not the electrophysiologic findings are normal and provide localization for the pathology, a suggested diagnosis, less likely etiologies, prognosis, and clinical management. Techniques employed include nerve conduction studies (electroneurography) and needle electromyography (EMG), somatosensory evoked potentials, and motor evoked potentials.

2. What is spontaneous activity?

After insertion of an EMG needle into normal muscle at rest, no electrical activity is seen. Spontaneous activity refers to electrical activity recorded in resting muscle after movement of the needle has ceased. Spontaneous discharges alone do not differentiate among neuropathic, myopathic, or neuromuscular transmission disorders.

3. Name the commonly observed spontaneous discharges and their characteristic "sounds."

Fibrillation potential—Clicking noises, like raindrops on the roof or static
Positive sharp waves—Pop, pop, pop, regular 2–20 Hz
Fasciculation potentials—Spontaneous, isolated, loud snaps
Myokymic discharges—Marching soldiers
Complex repetitive discharges—Motor boat or dive bomber that misfires occasionally, stops abruptly

4. Describe the EMG characteristics of a fibrillation potential.

Fibrillation potential is defined as a spontaneous action potential recorded from a single muscle fiber by a needle electrode located outside the endplate zone. The precise mechanism for generation of fibrillation potentials is not known, although the prevalent hypothesis is **"denervation hypersensitivity."** When a muscle fiber loses innervation, there is increased production of acetylcholine receptors and other membrane proteins, which are widely distributed on the muscle cell membrane. Fibrillations are also found in some myopathies, neuromuscular transmission disorders, metabolic disorders, and occasionally in healthy individuals.

5. What are positive sharp waves (PSWs)?

PSWs are spontaneous discharges usually seen together with or followed by fibrillations after motor nerve injury. A PSW is a spontaneous depolarization of a single muscle fiber recorded close to the stationary recording electrode tip.

6. What causes fasciculation potentials?

Fasciculation potentials result from the spontaneous discharge of a group of muscle fibers comprising either a whole or part of a motor unit. Fasciculations, when they occur in superficial muscles, are visible as twitches, but may not be seen if they occur in deep muscle. Their sources seem to be multiple and may be anywhere from the brain or spinal cord to terminal motor branches. Many study results indicate that most fasciculations originate distally.

Fasciculations can be seen in normal individuals and cannot be considered a pathologic finding unless accompanied by other EMG findings, such as fibrillation potentials and PSWs. EMG cannot differentiate between malignant and benign forms of fasciculations.

7. Describe the EMG characteristics of myokymic discharge.

Myokymic discharge is the electrical equivalent of the clinically observed **myokymia**, which is the undulating muscle movement observed on overlying skin or mucous membrane. Myokymic discharges are spontaneous bursts of a group of motor units potentials probably resulting from **ephaptic** transmission (muscle to muscle, axon to axon) between the motor units.

8. What are complex repetitive discharges (CRDs)?

These are continuous trains of polyphasic or serrated action potentials that may begin spontaneously or after needle movement. They have a uniform frequency, shape, and amplitude, with abrupt onset, cessation, or change in configuration. CRDs probably originate from ephaptic activation of groups of adjacent muscle fibers and are seen in both neuropathic and myopathic disorders. The term CRD is preferred to bizarre high-frequency discharges or pseudomyotonic discharges.

9. How can endplate spikes, fibrillations, and PSWs be differentiated? Why does a motor unit sometimes look like a PSW?

When a needle electrode records the **single muscle fiber action potential** inside the endplate zone, it will be recorded as an initially negative potential (endplate spikes), but outside the endplate zone, it will be recorded as a positive potential (fibrillation). There is no electrophysiologic difference between these two perspectives. Endplate spikes are caused by the irritating needle in the endplate. Therefore, when a electromyographer produces positive potentials after recording in several needle insertions at rest, they are more likely PSWs.

When recording a propagating **motor unit action potential** (MUAP) from the endplate zone with a monopolar electrode, the initial deflection will be negative because the potential is moving away from the recording electrode. However, if the recording electrode is placed near the tendon area, all oncoming potentials will be recorded as an initial positive deflection. A PSW will be spontaneous, recorded at rest, and independent of voluntary effort, while a positive MUAP will alter its firing rate with recruitment effort. If any doubt exists, the needle electrode should be repositioned away from the tendon or injured region of muscle. Also observe for consistency, firing pattern, and relationship to voluntary effort.

10. What is a motor unit? Describe its EMG characteristics.

The **motor unit** is the functional unit of centrally controlled muscle contraction. It includes the motor neuron, axon and branches, and all the muscle fibers innervated by that motor neuron.

Normally, each **single muscle fiber** is innervated by a single axon branch and produces an action potential of about 1–3 msec duration. This duration is almost the same as the fibrillation potential, although it may vary depending on the characteristics of the amplifier and recording electrode.

The diameter of the territory of a **motor unit** is usually about 5–10 mm. A monopolar EMG needle electrode typically records potentials from about 10–30 muscle fibers. The duration of a motor unit is about 6–15 msec and is primarily affected by conduction time along the axon branches and the muscle fiber spatial distribution. Motor unit durations become longer with monopolar needle recording, lower temperature, larger motor unit size advanced age, and neuropathy.

Motor units range in size from 10–1,500 fibers. The amplitude of the MUAPs is similar because the amplitude is primarily determined by fiber density (i.e., the number of muscle fibers
belonging to the same motor unit in close proximity to the recording electrode), not by the total
number of muscle fibers in that motor unit (size). Increased fiber density primarily contributes to
the increased amplitude of MUAP by bringing more fibers in close proximity to the electrode,
thereby inducing a greater potential with depolarization. The axons serving large motor units are
of larger diameter, and therefore their conduction velocities are faster than those of axons to the
smaller motor units.

11. Name the important parameters of motor units.

In order of decreasing clinical significance: duration, firing rate, consistency, amplitude, and
shape (i.e., phasicity).

12. Explain the motor unit recruitment pattern. What is the significance of the firing rate?

The primary mechanism for increasing muscle contractile force is the activation of more
motor units (**spatial recruitment**) rather than an increase in the firing rate (**temporal recruitment**) of the motor units. In slowly developing muscle contractions, motor units are recruited in
size order from small to large (**size principle**), allowing for fine adjustments in force. If the force
of muscle contraction is slowly increased, the motor units that initiated contraction will fire more
rapidly (5–8 Hz). The firing rate achieved by the first motor unit when the second is recruited is
termed the **recruitment rate** and is usually 10–12 Hz (< 15 Hz) in normal individuals. Single
motor unit firing rates can be driven up to 50 Hz.

Early recruitment signifies that too many MUAPs are activated upon initiating muscle contraction in proportion to the level of muscle contraction force. This condition is common in myopathic disorders, in which the force contribution of each motor unit is decreased relative to
muscle fiber numbers and size. This recruitment pattern may also present in end-stage neurogenic atrophy, when reinnervated motor units become smaller as muscle fibers are lost.

13. What do nerve conduction studies (NCSs) measure?

NCSs induce and detect the waves of depolarization along the nerve axons and the muscle
depolarization. The types of nerves tested are either sensory, motor, or mixed. Nerve conduction
velocity (NCV) is operationally defined by the velocity of the fastest fibers. *Velocity increases
with axon diameter, quality of the myelin sheath, internodal distance, and temperature.*

The NCV is decreased in demyelination, while the amplitude of the evoked sensory and
motor responses remains normal unless significant conduction block coexists. In contrast, in diseases with axonal degeneration, the NCV may remain in the normal range until the nerve trunk
loses most of the large fast fibers. The motor and sensory amplitudes are reduced.

14. What are the limitations of the conventional NCS and needle EMG examination?

NCSs selectively examine the large myelinated fibers and do not define the pathophysiology of the medium to smaller-sized nerve fiber populations, nor do they define the functional
deficit.

Routine needle EMG evaluates only early-recruited, relatively small motor units. Therefore,
pathology cannot be discerned for the later-recruiting, large motor units.

The needle electrode only detects signals up to several millimeters away from the tip.
Because this same area is not completely representative of the muscle, needle EMG sampling
needs to be extensive when analyzing motor unit parameters.

**15. What are the important questions to be considered when evaluating a patient with sus-
pected peripheral neuropathy?**

- Sporadic, diffuse, or localized?
- Old, new, or progressive
- Motor, sensory, or both?
- Axonal, demyelinating, or both?
- Neuromuscular junction, muscle, or both?
- Any combination of the above?

16. What is the blink reflex? What does it mean?

"Blink reflex" is an electrical analog of the corneal reflex. The afferent loop is the trigeminal nerve, and the efferent loop is the facial nerve. **R1** (motor response one) is probably disynaptic or oligosynaptic and ipsilateral only. **R2** is polysynaptic and bilaterally observed. This study has been used in the evaluation of cerebellopontine angle tumors, multiple sclerosis, demyelinating diseases, and facial nerve palsy. Synkinesis (involuntary movement of the muscle accompanying a voluntary movement of another muscle) can be identified by observing blink reflexes in facial muscles other than the orbicularis oculi; it results from aberrant reinnervation (late) or ephaptic axon-to-axon transmission (early).

17. When is a mixed nerve conduction study used?

When a mixed nerve trunk (which contains the motor, sensory, and autonomic fibers) is electrically stimulated, the propagating compound nerve action potentials (CNAPs) from all three fibers can be recorded from an active electrode proximally and distally along the nerve trunk. The study utilizes an **orthodromic sensory** and **antidromic motor** to avoid volume conduction from CMAPs. Mixed NCS studies are also used when distal motor or pure sensory responses cannot be obtained.

The amplifier sensitivity should be for the sensory conduction study mode because nerve potentials only are being recorded. The early part of the compound mixed nerve potential represents the large myelinated sensory and motor fibers.

18. Is the NCV of the proximal segment always faster than the distal?

In conventional electrodiagnosis, the conduction velocity represents the fastest fibers' velocity only, not the average or median velocity. As the distal nerve segments tend to be thinner, colder, and less myelinated, the NCV is expected to be slower than the proximal.

19. How does temperature affect electrodiagnostic measurements?

Nerve conduction velocities: Cooling results in a longer time for the action potential to propagate and a net slowing of conduction.

SNAP and CMAP amplitude: When cool, the duration of an action potential gets longer and the amplitude gets larger. In addition, when the duration of the action potential becomes longer, there will be less phase cancellation, resulting in a higher amplitude of sensory nerve action potential (SNAP) or CMAP. The degree of these effects may vary depending on whether cooling is local (a few Ranvier nodes) or general (major neural segment).

Conduction block: Prolongation of the action potential with cooling leads to an increase in the duration of current available for depolarization. This extra duration may be just long enough to excite or skip a short demyelinated segment. Therefore, conduction block can be overcome by cooling.

Neuromuscular transmission: Neuromuscular transmission improves with cooling because of complex mechanisms which include relative sparing of the neurotransmitter, enhanced sensitivity of the postsynaptic endplate, and decreased hydrolysis of acetylcholine.

Spontaneous and voluntary EMG potentials: Cooling leads to desynchronization, which results in an increase in the duration of the motor units and increased polyphasicity. The amplitude of the MUAP may or may not increase depending on which factor is more influential (local cooling effects for higher amplitude and desynchronization effects for lower amplitude). Fibrillations and positive waves decrease in frequency with cooling; fasciculations may increase.

Myotonia: In myotonic dystrophy, cold causes an increase in myotonia on EMG. In congenital myotonia and myotonia congenita, cold causes no significant changes. In paramyotonia congenita, there seems to be two different responses to cold. In patients with hypokalemic and hyperkalemic periodic paralysis, exposure to cold can precipitate weakness and/or myotonia.

20. How should the electrodiagnostician screen and monitor patients for low temperature of the limbs?

When you greet the patient, shake hands. If the patient's hand is cool, warm him or her up with a warm water bottle or warm tapwater followed by an infrared lamp. Continue the infrared lamp during your history and physical exam. Continuous monitoring of the temperature with a simple adhesive tape (Dermatherm) is also available.

Motor conduction study should be the first to be performed, rather than the sensory conduction or needle examination. Each report should include the temperature under which the study was performed. This allows for easy comparison with past or future values (as well as publication!).

21. How do you recognize and distinguish Martin-Gruber anastomosis from a Riche-Cannieu anastomosis?

These two are considered normal variants involving only **motor axons**. The **Martin-Gruber anastomosis** consists of motor axons that are normally destined for the ulnar nerve, but instead join up with the median nerve in the plexus, and then return to the ulnar nerve in the forearm. The forearm Martin-Gruber anastomosis may result in fibers crossing from the median to innervate various muscles, including first dorsal interosseous, hypothenar, and thenar "ulnar" muscles. Combinations are common.

Conversely, the **Riche-Cannieu anastomosis** occurs when the motor axons normally destined for the median nerve continue into the ulnar nerve, then return to the median nerve between the deep ulnar and recurrent median motor branches. The incidence and degree of ulnar to median nerve communication in the hand are difficult to assess with standard nerve conduction techniques. Several clues of Martin-Gruber anastomosis can alert the examiner who is investigating carpal tunnel syndrome:

- No clinical evidence of thenar muscle weakness or atrophy despite severely abnormal median sensory studies.
- Elbow stimulation elicits higher median nerve CMAP amplitude at the abductor pollicis brevis than wrist.
- The median motor conduction velocity across the forearm is excessively fast compared with that of the ulnar nerve.
- The CMAP of the median nerve with elbow stimulation has an initial positive deflection, while the CMAP on the wrist stimulation does not.

22. A surgeon calls for an emergency EMG for a patient who had a nerve injury yesterday. Should he wait for degeneration to be complete?

Wallerian degeneration takes at least 1 week to occur, and the denervation potentials may take 2–3 weeks; therefore, it is usually best to perform an electrodiagnosis 3 weeks after the injury. However, at this stage the surgeon is looking to see whether the lesion is complete (**neurotmesis**) or incomplete (**axonotmesis**). Neural continuity at a very early stage can be demonstrated by the presence of voluntary motor units on EMG and CMAP/SNAP on conduction studies across the injured segment.

23. Can electrodiagnosis help in assessing the prognosis in Bell's palsy?

In Bell's palsy, the neural compromise occurs mostly at the labyrinthine section of the fallopian canal in the intracranial portion of the facial nerve. Therefore, a conventional conduction study can only examine distal to the compromised section of the facial nerve, making latency values a poor instrument of prognostication.

The examiner should perform a side-to-side comparison of amplitude/area of the CMAPs after the occurrence of the wallerian degeneration, which occurs any time from 5–7 days after initial weakness. If within the first 14 days, the **evoked CMAP amplitude** remains > 10% of the nonaffected side, there is a 90% chance of satisfactory recovery. Some authors advocate the 30% CMAP amplitude criteria for excellent functional recovery within a 2-month period. Those with 10–30% CMAP amplitude may end up with some functional impairment.

Other methods of prognostication include needle EMG findings of good **voluntary motor unit recruitment**. Persistence or return of **R1 component** of the blink reflex has some value, but it tends to be less informative and does not accurately reflect the degree of the axonal loss. Similarly, the **motor latency values** poorly correlate with functional recovery. The needle EMG examination is an important follow-study in the early stages of recovery, as it is the only objective way to document reinnervation. Electrodiagnostic findings usually lag behind clinical recovery.

24. Where are dorsal root ganglions (DRGs)? Where do preganglionic lesions occur?

The DRGs are located within the middle zone (intraforaminal) of the lateral spinal canal. In most cases of radiculopathy, the pathology is proximal to this location (preganglionic). Since the postganglionic sensory fibers continue to be supplied by axoplasmic flow from the DRG, they remain intact, and routine sensory NCSs show no abnormalities despite sensory symptoms and signs. This is one reason why the routine NCS and EMG may fail to detect root pathology if the patient's complaint is "pain" without muscle weakness or atrophy.

25. What are the nondiscogenic radiculopathies?

Tumors: meningiomas, neurofibromas, metastases, leukemias, lymphoproliferative diseases, lipomas (cauda equina and conus medularis involvement)
Abscess, hemorrhage, cysts
Inflammatory: tuberculosis, Lyme disease, syphilis, HIV infection, cryptococcosis
Arachnoiditis: myelogram, surgery, anesthetics, steroid injections
Sarcoidosis, Guillain-Barré syndrome
Diabetes, herpes zoster
Many of these diseases may persist with polyradiculopathy.

26. How is electrodiagnosis useful in radiculopathy?

- Provides the only physiologic measures of root function available to diagnose radiculopathy. Such testing complements imaging studies.
- Confirms a diagnosis of radiculopathy in cases in which it is uncertain that the patient has any neurologic lesion.
- Distinguishes radiculopathy from other neurologic or nonneurologic lesions when they cannot be distinguished clinically.
- Confirms whether the anatomic lesion seen on imaging techniques (CT/MRI) is resulting in nerve root pathology.
- May help in estimating "age" of the lesion.
- Helps prognosticate motor recovery because the study can distinguish a neurapraxic lesion from a severe axonotmetic lesion.
- Defines the lesion in terms of the myotomal distribution but cannot define the specific anatomic etiology of a root lesion.

27. How is the diagnosis of radiculopathy made?

Basically, the electrodiagnostician has to demonstrate:
1. Normal sensory conduction study
2. Denervation potentials in the myotomal distributions
3. Denervation potentials in the paraspinal muscles

The needle EMG is the single most valuable tool in defining nerve root compromise. Look for **fibrillation potentials** and **positive sharp waves** in the specific root distribution. These potentials can be seen in limb muscles within 3 weeks after the acute neural insult but may require up to 5–6 weeks to develop in the most distal portion of the limb.

Motor conduction study carries little weight but may be done for completeness of study, and it may reveal CMAP changes in 5–8 days in severe cases. The CMAP provides a quantitative baseline to allow reassessment.

28. Why is the differentiation between motor neuron disease and multiroot lesions difficult for the electrodiagnostician?

On EMG, these conditions have the same characteristics. Both display normal sensory NCS findings, normal motor conduction velocities (with or without lower CMAP), and identical EMG findings except for the distribution. In particular, distinguishing between the cervical spondylitic myeloradiculopathy and amyotrophic lateral sclerosis can be more difficult. EMG of thoracic paraspinal, facial or tongue muscles, and other laboratory studies such as spinal imaging may be necessary to make the diagnosis.

29. How can you differentiate between C8–T1 radiculopathy and ulnar neuropathy at the elbow?

1. Positive Spurling's test, sensory involvement of the ring finger without splitting (difference from median to ulnar side), involvement of the sensation in the medial arm and forearm, entirely normal (R = L) ulnar SNAP, and concurrent involvement of the thenar and extensor indicis proprius muscles favor C8–T1 root pathology.

2. Sensory splitting of the ring finger, low-amplitude or absent ulnar SNAP, involvement in the dorsal ulnar sensation with intact medial forearm sensation, and atrophy of the ulnar intrinsic muscles without concurrent median thenar atrophy favor ulnar neuropathy at the elbow.

However, these oversimplified views can be complicated by thoracic outlet syndrome (thenar atrophy with ulnar sensory involvement), low trunk of the brachial plexus lesion, and ulnar neuropathy at the palm.

30. Is electrodiagnosis a useful tool in the evaluation of chronic low back pain?

Electrodiagnostic studies should not be used as a screening tool when there are no focal findings. Most chronic back pain is not a result of radiculopathy or nerve injury. Even if the pain originates from the root, when the patient's presenting problem is only "pain" rather than motor symptoms such as muscle atrophy, muscle weakness, or reflex changes, the chances of demonstrating EMG abnormalities are very low. Even in radiculopathy, depending on the stage, the process of terminal sprouting, and reinnervation, uncovering the denervation potentials in the muscles may be futile. Careful selection of patients and discreet education of the referring physicians may avoid this overuse.

31. Is the somatosensory evoked potential (SSEP) helpful in diagnosis and management of common low back pain or radiculopathy?

The theoretical advantage of SSEP over conventional NCS and needle EMG is that it allows evaluation of the preganglionic portion of the sensory pathways while conventional electrodiagnostic study does not. However, although SSEP has become almost routine in some electrodiagnostic laboratories, its clinical utility is yet to be fully demonstrated.

BIBLIOGRAPHY

1. Barry DT: Basic concept of electricity and electronics in clinical electromyography [AAEM minimonograph #36]. Muscle Nerve 14:937–946, 1991.
2. Perotto AO: Anatomic Guide for the Electromyographer: The Limbs and Trunk, 3rd ed. Springfield, MO, Charles C Thomas Publ., 1994.
3. Denys EH: The influence of temperature in clinical neurophysiology [AAEM minimonograph #14]. Muscle Nerve 14:795–811, 1991.
4. Dumitru D: Radiculopathies. In Dumitru D: Electrodiagnostic Medicine. Philadelphia, Hanley & Belfus, 1995, pp 523–584.
5. Ertas MM, Stalberg E, Falck B: Can the size principle be detected in conventional EMG recording? Muscle Nerve 18:435–439, 1995.
6. Gutmann L: Important anomalous innervations of the extremities [AAEM minimonograph #2]. Muscle Nerve 16:339–347, 1993.
7. Kraft GH: Fibrillation potential amplitude and muscle atrophy following peripheral nerve injury. Muscle Nerve 13:814–821, 1990.
8. Layzer RB: The origin of muscle fasciculations and cramps. Muscle Nerve 17:1243–1249, 1994.
9. McGonagle TK, Levice SR, Donofrio PD: Spectrum of patients with EMG features of polyradiculopathy without neuropathy. Muscle Nerve 13:63–69, 1990.
10. Parry GJ: Diseases of spinal roots. In Dyck P, Thomas PK, Griffin JW, et al: Peripheral Neuropathy, 3rd ed. Philadelphia, W.B. Saunders, 1993, pp 899–910.

32. ELECTROMYOGRAPHIC MANIFESTATIONS OF SYSTEMIC DISEASE

Charles E. Levy, M.D., Daniel M. Clinchot, M.D., and Theresa A. Oswald, M.D.

1. Describe the presynaptic storage and release of acetylcholine (Ach).

Ach storage occurs in three interrelated compartments. Ach in the largest compartment, the **main store**, is not immediately available for release across the synaptic cleft. This reserve supplies a smaller compartment, the **mobilization store**, which in turn supplies the smallest compartment, which contains Ach available for **immediate release** into the synapse. Here, Ach is packaged in vesicles approximately 300–500 Å in diameter, each vesicle containing 5000–10,000 Ach molecules, an amount known as a **quantum**. The main store contains approximately 300,000 quanta, the mobilization store holds 10,000 quanta, and the immediate-release store holds 1000 quanta. When an action potential reaches the presynaptic nerve terminal, it causes a voltage-sensitive influx of calcium ions, which signals the vesicles to pour their contents of Ach into the synaptic cleft.

2. What are the common disorders of neuromuscular transmission?

Myasthenia gravis (MG)
Lambert-Eaton myasthenic syndrome (LEMS)
Botulism
Congenital myasthenia
Tick paralysis
Toxic exposure (e.g., organophosphate insecticides)
Side effects of medications (e.g., aminoglycosides, procainamide, penicillamine)

3. How does a patient with a disease of neuromuscular transmission typically present?

With progressive weakness and fatigue, especially with repetitive activities. Strength is often restored with rest.

4. Do the major disorders of neuromuscular transmission differ in their clinical presentations?

In > 90% of the cases of **myasthenia gravis** (MG), the levator palpebrae (extraocular muscles) are involved. Drooping of the eyelids and intermittent diplopia result. The muscles of facial expression, mastication, swallowing, and speech are involved in 80% of cases, leading to altered facial appearance and difficulty in eating. Muscles of the neck, shoulder girdle, trunk, and hips may also be involved.

In **Lambert-Eaton myasthenic syndrome** (LEMS), the muscles of the trunk, shoulder girdle, pelvic girdle, and lower extremities are more likely to be initially affected. Unlike MG, patients may experience an increase in muscle power for the first few contractions.

Symptoms of **botulism** usually appear within 12–36 hours of ingestion of the tainted food. The typical neural symptoms of blurred vision and diplopia may be accompanied by anorexia, nausea, and vomiting. Unlike in MG, pupils are often unreactive in botulism. Other bulbar symptoms, such as a nasal or hoarse vocal quality, dysarthria, and dysphagia, follow rapidly and are soon joined by weakness of the neck, trunk, and limbs and respiratory insufficiency. This takes place over 2–4 days.

5. Are there any special electrodiagnostic procedures to help quantify and classify disorders of neuromuscular transmission?

Repetitive stimulation and **single fiber EMG** (SFEMG) are two specific techniques used to evaluate function of the neuromuscular junction. SFEMG employs a specialized needle electrode with a recording surface of 25–30 μm diameter located 3–4 mm along the shaft from the tip. This allows recording of two single fibers within a motor unit. SFEMG is one of the most sensitive (not specific) measures of neuromuscular transmission defects. SFEMG shows increased **jitter** (variation within consecutive discharges of the interpotential interval between two muscle fiber action potentials) and **blocking** (failure of the action potential to be propagated to one of the two fibers) in diseases of neuromuscular transmission. Repetitive stimulation allows the examiner to generate multiple stimulations in rapid succession to the same site. This allows inspection of the resultant compound muscle action potentials (CMAPs) for consistency of amplitude and duration.

6. How do LEMS and myasthenia gravis differ electrophysiologically?

MG is an autoimmune disease primarily affecting older men and younger women and is often seen in association with other autoimmune diseases, such as rheumatoid arthritis. The defect occurs when *antibodies bind to the postsynaptic Ach receptor*, resulting in destruction and reduction of the surface area of the postsynaptic membrane and fewer Ach receptors. Electrophysiologically, the CMAP amplitudes are usually normal. With 2–5 Hz repetitive stimulation, there is a > 10% decrement in the CMAP amplitude. This decrement is typically greatest between the first and second responses, with the maximum decrement occurring between the first and fourth to fifth responses (see figure). With continued stimulation the response amplitudes gradually return toward normal. A 10-second maximum isometric contraction usually will result in an increased response amplitude, but no > 50% above baseline.

LEMS occurs more often in men than women, usually presenting in the fifth decade. There is a high coexistence of malignancy, most commonly oat-cell carcinoma of the lung. LEMS appears to be due to *antibodies directed at the voltage-gated calcium channels* of the motor nerve terminal, which interfere with *release* of Ach. Electrophysiologically, the initial CMAP is usually low in amplitude. With 2–5 Hz stimulation, there may be a decremental response. With > 10 Hz stimulation or a 10-sec maximum isometric contraction (which approximates a 50-Hz stimulation), there is an increase in the CMAP amplitude that is usually much > 50%, often 200–400% above the single-stimulation CMAP (see figure).

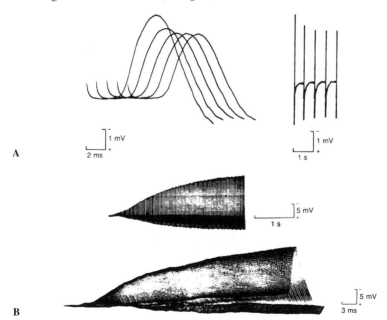

Repetitive nerve stimulation. *A*, Decrementing response in MG. *B*, Incrementing response in LEMS. (From Kimura J: Electrodiagnosis in Disease of the Nerve and Muscle: Principles and Practice, 2nd ed. Philadelphia, F.A. Davis, 1989; with permission.)

7. What is the "safety factor"?

Following depolarization of the terminal axon in normal persons, there is an overabundance of Ach released that is more than sufficient to bind Ach receptors available on the muscle membrane to accomplish neuromuscular transmission. This redundancy is called the "safety factor." In disease states such as MG, the neuromuscular transmission is much more tenuous. With fewer receptors available, a slight drop in Ach concentration may block transmission.

8. How is the course of events at the neuromuscular junction related to findings on repetitive stimulation?

Motor axonal discharge frequency affects neuromuscular transmission by modulating Ach availability and calcium concentrations at the synaptic cleft.

After depolarization of the nerve terminus causes the immediate release store to dump quanta into the synaptic cleft, 5–10 sec are required to replenish the lost Ach in the immediate release store from the mobilization store. Therefore, volleys arriving faster than every 5 sec progressively deplete the immediate release store. On the other hand, the calcium that is released with each depolarization requires 100–200 msec (or $\frac{1}{10}$–$\frac{1}{5}$ of a second) to diffuse away from the nerve terminal. Therefore, stimulation that arrives at rates > 5–10/sec (5–10 H) causes calcium to accumulate. Thus, MG repetitive stimulation at rates between 3–5 H shows a decremental response as smaller amounts of Ach are released into the neuromuscular junction, preventing some muscle fibers from reaching critical threshold. In LEMS, the CMAP may show a decremental response similar to MG at low stimulation frequencies. At frequencies of 20–50 H, however, facilitation is observed; successive CMAPs show increasing amplitude, often exceeding single-stimulation CMAPs by 200% of baseline, because rapid rates of stimulation result in accumulation of calcium at the presynaptic cleft of the neuromuscular junction, progressively allowing more Ach to be released.

9. Describe the components of a motor unit action potential (MUAP).

The MUAP is the recorded, summated electrical depolarization of the muscle fibers innervated by a single motor neuron (see figure).

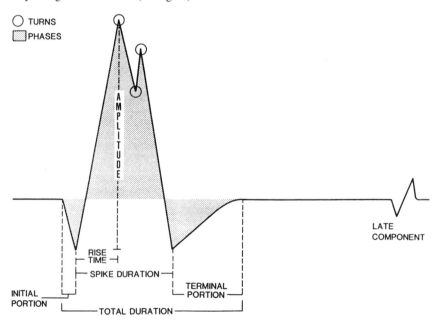

MUAP components and parameters. (From Johnson EW: Practical Electromyography, 3rd ed. Baltimore, Williams & Wilkins, 1988; with permission.)

Duration: The duration of an MUAP is proportional to the number of muscle fibers in the range of the active electrode. The duration is influenced by temperature and the specific muscle being examined. Normal values for duration have been established for individual muscles.

Amplitude: The amplitude of the MUAP is proportional to the size of the muscle and the synchronization of muscle fiber potentials. Fibers that are closest to the recording electrode play a significant role in the amplitude of the MUAP, as do temperature and the specific muscle being examined. As temperature declines, amplitude increases. Normal values for amplitude have been established for individual muscles.

Phases: The number of phases of a MUAP is determined by adding one to the number of baseline crossings. When this number is > 4 the MUAP is deemed polyphasic. The number of phases is proportional to the synchrony of fibers and the total number of fibers making up the MUAP.

10. What is the H-reflex?

The H-reflex usually refers to a potential recorded by surface electrodes overlying the calf after stimulation of the tibial nerve in the popliteal fossa. Submaximal stimulation of 1.0 msec (which is longer than the usual duration) preferentially activates the group IA afferents. The IA afferents synapse at the ventral spinal cord with the motor neuron pool to the calf, producing a late-occurring potential that is felt to be electrically similar to the ankle jerk. Because the H-reflex is dependent on the integrity and excitability of the spinal reflex arc, the H-reflex can be an important diagnostic tool in the evaluation of radiculopathy and neuropathy.

11. What is an F-wave?

The **F-wave** is a variable late response observed with supramaximal stimulation of peripheral motor nerves, resulting in antidromic depolarization of the stimulated motor neuron pool. This depolarization is not propagated for the majority of neurons because the axons, having just been fired antidromically, are refractory to an immediate second discharge. However, a small percentage (5%) of axons depolarize again and return an orthodromic volley. The F-wave provides a mechanism for the assessment of proximal nerve segments and motor neuron pool.

12. What is the A-wave?

The **A-wave**, or axon reflex, is a potential that usually occurs between the motor (M) response and the F-wave. This potential is due to an antidromic axonal depolarization that "crosses over" and returns orthodromically on another axon or axon group. A-waves have been observed in processes that include collateral sprouting or motor demyelination. Unlike the F-wave, this potential has a fairly constant configuration and latency. It is usually obtained with submaximal stimulation.

13. Can disorders other than denervation and myopathy lead to abnormal spontaneous potentials?

Fibrillation potentials and positive sharp waves can be seen in primary diseases of muscle such as muscular dystrophies; in congenital diseases such as myotonic dystrophy, myotonia congenita, and paramyotonia congenita; in neuromuscular junction diseases such as botulism; and with metabolic abnormalities such as hyperkalemia or hypokalemia. Curiously, abnormal spontaneous activity may be seen in CNS diseases such as stroke or spinal cord injury, particularly in the flaccid stage before tone returns. In CNS disease, lack of a necessary neuron-transported trophic factor has been offered to explain the appearance of fibrillation potentials and positive sharp waves. The upper motor neuron may provide some trophic support to the alpha motor neuron pool. Corticospinal tract damage can therefore result in alpha motor neuron damage as well, a phenomenon termed transsynaptic degeneration.

14. What is EMG disease? How was it discovered?

EMG disease, or more properly, the syndrome of diffuse abnormal electromyographic insertional activity, is an apparently benign condition characterized by diffuse positive sharp waves found in virtually any muscle tested in otherwise normal subjects. It was discovered accidentally by Dr. Ernest Johnson when a senior medical student volunteered to be examined electromyographically for a demonstration in front of his classmates. Much to Dr. Johnson's chagrin, every muscle explored showed diffuse spontaneous activity. Besides this, no other neurophysiologic abnormalities could be found. Patients with this "disease" have been followed for at least 3 years and remained clinically stable.

15. Describe the electrodiagnostic approach to the patient with a suspected peripheral neuropathy.

Motor and sensory latencies and amplitudes should be studied in at least three limbs. In addition, proximal and distal conduction should be evaluated, especially in early neuropathies. Assessment of conduction at different locations along the same nerve can identify areas of segmental demyelination. When an autonomic component to the neuropathy is considered, evaluation of the sympathetic skin response can be helpful. Every evaluation for peripheral neuropathy should include a needle exam, to help delineate the degree of axonal loss, clarify the pattern of involvement proximally and distally, and permit an assessment of chronicity.

Peripheral neuropathies are often classified according to their electrodiagnostic picture—i.e., according to the pattern of demyelination and axonal loss. It is a general rule of thumb that in the severely symptomatic patient, the assessment should begin in the least involved limb. In patients in whom the picture is milder, start in the most involved limb.

16. How can one differentiate pathophysiologic mechanisms of peripheral neuropathies based on nerve conduction studies and EMG?

From the electrodiagnostic findings, peripheral neuropathies can be classified according to their pattern of demyelination and axonal loss.

Sensorimotor, uniformly demyelinating: hereditary sensorimotor neuropathy types I, III, and IV; metachromatic leukodystrophy

Motor>sensory segmental demyelinating: Guillain-Barré syndrome, chronic inflammatory demyelinating polyneuropathy, leprosy, acute arsenic polyneuropathy, amiodarone neuropathy, AIDS neuropathy, ulcerative colitis neuropathy, hypothyroidism, diphtheria

Motor>sensory axonal: porphyria, hereditary motor sensory neuropathy types II and V, lead neuropathy, vincristine neuropathy, axonal Guillain-Barré syndrome

Sensory axonal: hereditary sensory neuropathy; Friedreich's ataxia; cisplatin, vincristine, isoniazid, and pyridoxine toxicity; Sjögren's syndrome; AIDS neuropathy; B12 deficiency

Sensorimotor axonal and demyelinating: diabetes, uremia

Sensorimotor axonal: amyloidosis, folate and thiamine deficiencies, alcoholic neuropathy, mercury and gold toxicities, rheumatoid arthritis, AIDS neuropathy

17. What is the most common treatable peripheral neuropathy in the world?

Leprosy (Hansen's disease), the most common treatable peripheral neuropathy, is caused by the microorganism *Mycobacterium leprae*. A typical presentation is one of multiple mononeuropathies with electrodiagnostic features of segmental demyelination. Leprosy can be thought of as a mononeuropathy of superficial sensory nerve branches within cutaneous lesions, with subsequent involvement of motor branches. *M. leprae* seems to have a predilection for ulnar, radial, peroneal, great auricular, facial and trigeminal nerves. Specific antileprosy treatment prevents or stops the progression of nerve damage.

18. What is the most common peripheral polyneuropathy in North America?

Diabetic polyneuropathy. Of the many forms of diabetic neuropathy, one commonly observed is diffuse, symmetric, primarily distal, sensorimotor polyneuropathy.

19. List the common patterns of peripheral nerve involvement seen in patients with diabetes mellitus.
Diabetic distal symmetric polyneuropathy
Hyperglycemic polyneuropathy
Diabetic autonomic neuropathy
Hyperinsulinic neuropathy
Diabetic polyradiculopathy (diabetic amyotrophy is an L2–L4 polyradiculopathy)
Diabetic cranial mononeuropathies
Diabetic limb mononeuropathies
Diabetic mononeuropathy multiplex

20. What generalized peripheral polyneuropathy may present initially with bilateral wrist drop?
Lead neuropathy may show predominant involvement of motor fibers innervating the upper-extremity extensors, presenting with bilateral radial neuropathy. The typical electrodiagnostic picture is distal, axonal, motor greater than sensory polyneuropathy.

21. Which etiologies of generalized peripheral polyneuropathy often have a pattern of demyelinating and axonal sensorimotor neuropathy?
Diabetic and uremic polyneuropathies.

22. Alcoholic neuropathy presents as which type of generalized peripheral polyneuropathy?
Axonal neuropathy, mostly of the distal nerves. The precise etiology of alcoholic neuropathy is controversial, involving either nutritional deficiency or a direct toxic effect of alcohol. Alcohol is one of the most common causes of peripheral neuropathy in the United States.

23. What are the cardinal features that allow discrimination of myopathy from neuropathy?
Myopathic processes usually present with proximal greater than distal weakness, whereas **neuropathies** usually present with distal greater than proximal weakness.
A **myopathy** results in the loss of individual muscle fibers, thus reducing the number of muscle fibers in a motor unit territory. The resulting MUAPs are lower in amplitude and shorter in duration. In addition, the MUAP usually becomes polyphasic due to the loss of muscle fiber action potentials. Loss of muscle fibers also results in earlier recruitment to generate any specified tension. In principle, recruitment interval is increased, although this may be difficult to observe clinically.
Neuropathic processes result in axon loss. Axon loss results in denervated muscle fibers which become reinnervated by remaining motor axons, thus producing fewer total motor units with larger muscle fiber territories. The increase in motor unit territory results in an MUAP with increased amplitude and duration and initially increased phases. As the reinnervation process proceeds, the number of phases decreases and the MUAP decreases in duration and increases in amplitude. In neuropathic processes, motor units take longer to recruit because individual motor units are able to generate more tension than normal; the recruitment interval is thus shortened.

24. What is Charcot-Marie-Tooth (CMT) disease?
CMT disease belongs to a spectrum of diseases referred to as **hereditary motor sensory neuropathies** (HMSNs). CMT disease is inherited in an autosomal dominant fashion. Persons with this disease have high arched feet (pes cavus) and weakness of the musculature of the distal lower limb. The legs have been described as stork-like or as an inverted "champagne bottle," due to the disproportionate wasting of the calf and feet in comparison to the thighs. Alterations in position and vibration sense are easily demonstrated. Interestingly, sensory complaints are mild. There is a hypertrophic (HMSN I) and a neuronal (HMSN II) form of CMT disease.

Differences Between HMSN I and HMSN II

DISEASE	MOTOR NCV	SITE OF MAXIMUM NCV SLOWING	AMPLITUDE OF CMAP	SENSORY NCV	HYPER-TROPHY OF NERVES	HISTOPATHOLOGY
HSMN I (hypertrophic)	↓↓	Distal	↓↓↓	↓↓	Present	Increase in fascicle size, onion bulb formation, segmental demyelination
HSMN II (neuronal)	Normal or ↓	None	↓↓	Normal or ↓	Absent	Preferential loss of large myelinated fibers

NCV, nerve conduction velocity. (Modified from Johnson EW: Practical Electromyography, 3rd ed. Baltimore, Williams & Wilkins, 1988.)

25. What is mononeuritis multiplex?

Mononeuritis multiplex represents a disorder with multiple lesions along multiple nerves. The etiology is believed to be thrombosis of the vasa nervorum (the small arterioles supplying the nerves) secondary to many underlying disease processes, such as vasculitis, malignancy, compression neuropathy, and AIDS. Typically, there is significant axonal loss along a nerve with minimal demyelination, usually resulting in normal nerve conduction velocities but reduced CMAP and SNAP amplitudes. The EMG should reveal evidence of denervation with positive sharp waves and fibrillation potentials as well as a loss of MUAPs. In addition, longstanding cases exhibit evidence of neuropathic MUAPs. Lastly, there should be no evidence of conduction block or temporal dispersion along the nerve, as this would indicate another disease process.

26. Describe the typical EMG changes seen in steroid myopathy.

Steroid myopathy is caused by excess corticosteroids, whether endogenous (Cushing's syndrome) or exogenous, resulting in proximal muscle weakness. Muscle biopsy reveals preferential atrophy of type II fibers, especially the fast-twitch glycolytic (type IIB) fibers. Accumulation of lipid droplets in type I fibers is also commonly found.

EMG examination shows normal insertional activity and no abnormal spontaneous activity. MUAP morphology may show the classic pattern seen in myopathies of short-duration, low-amplitude potentials, but frequently MUAPs are within normal limits. It is not unusual to find a normal electrophysiologic exam despite an abnormal muscle biopsy.

27. How can a steroid myopathy yield a normal electrophysiologic exam despite pathology of the type II fibers?

Routine analysis of MUAP morphology uses the initially recruited motor units, and these low-threshold motor units are usually of the type I, slow-twitch, oxidative fibers. It is only after the EMG instrument screen is filled with the activity of the type I fibers that the fast-twitch, glycolytic type II fibers are recruited. The activity of the type I fibers masks the absence of the type II fibers in steroid myopathy. Thus, MUAP morphology may be normal if type II fibers are predominantly affected.

28. What is a common distal myopathy?

In contrast to most other primary muscle disease, **myotonic dystrophy** has a pronounced distal pattern of weakness. In the **adult form**, the onset of muscle stiffness—with or without cramping, difficulty with release of tightly held objects, or opening tightly shut eyes—is first noted in adolescence or early adulthood. Progression of weakness eventually leads to wheelchair use, with death commonly in the fifth or sixth decade due to cardiopulmonary compromise. Physical exam may reveal the typical thin neck due to neck flexor wasting, frontal balding in men, and atrophy of the facial and masseter/temporalis muscles. The constellation of facial signs has been described as a "hatchet face" appearance.

The first signs of **congenital myotonia** may be reduced fetal movement in utero. Signs in the neonate include hypotonia and facial weakness or paralysis. Facial appearance is marked by an oddly shaped mouth with the lips forming an inverted V, known as "shark mouth." Club feet are also common. The appearance of myotonia is usually evident by age 5. As these children grow older, mental retardation is apparent.

One EMG finding in both the adult and childhood form is the **myotonic discharge**, provoked with pin electrode insertion, skin tapping adjacent to insertion, or voluntary contraction. This may produce a repetitive discharge of 20–80 Hz of either biphasic spike potentials < 5 msec in duration resembling fibrillation potentials, or positive waves of 5–20 msec in duration resembling positive sharp waves. The amplitude and frequency of these potentials wax and wane. These may be observed in affected infants as early as 5 days after birth. The myotonic discharge is not unique to myotonic dystrophy and can also be recorded in myotonia congenital, paramyotonia, myotubular myopathy, hyperkalemic periodic paralysis, and other metabolic muscle diseases.

29. What is McArdle's disease? What characteristic finding does it produce on EMG examination?

McArdle's disease (myophosphorylase deficiency) is a metabolic myopathy classified as type V glycogenosis and is one of 11 recognized disorders of glycogen metabolism. The lack of effective myophosphorylase blocks the rapid conversion of skeletal muscle glycogen to glucose. With vigorous exercise or under ischemic conditions, patients complain of painful muscle cramping. Many patients report a second-wind phenomenon, with return to exercise at or near previous levels for a prolonged period of time after a brief rest.

The signature of this disease is that an EMG electrode placed in the "cramping" muscle shows electrical silence, in contrast to ordinary muscle cramps with their abundant EMG activity. The cramp of McArdle's represents true muscle contracture; it is hypothesized that the lack of EMG activity signifies an electromechanical dissociation.

Diagnosis of McArdle's disease is supported by the relative lack of the normal elevation of lactate, the end product of glycogen metabolism, following exercise. Definitive diagnosis is achieved with muscle biopsy showing marked absence of myophosphorylase activity.

30. Name the varieties of motor neuron disease.

Motor neuron diseases usually arise from degeneration of the upper and/or lower motor neurons. This group of diseases is often conceptualized as a single disorder with variations classified by the sites in the spinal cord and brain most affected:

Progressive muscular atrophy—spinal anterior horn cell loss with little bulbar or upper motor neuron involvement

Progressive bulbar palsy—preferential degeneration of bulbar nuclei

Primary lateral sclerosis—preferential spinal white matter dysfunction without bulbar or spinal motor cell loss

Amyotrophic lateral sclerosis (ALS)—upper and lower motor neuron signs affecting both the bulbar and somatic musculature

Monomelic amyotrophy—upper and lower motor neurons findings restricted to one limb

These entities usually present with an insidious onset and eventual progression. In contrast, polio presents with an acute loss of alpha motor neuron function secondary to a viral infection and is usually static once the infection resolves.

31. Describe the electrodiagnostic evaluation of a person with suspected motor neuron disease.

A systematic approach to the evaluation is essential. To ensure that there is no evidence of peripheral neuropathy or conduction block (which would imply a different disease), the EMG examination should test the sensory and motor nerve latencies and amplitudes in three limbs. The

EMG exam also should include the paraspinals and cranially innervated muscles such as the tongue. In a patient with cranial nerve complaints, bulbar muscles should show denervation. This differentiation is essential since cervical stenosis with multilevel chronic radiculopathies can mimic the clinical picture of motor neuron disease.

32. Which potentially treatable disorders must be ruled out before diagnosing motor neuron disease?

Brainstem compression, cervical spinal cord compression, multifocal motor neuropathy, lead intoxication, and chronic mercurialism may resemble ALS clinically.

33. What is multifocal motor neuropathy (MMN)?

MMN is a rare disorder that presents with progressive limb weakness. It is important to be aware of this entity for two reasons. First, it has responded to immunotherapy, such as human immune globulin in several case series. Second, it may clinically resemble a motor neuron disease such as ALS. Multifocal conduction block is the cardinal feature of this syndrome. Although MMN has been characterized as a pure motor neuropathy, minor sensory symptoms and signs are often present.

34. What is the earliest electrodiagnostic change seen in patients with Guillain-Barré syndrome (GBS)?

Early studies often reveal only **prolonged** or **absent F-responses**. These early F-response abnormalities with normal distal conduction point to an increased susceptibility of the proximal/radicular part of motor fibers. The classic electrodiagnostic pattern is **segmental demyelinating, motor > sensory polyneuropathy**. Sensory conduction studies often show mild abnormalities. The sural nerve tends to be spared in GBS, while it is one of the first nerves to be affected in other polyneuropathies.

35. Are there electrophysiologic prognostic indicators in Guillain-Barré syndrome?

Estimation of the amount of axonolysis can provide insight into the prognosis of GBS. It is most accurate if the EMG is performed at the nadir of clinical function. When the amplitude of the distal CMAP is < 10% of normal, there is a great likelihood of a poorer outcome.

BIBLIOGRAPHY

1. Adams RD, Victor M: Principles of Neurology, 5th ed. New York, McGraw-Hill, 1993.
2. Albers JW: AAEM case report 4: Guillain-Barré syndrome. Muscle Nerve 12:705–711, 1989.
3. Auger RG: AAEM minimonograph 44: Disease associated with excess motor unit activity. Muscle Nerve 17:1250–1263, 1994.
4. Bodensteiner JB: Congenital myopathies. Muscle Nerve 17:31–44, 1994.
5. Brooke MH: A Clinician's View of Neuromuscular Diseases. Baltimore, Williams & Wilkins, 1977.
6. Brown WF, Bolton CF (eds): Clinical Electromyography, 2nd ed. Stoneham, MA, Butterworth-Heinemann, 1993.
7. Chaudhry V: Multifocal motor neuropathy: Electrodiagnostic features. Muscle Nerve 17:198–205, 1994.
8. Chokeroverty S: AAEE case report 13: Diabetic amyotrophy. Muscle Nerve 10:679–684, 1987.
9. Donofrio PD, Albers JW: AAEM minimonograph 34: Polyneuropathy: Classification by nerve conduction studies and electromyography. Muscle Nerve 13:889–903, 1990.
10. Dumitru D: Electrodiagnostic Medicine. Philadelphia, Hanley & Belfus, 1995.
11. Dyck PJ, Thomas PK (eds): Peripheral Neuropathy, 3rd ed. Philadelphia, W.B. Saunders, 1993.
12. Gutmann L: AAEM minimonograph 37: Facial and limb myokymia. Muscle Nerve 14:1043–1049, 1991.
13. Johnson EW: Practical Electromyography, 3rd ed. Baltimore, Williams & Wilkins, 1988.
14. Keesey JC: AAEM minimonograph 33: Electrodiagnostic approach to defects of neuromuscular transmission. Muscle Nerve 12:613–626, 1989.
15. Kimura J: Electrodiagnosis in Disease of the Nerve and Muscle: Principles and Practice, 2nd ed. Philadelphia, F.A. Davis, 1989.

33. ELECTRODIAGNOSIS AND THE CENTRAL NERVOUS SYSTEM

Jeffrey L. Cole, M.D.

1. How should you approach an electrodiagnostic consultation of the CNS?

Physiatric teaching and clinical orientation tend to focus on an individual's ability to perform a "function" or on a disability that limits activity. Begin your examination by studying the end organ or structure responsible for or limiting the desired performance or that area that is described as the most painful. *Each test must be directed toward a specific clinical problem* to produce the most efficacious answer for the patient.

2. What is meant by a CNS evoked potential (EP) study?

An EP is the true average of the electrical activity seen across the scalp at a given time relative to a stimulus delivered via a predetermined sensory pathway. Most commonly, the scalp potentials are recorded by looking at the voltage changes at a fixed point on the scalp plotted against time following a time-locked stimulus. The recorded scalp potential is the sum of some or all of the stimulus-evoked, event-related bioelectrical potentials from (depending on the area being studied) the peripheral nerve, retina, or cochlear mechanism, from the spinal cord or central conduction pathways, and from cortical and subcortical cerebral structures.

3. What is a somatosensory evoked potential (SEP) study?

An SEP is the electrophysiologic examination of sensory function, including the ability to perceive mechanoreceptive and proprioceptive stimuli. The SEP pathways can involve the body's longest axons with the greatest CNS span. SEP can be viewed simplistically as the CNS equivalent of the peripheral sensory nerve action potential (SNAP) study. The SEP technique traces the afferent impulses produced by peripheral nerve electrical stimulation through the plexus and root, through to the spinal cord, and into the brainstem and cerebrum.

4. Are only electrical stimuli used for eliciting SEP studies?

It is possible to evoke an SEP with mechanical skin tapping or muscle stretch, but one advantage of using electrical stimulation is that it permits synchronous activation of the majority of low-threshold large-diameter fibers, which produces a highly coherent transmission. When a mixed nerve is stimulated, this coherent action potential volley is conducted along the peripheral processes of the large-diameter, rapidly-conducting epicritic sensory system (discriminative tactile and kinesthetic information) and continues along the central processes in the ipsilateral spinal cord dorsal columns to synapse at the cervicomedullary junction in the dorsal column nuclei.

5. EP responses are often referred to as near-field or far-field potentials. What does that mean?

When extracellular activity is recorded near the generator site, as from electrodes placed on exposed primary sensory cortex, the EP can be obtained from individual stimulus trials. This is a **near-field** recording. Tracking an afferent signal along its spinal column course is also a relatively near-field recording, because the afferent volley approaches and then continues beyond the recording site. Near-field recordings are characterized by large spatial gradients in the potential field because there is less extracellular activity "spread" through the volume conductor between the generation and recording sites.

When the SEP is recorded at some distance from the source, the traveling extracellular negativity wave is always approaching but never reaching the electrodes; it is a **far-field** recording. Because the generator site is far from the accessible surface, the potential field (amplitudes) spatial gradients over the recording surface are low, and the extracellular distribution "spread" is broad. Far-field potentials must be recorded with widely separated electrodes to detect and sample the spatial gradient.

6. What are the usual nomenclature conventions for labeling the SEP peaks?

There are many variations in nomenclature, but the most typical labels for the upper-extremity SEP studies use the **polarity** (P or N, for positive or negative) and expected normal **latency** (in milliseconds), such as P_{14} or N_{20}. The lower-extremity peaks are more often marked with the polarity and their order, such as $P_{1(onset)}$, N_1, P_2, etc.

7. How many recording channels are required to do an SEP study?

There is no minimum number of channels required for clinical SEP studies. A single-channel, noncephalic referenced, upper-extremity study can contain all the needed data, or serial studies with recordings at different levels or paradigms can be obtained. The advantages of multichannel systems include more data acquisition per stimulus and per time, as well as better documentation of signal entry and transmission along the studied pathway. Multichannel recordings can be obtained from electrodes placed over the peripheral nerve (**afferent neurogram**), over different spinal levels (**electrospinographic potential**), or over relevant regions of the scalp.

8. Can the SEP be conclusively interpreted without any other testing?

No. To ascribe any SEP latency anomaly to a CNS lesion, we must know that there is no peripheral slowing (peripheral neuropathy or entrapment) along the nerve's afferent pathway.

9. What patient preparation is required before coming for an EP test?

For scalp electrode placement, the person's hair and scalp should be freshly cleaned to remove salts and other conductive contaminants and no conditioners applied that could reduce the signal by producing electrical "shunting" via a relatively low impedance bridging.

10. What is a visual evoked potential (VEP study)?

A VEP is the occipital cortex potential generated after a visual stimulus (usually alternating black-white checkerboard pattern). Light stimulates the retinal photoreceptors and transmits a signal to the bipolar cells and then to the inner retinal ganglion cells. These exiting ganglion cell axons make up the optic nerve fibers. Through the chiasm, retinal fibers from the nasal halves cross over to the opposite side to join the temporal field's ipsilateral fibers, thereby forming the optic tracts. Each optic tract's fibers synapse in the lateral geniculate bodies located in each lateral dorsum thalamus. The lateral geniculate body and retina neurons respond strongly to sharp contrasting borders, opponent colors, and spots of light. From there, the signals are relayed through the geniculocalcarine tract, or optic radiation, to the primary visual cortex in the calcarine fissure on the medial aspect of each occipital lobe. Binocular convergence occurs at the visual cortex. The shape recognition ability (edge perception) is responsible for the VEP.

11. Which VEP component is used primarily for clinical interpretation?

The wave usually has three peaks, which are labeled by their polarity and position (N_1, P_1, or N_2) or by latency (N_{75}, P_{100}, N_{140}). The most important VEP criterion is the P_{100} latency because of its normal stability and size and its clinical correlation with pathologies.

12. What are the normal value ranges and influences on the VEP peaks?

When all ages and genders are grouped together, the N_1 (N_{75}) generally has a normal range from 65–90 msec, the P_{100} (P_1) ranges from 88–116 msec, and the N_2 (N_{140}) can vary up to 151 msec in normal individuals. Visual acuity losses, even with use of corrective lenses, may attenuate the P_{100} amplitude but should have little effect on the latency. The P_{100} latencies shorten during the first year of life, reaching a plateau by 6 or 7 years of age, and then increase gradually after age 50–60. Females tend to have slightly shorter latencies. If the stimulus luminance and pattern contrast are not maximized, they may delay the latency and reduce the amplitude of the response.

13. What are some indications and applications for performing a VEP?

The VEP is particularly useful in clinical problems that are associated with mild or subclinical visual dysfunction. Conditions that affect **central retinal** or **macular function** can cause alterations in the VEP amplitude or waveform, rather than the latency, but may not be discovered unless a small check pattern is used. In fact, larger check patterns may fail to demonstrate several CNS pathologies. **Peripheral retinal diseases** will not significantly after the VEP until the macula is involved, and **central retinal artery occlusion** may not produce any VEP abnormality, while **ischemic** or **compressive optic neuropathies** can cause waveform and amplitude abnormalities which are out of proportion to the latency delay. **Papilledema**, in the absence of secondary ischemic atrophy, may not give any VEP abnormalities. Cortical blindness usually abolishes the VEP; however, it has been preserved in rare cases.

14. Do all demyelinating conditions produce an abnormal VEP?

The greatest utility of VEP is with optic nerve diseases giving latency prolongation (up to 250 msec), which can be a hallmark of demyelinating diseases. Of this group, evaluations for optic neuritis and multiple sclerosis are the most frequent indication. Paradoxically, toxic or nutritional amblyopias, which are considered demyelinating, are not usually associated with significant VEP alteration.

15. Can the VEP help identify the presence of a space-occupying CNS lesion?

Chiasmal lesions, which are usually space-occupying masses (pituitary adenoma, craniopharyngioma, meningioma, etc.), generally alter the VEP bilaterally. The resulting waveform distortion and amplitude losses are usually disproportionate to the modest latency delays observed (up to 25 msec), some of which are reversed following decompressive surgery. Post-chasmal focal lesions (tumors, cerebrovascular accidents, etc.) are best defined with partial or hemifield stimulation. A normal VEP is usually consistent with an intact pathway through the primary visual cortex, but lesions beyond area 17 require imaging studies.

16. What are the indications for doing an auditory brainstem (evoked) response (ABR) study in an adult?

In adults, the ABR has found utility in a variety of **audiologic problems**, including unexplained "central" losses on auditory tests and in the differential diagnosis of a sudden-onset unilateral deafness or severe hearing loss. The test has superb sensitivity in diagnosing **multiple sclerosis** and other demyelinating processes, looking for **acoustic neuromas**, for **intraoperative monitoring**, and for monitoring brainstem function during a **barbiturate coma** or in those who appear "**brain dead**."

17. When is an ABR study indicated in a child?

"Objective" audiometry using the ABR can be used in infants and neonates to detect the presence of early hearing loss. These studies should be considered in:

1. Infants and children suspected of hearing loss or hearing problems
2. Families with a history of metabolic or genetic diseases known to cause an early or congenital hearing impairment
3. Orofacial dysmorphic syndromes
4. All premature infants who have been in an ICU
5. Term infants who had hypoxic episodes which resulted in changes in consciousness lasting > 24 hours or unexplained impaired consciousness
6. Congenital infections or neonatal bacterial meningitis
7. Renal compromise after exposure to ototoxic drugs

18. What are the ABR peaks? What are their presumed anatomic correlates?

Anatophysiologic Processes	Peaks Produced

)))) → **Tympanic membrane** vibration
(Sound)   ↓

Auditory ossicle vibration
                    ↓

Traveling pressure wave along the **basilar membrane**
                    ↓

Stimulation of sensory **hair cells**
                    ↓

Depolarization (generator potentials) of **dendrites** and **spiral ganglion**
                    ↓

"All or none" **auditory nerve** action potential I
                    ↓

Cochlear nuclei (2nd-order neuron) in medulla II
                    ↓

Trapezoid body
Dorsal acoustic striae
Intermediate acoustic striae
                    ↓

Superior olivary complex (contralateral and ipsilateral 3rd-order neurons)
          in pons III
                    ↓

Lateral lemniscus (contralateral and ipsilateral) in pons IV
                    ↓

Inferior colliculus (primarily 4th-order, few 3rd-order neurons;
          contralateral and ipsilateral) in midbrain V
                    ↓

Medial geniculate body (5th-order neurone) in thalamus VI
                    ↓

Thalamocortical auditory radiations VII
                    ↓

Primary auditory area → **secondary** and **tertiary auditory area**

19. What clinical examination should be done before doing an ABR?

Review of the cranial nerves, and in neonates, a screening otoacoustic emissions test.

Gross assessment of hearing prior to establishing threshold values.

Otoscopic examination of the external auditory canal with tympanic membrane visualization to ensure that the canal is not blocked; if the auditory canal shows significant blockage, this should be removed before performing the studies.

Assessment of balance and other neurologic parameters if such data are not available.

20. What do rarefaction and condensation mean in ABR studies?

The click (stimulation) "polarity" is based on a mechanical phenomenon within the stimulating headset. **Rarefaction** means that the earphone diaphragm's initial movement is away from the tympanic membrane when the electric signal is delivered. **Condensation** implies that the electrical energy makes the diaphragm's first move toward the tympanic membrane. Rarefaction generally produces a shorter latency peak than does condensation when all other recording parameters are the same. Only one polarity should be used during any series of trials and compared to its baseline normal values.

21. Which ABR peaks are used for clinical data interpretation?

The **I–III interpeak latencies** have shown superb correlation with lesions in the peripheral auditory mechanism, auditory nerve, and lower pons. The **I–V interpeak latencies** have more widespread use in brainstem, thalamic, and cortical injuries when the I–III interpeak latencies are normal. There can be diffuse involvement both in the I–III and III–V interpeak latencies with multiple sclerosis and other demyelinating processes. Low stimulus intensity or hearing losses are suggested by a **wave I** peak delay.

22. What is an electrospinogram (ESG) study?

An ESG is the afferent nerve volley recorded over the spinal column produced from peripheral nerve stimulation. It can be used as a CNS entry marker or in conjunction with a SEP to shorten the segment being examined, to differentiate intracolumn pathology along the peripheral nerves versus spinal cord by level, help localize small segments of conduction disruption in multiple stenotic lesions (where imaging studies show diffuse involvement), or define latency data to the peripheral nerve's entry into the cauda equina. In pure sensory sacral radiculopathies, an asymmetrical ESG, by itself or in conjunction with abnormal H-reflex studies, may be the only evidence of pathology.

23. Is there an ideal time to do a CNS electrodiagnostic study?

No. These tests are ideally suited to augment our early examination after spinal cord or cerebral events, when the patient's ability to cooperate with examination is impaired. Such testing provides a repeatable continuous quantifiable measure of latency and amplitude for re-evaluation should the patient's clinical condition change.

24. What is a magnetically stimulated transcranial motor evoked potential (MEP)?

Cortical MEP studies were originally applied during intraoperative procedures to document efferent motor conduction that an SEP study could only imply. This was accomplished with transcranial (scalp to pallet) dipolar electrical stimulation. Because electrical stimuli could arouse seizure disorders, magnetic stimulation has replaced it. Mapping of the homunculus pattern stimulation is used to locate discrete motor areas. Ideally, with proper magnetic angular position, select subcortical arousal is possible.

25. What is the "silent period" that can follow a magnetic stimulus?

In addition to exciting corticospinal neural soma which produce the MEP, the magnetic stimulus delivered during voluntary activity produces a prolonged postexcitatory volitional activity inhibition, called the "silent period." The latency of this period usually increases slightly with age.

26. How else can electrical or magnetic stimuli be used to localize a lesion within the central conduction pathways?

ESG responses can be obtained, with more or less difficulty, at any interspinous vertebral level, giving "short" (CNS) segment information, and can be performed on patients who are unable to cooperate. Intervertebral space magnetic stimulation can also derive relatively short-segment information or can establish the peripheral motor latency (PML), but it is best used in patients who can voluntarily contract "target" muscles to obtain the best information. The central motor latency (CML), or conduction time, is the difference between the cortical and peripheral latencies: CML = MEP latency – PML.

27. Transcranial CML has been offered as a new tool for locating defining spinal cord lesions. Is it better in certain levels than in others?

In general, transcranial CML has not been a consistently valuable tool in diagnosing the presence of cervical spinal stenosis if there is not already clinical evidence of myelopathy. However, in cervical stenosis, magnetic stimulus may reduce the postexcitation silent period during which continued volitional activity is normally inhibited. The CML is more directly affected by lumbosacral stenotic lesions.

28. Where are transcranial MEPs helpful diagnostically?

Transcranial MEPs in Diagnosis

CONDITIONS	MOTOR EVOKED POTENTIALS		POSTSTIMULATION SILENT PERIOD
	LATENCY	AMPLITUDE	
Physiologic factors			
Normal aging	Linear ↑	Linear ↑	Slightly ↓
Increasing stimulation intensity	↓	↑	↑
With volition	↓	↑	Unchanged
Spinal cord lesions			
Cervical myelopathy	Normal or ↑	Normal	↓ (despite volitional contraction of target muscle)
Extramedullary cervical lesion	↑ in 60%	–	–
Intramedullary cervical lesion	↑ in 30%	–	–
Syringomyelia	Prolonged	↓ or absent	–
Lumbosacral myelopathy	↑	Normal	–
Various diseases			
Amyotropic lateral sclerosis	Minimally ↑	↓	–
Hemiparetic lesions	Normal	↓	↑ ↑
Huntington's disease	Normal	Normal	–
Peripheral neuropathy	↑	↓	Unchanged
Friedrich's ataxia	↑*	↓*	–
Hereditary spastic paraplegia			
Upper extremity	Normal	–	–
Lower extremity	Normal or ↑	–	–
Multiple sclerosis	↑ ↑	↓	↑
Myotonic dystrophy	Normal	Slight ↓	Unchanged
Parkinsonism	↓	↑	↓

* Proportional to disease duration.

29. What is the International 10–20 System for electrode placement?
The first prominent conference to standardize electroencephalography (EEG) electrode place-ments and their nomenclature was in 1947, which resulted in the 1958 proposal that produced the International 10–20 System for technique, scalp electrode placements, and standardized electrode site labeling. This scheme for scalp coverage uses a limited number of electrode sites whose lo-cations can be easily and accurately reproduced to permit good serial comparison and allow ex-change of comparative EEG data.

30. What are the 10–20 System landmarks?
All the electrode sites are derived by relative distances from four skull landmarks:
The nasion (the bridge of the nose)
The left and right preauricular points (the indentations above each tragus cartilate situated at the external auditory meatus openings)
The inion (the midline skull base ridge where it meets the neck)
The inion is commonly marked above its actual location, resulting in a measurement error that is carried through all subsequent measurements. In SEP applications, as in EEG, inaccurate or asymmetrical electrode location can prevent proper interpretation of the results.

31. Besides the 21 regularly used 10–20 sites, are there any other defined CNS scalp electrode areas?
Two nonscalp sets at the **ear lobes** (auricular, A_1/A_2) and **nasopharyngeal** (Pg_1/Pg_2) for temporal lobes, and two for **cerebellar** activity (Cb_1/Cb_2).

32. How are these noncephalic electrode sites recorded for SEP studies?

The 10–20 System was developed to answer EEG needs and gives an easily reproducible, fixed scheme for applying scalp electrodes. It is exactly this rigidity which is undesirable for SEP studies. A common SEP practice is to place an electrode "behind" a designated site and use a prime (′) mark per centimeter distance away (i.e., an electrode 2 cm behind C_Z, toward the inion, is designated C_Z''). This practice evolved in SEP because subtle site shifts were found to maximize the evoked amplitude and/or improve peak separation or identification. There is no ideal noncephalic site nomenclature that is used for reference electrode sites or for subcortical information. Designate precisely nonscalp recording sites with clear anatomic references.

33. Why do we test a scalp electrode impedance, but for peripheral sensory conduction studies, we do not?

Even though the preamplifier input impedances have improved over the years, the skin–electrode interface presents a formidable conduction barrier. Because CNS responses are so small relative to peripheral responses, the electrode site skin should be lightly abraded, an electrolyte applied, and the electrode well fixed. The resultant impedance from a properly applied cup or disc surface electrode should be 1–5 kOhms. Interdermal pin electrodes have inherently higher impedances because of the nature and size of their skin-electrode interface. If the tested surface electrode impedance is too low, it may be due to interelectrode conduction by perspired salts or conductive gel and could prevent proper signal acquisition. When using a digital meter, be certain that the lowest indicator actually represents a number above zero.

34. What can we conclude from an absent EP response?

Never interpret the absence of data! If an attempted study fails to evoke a response, one must correlate it to the clinical situation (i.e., Can the person feel or move the tested part? For an MEP study, is the movement from the target muscle or by substitution?). Check and re-set the electrodes and recording equipment. For SEPs, try a more rostral stimulus location until a response is obtained that can be compared to a normal database.

35. Is there a universally preferred minimum "reporting" format?

No, but a fundamental acceptable report should include the relevant aspects of the history and physical examination and the reason for the referral. The traces used for analysis and interpretation must show at least two clearly superpositionable runs to confirm the reliability. Include the printouts with the report to show the recording polarity, amplitude, and time-base calibrations. The stimulus site (type, intensity), active recording electrode site, reference location, equipment (settings), and recording parameters used for the test should be included with the data as well as a summary of the technique employed. Interpretation of latency, amplitude, and waveform morphology should always be based on size-to-site comparisons and statistical analysis (mean + 2.5–3 SD) for all the data criteria used. Also, when warranted or requested, include follow-up recommendations.

BIBLIOGRAPHY

1. Cole JL, Gottesman L: Anal electrophysiology and pudendal nerve evoked potentials. In Smith L (ed): Practical Guide to Anorectal Testing, 2nd ed. New York, Igaku-Shoin, 1995.
2. Cole JL, Pease W: Central nervous system electrodiagnostics. In DeLisa J (ed): Medicine: Principles and Practice, 2nd ed. Philadelphia, J.B. Lippincott, 1993.
3. Eisen AA, Shtybel W: AAEM minimonograph 35: Clinical experience with transcranial magnetic stimulation. Muscle Nerve 13:995–1011, 1990.
4. Little JW, Stiens SA: Electrodiagnosis in spinal cord injury. Phys Med Rehabil Clin North Am 5(3): 571–593, 1994.

34. ENTRAPMENT NEUROPATHY

Jaywant J. P. Patil, M.B.B.S., F.R.C.P.C.

1. How are nerve injuries classified?

Seddon has classified three categories of nerve injury, based on the severity of the injury:

1. **Neurapraxia.** There is loss of physiologic conductivity, and the axon is unable to propagate an action potential across the site of injury.

2. **Axonotmesis.** There is loss of anatomic continuity of the axon due to **irreversible damage**, with immediate conduction block across the site of the injury. Initially, the distal segment continues to remain excitable, making it difficult to distinguish between axonotmesis and neurapraxia on the basis of distal nerve excitability. **Wallerian degeneration** proceeds distal to the injury within a few days after the injury.

3. **Neurotmesis.** In addition to irreversible axonal damage, the supportive structures are damaged, including the **peri-neurium** that covers axon bundles and the **epineurium** that covers the nerve trunk.

2. List the common sites of nerve entrapment in the upper and lower limbs.

	Site of Entrapment	*Example*
Upper Limbs		
Median nerve	Wrist	Carpal tunnel syndrome
	Forearm	Anterior interosseous syndrome
Ulnar nerve	Elbow	Tardy ulnar nerve palsy
	Wrist	Guyon's canal syndrome
Lower Limbs		
Peroneal nerve	Knee or fibular head	Cross leg syndrome
Lateral femoral	Medial to anterior	Meralgia paresthetica
Cutaneous nerve of thigh (ASIS)	Superior iliac spine	
Tibial nerve	Under laciniate ligament	Tarsal tunnel syndrome

3. Which electrodiagnostic test demonstrates physiologic changes due to mixed nerve entrapment?

Sensory conduction studies are more sensitive in detecting mixed nerve entrapment. For example, the distal sensory latency of entrapped median nerves is twice as likely to be prolonged compared with median distal motor latencies. The sensory fibers, which are the fastest conducting (1A alpha) nerve fibers, are first to be affected. The conduction velocity increases with axonal diameter and density of myelination. Nerve compression results in demyelination along the segment of nerve, resulting in increased internodal distances at multiple levels, which in turn slows down saltatory conduction (where waves of depolarization jump from one node to the next). Techniques that compare latencies between short nerve segments are more sensitive to effects of focal compression than latencies measured over a longer segment (where there is a dilution of the abnormality).

4. What is Saturday night palsy? Honeymoon palsy?

Saturday night palsy is one of the "sleep palsies" that result from focal compression due to limb position. It occurs secondary to compression of the radial nerve at the brachium as it pierces the lateral intermuscular septum in the upper part of the arm and then continues to travel into the anterior compartment of the arm distally. Compression often occurs in patients who, in an alcoholic stupor, fall asleep with the arm resting against a firm edge of a chair or couch.

Honeymoon palsy is another "sleep palsy," in which the compression of the radial nerve occurs more distally in the arm. It results from the bed partner's head resting in the crook of the patient's arm.

Most of these lesions are no more severe than axonotmesis. Prognosis for recovery within a couple of months is fairly good.

5. Describe the anatomy of Guyon's canal and the entrapment of the ulnar nerve there.

In 1886, Phillip Guyon, a French physician originally described the Guyon's canal at the wrist. Guyon's canal is bordered medially by the **pisiform bone** and laterally by the **hook of the hamate**. This canal is covered on its volar aspect by the volar carpal ligament. The **ulnar nerve**, along with the **ulnar artery**, passes through this canal.

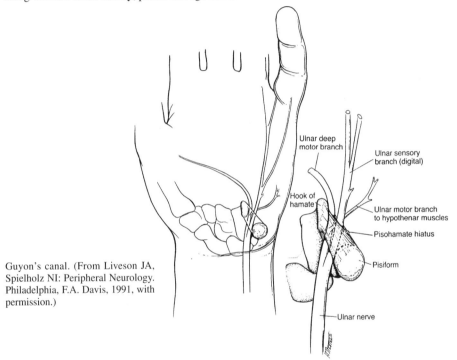

Guyon's canal. (From Liveson JA, Spielholz NI: Peripheral Neurology. Philadelphia, F.A. Davis, 1991, with permission.)

While in the canal, the ulnar nerve divides into a superficial and a deep branch. The **superficial branch** gives a twig to the palmaris brevis and continues as a sensory branch to the ring and little fingers, as well as supplying sensation to the area of the hypothenar eminence. The **deep branch** along with the ulnar artery winds around the hook of the hamate and runs between the adductor digiti quinti and the flexor digiti quinti brevis and eventually supplies the dorsal and palmar interossei, the third and fourth lumbricals, the adductor pollicis, the first dorsal interosseous, and the deep head of the flexor pollicis brevis.

Compression of the ulnar nerve in the Guyon's canal can occur secondary to a ganglion cyst, occupational trauma, local trauma, and less commonly, fracture, contracture scars, and ulnar artery pathology.

6. Describe the various clinical presentations of compressive ulnar neuropathy at the wrist.

There are three distinct compression syndromes:

1. Compression of the **superficial and deep branches** within Guyon's canal, resulting in weakness of the ulnar intrinsic muscles and loss of sensation over the little finger and ulnar half of the ring finger.

2. Compression of the **ulnar nerve** occurring after it exits Guyon's canal, resulting in weakness of the ulnar innervated intrinsic muscles with sensory sparing.

3. Compression of the **superficial branch of the ulnar nerve** in Guyon's canal, resulting in sensory deficit over the ulnar volar aspect of the palm and the volar aspect of the little and ring fingers.

7. What is the differential diagnosis of numbness of the little and ring fingers?

C8 and/or T1 root lesion: Examination may reveal hypoesthesia (decreased touch sensation) or hypoalgesia (decreased pain perception) along the ulnar aspect of the forearm. There also may be evidence of Horner's syndrome (myosis and anhydrosis of the involved side of the face) due to interruption of the preganglionic sympathetic fibers that exit with the T1 (C8) root on their way to the paravertebral sympathetic ganglia. In this situation, the patient is literally in trouble "up to their eyeballs."

Neurogenic thoracic outlet syndrome: This is often associated with vascular thoracic outlet syndrome. Vascular impingement is suggested by the Adson's test, which reproduces the symptoms and obliterates the radial pulse. This maneuver reduces the space in the triangle between the scalenus anticus, scalenus medius, and the dome of the pleura. Classically, neurogenic thoracic outlet syndrome is associated with numbness in the little finger and more thenar than hypothenar atrophy.

Ulnar nerve palsy at the elbow: This is associated not only with numbness in the little and ring fingers but also decreased sensation on the dorsum of the hand along the distribution of the ulnar dorsal cutaneous branch.

Ulnar nerve entrapment at the wrist: This results in sparing of sensation supplied by the dorsal cutaneous branch of the ulnar nerve on the dorsum of the hand.

8. List the three potential sites of entrapment of the neurovascular bundle in thoracic outlet syndrome.

Thoracic outlet syndrome often presents with discomfort in the shoulder/arm area that is often precipitated by elevation of the hand during work. This syndrome may present due to entrapment of the neurovascular bundle at the following sites:

Scalenus anticus syndrome—entrapment between the anterior and posterior scalenes and the first rib

Costoclavicular syndrome—entrapment between clavicle and first rib

Pectoralis minor syndrome—entrapment between the pectoralis minor, rib cage, and coracoid process

9. What is "double-crush syndrome"? Give an example.

The double-crush nerve entrapment syndrome was described in 1973 by Upton and McComas. In this syndrome, the sensory nerves or motor nerves of a particular root can be compressed proximally as well as distally. This commonly occurs in patients with a C6 or C7 radiculopathy who also have evidence of entrapment of the median nerve at the wrist. One must assess which of the two compressions is giving the patient more symptoms and treat it appropriately.

10. What clues from the patient's history help the clinician to differentiate between carpal tunnel syndrome and cervical radiculopathy?

The patient with cervical radiculopathy often complains of pain in the neck, anterior chest, shoulder area, and interscapular region or sneezing or Valsalva-associated pain. The symptoms of carpal tunnel syndrome are localized to the upper extremity and appear to be worse at night. In cervical radiculopathy, the patient is more likely to complain of numbness which starts proximally and moves distally. The electrodiagnostic examination should always explore the possibility of both lesions.

11. What are the clinical and electrodiagnostic features of anterior interosseous nerve entrapment?

Typically, the patient complains about vague aching pain of the forearm, which starts suddenly or gradually. The patient may be unaware of weakness, but physical examination reveals weakness in the muscles supplied by the anterior interosseous nerve (i.e., the flexor pollicis longus, flexor digitorum profundus (lateral head), and pronator quadratus). These muscles work together to make the okay sign with the hand. There is no sensory deficit. The anterior interosseous nerve can be entrapped at the forearm by a fibrous band. patients with sudden onset of this condition often give a history of prolonged focal compression or prolonged periods of repetitive pronation and supination.

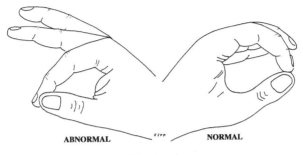

ABNORMAL   NORMAL

The okay sign.

12. How can one differentiate between a radial nerve palsy and a C7 radiculopathy?

Generally, the nerve conduction studies of the radial nerve are not affected significantly in C7 radiculopathy. In C7 radiculopathy, acute or chronic neurogenic alteration would be observed in the flexor carpi radialis, which is a median-innervated C7–8 muscle. Both conditions can co-exist as a result of the "double-crush syndrome." Paraspinous muscle EMGs of the segment at the C7–8 vertebral level may show membrane instability, confirming a C7 radiculopathy.

13. Differentiate between C5–6 radiculopathy and a lesion of the suprascapular nerve.

After suprascapular nerve impingement, the supraspinatus and infraspinatus muscles may show atrophy and weakness on clinical exam as well as membrane instability and/or chronic neurogenic alterations on EMG study. The deltoid, rhomboid, and biceps muscles would be normal.

14. How can you differentiate between lesions of the brachial plexus involving the posterior cord and those of the radial nerve?

In radial nerve palsy, the deltoid muscle (axillary nerve) is spared with a posterior cord lesion of the brachial plexus, where the lesion is at or above the takeoff of the axillary nerve, the deltoid muscle will show abnormalities.

15. How does one differentiate between C5–6 radiculopathy and long thoracic nerve palsy?

Long thoracic nerve (C5, 6, 7) palsy results in weakness of the serratus anterior muscle, which presents with scapular winging. In C5 radiculopathy, one may observe weakness of the deltoid muscle and, to a lesser degree, biceps muscle. In C6 radiculopathy, the weakness would be greater in the biceps and lesser in the deltoid muscle. With either isolated C5 or C6 radiculopathy, there is no significant winging of the scapula observed.

16. Describe the clinical features of meralgia paresthetica. How is it treated?

Meralgia paresthetica is secondary to compression of the lateral femoral cutaneous nerve of the thigh (purely sensory), which passes beneath or through the inguinal ligament approximately one fingerbreadth medial to the anterior superior iliac spine (ASIS). Often, this condition is associated with pregnancy or obesity, when a relatively large protuberant "belly" hangs over the ASIS. It can also be precipitated by the use of tight belts, corsets, and underwear. There may be tenderness, a positive Tinel's sign, or a positive compression test just medial to the ASIS. The patient usually complains of paresthesias and pain on the anterolateral aspect of the thigh where one can demonstrate evidence of sensory disturbance.

Treatment includes eliminating the causative factor, be it weight reduction, decreasing abdominal flabbiness, or increasing abdominal muscle tone. For symptomatic relief, a temporary block with a local anesthetic and a small amount of steroid around the lateral femoral cutaneous nerve can be helpful in reducing painful dysesthesias. Surgical release of the nerve might be considered if other methods of treatment fail.

17. What clinically distinguishes meralgia paresthetica and lumbosacral radiculopathy?

In **meralgia paresthetica**, the patient presents with a purely sensory syndrome on the lateral aspect of the thigh, further confirmed clinically by a positive Tinel's sign over the entrapment site which lies just medial to the ASIS.

In **lumbosacral radiculopathy** involving the L2, 3, or 4 root, the sensory symptoms and disturbances are not just limited to the lateral aspect of the thigh, but also involve the anterior aspect (femoral nerve). One may also find that the phasic stretch reflex (tendon tap reflex) in the iliopsoas (L1,2) or quadriceps (L3,4) may be decreased or absent. The sensory disturbance in the case of an L4 radiculopathy may extend below the level of the knee. The patient also may have symptoms of back pain, often radiating to the anterior aspect of the thigh, and a positive femoral nerve stretch test (with the patient prone, the hip is extended with the knee flexed, resulting in discomfort on the anterior aspect of the thigh). In addition to the clinical examination of the back, electrodiagnostic studies and appropriate imaging studies may confirm the diagnosis.

18. What are the common sites of entrapment in the sciatic nerve and the tibial nerve?

Though the sciatic nerve can be injured as a result of neoplasm, pelvic fractures, pelvic infection, gravid uterus, penetrating injuries, surgical trauma, or intramuscular injection, entrapment of the nerve is uncommon. The sciatic nerve can be entrapped especially by the piriformis muscle (piriformis syndrome). In this situation the gluteus medius, gluteus minimus, and tensor fasciae latae muscles are generally not affected. The sciatic nerve can also be compressed between the greater trochanter and the ischial tuberosity or between the hamstring muscle and adductor magnus. A large cystic swelling, such as a Baker's cyst, in the popliteal fossa can compress the sciatic nerve after it bifurcates into the tibial and peroneal nerves. Tibial nerve can be entrapped at the ankle in the tarsal tunnel.

19. Where does entrapment of the tibial nerve commonly occur?

The tibial nerve travels into the posterior compartment of the calf and is protected from trauma until it reaches the medial ankle. Entrapment of the tibial nerve occurs under the flexor retinaculum or just posterior to the medial malleolus. This is popularly known as **tarsal tunnel syndrome** and can occur as a result of tenosynovitis, venous stasis, edema, trauma, pronated foot (pes planovalgus), arthritis of the subtalar joint, or ganglia arising around the area of the medial aspect of the ankle. Lesions distal to the flexor retinaculum can either compress the medial or lateral plantar branches of the tibial nerve.

20. Describe the clinical presentation of tarsal tunnel syndrome.

- Presents in middle age
- Painful dysesthesias of the soles and toes, associated with sensory deficit on the plantar aspect of the foot and toes and with weakness in the intrinsic muscles of the feet
- Pain occurs at rest, while the patient is sitting or in bed
- Positive Tinel's sign (paresthesias in the nerve distribution with percussion over the nerve at the entrapment site) posterior to the medial malleolus
- Latencies of medial and/or lateral plantar branches may be prolonged
- Possible membrane instability of the abductor hallucis and/or abductor digiti quinti

21. How can you differentiate between scapular winging secondary to long thoracic nerve injury as opposed to spinal accessory nerve injury?

In **long thoracic nerve** injury or neuropathy, the serratus anterior weakness allows the vertebral border of the scapula to drift closer to the midline and the inferior angle to rotate medially. The winging increases with protraction of the scapula when the patient forcefully pushes forward with his or her arm against resistance; however, attempts at abduction of the shoulder decrease the winging.

Injury to the **spinal accessory nerve** which supplies the trapezius muscle is associated with a lesser degree of winging at rest, with the inferior angle of the scapula becoming more prominent. The inferior angle of the scapula is rotated medially as in serratus anterior weakness, but the scapula drifts away softly from the midline. The shoulder in this condition droops down due to atrophy of the superior part of the trapezius muscle. Attempts at shoulder abduction tend to increase winging initially, but as the shoulder approaches 90°, the winging diminishes.

22. How can one clinically differentiate between peroneal nerve palsy and L5 radiculopathy?

In **peroneal nerve palsy**, one may find weakness of the dorsiflexors and the evertors of the foot. Unlike in L5 **radiculopathy**, generally there should also be weakness of significance detected in the inverters of the foot as a result of weakness in the posterior tibial muscle.

23. How does one differentiate between L3 radiculopathy and femoral neuropathy?

In **L3 radiculopathy**, one detects abnormalities in the hip adductors (supplied by the obturator nerve L2,3,4 roots) as well as in the quadriceps muscle. In **femoral neuropathy** these abnormalities are confined to the quadriceps muscle.

24. What is Morton's neuroma?

Entrapment of the interdigital nerve between either the third and fourth or second and third metatarsal heads. The symptoms include shooting pain and buring of the second, third, or fourth toes. There is a cramping sensation at the metatarsal heads that is relieved with massage. Examination reveals tenderness of the sole and affected web spaces. Dorsal tenderness of the metatarsophalangeal joints may be indicative of extensor tendinitis or synovitis. Conservative treatment of Morton's neuroma includes a pad just proximal to the metatarsal heads and/or an injection of bupivicaine and corticosteroid.

25. Outline the approach to treatment of entrapment neuropathies.

Prevention

Avoid sustained or intermittent extreme pressure or tethering at the entrapment sites.

Avoid vitamin deficiencies, especially with B12, folic acid.

Monitor and optimally control diabetes. (Diabetics are more vulnerable to developing not only polyneuropathy or peripheral neuropathy but also entrapment neuropathies.)

Treatment

Nonoperative

Splint the limb in a neutral position that maximizes space for the entrapped nerve. Maintain good blood flow to the limb and reduce swelling and edema in order to prevent further compression.

Modify activity, and avoid positions that can be a source of nerve trauma.

Reduce inflammation and consider the use of ice, NSAIDs, and corticosteroid injections in structures around the nerves that may be inflamed.

Operative

If, despite nonoperative treatment, there is evidence of continuing axonal degeneration in the entrapped nerve, consider referral for surgical decompression.

BIBLIOGRAPHY

1. Liveson JA, Spielholz NI: Peripheral Neurology: Case Studies in Electrodiagnosis. Philadelphia, F.A. Davis, 1991.
2. Upton ARM, McComas AJ: The double crush in nerve-entrapment syndromes. Lancet 2:359, 1973.

35. CARPAL TUNNEL SYNDROME AND/OR MEDIAN NEUROPATHY AT THE WRIST

Janet C. Limke, M.D., and Steven A. Stiens, M.D.

1. What is the carpal tunnel?

The carpal tunnel is the small, oblong pathway in the wrist through which the median nerve and 9 tendons pass (4 tendons each from the flexor digitorum superficialis and profundus muscles and 1 from the flexor pollicis longus). On the volar side, it is bounded by the taut transverse carpal ligament, or flexor retinaculum, and on the dorsal side by the carpal bones.

2. How does carpal tunnel syndrome (CTS) present?

Carpal tunnel syndrome is the most common focal nerve entrapment syndrome. The presentation includes major specific symptoms of pain and paresthesias (tingling, burning, and numbness) in the median nerve distribution. In advanced cases, weakness of the median-innervated hand musculature is present. Minor, nonspecific symptoms include: wrist pain, clumsiness, tightness, and complaints of dropping things easily. Pain commonly involves the hand or wrist but may also be felt proximally in the forearm, elbow, or shoulder. Symptoms are often brought on by overuse of the hand, especially forceful

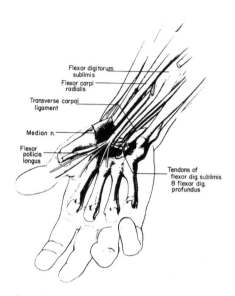

Carpal tunnel. (From Liveson JA, Spielholz NI: Peripheral Neurology: Case Studies in Electrodiagnosis. Philadelphia, F.A. Davis, 1991, p 20; with permission.)

gripping or repetitive hand/wrist motion. Nocturnal symptoms are frequently reported and are associated with the characteristic **"flick" sign** (shaking the hand to relieve paresthesias).

3. How is the diagnosis of CTS made?

Median nerve impingement, which produces the spectrum of pathophysiologic changes known as CTS, can be discerned with nerve conduction studies, magnetic resonance imaging, or open surgical exploration. The clinical evaluation includes a systematic history, eliciting of signs with provocative maneuvers, as well as confirmatory physiologic and anatomic tests.

Some clinicians rely solely on clinical history and physical exam and recommend surgery after conservative measures have failed. However, because many conditions can be confused with CTS, treating solely on the basis of physical signs and symptoms can be problematic. Whereas some researchers define CTS as a clinical diagnosis, others define it with combined clinical and electrodiagnostic changes supportive of CTS. It may be argued that more stringent criteria, i.e., nerve conduction abnormalities, should be present before surgery is considered.

4. List the differential diagnosis of CTS.

Neurologic: cervical radiculopathy (C5,6,7,8); ulnar, radial, or proximal median nerve lesion or generalized neuropathies; brachial plexus lesions, including thoracic outlet syndrome; syringomyelia or other central sensory and motor phenomenon

Musculoskeletal: tenosynovitis including deQuervain's (inflammation of synovial tendon sheaths), osteoarthritis of the metacarpal-trapezial joint (thumb carpometacarpal arthritis), Kienböck's disease (avascular lunate necrosis), scaphoidal-trapezial arthritis, digital neuritis
Vascular: Raynaud's phenomenon, radial artery thrombosis

5. What is the difference between CTS and median neuropathy at the wrist?

Definite CTS is confirmed when the clinical syndrome is present *along with* physiologic, anatomic, or pathologic evidence of median nerve impairment. When neurophysiologic evidence of median nerve impairment is present *without* signs and symptoms, the situation is best termed asymptomatic median neuropathy, not CTS. Median entrapment neuropathy is often discovered in the process of an electrodiagnostic consultation precipitated by another question or while doing research on an asymptomatic population.

6. Do tests that attempt to objectify sensory impairment have utility in screening for CTS?

Yes, but none are substitutes for NCS, currently the only truly objective measurement of nerve impairment. Tests of sensibility (sensory perception) can be divided into two general categories: threshold tests and innervation density tests.

The **thermal threshold test** quantifies dysfunction in the small myelinated and unmyelinated axons, whereas NCS tests large myelinated fibers. When compared to NCS as the gold standard, thermal threshold measurements are sensitive but not specific in early CTS.

Like NCS, **vibrometry** evaluates larger myelinated fibers. However, in an excellent recent study, vibrometry was not sensitive in picking up early CTS in an industrial population. According to the researchers, axonal injury must be present, as in more severe CTS, before abnormalities will be detected.

Another threshold test, the **Semmes-Weinstein monofilament test**, assesses touch perception of the thinnest detected filament applied to the digit. In general, the threshold tests are more sensitive than innervation density tests, such as the **Weber two-point discrimination**. Normal two-point discrimination is 5 mm or less and can be determined with the use of ECG calipers and a ruler. All of the sensibility tests have been used in documenting recovery of CTS, particularly after surgery.

7. Name the important components of the electrodiagnostic consultation in suspected CTS.

The electrodiagnostic medical consultation evaluates nerve and muscle function as an extension of the clinical neuromuscular examination. The role of the electromyographer in management of CTS varies with referral requests. At the least, the consultative record should render an interpreted review of the patient's history (family history of CTS, diabetes, thyroid disease, employment), symptoms (acroparesthesias, weakness duration, distribution and symptoms, exacerbating/relieving facts), physical findings (temperature, sudomotor changes, atrophy, edema, reflex, strength sensation, evocative maneuvers), and electrodiagnostic data. Neuromuscular or systemic conditions that could masquerade as CTS or predispose the patient to CTS should be uncovered, studied, and reported (i.e., diabetes).

8. How is the Phalen wrist flexion test carried out?

Dr. George S. Phalen, former Chief of Hand Surgery at the Cleveland Clinic and a founding member of the American Society for Surgery of the Hand, recommended that the patient place his or her flexed elbows on a table and allow the wrists to fall freely into maximum flexion (no forced flexion by patient or examiner). The median nerve is compressed between the proximal edge of the transverse carpal ligament and the flexor tendons. This position is expected to elicit numbness and tingling in a median distribution in 75% of persons with CTS symptoms and median neuropathy within 1–2 minutes and in > 25% of normals at 10 minutes.

9. What are other commonly used provocative tests?

The examination should include a bilateral directed evaluation of the cervical, shoulder, forearm, wrist, and hand regions. Provocative tests complement the examination by demonstrating a relationship between symptoms and mechanical manipulation of the median nerve. All are plagued with false-negative and false-positive results.

1. **Tinel's sign**—Percussion over the nerve produces tingling sensations in the distribution of a regenerating injured nerve. Light percussion with a reflex hammer along the nerve while the wrist is extended increases sensitivity, but false-positives have been reported to range from 6–45%.

2. **Tethered median nerve stress test**—Hyperextend the index finger at the DIP joint with the wrist extended and supinated to pull or stretch the nerve. A positive test produces median dysesthesias or forearm pain.

3. **Carpal compression test**—Apply 150 mmHg pressure over the volar wrist at the median nerve for 30 seconds. The test is positive if median dysesthesia is reported.

4. **Reverse Phalen test**—Extend the wrists to 90° in a praying-hands position for 60 seconds. Paresthesis in the median distribution indicates a positive result.

10. If median neuropathy of the wrist is suspected, what is the current standard electrodiagnostic approach?

A combined committee of the American Association of Electrodiagnostic Medicine, American Academy of Neurology, and American Academy of Physical Medicine and Rehabilitation published a practice parameter for electrodiagnostic studies in CTS. After a thorough review of the literature, recommendations include:

1. Sensory NCS of the median nerve across the wrist, and if the latency is abnormal, comparison to one other sensory study in the symptomatic limb.

2. If the initial median sensory NCS across the wrist has a conduction distance > 8 cm and the results are normal, additional studies as follows:
   • Median sensory NCS across the wrist over a short (7–8 cm) conduction distance *or*
   • Comparison of median sensory NCS across the wrist with radial or ulnar sensory conduction across the wrist in the same limb.

The practice parameter also recommends motor NCS of the median nerve with comparison to one other motor nerve in the symptomatic limb and an option for EMG study of the limb.

11. How do imaging studies contribute to the clinical data?

MRI reveals anatomic as well as chemical changes. Morphologic changes suggesting median nerve impingement include enlargement with edema, flattening, narrowing, and loss of normal fat in the carpal tunnel. Postsurgical changes may include hematomas, abscesses, and excess scar formation. Recent studies have demonstrated that MRI may reveal peripheral nerve lesions involving axonotmesis as early as 4 days after the onset of symptoms or injury by picking up an altered signal from denervated muscle. Neurapraxic injuries (conduction block without axon loss) result in normal signal from median innervated muscles. Despite these capabilities, MRI is not part of a routine workup for CTS.

12. What are patient factors that are associated with false-positive results in CTS?

Cold temperature of the hand will slow the conduction, prolong distal latencies, and increase the amplitude of a response.

Increasing age is correlated with slower conduction times and smaller amplitude responses. Median digital amplitudes recorded antidromically fall slightly more than 2 μV per decade.

Height, and therefore **axon length**, is directly correlated with latency and inversely related to amplitude.

Finger circumference is inversely related to the amplitude, as the intervening soft tissue causes attenuation of the recorded response on the skin surface.

Gender does not appear to play as much of a role when the above factors are considered.

13. What technical problems can result in inaccurate results?

Proper technique is essential to ensure the accuracy of NCS. The extremity should be warmed to > 32°C. A submaximal stimulus intensity may lead to an erroneously small amplitude response. Exact distances should be measured and rechecked if abnormal values are noted.

Consistent amplifier gain, sweep speeds, and filter settings should be utilized that are appropriate for the given study and allow for comparison to reference values. Techniques to minimize stimulus artifact interference and overcome electrode and skin resistance should be adhered to.

For sensory studies < 4-cm electrode separation during bipolar recordings may result in an abnormally small amplitude due to a smaller potential difference between the active and reference electrodes. For motor studies, the recording electrode must be centered over the main muscle belly or motor point and the reference over the tendon or adjacent joint. If the recording electrode is not properly centered, a positive deflection will be recorded before the negative deflection and may confuse the latency measurement.

14. Describe anomalous innervations affecting the NCS and interpretation in CTS.

The **Martin-Gruber anastomosis**, a median-to-ulnar connection in the forearm motor fibers via the anterior interosseous nerve, occurs in 15% of individuals and affects both median and ulnar recordings. In an individual without median neuropathy, this variation will result in a larger than expected CMAP amplitude when stimulating the median nerve at the elbow. In median neuropathy, the anastomosis causes an initial positive deflection when stimulating over the elbow, despite proper centering of the recording electrode over the belly of the thenar muscles. The same deflection is not noted on distal wrist stimulation. The early positive deflection represents volume conduction from the stimulation of the anomalous ulnar axons that are conducting the impulse quicker since they do not pass through the carpal tunnel.

15. How do various innervations of hand muscles affect EMG interpretation of MN?

Many variations exist in the innervation of the thenar muscles. Approximately one-third of patients have all median-innervated thenar muscles: flexor pollicis brevis, abductor pollicis brevis, and opponens pollicis. Another third show median innervation to opponens pollicis and abductor pollicis brevis and ulnar innervation to the entire flexor pollicis brevis, while 15% show dual innervation of flexor pollicis brevis. Up to 2% of hands show an all-ulnar-innervated pattern. This knowledge of anatomy calls for caution in interpreting EMG abnormalities in thenar muscles, since ulnar lesions may account for changes in some patients.

16. What does the needle EMG exam contribute to the diagnosis of CTS?

1. It provides evidence of motor axon injury and/or reinnervation of the thenar muscles. Thus, along with NCS abnormalities consistent with a median nerve process at the wrist, it confirms axon loss in severe CTS and may help to determine chronicity.

2. It is useful in assessing separate or concomitant pathology, such as proximal median neuropathy, cervical or thoracic radiculopathy, plexopathy, or polyneuropathy. Proximal lesions along any part of the origins of the median nerve from the cervical spine and distal, in addition to median neuropathy at the wrist, represents a **"double-crush" syndrome**. The distribution of abnormalities will lead the skilled electromyographer to the correct diagnosis or diagnoses.

17. What other lower motor neuron problems may present with similar symptoms?

The sensory dermatomal distribution of the hand is C6–8 going lateral to medial, while motor innervation to thenar muscles is C8–T1. A cervical radiculopathy will typically show abnormalities in the muscles innervated by the corresponding nerve root *without* sensory conduction changes since the dorsal root ganglion is typically spared. A plexopathy may present with a variety of patterns affecting the median nerve, since it arises from all three trunks of the brachial plexus. Tracing the changes back through the plexus will usually reveal the point or points of plexus involvement. A polyneuropathy results in multiple NCS findings in more than one limb.

18. What other common sites of median nerve compression should be considered in the evaluation of CTS?

1. At the **supracondylar ligament** before it enters the pronator canal in the distal upper arm

2. Between the **pronator teres** and the edge of the flexor sublimis (pronator syndrome), which spares the innervation to pronator teres

3. At the **anterior interosseous branch**, a pure motor branch of the median nerve in the forearm.

Proximal motor stimulation, transcarpal assessment, and careful EMG of median-innervated muscles help demonstrate these other entrapments.

19. Describe a practical severity rating scale for CTS and median neuropathy (MN) for use when reporting electrodiagnostic findings.

There are different ways to report severity. One logical system which incorporates both latency and amplitude changes follows:

Mild MN: Median sensory nerve conduction slowing without motor nerve conduction slowing *and/or* loss of median sensory amplitude of < 50% of the reference value.

Moderate MN: Median sensory and motor slowing *and/or* loss of median sensory amplitude of > 50% of the reference value.

Severe MN: Absence of median sensory potential along with median motor slowing, *or* median motor slowing along with reduction of median motor amplitude, *or* median NCS abnormalities along with evidence of axonal injury on EMG of the thenar muscles.

20. Discuss the nonoperative treatment of CTS.

Once CTS has been confirmed, basic laboratory tests for thyroid or renal disorders and diabetes should be obtained. Any underlying disorders should be treated. Appropriate radiologic studies should be obtained.

Nonoperative therapy may include **hand splinting** in 0–30° extension, medications such as **diuretics** and **NSAIDs**, **ergonomic modifications**, and **steroid injections** in the wrist. Modest doses of pyridoxine (vitamin B6) have been advocated, although no well-designed study has demonstrated its efficacy.

21. List five identified factors that predict failure of nonoperative treatment.

Age > 50 years
Duration > 10 months
Constant paresthesias
Stenosing flexor tenosynovitis
Positive Phalen test in < 30 seconds
Less than 10% of persons with 3 of 5 risk factors improve with medical management alone

22. What are ergonomic risk factors for CTS?

Increased force, repetition, vibration, awkward posture, and temperature extremes have all been implicated as ergonomic risk factors for occupational hand and wrist disorders, including CTS.

23. What surgical treatments are possible for CTS?

The most widely accepted technique for CTS release is an **open procedure** using a 4–5-cm, curved, longitudinal incision with good exposure of the transverse carpal ligament to minimize nerve injury. Occasionally, the palmar branch of the medial nerve and rarely the motor branch to the thenar muscles are transligamentous. When these variations are present, the branches are identified and dissected free from the ligament.

Endoscopic techniques have been described for release of the transverse carpal ligament. A preliminary, prospective, randomized study suggested that functional recovery is achieved sooner but that a higher incidence of nerve injury complications is observed after the endoscopic technique as compared with the open method. A redesign of the one form of instrumentation has attempted to solve this problem. Further longer-term studies are needed to evaluate not only the complications but also the long-term efficacy of the endoscopic approach.

24. What are the possible complications of surgery?

Surgical complications occur in about 2% of cases and include excessive scar formation (particularly with longitudinal incision proximal to the palmar flexor crease), infection, nerve injuries (including the motor branch or palmar cutaneous branch of the median nerve or the digital sensory nerves), pain (at the scar or reflex sympathetic dystrophy), and bowing of the tendons of the wrist with loss of grip strength.

25. Discuss follow-up after CTS surgery. How quickly does nerve function recover and NCS abnormalities resolve?

After surgery, the wrist is splinted in extension for 1–3 weeks, and the fingers are gently exercised. A patient having an open surgery may be excused from work for 1–6 weeks (most would return to light duty much earlier) depending on the demands of the job, and those having the endoscopic technique may return to work in 1–3 weeks. Pain and paresthesias usually improve in the first several weeks, while numbness and weakness may require 6–9 months for optimal recovery. Patients with preoperative thenar involvement are less likely to have resolution of paresthesias after surgery. With a median follow-up of 5.5 years, 86% of patients with surgical decompression showed at least partial improvement of NCS. Pain is the most significantly improved symptom. Poorer outcome has been observed in patients who have strenuous work activities. Nonoperative approaches also show a poor outcome in the heavy labor population, suggesting a need for ergonomic or vocational adjustments if CTS is to be relieved. Following surgery, NCS abnormalities typically improve, although complete normalization does not always occur.

BIBLIOGRAPHY

1. Agee JM, McCarroll HR, North ER: Endoscopic carpal tunnel release using the single proximal incision technique. Hand Clin 10:647–659, 1994.
2. American Association of Electrodiagnostic Medicine, American Academy of Neurology, and American Academy of Physical Medicine and Rehabilitation: Practice parameter for electrodiagnostic studies in carpal tunnel syndrome: Summary statement. Muscle Nerve 16:1390–1391, 1993.
3. Franzblau A, et al: Workplace surveillance for carpal tunnel syndrome: A comparison of methods. J Occup Rehabil 3:1–14, 1993.
4. Katz RT: Carpal tunnel syndrome: A practical review. Am Fam Physician 49(6):1371–1378, 1994.
5. Kaplan SJ, Gickel SZ, Eaton RG: Predictive factors in the non-surgical treatment of carpal tunnel syndrome. J Hand Surg 15B:107, 1990.
6. Kuschner SH, Brien WW, Johnson D: Complications associated with carpal tunnel release. Orthop Rev 20:346–352, 1991.
7. Rosenbaum RB, Ochoa JL: Carpal Tunnel Syndrome and Other Disorders of the Median Nerve. Stoneham, MA, Butterworth-Heinemann, 1993.
8. Stetson DS, Albers JW, Silverstein BA, Wolfe RA: Effects of age, sex and anthropometric factors on nerve conduction measures. Muscle Nerve 15:1095–1104, 1992.
9. Werner RA, Alberts JW: Relation between needle electromyography and nerve conduction studies in patients with carpal tunnel syndrome. Arch Phys Med Rehabil 76:246–249, 1995.
10. West GA, et al: Magnetic resonance imaging signal changes in denervated muscles after peripheral nerve injury. Neurosurgery 35:1077–1086, 1994.

V. Rehabilitation of System-Based Disorders
A. Cardiac, Pulmonary, and Circulatory Systems

36. CARDIAC REHABILITATION

*Jeffery A. Lehman, M.D., Steven A. Stiens, M.D.,
and Eugen M. Halar, M.D.*

1. Define cardiac rehabilitation (CR).
A series of definitions should provide perspective:
- The **American Association of Cardiovascular and Pulmonary Rehabilitation** (AACPR) defines CR as "the application of rehabilitative services to *improve* and *maintain* a patient's physiologic, physical, psychosocial, and vocational functioning at an optimal level."
- The **U.S. Department of Health and Human Services** defines CR services as comprehensive, long-term programs involving medical evaluation, exercise prescriptions, cardiac risk-factors modification, education, and counseling to *limit* the physiologic and psychological adverse effects of cardiac illness.
- We define the CR similarly but emphasize the person as the center for rehabilitation goals and the key to success. CR is a patient-participative interdisciplinary process that seeks to enhance the patient's personal effectiveness through cardiac disease prevention, cardiovascular and psychosocial adaptation, functional improvement, and role reintegration.

2. Who can benefit from CR?
Patients who have functional, physiological, and psychosocial deficits related to impairments of the cardiovascular system can benefit from CR. This includes patients with the following diagnoses or therapeutic interventions: ischemic heart disease, recent myocardial infarction, post-coronary artery bypass surgery, post-percutaneous transluminal coronary angioplasty (PTCA), post-cardiac transplant, post-heart valve replacement, and congestive heart failure.

3. What is the incidence and significance of coronary heart disease (CHD) in the United States?
The 1993 statistics indicate that CHD affects 13.5 million Americans. Seven million suffer from stable angina and could benefit from CR. One and one-half million suffer myocardial infarction each year, and almost 1 million survive. Forty-five percent of all myocardial infarctions are in persons under age 65. In addition, 309,000 coronary artery bypass graft and 362,000 PTCA procedures are done annually, and 54% of these patients are under age 65. All of these people could benefit from CR services, but only 11–20% of them do participate.

4. What are the overall goals of the CR process?
To prevent and reverse atherosclerosis
To reduce myocardial ischemia and the risk of infarction or sudden death
To maximize cardiovascular function and capacity
To maximize exercise tolerance and ADL performance
To establish a patient-controlled and safe aerobic exercise program
To provide guidelines for safe activities and work
To control risk factors for CHD

To help patients cope with perceived stressors
To utilize energy conservation and work simplification
To improve quality of life

5. Describe the phases of the CR process.

The CR intervention sequence integrates into the classic medical continuum of intervention with any illness:

prevention → acute care (medical/surgical) → rehabilitation

The typical patient referred for CR has sustained a myocardial infarction and/or undergone coronary artery bypass surgery. CR has therefore typically been divided into 3 sequential phases that bring the patient out of acute care:

Phase I—Inpatient phase from hospital admission to hospital discharge.

Phase II—Outpatient training phase including aerobic conditioning, reacquisition of full activity, integration of diet and lifestyle changes.

Phase III—Maintenance phase, with patient-monitored continuation of the aerobic exercise program, risk-reduction strategies, and activity/work modifications.

These phases represent a time line for the process of intervention. It is important to recognize many interventions continue through the phases on an ongoing basis and that the application of CR interventions should be tailored to the need of each individual.

6. How is cardiovascular impairment estimated by the rehab team through chart review and bedside exam?

The history, physical examination, EKG, and chest radiograph can predict coronary artery disease seen by catheterization and eventual mortality. The following components are to be included in each evaluation.

History: angina (typical, atypical, nocturnal, progressive, as well as activity limits and intensity required), risk factors, dyspnea (exertional), paroxysmal nocturnal dyspnea (1–5 hours after recumbent), fatigue level (exercise tolerance), and premorbid level of functioning (walking stairs, ADLs, etc.).

Physical exam: vital signs, orthostatics (pulses and BP while supine, sitting, and standing, if possible), pulses, jugular venous distention, cardiac auscultation (murmurs, gallops), pulmonary assessment (rales), abdominal exam (hepatojugular reflux, bruits), edema, and tolerance of functional activities.

Functional clinical evaluations (to assess tolerance): grooming, bathing, dressing, bed mobility, transfers, ambulation with or without device, stairs, aerobic exercises, work simulation, etc. Musculoskeletal and neurologic exams are also essential to determine impairments that may affect functional and exercise training.

Laboratory tests: total creatine kinase-MB, hematocrit, chest x-ray (cardiac silhouette), EKG (arrhythmias, Q waves, estimate MI severity, ST-T wave changes, voltage), BUN/CR ratio, echo/MUGA (ejection fraction), cardiac exercises stress tests, or other cardiac imaging tests or studies.

From the above findings, patients are stratified as low, moderate, or high risk and their level of required supervision is determined. The patient's prescriptions and CR program are also tailored to the above findings.

7. What are possible contraindications for entry into inpatient or outpatient exercise programs?

According to the American College of Sports Medicine, they are:
Unstable angina
Resting systolic BP > 200 mmHg
Resting diastolic BP > 100 mmHg
Orthostatic BP drop or drop during exercise training of ≥ 20 mmHg
Moderate to severe aortic stenosis

Acute systemic illness or fever
Uncontrolled atrial or ventricular dysrhythmias
Uncontrolled sinus tachycardia (120 bpm)
Uncontrolled congestive heart failure
Third-degree A-V block
Active pericarditis or myocarditis
Recent embolism
Thrombophlebitis
Resting ST displacement (> 3 mm)
Uncontrolled diabetes
Orthopedic problems that prohibit exercise

8. What are the foci of intervention during Phase I, the inpatient phase of CR?
Interventions include:
Alleviation of anxiety and depression through explanation of the cardiac event
Reestablish patient's control of self
Patient education regarding rationale for treatment and exercises
Medical evaluation of cardiac anatomy, injury severity, EKG changes and rhythm stability
Development of a team knowledge base of the patient's previous activities and life roles as
     well as current personal goals
Risk factor quantification, stratification, and reduction strategies
Assessment of cardiovascular function and impairments
Early remobilization (a combination of functional activities and exercises)
Reachievement of basic ADL function (self-care activities)
Prescription and education with guidelines for activity and work after discharge

**9. Describe the relationship between heart rate, stroke volume, cardiac output, aerobic
capacity, and the anginal threshold.**
The maximum **heart rate** (HR) is defined as the maximum obtained on an exercise stress
test. It decreases with age and can be estimated for the normal population by subtracting the patient's age in years from 220. **Stroke volume** (SV) is the amount of blood ejected with each ventricular contraction and increases with exercise to become maximum at 50% over the basal heart
rate (resting HR). **Cardiac output** (CO) equals HR × SV and relates directly to the total body
oxygen consumption (VO_2) because all O_2 consumed is delivered to the body tissues via the
blood. **Maximum aerobic capacity** (VO_2 max) is the greatest rate (VO_2 ml/kg body mass/min)
of O_2 consumption a person is capable of metabolizing; it relates directly to maximum work
output in watts. One way to understand and calculate VO_2 max is to use the formula SV × HR ×
$(a - V\ O_2$ difference), which integrates the delivery and extraction of O_2. Thus, an increase in CO,
the product of SV × HR, and/or increase in arteriovenous O_2 difference increases in VO_2 maximum. The **anginal threshold** is defined as the CO at which myocardial O_2 demand exceeds O_2
delivered. An ischemic myocardium is not capable of maintaining the same cardiac work load,
which results in a fall in CO, HR, and/or BP.

10. What are the modifiable risk factors for atherosclerotic coronary artery disease?
According to the Framingham studies of 1984, the significant risk factors for developing
coronary heart disease are age, male sex, elevated total cholesterol, elevated low-density lipoprotein (LDL) cholesterol, low level of high-density lipoprotein (HDL) cholesterol, elevated systolic
or diastolic BP, diabetes, obesity, sedentary lifestyle, cigarette smoking, stress, family history of
premature coronary disease, and EKG evidence of left ventricular hypertrophy. From the risk
factors reported in the Framingham study of 1984, one can define the **modifiable risk factors**
as hypertension, cigarette smoking, hypercholesterolemia (> 200 mg/dl), inactivity, low HDL
cholesterol (< 35 mg/dl), obesity, hypertriglyceridemia, diabetes mellitus, and stress. There is
strong evidence that modification can cause regression of pathology. Recent prospective studies

of patients randomized to control groups of monotherapy with simvastatin, lovastatin, colestipol, or niacin for cholesterol control have demonstrated coronary atheroma regression, lower rates of coronary artery bypass grafting, and reduced mortality. Meta-analysis of data from randomized control trials of CR programs consisting of exercise training and risk factor management has demonstrated at least a 10% reduction in the 3-year mortality rate.

11. Which types of cardiac stress tests are used to evaluate for cardiac ischemia or dysrhythmias?

EKG testing: Risk stratifies and determines safe work output. The test includes EKG monitoring for heart rate, arrhythmia, ischemia (ST depression > 1 mm), and monitoring for symptoms and BP. Protocols include 3–5-min stages, Bruce inclined treadmill stages 1–5 (incline degrees 10, 12, 14, 16, and 18°); speeds 1.7, 2.5, 3.4, 4.2, and 5.0 mph), bicycle ergometry, upper-extremity ergometry (increase work by increasing arm crank resistance), wheelchair ergometry, or arm-leg ergometry utilized by hemiplegics.

Nuclear stress testing: Thallium-201 perfusion scintigraphy depends on coronary vasodilation from exercise or vasodilators (dipyridamole, adenosine), which increases the **cardiac steal phenomenon** (stiff, narrowed vessels dilate less). Immediate post-first-pass perfusion indicates myocardial blood flow in various vessel territories. Delayed images 2–24 hours later demonstrate viable myocardium.

Dobutamine HCl echocardiography: Can be used to access areas of cardiac ischemia by determining regions of wall motion abnormalities. The cardiac demand is increased by dobutamine, which increases both HR and BP. Therefore, in contrast to the dipyridamole thallium tests, dobutamine stress echocardiograms not only identify coronary ischemia (sensitivity 95%, specificity 82% vs catheterization) but also the ischemic anginal threshold, the maximum HR and BP, or rate-pressure product. This additional information helps prescribe the patient's cardiac guidelines for exercises, activities, and work.

12. What are the major goals during Phase II, the outpatient training phase of CR?

Besides continuing the goals of phase I CR, the major goals of Phase II are:

To achieve cardiovascular conditioning via an aerobic exercise training program

To modify risk factors using psychosocial and pharmacologic interventions

To diagnose etiologies for exercise intolerance and to adjust treatments to improve exercise tolerance

To provide upgraded guidelines for ADL and work

To educate the patient to self-monitor the appropriate level of exercise, work, or activities via HR and/or rating of perceived exertion

To further improve positive behaviors

To continue psychosocial support

The CR training phase should result in improvements in VO_2 max; lower resting and submaximal HRs for a given workload; reduced systolic BP; beneficial peripheral effects (improved O_2 extraction/utilization by skeletal muscle); risk factor reduction; diminished anxiety, stress, and depression; and improved coping with new deficits and psychosocial stressors.

13. List the five major parts of a CR exercise prescription.

1. **Modality**—The American College of Sports Medicine recommends that the exercise modality be "any activity that uses large muscle groups, that can be maintained for a prolonged period, and is rhythmic and aerobic in nature."

2. **Intensity**—Either prescribed by HR, rating of perceived exertion (RPE), or metabolic equivalents (METs).

3. **Duration**—Depends on the mode and intensity of exercise. Usually it is 20–30 minutes initially and later may increase to 60-minute sessions.

4. **Frequency**—Daily while in the hospital, and at least 3 times weekly while in the aerobic training and maintenance phases, usually skipping a day between intensive sessions.

5. **Rate of progression**—Depends on the patient's individual tolerance, progress, endurance, needs, and goals.

14. What is the purpose of a warm-up period?

The warm-up period, usually lasting 5–10 minutes, increases the intensity of exercise gradually from rest to the desired intensity level and also stretches the major muscles that will be used. This warm-up decreases the risk of cardiovascular problems (i.e., delay in onset of angina) and prevents sprain or strain injuries. Some patients, such as those with cardiac transplants and CHF, need longer periods of warm-up before proceeding to the more intensive aerobic exercises.

15. What is the purpose of a cool-down period?

It allows gradual reduction of cardiac work and redistribution of blood from muscles and extremities to internal organs. A gradual reduction of work intensity with continued body movement maintains venous return; prevents cardiovascular injuries, musculoskeletal problems, postexercise hypotension, or end-organ insufficiencies; and promotes dissipation of heat.

16. What are the major interventions of Phase III, the maintenance phase of CR?

Phase III has the same goals as Phase II (the training phase), except that the program is monitored by the patient and/or family. The program continues outside the CR center, in a community-based setting or wherever the patient feels comfortable. The members of the CR team (i.e., physician, therapist, nutritionist, psychologist, social worker, etc.) then may be available to assist and advise the patient as needed. The patient continues the level of exercise program achieved and self-monitors his or her own exercises, activities, and work to avoid overexertion. Periodic evaluations should be done to monitor the patient's progress and tolerance and maintenance of previously achieved goals. Before beginning or changing the exercise program, the patient should check with his or her doctor.

17. Which changes in lifestyle after symptomatic coronary artery disease are beneficial?

Aggressive lifestyle changes, including a vegetarian diet with < 10% of total calories from fat combined with 3 hours of aerobic exercise per week and stress management, have been demonstrated to produce clinically significant regression in coronary atherosclerosis documented by arteriography. In the lifestyle Heart Trial Study, patients on the American Heart Association-recommended diet of < 30% fat showed progression of their coronary atherosclerosis on repeat catheterization. Such studies suggest that conventional recommendations for patients with coronary artery disease are not sufficient to abate or reverse the disease process.

A CR dietary program should provide the metabolites needed for muscle adaption with exercise, reduce risk factors associated with lipids and body fat content, and establish a body habitus that minimizes cardiac work, thus maximizing functional independence. In an attempt to approach this dietary ideal, the amount as well as the content of the diet need to be calculated. The incidence of myocardial infarction (MI) in depressed patients is significantly greater, and depression after MI increases morbidity and mortality; thus, pharmacologic and psychological intervention are important components of CR. Adequate social support enhances recovery of MI patients and is a buffer against stress.

18. What factors cause reduced exercise capacity after spinal cord injury (SCI)?

Reduced exercise capacity in SCI patients is multifactoral. These factors include impaired autonomic nervous system control of the cardiovascular system, altered hormonal effects on the cardiovascular system, loss of the muscle pump causing decreased venous return, muscle weakness and/or atrophy, altered respiratory system, small size of cardiac chambers, greater use of type II over type I muscle fibers, and sedentary lifestyle.

19. What modes of aerobic exercise training can be used in SCI patients?

Wheelchair propulsion, arm ergometry, wheelchair cycling using an arm crank, functional electrical stimulation (FES), and hybrid exercise (arm ergometry combined with lower-extremity FES).

20. Should patients with congestive heart failure be excluded from CR?

No, stabilized and compensated patients with congestive heart failure are capable of achieving an increase in functional capacity of 20% with slowly progressive intensity and duration of each exercise session, provided the program lasts at least 3 months and is continued with a maintenance CR program.

21. What about cardiac transplant?

Due to denervation of the heart, the HR increases only in response to circulating catecholamines. Intervention in transplant recipients includes a longer warm-up, slowly progressive endurance exercise, followed by longer cool-down periods. Cardiac transplant patients are characteristically very deconditioned and need conditioning and CR programs.

22. What about other patients under rehabilitative care who may have risk factors for coronary disease and cardiac complications?

The list of patients is enormous and includes geriatric patients, those with stroke, those with a previous history of cardiac abnormalities, etc. These patients should be rehabilitated within the guidelines of cardiac precautions.

BIBLIOGRAPHY

1. American Association of Cardiovascular and Pulmonary Rehabilitation: Guidelines for Cardiac Rehabilitation Program. Champaign, IL, Human Kinetics Books, 1991.
2. American College of Sports Medicine: Guidelines for Exercise Testing and Prescription, 4th ed. Malvern, PA, Lea & Febiger, 1991.
3. Cardiac Rehabilitation Guidelines Panel: Cardiac Rehabilitation [Clinic Practice Guidelines no. 17. AHCPR pub no. 96-0672]. Rockville, MD, Agency for Health Care Policy and Research, 1995.
4. Halar EM (ed): Cardiac Rehabilitation, Parts I and II. Phys Med Rehabil Clin North Am. Philadelphia, PA, W.B. Saunders, 6:1–224, 1995.
5. Lakkat T, Venalainen J, Rauramma R, et al: Relation of leisure-time, physical activity, and cardiorespiratory fitness to the risk of acute myocardial infarction in men. N Engl J Med 330:1549–1554, 1994.
6. Oldridge NB, Guyatt GH, Fischer NE, et al: Cardiac rehabilitation after myocardial infarction: Combined experience of randomized clinical trials. JAMA 260:945–950, 1988.
7. Ornish D, Brown S, Scherwitz L, et al: Can lifestyle changes reverse coronary heart disease? The Lifestyle Heart Trial. Lancet 336:129–133, 1990.
8. Pederson TR, et al: Randomized trial of cholesterol lowering in 4444 patients with coronary heart disease: The Scandinavian Simvastatin Survival Study. Lancet 344:1383–1389, 1994.
9. Skerker R: Review and update. The aerobic exercise prescription. Crit Rev Phys Med Rehabil 2:257–271, 1991.

37. RESPIRATORY REHABILITATION

John R. Bach, M.D.

1. Describe the two basic categories of respiratory diseases.

All respiratory disease can be categorized as intrinsic versus mechanical, or obstructive versus restrictive. Patients with intrinsic or obstructive disease have lung disease that results in **oxygenation impairment** of the blood. These patients are normally eucapnic or hypocapnic despite hypoxia. Patients with mechanical dysfunction of respiratory muscles, lungs, or chest wall have **ventilatory impairment**, from which hypoxia occurs secondarily.

2. What are the goals of pulmonary rehabilitation?
- Supporting or improving cardiopulmonary function
- Preventing or treating complications by physical medicine (noninvasive) measures

- Fostering compliance with optimal medical care
- Reducing numbers of exacerbations, emergency room visits, and hospitalizations
- Educating the patient to confront the disease realistically
- Preparing the patient to take responsibility for his or her rehabilitation and well-being
- Optimizing psychosocial functioning and coping mechanisms
- Returning the patient to a more active, productive, and emotionally satisfying life

OBSTRUCTIVE DISEASES (OXYGENATION IMPAIRMENT)

3. What causes chronic obstructive pulmonary disease (COPD)?

Chronic bronchitis, emphysema, asthmatic bronchitis, and cystic fibrosis are the most common causes. COPD often results from a combination of genetic predisposition and environmental factors in which allergic diseases (e.g., asthma), respiratory infections (e.g., bronchopneumonitis), chemical inflammation (e.g., cigarette smoke, asbestosis), and metabolic abnormalities (e.g., α_1-antitrypsin deficiency) can play a role. Cigarette smoking is the main cause of chronic bronchitis-emphysema. Smokers are 3.5–25 times more likely (depending on the amounts smoked) to die of COPD than nonsmokers.

4. What is the difference between emphysema and bronchitis?

Emphysema is characterized by distention of air spaces distal to the terminal nonrespiratory bronchiole with destruction of alveolar walls. There is a loss of lung recoil, excessive airway collapse on exhalation, and chronic airflow obstruction. Chronic **bronchitis** and cystic fibrosis are characterized by enlargement of tracheobronchial mucous glands and chronic mucous hypersecretion and chest infections. Chronic bronchitis is distinguished from asthmatic bronchitis by its irreversibility, lack of bronchial hyperreactivity, lack of responsiveness to bronchodilators, and distinctive abnormalities in ventilation-perfusion.

5. How can you determine the prognosis for patients with COPD?

The extent of pulmonary function abnormalities correlates with prognosis: 30% of COPD patients with $FEV_1 < 750$ ml die within 1 year and 50% within 3 years. However, pulmonary function abnormalities do not predict the extent of the patient's functional impairment.

6. Who are candidates for pulmonary rehabilitation?

Any motivated nonsmoker or patient who has quit smoking, whose activities are limited by dyspnea due to COPD, and who has adequate medical, neuromusculoskeletal, financial, and psychosocial resources to permit active participation. Patients who benefit the most usually have a respiratory limitation to exercise at 75% of predicted maximum oxygen consumption and irreversible airway obstruction with a $FEV_1 < 2000$ ml or FEV_1/FVC ratio $< 60\%$. Ventilator users should be managed and possibly weaned in inpatient programs.

7. Why use clinical exercise testing?

Clinical exercise testing, whether done with a treadmill, stationary bicycle, or upper extremity ergometer, includes monitoring of oxygen consumption, CO_2 production, minute ventilation, and metabolic rate. It permits the differentiation of impairment due to cardiac disease or exercise-induced bronchospasm from pulmonary disease. It indicates the reasons for exercise-related symptoms and documents the patient's progress during rehabilitation by demonstrating changes in symptom-limited oxygen consumption and other physiologic parameters.

8. When do you terminate a clinical exercise test?

The test should continue until oxygen consumption fails to increase, maximum allowable heart rate for age is reached, or electrocardiographic changes, chest pain, severe dyspnea, or fatigue occur. A minute ventilation 35 times the patient's FEV_1 is often attainable.

9. What medical strategies are used to manage patients with lung disease and primarily oxygenation impairment?

Pulmonary function should be optimized medically and by facilitating airway secretion elimination. Hypoxic (PaO_2 < 60 mm Hg) patients benefit from oxygen therapy with decreased dyspnea, enhanced performance, and prolonged survival. Medications such as bronchodilators (β_1-adrenergics, anticholinergics, and methylxanthines) and, occasionally, glucocorticoids, expectorants, mucolytics, antibiotics, and mast-cell membrane stabilizers may also be helpful.

10. Outline a sample rehab prescription for a COPD patient. Name its seven major components.

Goals

Improve endurance

Optimize medication delivery, oxygen utilization, and airway secretion elimination

Increase walking capabilities and independent functioning

Reduce anxiety and improve self-esteem

Precautions

Maintain oxyhemoglobin saturation (SaO_2) > 90%

Discontinue exercise and notify physician if chest pain, severe dyspnea, or ventricular premature beats > 6/min occur during exercise

Maintain heart rate < 120 bpm

Respiratory therapy

With oximetry, titrate oxygen flows to maintain SaO_2 > 90% during exercise

Instruct in diaphragmatic and pursed-lip breathing

Instruct in inhaler use

Evaluate and instruct in methods to eliminate airway secretions

Instruct in home portable oxygen use

Instruct in respiratory muscle resistive exercise training and log use

Physical therapy

Assess baseline 12-minute walk, instruct in using log

Supervise incremental exercise program with stationary bicycle or treadmill three times daily, instruct in making log entries

Review body mechanics and coordinate with breathing patterns

Supervise use of diaphragmatic and pursed-lip breathing as appropriate

Occupational therapy

Assess upper body mobility, strength, and endurance

Develop an upper-extremity exercise program

Evaluate and facilitate activities of daily living (ADL) and use of adaptive aids as appropriate

Train in energy and work conservation

Evaluate the home, recommend modifications and equipment to improve safety, efficiency, and independence

Relaxation exercise training

Nutrition

Assess nutritional intake, advise modifications as appropriate

Psychology

Evaluate cognitive status and adjustment issues, intervene as needed

11. What methods can be used to assist the patient in airway secretion elimination?

Inexpensive methods: huffing, chest percussion and postural drainage, autogenic breathing, positive expiratory pressure masks, use of flutter valves that create positive back pressure and oscillate airflow.

Expensive methods: vibrating vests, vibrating air under chest shells, high-frequency oscillations (40–200 times/minute) of the air column delivered via mouthpiece or endotracheal tube.

The expensive methods have not been shown to be more effective than the less expensive approaches.

12. Should the respiratory muscles of COPD patients be rested?

Diaphragm rest can be achieved by assisting ventilation noninvasively with the use of body ventilators, mouthpiece or nasal intermittent positive-pressure ventilation (IPPV), or tracheostomy IPPV. Although assisting ventilation can exacerbate air trapping in COPD patients, the benefits of resting respiratory muscles and decreasing oxygen consumption may outweigh this in importance. Some studies suggest that use of ventilatory assistance daily, usually delivered overnight, can improve daytime blood gases, vital capacity, dyspnea, 12-min walking distance, respiratory muscle strength and endurance, functional activities, and quality of life, while decreasing hospitalizations. Patients with some combination of maximal inspiratory force < 50 cm H_2O, FEV_1 < 25% of predicted normal, PCO_2 > 45 mm Hg, respiratory rate > 30/min, and chest/abdomen dyssynchrony might be considered for nocturnal ventilatory assistance.

13. When should supplemental oxygen therapy be used?

For patients with PO_2 < 55–60 mm Hg, whether daytime or nighttime. Home oxygen therapy, when indicated, decreases reactive pulmonary hypertension, polycythemia, and perception of effort during exercise and prolongs life. Cognitive function may be improved, and hospital needs reduced. It should be given with caution to patients who retain CO_2.

14. Should supplemental oxygen be used by COPD patients on commercial airlines?

It should not, unless it is already being used on a regular basis, and then an increase of 0.5 l/min is generally sufficient.

15. Are nutritional supplements necessary?

As many as 50% of inpatients with COPD are malnourished. Inadequate or inappropriate nutrition (e.g., increased carbohydrate intake can increase PCO_2) can impair lung repair, surfactant synthesis, pulmonary defense mechanisms, control of ventilation and response to hypoxia, respiratory muscle function and lung mechanics, water homeostasis, and the immune system. Patients with significant nutritional impairment have more tracheal bacteria and are more frequently colonized by *Pseudomonas* species. Malnutrition can lead to hypercapnic respiratory failure, difficulty in weaning from mechanical ventilation, and infection. Short-term refeeding of malnourished patients leads to improved respiratory muscle endurance and, in some patients, increases in respiratory muscle strength in the absence of demonstrable changes in peripheral muscle function.

16. Can respiratory muscles be trained?

Maximum sustained ventilation exercises and inspiratory resistive exercises, including inspiratory resistive loading and inspiratory threshold loading, have been shown to improve respiratory muscle endurance. With a few exceptions, studies have not shown improvements in other pulmonary function parameters, and respiratory muscle exercise does not appear to carry over to improve general exercise tolerance or ADL capabilities. However, the combination of respiratory muscle exercise and rest, which appears to be especially effective for ventilator weaning, has not been adequately explored for the COPD patient.

17. How should reconditioning exercises be prescribed?

The intensity of reconditioning exercises may be guided by clinical exercise testing, e.g., 80–85% of maximum achievable heart rate or heart rate at ventilation levels of 35 times FEV_1. Walking, stair climbing, calisthenics, bicycling, and pool activities may be used. Upper extremity reconditioning should also be part of the program. A stationary bicycle should be purchased for the patient's home and used twice a day. In addition, a daily 12-minute walk can be used as well as several 15-minute sessions daily of inspiratory muscle training. A log should be kept of time and distance bicycled, distance walked, and inspiratory resistance tolerated during

15-minute inspiratory training sessions. In general, the pulse should increase at least 20–30% and return to baseline 5–10 minutes after exercise. The program should consist of weekly re-evaluations for several months, after which the patient should continue the home program and maintain the logs.

18. Should exercise reconditioning be used for advanced patients with marked hypercapnia?
There is evidence that even advanced patients with hypercapnia can benefit from an exercise reconditioning program, showing significant improvement in walking distance, ADL, and, possibly, certain pulmonary parameters.

19. What are the benefits of rehabilitation?
1. Reduction in dyspnea and respiratory rate
2. Increased exercise tolerance, symptom-limited oxygen consumption, work output, and mechanical efficiency
3. Improvement in ADL
4. Decreased anxiety and depression
5. Increased cognitive function and sense of well-being
6. Decreased frequency of hospitalizations for respiratory impairment

GLOBAL ALVEOLAR HYPOVENTILATION

20. List the diseases causing alveolar hypoventilation amenable to respiratory rehabilitation.
GAH can result from any neuromuscular or skeletal disorder that causes respiratory muscle dysfunction. Patients with diagnoses listed in the table are often candidates for physical medicine alternatives to endotracheal intubation or ventilatory support via an indwelling tracheostomy tube.

Conditions Leading to GAH Amenable to Physical Medicine Intervention

Myopathies	Neurologic disorders
Muscular dystrophies	Spinal muscular atrophies
Dystrophinopathies (Duchenne and Becker dystrophies)	Motor neuron diseases
	Poliomyelitis
Other muscular dystrophies (limb-girdle, Emery-Dreifuss, facioscapulohumeral, congenital, childhood autosomal recessive, and myotonic dystrophy)	Neuropathies (phrenic neuropathies, Guillain-Barré syndrome)
	Multiple sclerosis
	Traumatic tetraplegia and other myelopathies
Non-Duchenne myopathies (congenital and metabolic myopathies, polymyositis, myasthenia gravis)	Sleep disordered breathing (including obesity hypoventilation)
	Kyphoscoliosis
	Chronic obstructive pulmonary disease

21. Which patients with GAH can benefit from noninvasive respiratory rehab interventions?
Patients who can most benefit from physical medicine and general rehabilitation interventions must (1) have the ability to learn and (2) have adequate bulbar muscle function to use equipment and techniques that can optimize general physical functioning, including the various inspiratory and expiratory muscle aids and biofeedback approaches that can optimize pulmonary function. Some patients whose bulbar muscle weakness precludes safe use of noninvasive inspiratory aids may still benefit from mechanical cough-assist methods.

22. Name the eight most common errors in managing patients with ventilatory impairment.
1. Misinterpretation of symptoms due to GAH
2. Failure to do spirometry with the patient supine

3. Failure to monitor sleep
4. Use of arterial blood gas analyses instead of oximetry and noninvasive CO2 monitoring
5. Administration of oxygen, periodic intermittent positive-pressure breathing (IPPB), continuous positive airway pressure (CPAP), or inadequate bi-level positive airway pressure (BiPAP) when noninvasive respiratory muscles aids are indicated
6. Use of methylxanthines and any other respiratory medications on an ongoing basis
7. Failure to prevent acute respiratory failure and hospitalization
8. Resort to tracheostomy when peak cough expiratory flows exceed 3 l/sec

23. Name the clinical parameters critical for monitoring patients with advanced neuromuscular disease.
- Vital capacity
- Peak cough flows, unassisted and assisted
- Oxyhemoglobin saturation
- Pulse rate
- SaO_2 (via oximetry)

24. What are respiratory muscle aids?
The respiratory muscles can be aided by applying manual or mechanical forces to the body or intermittent pressure to the airway. The devices that act on the body include the negative-pressure body ventilators (NPBVs) and oscillators that assist respiratory muscles by creating atmospheric pressure changes around the thorax and abdomen, body ventilators and exsufflation devices that apply force directly to the body to mechanically displace respiratory muscles, and devices that apply intermittent pressure changes directly to the airway.

25. What are the ideal inspiratory muscle aids for daytime use?
Mouthpiece IPPV and the intermittent abdominal-pressure ventilator (IAPV) are the ideal inspiratory muscle aids (ventilatory support methods) for long-term daytime ventilatory support. For **mouthpiece IPPV**, a mouthpiece is set up near the mouth, adjacent to the sip-and-puff, tongue, or chin controls of a motorized wheelchair, where the patient can easily grab it up to 6–8 times a minute for full ventilatory support.

The **IAPV** intermittently inflates an air sac contained in a corset or belt worn beneath the patient's outer clothing. Inflation by a positive-pressure ventilator moves the diaphragm upward, causing a forced exsufflation; during deflation, the abdominal contents and diaphragm fall to the resting position, and inspiration occurs passively. A trunk angle of ≥ 30° from horizontal is necessary for the IAPV to be effective. The IAPV augments tidal volumes by 250–1200 ml. Patients with < 1 hour of ventilator-free breathing time often prefer to use the IAPV when sitting than to use noninvasive methods of IPPV.

26. What are the ideal inspiratory muscle aids for nocturnal use?
- **Nasal IPPV with CPAP masks or custom-molded nasal interfaces** has become the most popular method of noninvasive nocturnal ventilatory support. At least three or four different nasal interfaces should be tried by each patient to find which one will be preferred by that patient. Many patients use different styles on alternate nights to vary skin contact pressure.
- **Mouthpiece IPPV with lipseal retention** is a more effective but generally less preferred method of nocturnal ventilatory support. Using the lipseal, mouthpiece IPPV can be delivered during sleep with less insufflation leakage and with little risk of the mouthpiece falling out. However, speaking clearly is difficult.

27. How can airway secretions be best eliminated in this population?
At least 3 l/sec of expiratory flow is necessary to bring airway secretions out of the airway and into the mouth. However, whether using a ventilator or not, patients with GAH are often unable to generate as much as 2 l/sec of peak cough flows (PCF). With the use of an insufflation

to > 1.5 liters and a properly timed abdominal thrust, PCF can usually be increased to 3–7 l/sec. When scoliosis, abdominal distension, trauma, or obesity interfere with manually assisted coughing, a mechanical insufflator-exsufflator can be used to provide 10 l/sec of expiratory flow.

28. Which factors decrease blood oxyhemoglobin saturation (SaO$_2$)?
1. Hypoventilation (hypercapnia)
2. Mucous plugging (usually sudden)
3. Intrinsic lung disease (such as pneumonia or other pulmonary pathology)

Oximeters that measure pulse and blood SaO$_2$ are increasingly less expensive, and oximetry should be considered a fourth vital sign. If bronchial mucous plugs are not cleared in a timely manner, pneumonia develops.

29. Discuss the use of oximetry in starting noninvasive IPPV.
Introduction to and use of mouthpiece or nasal IPPV is facilitated by oximetry feedback. An SaO$_2$ alarm may be set at 93–94%. The patient sees that by taking deeper breaths the SaO$_2$ will exceed 95% within seconds. The patient should be instructed to maintain the SaO$_2$ > 94% all day and can achieve this by unassisted breathing, followed by mouthpiece or nasal IPPV delivered by a portable ventilator once he tires. With time, the patient will require increasing periods of noninvasive IPPV to maintain adequate ventilation (SaO$_2$ > 94%). In this manner, an oximeter may also help to reset central ventilatory drive and facilitate optimal daytime use of noninvasive IPPV.

30. How is SaO$_2$ useful in managing acute respiratory tract infections?
During acute respiratory infections, respiratory muscle weakness is exacerbated, which along with bronchial mucous plugging, causes a diminution in the patient's vital capacity. Plugging and hypoventilation, compounded by patient fatigue, cause decreases in SaO$_2$. The patient is instructed to augment ventilation and maintain a normal SaO$_2$ by taking mouthpiece-assisted insufflations as necessary. When mucous plugging causes a sudden decrease in SaO$_2$, manually and mechanically assisted coughing is used until the mucus is eliminated and the SaO$_2$ returns to normal. When the SaO$_2$ baseline decreases to 92–94% despite optimal ventilation and mucous clearance, microscopic atelectasis is present, but this generally clears with continued treatment. Lower baseline SaO$_2$s occur when airway secretion management is inadequate and either pulmonary infiltrations or some other serious pulmonary complications have occurred. This event justifies hospitalization, diagnostic work-up, supplemental oxygen therapy, and other intensive measures.

31. How is glossopharyngeal breathing (GPB) accomplished?
The patient is instructed to take a deep breath, and then augment it by projecting boluses of air past the glottis with the tongue and pharyngeal muscles. The glottis closes with each "gulp." One breath usually consists of 6–8 gulps of 60–100 ml each. During training, GPB efficiency is monitored by spirometrically measuring the milliliters of air per gulp, gulps per breath, and breaths per minute. A GPB rate of 12–14 breaths per minute can provide patients with little or no vital capacity with normal tidal volumes, minute ventilation, and hours of ventilator-free breathing time.

32. What is GPB good for?
GPB is most commonly used as a method for providing maximal insufflations and as a noninvasive method for supporting ventilation. It is an excellent back-up in the event of ventilator failure. Deep GPB is also useful for manually assisted coughing and to prevent microatelectasis. GPB can normalize the volume and rhythm of speech and permit the patient to shout. A tracheostomy virtually precludes use of GPB, because even with the tube plugged, gulped air leaks around the tube and out the tracheostomy site.

33. When is endotracheal intubation or tracheostomy indicated?
Respiratory failure and:

A mentally incompetent or uncooperative patient, or one who is using heavy sedation or narcotics

Intrinsic lung disease that necessitates supplemental O_2

SaO_2 that cannot be maintained > 90% by aggressive airway secretion elimination (PCF < 3 l/sec) and normal alveolar ventilation

Substance abuse or uncontrollable seizures

Conditions interfering with the use of IPPV interfaces, such as facial fractures, inadequate bite for mouthpiece entry, or nasogastric tube.

34. Does oxygen therapy ease symptoms of hypoventilation?
Although oxygen therapy is given to virtually all ventilator users, whether or not they are hypoxic, for patients with GAH, its use is tantamount to putting a BandAid on a cancer! Oxygen therapy depresses ventilatory drive, exacerbating GAH; prevents the use of oximetry biofeedback; increases fatigue, daytime drowsiness, nightmares, and depression; and renders the nocturnal use of nasal or mouthpiece IPPV ineffective. In addition, patients with GAH who are treated with oxygen therapy have a higher incidence of pulmonary complications than patients not treated at all. A cardinal rule is to always first attempt to normalize SaO_2 by providing adequate ventilation and assisted coughing before considering the use of oxygen. Assiduously removing the airway secretions that are causing the desaturations will help prevent the development of pneumonia.

35. What is the difference between CPAP and BiPAP?
Continuous positive airway pressure (CPAP) delivered via a CPAP mask provides a pneumatic splint that maintains airway patency during sleep and allows the patient with obstructive sleep apneas to breathe using his or her own muscles. **Bi-level positive airway pressure** (BiPAP) permits independent adjustment of inspiratory (IPAP) and expiratory positive airway pressures (EPAP): the greater the IPAP/EPAP difference (span), the greater the inspiratory muscle support. Spans of ≥ 20 cm H_2O are often required to ensure adequate ventilation.

36. Pressure support ventilation, synchronized intermittent mandatory ventilation (SIMV), positive end-expiratory pressure (PEEP), and oxygen administration are necessary for ventilator weaning? Right?
No. In our ventilator unit, virtually every ventilator user arrives using a combination of all of the above. When we turn off the oxygen, the SaO_2 plummets until we exsufflate the patient through the tracheostomy tube. This clears the airway secretions and often normalizes the SaO_2, and the patient can continue to breathe room air. We then often turn off the SIMV, PEEP, and pressure support and place the patient on a portable volume ventilator from which he or she can take assisted breaths via a mouthpiece whenever needed to prevent dyspnea and maintain normal SaO_2. Thus, the patient takes fewer assisted breaths and weans himself or herself without resort to complicated and unnecessary technology.

37. List five maxims regarding use of intubation and tracheostomy in the rehabilitation of ventilatory failure.
1. Intubation and tracheostomy are neither needed nor desired by most patients with GAH who require 24-hour/day ventilatory support.
2. Oxygen should never be used as a substitute for assisted ventilation.
3. Rehabilitation is not complete for any patient who has not been evaluated for tracheostomy tube removal and had the tube removed when peak cough flows permit, irrespective of extent of ventilatory failure.
4. Endotracheal intubation is unnecessary for managing many cases of acute ventilatory failure.

5. Endotracheal suctioning is often less effective than insufflation-exsufflation via an endotracheal tube (exsufflation creates high expiratory flows to clear both lung fields, preventing pneumonia).

Physical medicine alternatives to the invasive measures of endotracheal intubation, tracheostomy, and airway suctioning are cheaper, safer, more comfortable, and greatly preferred by patients with GAH. They deserve wider application.

BIBLIOGRAPHY

1. Aldrich T: Respiratory muscle training in COPD. In Bach JR (ed): Pulmonary Rehabilitation: The Obstructive and Paralytic Conditions. Philadelphia, Hanley & Belfus, 1996.
2. Bach JR: A comparison of long-term ventilatory support alternatives from the perspective of the patient and care giver. Chest 104:1702–1706, 1993.
3. Bach JR: Pulmonary rehabilitation. In DeLisa JD (ed): Rehabilitation Medicine: Principles and Practice. Philadelphia, J.B. Lippincott, 1993, pp 952–972.
4. Bach JR, Alba AS, Saporito LR: Intermittent positive pressure ventilation via the mouth as an alternative to tracheostomy for 257 ventilator users. Chest 103:174–182, 1993.
5. Bach JR: Update and perspectives on noninvasive respiratory muscle aids: Pt 1. The inspiratory muscle aids. Chest 105:1230–1240, 1994.
6. Bach JR: Update and perspectives on noninvasive respiratory muscle aids: Pt 2. The expiratory muscle aids. Chest 105:1538–1544, 1994.
7. Bach JR (ed): Pulmonary Rehabilitation: The Obstructive and Paralytic Conditions. Philadelphia, Hanley & Belfus, 1996.
8. Casaburi R, Petty TL (eds): Principles and Practice of Pulmonary Rehabilitation. Philadelphia, W.B. Saunders, 1993.
9. Dail C, Rodgers M, Guess V, Adkins HV: Glossopharyngeal Breathing Manual. Downey, CA, Rancho Los Amigos Hospital, 1979.
10. Dail CW, Affeldt JE: Glossopharyngeal Breathing [video]. Los Angeles, College of Medical Evangelists, 1954.
11. Hardy KA: A review of airway clearance: New techniques, indications, and recommendations. Respir Care 39:440–455, 1994.
12. Sortor S, McKenzie M: Toward Independence: Assisted Cough [video]. Dallas, BioScience Communications of Dallas, 1986.

38. REHABILITATION FOR PERIPHERAL VASCULAR DISEASE

Heinz I. Lippmann, M.D.

1. What is peripheral vascular disease (PVD)?

PVD includes the diseases of the arteries (macrovascular), arterioles, and capillaries (microvascular); venous system (phlebologic); lymphatic system (lymphologic); and blood flow (rheologic) and their effects on cellular, organ, or body nutrition, metabolism, and health.

2. Who gets PVD?

Peripheral arterial disease, or **atherosclerosis obliterans** (ASO), correlates in prevalence with coronary artery disease; it is found in over 2% of individuals > 65 years of age in the United States. Intermittent claudication affects nearly 2% of the people under age 60 and increases to 4% in the 7th decade and to > 5% in the 8th decade and later.

The distribution of claudication pain is a reasonable clue as to the expected immediate proximal occlusion, but very proximal occlusions can produce ischemia via the "steal" phenomenon with circulatory shunting. Claudication can occur suddenly due to a proximal occlusion, then disappear over months due to collaterals and recanalization.

3. Are there known markers for ASO?

Known risk factors are hypertension, low-density lipoprotein (LDL) cholesterol, genetic trends, diabetes mellitus, and smoking. Other conditions such as obesity and psychologic and behavioral stresses are less certainly implicated.

4. Any established principles of management, or any cure?

In an early stage, ASO is reversible, but structural tissue damage is permanent. Management aims at securing arterial perfusion (i.e., a blood supply) adequate for the demands of tissues and organs.

Treatment methods have changed in the past 7 decades, with a watershed in 1952, when surgical revascularization techniques became established. Before 1952, management of limb ischemia was only supportive, because ASO was believed to lead inexorably from an asymptomatic stage, to intermittent claudication, to rest pain, to necrobiosis (gangrene), ending in loss of limb. The past 40 years have taught us that the last two stages are complications rather than manifestations of ASO, that rest pain is often reversible, and that chronic ASO does not necessarily lead to loss of limb.

5. Why does rest pain occur in ASO?

It means that the blood supply to the limbs at rest does not quite catch up with tissue demand, but the deficit may be minimal and is often correctable. The most common type of rest pain is due to tissue ischemia exacerbated by the edema of dependency, usually aggravated by a weak or idle muscle pump. Edema may be reversed by leg elevation, but this maneuver is badly tolerated since it opposes arterial perfusion. As a compromise, an 8-inch block placed under the head of the bed often allows the patient to sleep with minimum edema and tolerable pain. During the day, the muscle pump clears ischemic waste of metabolism (lactate, etc.) and the upright position adds to perfusion pressure, avoiding the problems that cause rest pain.

6. At what level of blood flow does permanent tissue damage result?

Blood flow demands vary from tissue to tissue and from organ to organ, as well as with activity and environment. Normal skin needs only 0.5 ml/100 gm/min at room temperature, while at 44°C, its needs may rise to > 11 ml/100 gm/min and inflamed skin may demand 25 ml or more! The brain requires 46 ml/100 gm/min, and when its demands are not met, damage will be permanent after a few minutes. Skin ulceration that eventually progresses to gangrene starts at perfusion pressures < 40 mmHg at the ankle or digit.

Resting muscle needs 3 ml/100 gm/min, and its needs rise with work up to 60 ml/100 gm/min. Skeletal muscle has the ability to work anaerobically but will stop contracting (claudicate) after awhile. It will recover when the tardy blood arrives through narrow vessels to repay the oxygen debt, and no damage will be done.

7. Will natural collateral circulation prevent tissue damage in a leg whose arteries gradually close?

Yes, for low demands in chronic ASO, when arteries are gradually obstructed. But on sudden disruption of arterial inflow, e.g., after a major trauma, an embolus, or ruptured aneurysm, collaterals take weeks to open adequately, and the limb can be salvaged only by revascularization.

8. How is sudden arterial occlusion recognized?

Acute arterial occlusion must be diagnosed and treated rapidly. The clinical constellation can be summarized as the **6P's**:

Pain	Pallor
Paresthesia	Polar (asymmetric temperature)
Paralysis	Pulselessness

Look for an embolic source. Seek revascularization.

9. When were the surgical revascularization techniques used in AOS first described?

Alexis Carrel, in a series of experiments published from 1902 through 1912, laid the ground-work for vessel anastomoses (end-to-end, side-to-side, artery-to-artery, artery-to-vein), patch grafts, homografts, and autografts using tubes, glass, resorbable manganese tubes, artery banks, etc. Also, E. Jaeger described the anastomoses created for congenital heart disease.

All of these techniques were forgotten until 1952, when Hufnagel reminded the surgical community of this treasure buried in the literature. Within a few years after 1952, novel methods in microsurgery, internal cleansing of obstructed arteries using thrombolysis and even roto-rooter, and other daring methods appeared on the scene.

10. So, is vascular surgery now the definitive treatment for AOS?

Not quite! Surgical revascularization has become a blessing for patients whose limbs can be salvaged after a sudden major artery occlusion, but in ASO, surgical revascularization is just one alternative—and the less common one—of two therapeutic options. The second approach, the nonoperative one, is to follow the patient closely. By following elderly individuals with ischemic limbs for years, we have learned that the low demands for blood in tissues distal to the arterial obstruction (mainly skin) afford significant long-term protection against limb loss. Both ap-proaches, the surgical and the physiatric, see a functioning human protected against loss of limb.

11. How do you approach a new patient?

The patient's initial complaint, typically pain on walking, is nonspecific for intermittent claudication (IC). Further questioning as to the duration of leg pain and the leg involved seeks to find out whether it is IC or shortness of breath or insuperable weakness (both cardiac symptoms) that stops him or her. Once this is established, ask for the patient's activities—can she or he ne-gotiate steps at home, work at home, shop, cook, do gardening, etc.—to find out the level of in-dependence and diurnal frequency of activities of daily living (ADL). The goal is to determine, is this individual's IC disabling?

12. Is IC a symptom specific for ASO?

Yes, with exceptions. For example, there are rare cases of severe anemia (Hgb < 6 gm/dl) in cases of slow blood loss. **Pseudo-claudication** (spinal stenosis, decreases with forward flexion), like IC, stops the patient after some distance but, unlike IC, causes pain that lasts longer than a few seconds, with recovery only after sitting down. In addition, other diagnostic signs for radicu-lopathy, lumbar stenosis, or similar conditions are present.

13. How do you use your senses to diagnose and clinically quantify ASO?

You look, feel, touch, and use your sense of smell as follows:

1. **Look for pallor on elevation.** With the patient supine and both legs lifted high, pressing the soles against your palms for 25 seconds, then release the pressure and count seconds until flush appears (**capillary refill**). Normally this occurs in < 9 seconds. Delay is due to drop in arte-rial pressure due to ASO.

2. Have the patient sit with legs dependent. **Rubor of dependency** is a dusky-red discol-oration of cold skin that occurs within 3 minutes due to precapillary sphincter failure of normal sympathetic-mediated constriction. Rubor is elicited in the normal person for some hours after weeks of bedrest or in healthy astronauts, but it is permanent due to anoxic irreversible damage of the sphincters, meaning that ASO has been present for at least 3 months. **Hair distribution** has a wide normal range and offers little information. **Unilateral edema or atrophy** can be used to rule out deep vein thrombosis or coexistent neuropathy.

3. Check the quality of **skin on the feet**, between toes, and on the heels (intact, maceration, calluses, etc.). With the patient supine, check the four ankle pulses—the posterior tibial, anterior tibial (upper ankle medial to extensor hallicus longus), dorsalis pedis, and perforating peroneal (on top of external malleolus). The last two may be absent normally. Also check the popliteals, femorals, external iliacs, and abdominal aorta, the last to rule out a pulsating aneurysm. If one

pulse is finger-palpable in the foot, perfusion is likely adequate for viability. **Skin temperature** is used for diagnosing ASO only after taking into account sympathetic tone (e.g., in peripheral neuropathy, the warmer foot may even be the more ischemic one.) Check the skin of the foot for **dryness** (autonomic neuropathy) or **humid skin** (wetting dermatitis), as well as for **tender areas**, pressure signs, injuries, and tendinitis.

4. **Listen for bruits** from the inguinal region along the legs, in the abdomen (abdominal aneurysm), carotids, vertebrals, and temporal arteries. In addition, the instruments used in clinical practice are the **oscillometer** and, when available, the **pulse volume recorder**, both of which estimate the volume of pulsatile blood passing the segment under the cuff between systole and diastole. However, these instruments do not register collateral flow, and the **ultrasonic Doppler** pinpoints systolic pressure, when the flow signal starts during deflation of a proximal cuff.

14. What is the ankle-brachial index (ABI)?

Normal systolic pressure in the foot arteries of a supine person exceeds the brachial artery pressure by 10–20 mmHg. Thus, the **ABI** is the systolic pressure quotient of the ankle divided by the arm and is normally 1.1–1.2. A drop to an ABI < 0.5 is considered by some an indication for surgical revascularization. A ratio of 0.3 or less indicates poor viability of foot tissues and poor prognosis for wound healing. **Transcutaneous oxygen tension** is another noninvasive measurement of the PO_2 delivered to the skin ($TcPO_2$). $TcPO_2$ obtained on the skin of ischemic limbs predicts healing if > 40 mmHg and nonhealing if < 20 mmHg.

15. What is the vanishing exercise pulse phenomenon?

This test is highly informative as to the presence of ASO in early stages and with an uncertain history. The oscillometric index is performed, and with the cuff in place at the ankle, it is repeated after 30 seconds of vigorous dorsiplantar flexions (2 seconds' duration for full range). In the normal person, postexercise readings equal or exceed the preexercise readings. Lower readings indicate a proximal arterial bottleneck, delaying flow due to obstruction (or to compression, such as a tumor) and causing diminution of arterial reserve, even in the presence of normal resting values. Normal oscillometric indices are 2–6 at the ankle, 4–11 at the upper calf, 5–15 at the low thigh levels (1 to 2 to 2.5 × at these three levels).

16. What are reactive hyperemia tests?

Reactive hyperemia tests are part of routine ASO workup. They assess total blood flow (pulsatile + collateral).

Lower extremities—**Lewis-Pickering test**—A cuff at the high leg level, inflated to 20 mmHg higher than systolic pressure, is suddenly released exactly after 300 seconds, and the return of full flush in the feet and soles is timed in seconds. The normal time for maximum flush in the soles is 12 seconds. Occluded segmental areas or digits show no or delayed flush.

Upper extremities—**Allen test**—This test has two parts. First, compress both ulnar and radial arteries while the patient squeezes out blood by making a fist. Release the radial after 2 minutes. Flush over the radial side is immediate in normal persons. Then do the same for the ulnar. For the second part, repeat the test by releasing both pulses after 2 minutes simultaneously and look for ischemic segments (e.g., digits).

With experience, all of these tests yield reliable data in < 30 minutes on pulsatile and collateral local blood supply, the site of arterial bottlenecks, and skin viability.

17. How do we manage the patient with chronic ASO?

The physiatrist's main goals are prevention of loss of limb, prevention of disabling complications (injuries or infections), and maintenance of function.

18. How do you determine the need for revascularization?

All surgical or angioplastic reopenings of mainstream flow close the collaterals in short order. The best long-term results carry a 5-year patency rate of 74%. If the bypass closes, the limb is in immediate danger of loss, since it takes weeks for collateral flow to return. This risk is not acceptable to most well-informed patients who claudicate, unless surgical intervention is proposed for immediate limb salvage.

19. Is IC disabling only if the patient takes it too seriously?

Correct! Our experience shows that most ASO patients of middle-age can live with IC, including letter carriers we treated who did not want to jeopardize their pension benefits by submitting to surgery in the risky hope of working without IC.

20. How disabling is IC really?

That depends on the patient's self-reliance and self-image, a proper job, reliable information of the risks of action or inaction, some serenity, and a capacity to reason and communicate with family and friends. A person who believes that IC can be cured will feel disabled at the first forced stop, but will adapt to IC as a nuisance when he or she knows that revascularization increases the danger of loss of limb.

21. How do we reduce blood flow demands?

By keeping the skin in good condition, early treatment of infections, and avoiding injuries.

22. Outline a good skin and foot care program.

It includes daily washing with lukewarm water and soap, daily application of skin cream, and daily examination of the feet for red spots.

Nothing warmer than 92°F should be applied to the feet—no sun in the summer, no radiators or heating pads in winter. Severely ischemic skin is endangered by first-degree burns.

Local necrobiosis may start the downhill course to an amputation. The feet should not be soaked. It defats the skin, which then tends to crack and split, and increases the risk of infection.

23. Which creams are preferable?

Lanolin, eucerine (Nivea cream), mink oil, olive oil, and some preparations containing mineral oil (Alpha Keri), but not vaseline or heavy mineral oil, which is badly absorbed.

24. Does this regimen truly protect against loss of limb?

It is difficult to prove without long follow-up of many patients. However, in an old-age home and infirmary with 500-plus residents (average age, 86 years), before I started a foot care program, prior history described 8–15 major amputations yearly. None of the 270 residents who participated in the foot care program ever lost a leg during the 35 years of that program. Foot care is a continual ongoing task. Some participating residents whose foot care routine was interrupted by hospitalization for medical, orthopedic, or surgical unrelated disease promptly developed pressure sores and gangrene and required amputation.

25. Can circulation in ASO be improved by medication?

Pentoxifylline (Trental) is marginally effective by reducing blood viscosity, and it increases walking distance thresholds for claudication slightly in some patients. **Rheologic agents** are costly and are seldom of benefit in clinical practice. **Vasodilators**, administered intra-arterially, increase local blood flow for a limited time; their study predates the availability of vascular surgical procedures. Oral vasodilators are ineffective in ASO because all collaterals have previously opened during the long course of the disease. Platelet inhibition to prevent arterial occussion with **aspirin**, 325 mg once daily to three times daily, is prudent.

26. What, if any, effect does exercise have on IC?

Exercise probably increases perfusion due to more and larger diameter collaterals, redistributes blood flow (improves autoregulation), improves walking efficiency, increases pain tolerance, and brings about metabolic changes in the calf muscles.

We ask the patient with an ischemic leg to walk up to the onset of IC in an attempt to secure optimal aerobic homeostasis, to prevent disuse, and to enjoy endorphin-enriched ambience. Currently, exercise regimens recommend prescreening for coronary disease, physical-therapist-supervised initial sessions, and baseline walking distance with pain assessment. Patients are encouraged to walk up to pain and to exercise for 30–45 minutes/day at least three times per week for a period of at least 3 months before formal reassessment.

27. How about patients with trophic changes in ischemic limbs?

Here, clinical decisions regarding surgical vs. medical management, are guided by watching for signs of healing or deterioration and close patient follow-up. Trophic changes include phlegmons, abscesses, ulcerations, osteomyelitis, and gangrene.

Abscesses and **phlegmons**, regardless of site or size, require surgical drainage, especially when the area is ischemic. **Osteomyelitis**, particularly in digits, may respond to medical treatment which ends in extrusion of sequesters and digital shortening. An infected sinus may then develop, which can be drained with a small catheter and perfused with Elase and an antibiotic, resulting in cleaning and healing.

Protruding phalanges with kissing interdigital ulcers are separated by gauze or lamb's wool. Patients with massive **gangrene** of a digit that does not extend into the foot are encouraged to ambulate, provided the gangrene does not progress or no edema develops.

Any open skin lesion in an ischemic leg presents a dilemma, including infection and a long morbidity. **Ulcerations** are caused by extraneous injury, bruises, burns, malfitting shoes, pressure sores in bed, bad pedicure, and an almost infinite array of noxious encounters with the environment; these should be prevented, promptly diagnosed, and controlled. Almost all ulcers culture some bugs, although the invasion into adjacent tissues is not always present. Antibiotics are given by systemic administration, since the occasional case of hypersensitivity to topical antibiotics in an ischemic leg may endanger the limb by steep increases in the demand for blood.

Gangrene of any size carries an uncertain prognosis and requires closest follow-up. A lesion the size of one petechia can spread ending with loss of limb, while a massive gangrenous forefoot can demarcate cleanly at midfoot level. If demarcation is visible, end results are not infrequently better when surgical debridement is postponed. Again, proper timing is essential and mandates ongoing observation.

The recognition of progression of a trophic lesion, especially gangrene or an infection, requires clinical experience and special training (or where obtainable, the advice of an angiologist or vascular surgeon) to decide whether revascularization or debridement is needed or whether the limb is salvageable.

28. Why should a physiatrist be concerned with venous diseases?

Venous disease, a component of peripheral vascular disease, includes a spectrum of disorders including varicose veins, chronic venous insufficiency (CVI), deep vein thrombosis (DVT), and pulmonary embolism (PE). Venous disease is a major cause of disability, while thromboembolism is a leading cause of mortality in the United States.

29. How common and how dangerous is pulmonary embolism?

Pulmonary embolism in the United States is fatal in 12% of all patients diagnosed with pulmonary embolism. Most pulmonary emboli depart from the deep veins of the thigh, proximal to the popliteal vein, less often from the pelvis or the right heart. The clinical outcome depends on hemodynamic factors and on the size of the embolus. "Massive" pulmonary emboli are defined by the National Heart, Lung and Blood Institute as causing a filling deficit in two or more pulmonary lobar arteries and are fatal.

30. What is Virchow's triad?

Stasis (reduced blood flow velocity), venous endothelial damage, and hypercoagulability (tendency for blood to clot). These three elements produce a DVT.

31. Name several populations at increased risk for developing DVT.

Surgical patients, parturients, cigarette smokers, geriatric patients, patients with prior history of DVT, patients on prolonged bed rest, and patients after anesthesia. Also at risk are persons with cardiac disease, limb trauma, neoplasms, obesity, and immunologic problems.

32. Specify four tests used to diagnose DVT.

Contrast venography (phlebography)

Doppler ultrasound techniques (Duplex imaging, Doppler flow test)

125-Iodine-labeled fibrinogen uptake test

Impedance plethysmography. A useful algorithmic method to diagnose DVT in a clinical setting is available.

33. Indicate five suggested methods of preventing stasis.

Leg elevation, isotonic exercise, elastic hosiery, sequential compression pumping, and electric stimulation.

34. What pharmacologic options are available for dealing with hypercoagulability?

Low-dose heparin activates antithrombin III, which prevents the start of the coagulation cascade by inhibiting Stuart factor Xa needed to form thrombin. It is given at 5000 units 2 hours preoperatively, followed by 8–12-hour intervals for 7 days. Low-molecular-weight heparins (LMWH) are depolymerized fragments of standard heparin (SH). Their half-life exceeds that of SH, and bleeding complications are less common. Nadroparin calcium, an LMWH, has been well studied. Several other LMWHs are available for clinical use. When in a clinical situation thrombin is already circulating (e.g., after hip fracture or major trauma), higher doses of SH rather than LMWHs are used to render safer protection against fibrin formation and PE.

Dihydroergotamine (DHE), 0.5 mg by subcutaneous injection b.i.d. or t.i.d., constricts veins and venules of the lower extremities and accelerates venous return. In combination with low-dose heparin, it improves DVT prevention.[6]

Dextran, a polysaccharide bacterial product, decreases blood viscosity, weakens the interaction of platelets with the damaged endothelium, and renders fibrin more susceptible for lysis. There is some evidence that its use in high-risk patients (e.g., those with cancer or during orthopedic procedures) protects against DVT and PE, but its effect in lower-risk patients has not been established. Dextran has important side effects. It causes fluid retention and its use in heart pump failure or advanced renal disease is contraindicated. It often produces allergic reactions and may be associated with a higher risk of bleeding. Aspirin or dipyridamole, both of which affect platelet function, are only moderately effective in preventing DVT (documented only in male patients undergoing orthopedic procedures).

Oral coumadin (warfarin sodium) is used for anticoagulation of longer duration and is taken up later. It should not be used in hypercoagulable states, but in heparin-induced thrombocytopenia, nadroparin may work.

35. What is chronic venous insufficiency?

Chronic venous insufficiency (CVI) is defined as a structural trophic damage of skin and subcutis due to increased venous pressure.

36. Name the clinical manifestations of CVI.

Discoloration (due to hemosiderin deposition), fibrosis, sclerosis, lipodermosclerosis, subcutaneous ossification, and ulceration.

37. State three interrelated processes needed for successful healing of a venous ulcer?

Granulation, contraction, and epithelialization.

38. What is Unna's boot?

Unna's boot (UB) is a gauze roller bandage impregnated with a mixture of gelatine, zinc oxide, glycerine, and water. The moist bandage is applied to the leg from the base of the toes to the lower edge of the popliteal area without interposition of any material. It covers the ankle. The dried bandage forms an adherent, nonelastic, pliable, porous, nonallergenic precise contour of the limb. Because it is nonelastic and adheres to the skin, it is circumferentially stable along all segments of the leg. It transforms the leg muscle bulge during ambulation into pressure gradients like a muscle fascia. It also transforms the forces that move the ankle (the body weight during active and a motorized foot plate during passive ankle motion) into circumferential compressive forces by virtue of ankle joint kinetics. In an average adult, the ankle moves up and 4 cm forward during dorsiflexion and down and 4 cm backward during plantar flexion. The nonelastic adherent Unna cover, by resisting both dorsiflexion and plantar flexion, exerts a strong posterior pressure during dorsiflexion and an equally strong anterior pressure during plantar flexion. Both forces develop gradually in correlation with the ankle motion regardless of whether the joint moves actively or is moved passively. This is why the differential pressures and their timing equal those developed by a normal MP during ambulation. Measurements show transient values higher than mean arterial pressure at extreme dorsiflexion and extreme plantar flexion, and down to base value when the foot plate is straight at base, but always correlating with the angle of the foot plate during motion. It controls edema by creating the ankle pump, which replaces a failing muscle pump in CVI.

BIBLIOGRAPHY

1. Abramson DI: Circulation in the Extremities. New York, Academic Press, 1967.
2. Barradel LB, Buckley MM: Nadroparin calcium: A review of the pharmacology and clinical applications in the prevention and treatment of thromboembolic disorders. Drugs 44(5):858–888, 1992.
3. Fontaine R, et al: Long-term results of restorative arterial surgery in obstructive diseases of the arteries. J Cardiovasc Surg 5:463–472, 1964.
4. Gardner AW, Poehlman ET: Exercise rehabilitation programs for the treatment of claudication pain. JAMA 274:975–980, 1995.
5. Kannel WB, McGee DL: Update on some epidemiologic features on intermittent claudication: The Framingham Study. J Am Geriatr Soc 33:13–18, 1985.
6. Lindgarde F, Jelmes R, et al: Conservative drug treatment in patients with moderately severe chronic occlusive arterial disease. Circulation 80:1549–1556, 1989.
7. Lippmann HI: Medical management of occlusive arterial disease. J Med Soc NJ 79:29–32, 1982.
8. Lippmann HI, Briere JP: Physical basis of external supports in chronic venous insufficiency. Arch Phys Med Rehabil 52:555–449, 1970.
9. Lippmann HI, Fishman L, Farrar R, et al: Edema control in the management of disabling chronic venous insufficiency. Arch Phys Med Rehabil 75:436–441, 1994.
10. Rosenow EC III: Venous and pulmonary embolism: An algorithmic approach to diagnosis and management. Mayo Clin Proc 70(1):1–8, 1995.
11. Tunis SR, Bass EB, Steinberg EP: The use of angioplasty, by-pass surgery and amputation in the management of peripheral vascular disease. N Engl J Med 325:556–562, 1991.
12. Vogt MT, Wolfson SK, Kuller LH: Lower extremity arterial disease and the aging process: A review. J Clin Epidemiol 46:529–542, 1992.

39. LYMPHEDEMA

Elizabeth Augustine, P.T., M.S.

1. Describe the lymphatic system.
The lymphatic system is a one-way-valved drainage system from the interstitial space to the subclavian vein that transports 2–4 liters of lymph daily. Once the interstitial fluid enters the **lymph capillary** (consisting of overlapping one-cell-thick endothelial cells), the fluid is then referred to as lymph. The lymph capillaries drain into **lymphangions** (larger bicuspid valved conduits with smooth muscle within its walls), which empty into a larger vessel called the **lymphatic trunk**, which finally empties into the **lymphatic duct**. Periodically throughout the lymphatic

system, the lymph fluid is filtered and concentrated by the **lymph nodes**, which removes any foreign substances or initiates an immune reaction when indicated.

The **thoracic duct** is the largest lymph vessel in the body, while the **cisterna chyli** is the most expandable. Three-fourths of the body's lymph fluid drains into the juncture of the left internal jugular vein and subclavian vein via the thoracic duct. The other one-fourth drains from the body's right quadrant into the juncture of the right subclavian vein and internal jugular vein via the right lymphatic duct.

2. What is lymphedema?

Lymphedema is a high-protein edema (protein concentrations of 1 gm/dl or more in the interstitium), as compared to a low-protein edema caused by renal failure or congestive heart failure.

3. What causes lymphedema?

Whenever the lymphatic system is damaged or blocked, a build-up of protein occurs between the tissue cells in the interstitium, which attracts fluid due to a change in the colloid osmotic pressure. Up to one-third of women who require surgery for breast cancer will develop lymphedema in the arm following surgery. Without appropriate intervention, the condition only progresses to limb enlargement, with interstitial fibrinoid material causing a firm nonpitting, brawny (muscle-like) edema. Worldwide, infections caused by **parasites** (e.g., filarial worms) are the leading cause of lymphedema.

4. How many types of lymphedema are there?

There are two types: primary and secondary.

Primary lymphedema (from too few lymphatics): appears at birth (congenital), during puberty (praecox), or after age 35 (tarda).

Secondary lymphedema: due to damage or blockage of the lymphatics, caused by:
Surgery—lymph node resection
Radiation therapy—damages lymph nodes and vessels
Fibrotic tissue—constricts vessels
Traumatic accidents—lymphatic vessels are torn
Chronic venous insufficiency—overloads lymphatics
Paralysis—lymph stasis due to ineffective muscle pump

5. How is lymphedema graded?

Grade 1: pitting edema which is partially reversible with elevation.

Grade 2: nonpitting (brawny) edema which is not reduced by elevation. The skin hardens due to excess fibrotic tissue from a chronic excess of protein in the interstitium.

Grade 3: elephantiasis—an enormous swelling of the involved extremity!!

6. How can you identify the etiology for lymphedema?

The physician can usually distinguish lymphedema from other edemas caused by medical conditions such as congestive heart failure, renal failure, venous insufficiency, or embolus with a good medical history, observations, and, if necessary, special radiologic studies MRI, CT scan, and lymphoscintigraphy. Lymphangiography should *never* be used because the oily contrast medium can cause additional blockage of the lymphatics.

7. How do you measure lymphedema?

There are several methods: volume, circumference, tonometry, and bioelectrical impedance. **Circumferential** measurements (with three marked sites to guide the tape measure around the extremity) is the most frequently used method in the clinic for measuring lymphedema. The uninvolved extremity is always measured as the control. The upper extremity is measured proximal every 5 cm beginning with the ulnar styloid to the axilla. The lower extremity is measured proximal every 10 cm beginning with the lateral malleolus to the groin. A **delta value** can be obtained by subtracting each corresponding measurement (involved – uninvolved = n1) and adding up all the differences (delta = n1 + n2 + n3 + ...). These measurements can be taken daily, weekly, monthly, and yearly, and by tracking the delta value, the therapist or physician can monitor the patient's progress or regression.

8. How is lymphedema treated?

For the past 15 years the mainstay of lymphedema treatment in the United States has been elevation of the extremity, diuretics, pneumatic pumps (external pneumatic compression devices), compression garments, massage, and surgery.

9. How do pneumatic pumps work?

Pneumatic pumps come in several different designs, and you should read the instruction manual before applying one to a patient. There are **compression pumps** with either a single compartment sleeve, which inflates in a uniform or nonsequential manner, or a multicompartment sleeve, which inflates in a sequential or distal to proximal manner. A review of the medical literature indicates that use of sequential and multipressure or graded pumps obtain better limb reduction. Recent research indicates that pneumatic pumps are very effective in the reabsorption of water from the interstitial fluid into the venous capillaries, causing a reduction in the size of the lymphedematous limb. However, the large protein molecules still remain in the interstitial fluid, which can cause a Grade 1 (pitting) lymphedema to develop eventually into a Grade 2 (nonpitting) lymphedema.

When the sole treatment modality for lymphedema is a pneumatic pump, the patient is required to use it daily (2–6 hours depending upon the severity) for the rest of that patient's life. The patient will also be required to wear a compression garment daily to prevent the limb from refilling with fluid.

10. What is lymph massage?

Manual lymph drainage is a specialized massage technique that stimulates the lymphatic system to remove the large protein molecules from the interstitial fluid via the lymph capillaries. It should be performed *prior* to administering an external compression device. In it, the massage is applied from proximal to distal with circular movements, in which pressure is applied during 50% of the cycle in the direction of lymphatic flow followed by no pressure. This technique emphasizes manual pressure around 30–40 mmHg. Manual lymph drainage is *contraindicated* when an infection is present.

11. When are compression garments worn?

Once the size of the lymphedematous extremity has plateaued, a compression garment is issued to maintain the reduction. Different manufacturers of compression garments have different grades of pressure. Usually, the patient is issued a graded compression garment within the 30–40 mmHg range. Two pairs should be issued, one to wear while the other one is being cleaned. If the patient has good daily compliance in wearing the compression garment, the garments should be worn out and replaced in 4–6 months.

12. What is complex physical therapy (CPT)?

CPT is a combination of advanced techniques used by physical therapists to reduce lymphedema. It consists of five components:

1. **Skin care**—Daily cleansing, moisturizing the skin with a low-pH lotion, and monitoring for rashes and infections.
2. **Manual lymph drainage**—Done by a trained professional.
3. **Compression bandages**—The involved extremity is wrapped with a low elastic bandage (versus a high elastic bandage like an Ace wrap) to provide support and compression.
4. **Exercises**—Stimulate the lymphatics by using muscle contractions as a pump.
5. **Compression garment**—The size of the involved extremity should plateau by 4 weeks.

To maintain this reduction, the patient needs to wear the compression garment during part or all of the day.

In some instances (i.e., mild secondary lymphedema) when CPT has been initiated early enough, there is a possibility that collateral remodeling within the edematous limb will occur to create new lymphatic vessels, and further CPT will not be needed.

13. What are the precautions and contraindications for a compression pump used on a lymphedematous extremity?

Precautions

1. It should be used *only* after manual lymph drainage has been done to clear the lymphatics for the production and transportation of more lymph fluid.

2. Avoid exceeding 40–45 mmHg to prevent collapse of the superficial lymphatic vessels.

3. Discontinue pumping with an increasing limb circumference above the pump's sleeve.

Contraindications

1. Primary lymphedema—adjacent areas can become edematous due to poor fluid transportation.

2. Bilateral mastectomy—truncal edema can result.

3. Following pelvic surgery when bilateral proximal swelling is present in the legs—it can create genital and/or truncal edema.

4. When more than one lymphedematous area is involved—there is no place for the additional fluid to go, and another edematous area can be created or made worse.

5. Genital lymphedema—if it is already present, it can get worse (especially in men).

14. Are any drugs effective in treating lymphedema?

Diuretics are *not effective* for high-protein edema. They tend to remove only the water and concentrate the protein in the interstitium. The protein osmotically attracts fluid, and once the diuretic is stopped, the fluid returns and the limb swells again.

Benzopyrone increases the number of macrophages with the capacity for phagocytosis and proteolysis. The resulting smaller molecules can easily diffuse through the capillary wall and be removed by the blood flow. 5,6-Benzo-α-pyrone has not yet been approved by the FDA, though clinical trials are in progress. However, **flavonoids** (benzo-γ-pyrone) are available and can be beneficial in treating lymphedema. One of the side effects can be gastric irritation. Significant reductions in an edematous extremity can be achieved when the use of benzopyrone is combined with the use of a compression pump and CPT.

BIBLIOGRAPHY

1. Bastien MR, Goldstein BG, Lesher JL, Smith JG: Treatment of lymphedema with a multicompartmental pneumatic compression device. J Am Acad Dermatol 20:853–854, 1989.
2. Boris M, Weindorf S, Lasinski B, Boris G: Lymphedema reduction by noninvasive complex lymphedema therapy. Oncology 8(9):95–106, 1994.
3. Casley-Smith JR, Morgan RG, Piller NB: Treatment of lymphedema of the arms and legs with 5,6 benzo-[alpha]-pyrone. N Engl J Med 329:1158–1163, 1993.
4. Callam MJ, Ruckley CV, Dale JJ, Harper DR: Hazards of compression treatments of the leg: An estimate from Scottish surgeons. BMJ 295:1382, 1987.
5. Morgan RG, Casley-Smith JR, Mason MR, Casley-Smith JR: Complex physical therapy for the lymphoedematous arm. J Hand Surg 17B:437–441, 1992.
6. Olszewski W: Lymph Stasis: Pathophysiology, Diagnosis and Treatment. Boca Raton, FL, CRC Press, 1991.
7. Piller NB, Swedborg I, Norrefalk JR: Lymphoedema rehabiliation programme: An application of anatomical, physiological and pathophysiological knowledge. Eur J Lymphol 3(2):57–71, 1992.
8. Wittlinger G, Wittlinger H: Textbook of Dr. Vodder's Manual Lymph Drainage, 5th ed. Brussels, Haug International, 1992.

40. AMPUTATION REHABILITATION

Nasser Eftekhari, M.D.

1. What is the incidence and prevalence of limb loss in the United States?

The incidence of major amputations is estimated to be at least 70,000 new cases annually. Prevalence is estimated to be over 500,000 cases for major amputation and nearly 2 million for finger and toe amputations. The majority of new amputations are of the lower extremity related to diabetes with an average cost of $40,000 each!

2. What are the major reasons for amputation in the United States? Which limb is amputated more often, the upper or lower?

The greatest cause of limb loss is **peripheral vascular disease** (65%), often associated with diabetes. These patients are generally in the 60–75-year age group, with mean age of 62. Nearly half of diabetic lower-extremity amputees will eventually lose the other leg within 5 years.

Trauma accounts for 25% of all amputations and occurs most commonly in the 17–55-year age group, with most cases involving the lower extremity. **Malignancy** accounts for 5% of all amputations and is frequently seen among 10–20-year-olds. Approximately 5% of amputations are due to **congenital limb deficiency**, which accounts for 60% of all amputations in children.

Lower-extremity amputations (excluding digits) account for 80–85% of major limb amputations. More than two-thirds of cases are caused by vascular and infectious complications, with or without diabetes. Right and left occurrence is about equal.

3. What special concerns are faced in the elderly patient undergoing an amputation?

Geriatric amputation deserves special attention due to the continuous increase in the aging population with their higher incidence of diabetes and peripheral vascular diseases. Elderly patients are more likely to require higher levels of amputation. About 80% of all amputations performed at age 80 or later are above the knee. Long-term survival for elderly amputees has been increasing in the past few decades, but elderly amputees continue to remain at considerable risk. In most major series, the 2-year survival rate after bilateral amputation is < 50% and decreases steadily with age at the time of amputation. As expected, the common causes of death are coronary, stroke, and malignancy. The more proximal the amputation, the higher the mortality rate.

4. How common are amputations due to PVD among patients with diabetes mellitus?

Many of the estimated 14 million persons in the U.S. with diagnosed or undiagnosed diabetes will experience pathologic changes in their lower extremities, which when combined with minor trauma and infection may lead to serious foot problems. The most commonly described diabetic foot conditions include neuropathy, structural deformities, calluses, skin and nail changes, foot ulcers, infection, and vascular disease (See figure, following page).

An estimated 20% of diabetic patients will develop an ulcer on the feet or ankles at some time during the disease course. At least 50% of diabetic patients with PVD in the U.S. population eventually undergo nontraumatic lower limb amputation.With the increasing number of diabetics it is estimated that the total number of diabetic patients could exceed 20 million by the year 2000.

5. Is there a link between glycemic control and amputation risk in diabetics?

Many investigations have postulated that the presence of chronic hyperglycemia accelerates development of chronic complications of diabetes. The relationship between glycemic control and amputation was addressed by West, who found among patients with diabetes and higher blood glucose levels, a twofold increased risk for leg lesions, including gangrene, than in those with lower blood glucose concentrations. In the population-based Rochester study, amputation risk was higher for non-insulin-dependent diabetics than for insulin-dependent diabetics (35.6 vs. 28.3 per 10,000 patients).

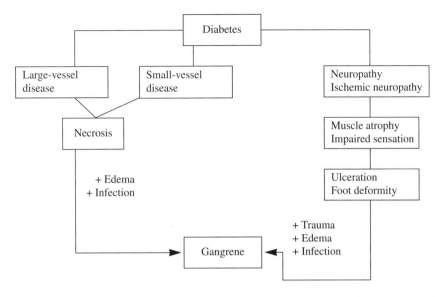

6. Name the most significant signs and symptoms of acute arterial occlusion in diabetic patients.

In the diabetic patient, most ischemic changes occur slowly, although sudden occlusion from emboli or acute complete thrombosis can occur with atherosclerosis as the underlying cause. More than 70% of the emboli originate in the heart (underlying conditions such as atrial fibrillation or myocardial infarction with mural thrombi usually exist). The signs and symptoms of acute arterial occlusion are commonly referred to as the **five Ps**:

Pain (sudden onset)   **Pulselessness** (no pulse below the block)

Pallor (waxy)   **Paresis** (sudden weakness)

Paresthesia (numbness)

7. What are the levels of amputation?

In 1974, the Task Force on Standardization of Prosthetic-Orthotic Terminology developed an international classification system to define amputation level. The major terms in common use today are as follows:

Levels of Amputation

Partial toe—Excision of any part of one or more toes	Short below-knee (transtibial)— < 20% of femoral length
Toe disarticulation—Disarticulation at the MTP joint	Knee disarticulation—Amputation through the knee joint, femur intact
Partial foot/ray resection—Resection of the 3rd, 4th, 5th, metatarsals, and digits	Long above-knee (transfemoral)— > 60% of femoral length
Transmetatarsal—Amputation through the mid-section of all metatarsals	Above-knee (transfemoral)—35–60% of femoral length
Syme's—Ankle disarticulation with attachment of heel pad to distal end of tibia; may include removal of malleoli and distal tibial/fibular flares	Short above-knee (transfemoral)— < 35% of femoral length
	Hip disarticulation—Amputation through hip joint, pelvis intact
Long below-knee (transtibial)— > 50% of tibial length	Hemipelvectomy—Resection of lower half of the pelvis
Below-knee (transtibial)—20–50% of tibial length	Hemicorporectomy—Amputation of both lower limbs and pelvis below L4,5 level

8. How many types of transtibial below-knee (BK) amputations are performed?

1. Closed amputation
   - Long posterior flap (Burgess technique)
   - Equal anterior and posterior flaps (fishmouth)
   - Equal medial and lateral (sagittal) flaps
   - Skew flaps
2. End-weight-bearing amputations (osteomyoplasty, Ertl procedure)
3. Open amputations
   - Guillotine
   - Open circumferential
   - Open flap(s)

9. Describe the major criteria in determining amputation level in the dysvascular limb.

Patients about to undergo an amputation are informed that the amputation will be performed at the lowest possible level, but the exact level will have to be determined in the operating room. Clinical features that have bearing on the selection of the amputation level include:

1. Palpable pulses at the next more-proximal joint have clinical significance only when present, and their presence is a very positive indication of the likelihood of healing at any given level.

2. Skin temperature is a representative measure of collateral circulation. Skin temperature should always be compared to the opposite limb and evaluated throughout the diseased limb.

3. Dependent rubor indicates marginal viability of the skin. Incision through ruborous tissue may not heal, and dependent rubor should be considered an absolute contraindication to amputation at that level.

4. Degree of sensory loss is of significance in the diabetic patient whose ischemic process is frequently accompanied by peripheral neuropathy. The etiology of the diabetic ulcer or infection is frequently on a neuropathic as well as an ischemic basis.

5. Bleeding of the skin edges at the time of surgical incision is probably the best clinical sign available to predict healing at intended level.

10. What are the limb-salvage decision-making variables?

Certain criteria can predict amputation of the limb in patients with severe skeletal or soft tissue injuries of the lower extremities with vascular compromise. These data might discriminate the salvageable from the unsalvageable limb.

Patient variables
   Age (usually unfavorable result after age 50)
   Occupational considerations
   Patient and family desires
   Underlying chronic disease (e.g., diabetes)
Extremity variables
   Mechanism of injury (soft tissue injury kinetics); massive crush or high-energy soft tissue injuries have poor prognosis)
   Arterial/venous injury location (e.g., poor prognosis with infrapopliteal arterial injury)
   Neurologic (anatomic) status
   Injury status of ipsilateral limb
   Intercalary ischemic zone after revascularization
Associated variables
   Magnitude of associated injury
   Severity and duration of shock (poor prognosis with prolonged severe hypovolemic shock)
   Warm ischemia time (unfavorable prognosis if warm ischemia time is > 6 hours)

11. Which type of flap technique is preferable for dysvascular BK amputation?

The long posterior flap (Burgess technique) is preferable because the muscle padding in the long posterior flap facilitates true total contact fitting. The anterior and posterior flaps meet in a small half circle that eliminates the "dog ear." Skin overlying the muscles is supplied by vessels coming through the muscles, while skin overlying bones depends on collateral skin circulation arising proximally. Thus, in the dysvascular limb, any skin overlying muscle has a far better chance of surviving than does skin overlying bone.

12. What is myoplasty?

In myoplasty, opposing muscle groups are simply joined to each other by sutures through myofascia and investing fascia over the end of the bone. In a severely dysvascular residual limb with marginal muscle viability, myoplasty is probably the preferable method, but it should be done with little closure tension. Tapering of the muscle mass avoids excessive distal bulk.

13. What is myodesis?

The most structurally stable residual limbs are achieved with **myodesis**, in which the surrounding muscles and their fasciae are sutured directly to the bone through drill holes. In the case of transfemoral amputation, the additional advantages of myodesis are stabilization of the femur in adduction by the adductor magnus, enhanced hip flexion by the rectus femoris, and enhanced hip extension by the biceps femoris, all three being muscles that cross the hip joint. In this method, tapering of the muscle mass prevents excessive distal bulk. Myodesis is contraindicated in cases of severe dysvascularity in which the blood supply to the muscle appears compromised. In patients with normal blood supply to the stump, myodesis may be combined with myoplasty.

14. What are the options in postoperative dressing in lower-extremity amputation?

Immediate postoperative fitting prosthesis (IPOP) or **rigid dressing** using elastic plaster bandage with minimal tension starting on the distal lateral aspect of the residual limb. In BK amputation, IPOP is done easier than at the above-knee level, since the use of rigid spica, particularly in elderly people, causes physical difficulties and hygienic problems.

Semirigid postoperative dressing. A variety of semirigid dressings have been used to provide wound support and pressure. The **Unna paste dressing**, a compound of zinc oxide, gelatin, glycerin, and calamine, may be used as a wrapping over conventional soft dressings. It allows limited joint movement.

Controlled environment and **air bags.** The equipment for controlled environment treatment is designed to provide a controlled wound-healing environment. Pressure humidity, temperature, gas, sterility, visualizations of the wound, and some degree of immobilizing are obtained with a flow-through air bag attached to a portable mechanical console unit. There will be no dressing directly over the wound or operative site, which can be inspected until the bag is removed (usually 10–14 days postoperatively).

Soft dressing. This is the oldest method of postoperative residual limb management and includes two forms: elastic shrinker and elastic bandages. Soft dressings are inexpensive and lightweight, and they can be reapplied several times daily. Their disadvantages include poor control of edema; they require a skilled individual to wrap the residual limb properly.

15. What are the benefits of IPOP?

1. Rapid wound healing by controlling postoperative edema without restricting circulation
2. Earlier ambulation and shorter hospital stay
3. Minimizing inflammatory reaction
4. Reducing phantom pain
5. Psychological benefit

16. What are the major factors in prognosis of a dysvascular limb?

Symptoms	Better Prognosis	Poor Prognosis
Pain	Slow onset	Rapid onset
Vibratory sensation	Present	Absent
Deep tendon reflexes	Present	Absent
Gangrene	Slow onset	Rapid onset
Infection	Absent	Present and spreading
Edema	Absent	Present
Diabetes	Absent or well-controlled	Present
Smoking	Nonsmoker	Smoker

17. Name the major vascular complications of smoking?
Acceleration of atherosclerosis
Increased blood viscosity and clotting factors
Inhibition of prostacyclin production
Increased VLDL and decreased HDL cholesterol
Increased platelet aggregation, fibrinogen, and von Willebrand factor
Decreased plasminogen
Increased carboxyhemoglobin and carbon monoxide

18. What is the ischemic index?
The pulse signal can indicate the degree of collateral circulation by pulsatility. An ischemic index is calculated for each level by dividing the systolic pressure measured in the limb by the brachial artery pressure. For example, the systolic pressure may be 120 mmHg at the arm and thigh, 90 mmHg at the calf, 60 mmHg at the ankle, and 20 mmHg at midfoot. The ischemic index would be 1 at the arm and thigh, 0.75 at the calf, 0.50 at the ankle, and 0.17 at the midfoot. The lowest level of healing is at 0.45 in the diabetic and at 0.35 in nondiabetics.

19. Define phantom limb pain.
Phantom pain can be defined as pain referred to a surgically removed limb or portion of the limb. **Stump pain** is a different entity and should be distinguished from phantom pain. There are three most commonly described painful sensations:
Postural type of cramping or squeezing sensation
Burning pain
Sharp, shooting pain
Many patients may complain of a mixed type of pain, but often the major sensation falls into one of the above categories. Other unpleasant sensory occurrences, such as paresthesia, hypothesia, and dysesthesia, should be excluded from the definition (they may coexist with phantom pain).

20. What is phantom sensation?
This term is usually reserved for individuals who have an awareness of the missing portion of their limb in which the only subjective sensation is **mild tingling**. It is rarely unpleasant or painful. The incidence of phantom sensation is 80–100% in amputees immediately after amputation. Only 10% develop it after 1 month. Phantom sensation may appear in children with congenitally missing limbs and those who had amputations in early childhood.

Most of the available data indicate that nonpainful phantom sensation seems to be the normal experience of the body, encoded (neurosignature) over a precise brain region (neuromatrix) from birth. Phantom sensation experience is produced by networks in the brain that are normally triggered by the continuous incoming modulated flow from the periphery. As soon as this flow ceases, nonpainful phantom sensation replaces the lost organ. To most patients, the limb feels perfectly normal or somewhat shortened. Patients can "move" this phantom limb normally into various positions. Sometimes, the phantom limb stays in a single position, the position of the limb at the time of the accident and before the amputation (e.g., in the case of prior peroneal palsy the patient may experience phantom drop foot!).

21. What is the incidence of phantom pain?
Older studies show a lower incidence (0.5%–10%), but they seem to be flawed by a sampling bias and by difficulties in clinical differentiation between phantom and stump pain. More recent studies show much higher rates, at least 50%.

Interestingly, in a surveyed population of 2700 veterans, 69% were told by their physicians that the pain was just "in their heads," and only 20% were offered any treatment for their pain. However, in a survey of 5000 veteran amputees, phantom pain prevented 18% from working and interfered with the work of 33.5% who were employed; 36% found it hard to concentrate due to pain, 82% had sleep disturbances, and 45% could not carry out social activity. All this implies that the true reported incidence could be higher than 50% (maybe up to 85%). Many are afraid to tell their physician about the phantom pain for fear that physician will think them "insane."

The incidence of phantom pain is the same in civilian and war-related amputations. Pain may occur immediately after the amputations, and 50–75% of patients have pain within 1 week postoperatively. Pain may be delayed weeks, months, or years after the amputation.

22. Is there any treatment for the phantom pain?

Therapeutic regimens have had < 30% long-term efficacy in the treatment of phantom limb pain. Although at least 68 methods of treatment have been identified, most report varying success. Treatment methods include TENS, tricyclic antidepressants, anticonvulsants, beta-blockers, chlorpromazine, chemical sympathectomy, neurosurgical procedures, analgesics, anesthetic procedures, and sedative/hypnotic medications. Usually, treatments reducing stump problems (neuroma, infection, etc.) also decrease phantom pain.

Treatment measures that create increased peripheral control input may provide at least temporary relief of the phantom pain. One of the more effective adjuncts is extensive use of the prosthesis. Other treatments include gentle manipulation of the stump by massage or a vibrator, stump wrapping, baths, ultrasound, and application of hot packs if sensation is intact. No single drug has been proved effective in long-term control of phantom pain (narcotics should be avoided). Trigger point injection on or near the stump may be useful (aqueous steroid and local anesthetic agents).

23. What are the common skin problems of amputees?

Amputation at any level is accompanied by distinct problems of functional loss, prosthetic fitting and alignment problems, and medical conditions such as skin disorders that are secondary to the use of the prosthesis. Skin lesions, however minute they may appear, are nevertheless of great importance since they can be the beginning of an extensive skin disorder that may be physically, mentally, socially, and economically disastrous.

Commonly Occurring Skin Problems in Amputee Stumps and Their Treatment

PROBLEM	CAUSE	TREATMENT
Maceration	Moist skin	Cornstarch in socket and on stump Absorbent stump socks More frequent sock changes
Folliculitis, cysts, boils	Hair follicle and sweat gland occlusion	Eliminate high-pressure points in socket
Open wound/ulcer	Multiple causes, e.g., high-pressure area is common cause	Remove prosthesis until healed Local wound care
Friction and skin stretch	Secondary to socket design	Elasto-Gel Thin nylon stump sock
Excessive sweating	Lack of evaporation	Antiperspirants
Hypersensitivity	Failure to desensitize	Massage and handling
Skin adherence	Scar tissue	Massage Socket modifications Plastic surgical revision
Poor hygiene	Bacterial and fungal infections, dermatitis, odor	Wash stump and socket, and wash stump socks with sudsing detergent at night
Contact dermatitis	Secondary to prosthetic parts and finishes	Patch test; remove contact Cool compress Topical corticosteroids
Epidermoid cysts	Follicular keratin plugs very sensitive (usually found along upper margins of prosthesis)	Surgical incision and drainage or excision
Fungal infections inside socket	Secondary to moisture	Fungistatic creams
Painful neuromas		Desensitize by tapping local injection Surgical removal

24. What is "choked stump syndrome"?

This problem consists of a painful verrucous hyperplasia, often associated with cracking and weeping of the skin. "Chocked stump" is the result of a combination of insecure suspension and lack of total contact distally. Circumferential pressure proximally contributes to distal edema, and the lack of suspension allows the skin to piston or slide on the underlying soft tissues, thus stretching the skin over the end of the bone with each step.

Chronic edema encourages the development of stasis pigmentation and hemorrhagic papules and nodules of the distal portion of the stump. In diabetic and dysvascular individuals, progressive lymphatic and venous outflow obstruction may produce a stasis ulcer at the distal end of the stump.

Treatment includes removal of the ill-fitting socket and application of appropriate topical treatment combined with continuous stump wrapping. Refitting with the new total-contact prosthesis usually solves the problem, and skin changes gradually revert to normal.

25. Is there a difference between energy expenditure of dysvascular and traumatic amputees during ambulation?

Older dysvascular amputees use more energy during walking than their younger, usually traumatic counterparts. A comparison of the two etiologies of amputation at the below-knee (BK) and above-knee (AK) levels reveals that comfortable walking speed is slower and the O_2 consumption higher for the dysvascular BK amputee than for the traumatic BK amputee (45 m/min and 0.20 ml/kg/m vs. 71 m/min and 0.16 ml/kg/m, respectively). The same differences were observed at the AK level between dysvascular and traumatic amputees (36 m/min and 0.28 ml/kg/m vs. 52 m/min and 0.20 ml/kg/m). Most older patients who have AK or higher amputations for vascular disease are not successful prosthetic ambulators. Very few are able to walk with a prosthesis without crutch assistance. If able to walk, they have a very slow walking speed and an elevated heart rate if crutch assistance is required.

26. How is the energy expenditure different between crutch and prosthetic ambulation?

Direct comparison of walking in unilateral traumatic and dysvascular amputees at the Syme's, BK, and AK levels using a prosthesis or a swing-through crutch-assisted gait without a prosthesis reveals that almost all amputees have a lower rate of energy expenditure, heart rate, and O_2 cost when using a prosthesis. This difference is insignificant in dysvascular AK patients and is related to the fact that even with a prosthesis, most of these patients require crutches for some support, thereby increasing the O_2 rate and heart rate. It can be concluded that a well-fitted prosthesis that results in a satisfactory gait not requiring crutches significantly reduces the physiologic energy demand. Since crutch-walking requires more exertion than walking with a prosthesis, crutch-walking without a prosthesis should not be considered an absolute requirement for prosthetic prescription and training.

27. Is there any correlation between length of residual limb and energy expenditure during ambulation?

Studies have examined the relationship of stump length and gait performance in BK patients (stump length ranging from 9–24 cm). No significant correlations were noted between comfortable walking speed and energy expenditure in the studies. Of particular clinical importance, a stump as short as 9 cm results in BK performance (lower O_2 cost and higher walking speed) that is superior to knee disarticulation and AK levels.

28. What is the goal in rehabilitation of the geriatric bilateral amputee?

The great majority of bilateral lower-limb amputees today are elderly who lose their limbs secondary to diabetes and peripheral vascular disease. In general, dismissing these patients as poor prosthetic candidates is a grave mistake, and it compromises their rehabilitation potential when immediate postsurgical treatment is delayed. Lack of exercise and mobility will encourage joint contractures, weaken the patient, cause loss of independence, bring on depression, and maybe even become life-threatening. Unfortunately, the challenge of rehabilitating these patients is frequently complicated by the presence of other illnesses, such as diabetes, chronic infection, kidney disease, cardiovascular disease, respiratory disease, arthritis, impaired vision, delayed wound healing, and neuropathy. These coexisting diseases warrant additional consideration and precautions, but chronologic age *alone* should not determine whether an amputee is a prosthetic candidate.

29. What are the advantages and disadvantages of wrist disarticulation?

Generally, wrist disarticulation is considered to be a very useful and functional level of amputation.

Advantages
- Preservation of distal radial ulnar joint, which allows full pronation and supination.
- Square-ended, bony, and flattened stump can transmit up to two-thirds of the pronation and supination to the prosthesis.
- The prosthetic socket can be short, and no auxiliary suspension is necessary.
- The bulbous end of the stump aids in attachment of the socket.
- Long lever arm makes it easier to lift terminal device and load.

Disadvantages
- Cosmetically, prosthesis is bulky at its distal end, and its length makes it difficult to fit a terminal device that does not appear to be too long.
- Socket fit must be very precise because of the lack of subcutaneous soft tissue or muscle bellies to cushion the bony end.
- Neuroma can be troublesome, mainly because of lack of soft tissue cushion.
- Myoplasty is difficult since tendons over the end of the bone have tendency to displace.

30. Does lumbar sympathectomy offer any help in limb ischemia?

Lumbar sympathectomy was often attempted to improve the blood flow of the lower portion of the leg in critical leg ischemia. Although a perception of increased flow is achieved in some patients because of an apparently warmer foot, this warmth is due to opening of nonnutritional arteriovenous shunts and does nothing for the flow in the nutritional capillary bed unless the perfusion pressure is already reasonably good. In a small number of patients with isolated rest pain, chemical or operative lumbar sympathectomy may help to relieve this pain by direct inhibitory effect on pain perception pathways.

31. What is the segmental weight of the limbs and its percentage of total body weight?

In a typical rehab setting, knowing the approximate segmental weight of each limb at different levels can be helpful in managing various clinical situations, including nutritional assessment of an amputee. Following are segmental weights of the limbs and percentage of the total body weight for a 150-lb man:

Lower limb (entire length)	23.4 lb	15.6%	Upper limb (entire length)	7.3 lb	4.9%
Thigh	14.5 lb	9.7%	Arm	4.0 lb	2.7%
Leg	6.8 lb	4.5%	Forearm	2.4 lb	1.6%
Foot	2.1 lb	1.4%	Hand	0.9 lb	0.6%

32. To what degree does malnutrition affect the healing of lower-extremity amputations?

The significant incidence of malnutrition in hospitalized patients has been well documented. Patients undergoing lower-limb amputations are frequently elderly and debilitated. Diabetics with dysvascular limbs often have open wounds and systemic sepsis, causing increased metabolic demands and an increased energy requirement 30%–55% above basal values. Protein malnutrition, in general, has an adverse effect on mortality in hospital patients.

Dickhaut demonstrated that in Syme's amputations, even subclinical malnutrition makes wound healing almost impossible. Despite the technical expertise that yielded an 86% success rate in his nourished patients, Dickhaut had an 85% failure rate in malnourished amputees (Syme's).

Serum albumin levels and total lymphocyte counts are excellent ways to gauge the nutritional status of the patient. They are easy to obtain and have great predictive value for complications in the hospitalized patient. Serum albumin of < 3.4 g/dl and total lymphocyte counts < 1,500 cells/mm³ are considered abnormal. Surgical procedures on these patients should be delayed until their nutritional status is improved.

33. Why is preoperative amputee assessment an important part of the rehab program?

Amputees at various levels have distinctive problems of anatomic and functional loss, fitting and alignment of the prosthesis, gait abnormalities, and medical issues that require continued care for the remainder of their lives. A neglected part of total patient management is the pre-amputation stage. When amputation is anticipated or planned, rehabilitation clinicians have the opportunity to help prepare the patient physically and psychologically.

Questions can be answered and instructions given to alleviate anxieties of the unknown. Patients want to know what a prosthesis looks like, of what it is made, and how much it costs. The patient should be shown what type of exercise program is expected and how ambulation is performed with crutches or a walker on flat surfaces and stairs. Addressing these issues before amputation not only shortens the recovery time but also gives the patient a psychologic edge.

34. What is the risk categorization for injury prevention of insensate foot?

Risk and Management Categories

RISK	MANAGEMENT
Category 0	
Protective sensation present	Foot clinic once/year
No history of plantar ulcer	Patient education to include proper shoe style
May have foot deformity	selection
Has a disease that could lead to insensitivity	
Category 1	
Protective sensation absent	Foot clinic every 6 months
No history of plantar ulceration	Review all footwear the patient wears
No foot deformity	Add soft insoles
	Also consider leprosy
Category 2	
Protective sensation absent	Foot clinic every 3–4 months
No history of plantar ulcer	Custom-molded orthotic devices are usually
Foot deformity present	necessary
	Prescription footwear often required
Category 3	
Protective sensation absent	Foot clinic every 1–2 months
There is a history of foot ulceration and/or	Custom orthotic devices are necessary
vascular laboratory findings indicate	Prescription shoes are often required
significant vascular disease	

BIBLIOGRAPHY

1. Bowker J: Atlas of Limb Prosthetics. St. Louis, Mosby, 1993.
2. Kostnik J: Amputation Surgery and Rehabilitation. New York, Churchill Livingstone, 1981.
3. Lange R: Limb reconstruction versus amputation: Decision making in massive lower-extremity trauma. Clin Orthop 96:1–243, 1989.
4. Levin M, O'Neal L, Bowker J (eds): The Diabetic Foot. St. Louis, Mosby, 1993.
5. O'Sullivan S, Schmitz T: Physical Rehabilitation: Assessment and Treatment. Philadelphia, F.A. Davis, 1994.
6. Sherman R, Arena J: Phantom limb pain. Crit Rev Phys Med Rehabil 4:1–26, 1992.
7. Varda G, Friedmann L: Postamputation phantoms. Phys Med Rehabil Clin North Am 1:334, 1991.
8. Waters R: Energy expenditure. In Perry J (ed): Gait Analysis: Normal and Pathological Function. Thorofare, NJ, Slack, 1992, p 477.

V. Rehabilitation of System-Based Disorders
B. The Nervous System

41. RESTORATIVE NEUROREHABILITATION

Charles E. Levy, M.D., Elizabeth Walz, M.D., and Lisa Fugate, M.D., M.S.

1. Define restorative neurology.

Restorative neurology refers to the natural mechanisms of recovery from CNS insult, as well as interventions to preserve and promote brain and spinal cord recovery and function. Strategies exist to contain the initial injury in the first minutes and hours after an event and to promote healing and adaptation in the postacute period.

2. Why get excited about amino acids? What is their role in neuronal injury?

In many neurologic diseases, including stroke and traumatic brain injury (TBI), the total territory of injury is likely to result from two processes. First, an initial zone of neuronal death is caused by the underlying pathologic process. Death of individual neurons then causes release of stored excitatory amino acids such as glutamate, normally a highly regulated neurotransmitter. This excess glutamate binds to *N*-methyl-*D*-aspartate (NMDA) and α-amino-3-hydroxy-5-methyl-4-isoxazolepropionate (AMPA) receptors on neighboring healthy neurons, which allows excess calcium to enter them. This incites neuronal membrane depolarization, which results in activation of voltage-sensitive Ca^{2+} channels, allowing influx of even more Ca^{2+}. In the final step of this cascade, the excess Ca^{2+} activates numerous intracellular enzymes, such as protein kinases, proteases, phospholipases, and nitric oxide synthase, and uncouples oxidative phosphorylation, leading to neuronal death. Thus, a second zone of injury is created.

Besides stroke and TBI, overstimulation is thought also to mediate cellular death in epilepsy and degenerative diseases such as Huntington's disease, amyotrophic lateral sclerosis (ALS), AIDS dementia complex, Parkinson's disease, and Alzheimer's disease.

3. Does this cascade allow any clinical interventions?

Yes, potentially. Drug trials are ongoing with agents that act on various parts of the cascade in hopes of decreasing neurologic damage and/or slowing progression of disease. The following agents have shown promise for diseases such as stroke, subarachnoid hemorrhage, amyotrophic lateral sclerosis, and spinal cord injury.

Riluzole, an antiglutamate agent
NMDA and AMPA receptor antagonists
Cerebroselective calcium channel blockers
Tirilazad, an antioxidant
Lamotrigine, an anticonvulsant
Phenytoin, an anticonvulsant

4. How does neuronal injury to the peripheral nervous system (PNS) differ from that to the CNS?

In the PNS, an injured axon often regenerates to reinnervate its original target. This is not true of the CNS, where regeneration is severely restricted, especially if the affected structure has reached maturity.

5. If CNS regeneration is so limited, why does recovery happen at all?

While regeneration to the original target by the original axon is rare, other modes of neuronal rearrangement are more common.

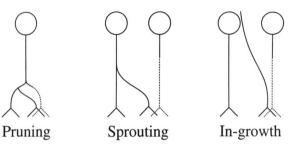

Modes of neural regeneration.

1. **Pruning** occurs in neurons with highly collateralized axons. Here, an injured axon grows a new branch to reinnervate the abandoned target. Animal data suggest that when this process occurs, it takes months to complete.

2. **Collateral sprouting** involves a neighbor axon branching to assume the territory of the injured axon. This process is widespread. It can aid in recovery if the contributing neuron is similar to the lost neuron, but may lead to dysfunction if the new sprout transmits signals of significant variance to the original. Collateral sprouting is evident within 8 hours of injury in experimental animals and is usually complete within 1 month.

3. **Ingrowth**, which takes months to complete, differs from collateral sprouting in that the contributing axon is remote from the injured axon. Because of the distance, the contributing neuron innervates a foreign target, leading to maladaptive and worsened functional deficits.

6. Are there other models of early recovery of function after brain injury?

In the hours and days immediately following a brain injury, some recovery may be attributed to the resolution of cerebral edema and arterial spasm. **Unmasking** and **functional reorganization** are two models of recovery beyond the immediate postinjury period.

7. Describe the role of unmasking in early recovery.

Unmasking involves activation of previously "silent" synapses which begin to function only after injury to primary functional synapses. With time and increased demand, these new routes might gain efficiency that rivals the original. It has also been postulated that intact primary functional structures inhibit or "mask" the activity of potentially useful parallel synapses, and with injury to the primary structures, these parallel routes are free to flourish.

8. Give an example of neurologic restoration due to functional reorganization.

An example of this concept is teaching patients with visual agnosia to read by having them trace large letters while phonating, thus using motor and sensory pathways to compensate for the damaged visual pathways.

9. What is neuronal plasticity?

Neuronal plasticity refers to the potential of the CNS to reorganize in structure and function. The term *plasticity* has been used in the following contexts:

- Normal differentiation and specialization that take place as the human brain and spinal cord mature from the prenatal period throughout childhood
- Changes evoked by the effects of environmental exposure and experience (learning) or environmental deprivation
- Response of the CNS to lesion or other injury

Implicit in all these examples is a responsive, flexible, and dynamic CNS, as opposed to the picture often presented of the CNS as a fixed structure incapable of repair or adaptation.

10. Explain the interaction between maturation and plasticity in animals deprived of stimulation.

Deprivation of sensory stimulation, sleep, warmth, and nutrition reduce the number of dendritic spines, and hence synaptic input, to a given neuronal cell body. For example, blindfolding newborn kittens for a prolonged time during a critical period will induce the inability to process visual input even after the blindfold is removed, despite an intact retina and optic neural pathways. The cell bodies of the lateral geniculate nucleus, which form the first extraretinal synapse in the visual pathways, shrink. The number of cells is also reduced; likewise, there may be a reduction in the number of synapses these cells form.

The persistence of deficits caused by deprivation depends on when the deficit occurs developmentally (i.e., the critical period), the duration of deprivation (a longer time causes deficits more resistant to change), the completeness of the deprivation, and the environment the animal is exposed to following the deprivation.

11. Is it possible to regain function after deprivation?

Strategies to retrain the damaged functions can promote some restitution of lost function. Of course, many functions are more easily remediated if the injury occurs at an earlier age. A commonly cited example is the ability of children to recover language function after dominant hemispheric damage, whereas an anatomically similar lesion in an adult would leave permanent language impairment. The language function appears to be transferred to the formerly nondominant hemisphere, though with the cost of lowered verbal and nonverbal IQ scores.

12. What is a "brain attack"?

This term is now being used for **acute ischemic stroke** in hopes of relaying its acute nature and need for active intervention, like in "heart attack."

13. What type of acute intervention is possible in a stroke?

When an artery is occluded, a central core area of brain tissue undergoes severe ischemia and infarction, but the surrounding area (ischemic penumbra) may continue to have some perfusion via collateral vessels and may be salvageable for at least several hours if reperfusion occurs.

In hopes of salvaging this ischemic penumbra in the early hours after stroke, **thrombolytics**, such as urokinase, streptokinase, and tissue plasminogen activator (tPA), are being studied. Agents that blunt the excitatory amino acid cascade are also being studied in hopes of decreasing cell death while reperfusion is being established. **Ancrod**, a purified snake venom which acts on the coagulation cascade, is also being investigated. The penumbra may also be preserved by preventing relative hypotension and hypoxemia. Hyperglycemia, which can increase edema, should be avoided to preserve the penumbra.

14. Who was Constantin von Monakow?

Von Monakow (1853–1930) was a Russian-born German neurologist. He was described as a "huge bearded figure with a shrill voice" given to boisterous and eccentric behavior in his youth. He noted the atrophy of the superior colliculus after the removal of the contralateral eye and the complete degeneration of the lateral geniculate nuclei following the excision of the occipital lobes in newborn experimental rabbits. This work formed the background for his concept "diaschisis."

15. What is diaschisis?

Diaschisis (from the Greek, meaning *shocked throughout*) is a term coined by von Monakow to explain functional deficit and recovery from a brain injury. In 1914, he postulated that following focal brain injury, sites distant to the primary injury may be affected by loss of neural input from the injured portion of the brain. Thus, the original deficit reflects not only loss of function attributable to cell death, but also to dysfunction of distant brain sites dependent on input from the now-dead tissue. Gradually, this effect regresses, and function returns to the undamaged neural tissue. Von Monakow described an active brain struggling to recover function in a way that somewhat mirrors modern concepts of dynamic neural recovery and plasticity.

16. What objective data support the existence of diaschisis?

Patients with cortical strokes have shown ipsilateral thalamic and/or basal ganglia metabolic depression. Patients with frontal lobe infarcts show decreased blood flow and oxygen metabolism in the contralateral cerebellum on PET scans as compared with controls. In rats, a small thrombotic infarction of the left frontal pole causes a decrement of activity of the ipsilateral ventrobasal thalamus, even when the rat receives stimulus that would ordinarily excite this area. Experimentally induced right middle cerebral artery ischemia in rats causes widespread reduction of brainstem neurotransmitters, particularly norepinephrine (NE).

17. Cite an experiment suggesting that haloperidol might inhibit recovery from stroke.

Various evidence indicates that widespread catecholamine depletion is a consequence of localized sensorimotor brain insult such as stroke and thus supports the existence of diaschisis. Feeney et al.'s work further demonstrates that, at least upper certain circumstances, treatment with amphetamines (AMP) speeds recovery, whereas haloperidol (a catecholamine antagonist) impedes recovery, particularly for motor skills. In a commonly cited experiment, Feeney et al. subjected rats to unilateral sensorimotor cortex ablation, causing pronounced but transient hemiplegia as reflected in a beam-walking task. When the rats were exposed to AMP after ablation, their performance markedly improved over the saline-treated animals. However, this improvement was abolished if haloperidol was given 2 minutes after the administration of AMP.

Another interesting finding was that neither haloperidol nor AMP had any significant effect if the rat was confined for 8 hours, unable to walk the beam. Clearly, behavior in this study was under both pharmacologic influence and environmental control. Feeney postulated that the combination of physical therapy plus stimulation of the catecholamine systems might facilitate recovery in brain-injured humans.

18. What medications are CNS stimulants?

The three stimulants usually discussed as potentially beneficial in a rehabilitation setting are:
• Dextroamphetamine (Dexedrine)
• Methylphenidate (Ritalin)
• Pemoline (Cylert)
The stimulant class also includes cocaine and nicotine, drugs more commonly cited for their abuse potential, as well as caffeine. Dextroamphetamine and methylphenidate are often grouped together in terms of mechanism of action and effect.

19. Discuss the history and uses of the three potentially useful stimulants.

Amphetamine (AMP) was first synthesized by Edeleano in 1887, but its sympathomimetic effect went largely unappreciated until it was resynthesized by Alles in 1927 in an effort to find substitutes for ephedrine in the treatment of asthma. AMP was commonly used in the 1930s to treat a wide variety of illnesses, including narcolepsy and depression; benzedrine was available over the counter in 1936. World War II saw the expansion of the use and abuse of amphetamines. German Panzer troops used "huge amounts of methamphetamine" during the invasions of Poland, Belgium, and France. American, British, and Japanese forces also used these substances. After World War II, medical enthusiasm and interest in AMP waned as its abuse potential became better understood. A further blow to the use of amphetamines was the development of tricyclic antidepressants, starting with imipramine in 1957 and amitriptyline in 1961. Currently, AMP is a highly restricted drug whose only FDA-approved indications are for the treatment of narcolepsy and attention deficit hyperactivity disorder. AMP has a half-life of 7–10 hours and reaches peak effect in 2–4 hours.

Methylphenidate (MPH) was marketed in 1954 as a mood elevator. This stimulant was reported to induce less euphoria, addiction, and "rebound letdown" than AMP. However, by 1960, cases of abuse and addiction were noted, and by 1962, cases of MPH psychosis were reported. MPH has a half-life of 2–4 hours and reaches peak effect in 1–2 hours.

Pemoline, developed in 1974, is the least potent of the three stimulants. Its mechanism of action is unclear, but it is thought to enhance the release of dopamine and reduce catecholamine turnover. Its half-life is 12 hours, and it takes days to weeks to reach its peak.

20. What are the mechanisms of action of AMP and MPH? Are there any differences?

Much more is known about AMP. Both cause increases in the availability of dopamine (DA) and norepinephrine (NE). AMP causes direct release of DA and NE as well as blockade of catecholamine uptake. Evidence suggests that with AMP, the release of DA is from a newly synthesized pool that is not calcium-dependent. It is believed that the DA released by MPH exists in a calcium-dependent storage pool. Further, both drugs may affect serotonin in distinct manners.

21. Why is it important to know that there are differences between MPH and AMP?

Because these two medications have many similarities, it is often assumed that what is true for one is true for the other. In fact, reaction to MPH often fails to predict the reaction to AMP, and vice versa. This is true whether the subjects were normal controls, sufferers of depression, schizophrenics, or children with attention deficit disorder. It is important to resist classifying a patient as a stimulant-treatment failure based on a trial of a single stimulant.

22. What are the current established applications of stimulants in general medical practice?

• Attention deficit/hyperactivity disorder
• Depression accompanying medical illness
• Narcolepsy

23. Is there evidence that AMP is actually helpful to brain-injured patients?

Lipper and Tuchmann's 1976 case study demonstrated a diminution in confusion and paranoia and an improvement in short-term memory in a TBI patient treated with AMP.

Crisostomo et al. randomized 8 patients with hemiplegia due to stroke to receive either a single dose of AMP or placebo in a double-blinded study. The four who received AMP showed a statistically significant improvement in Fugl-Meyer motor scale scores as compared with the controls one day after patients received the drug.

Bleiberg et al. studied a single TBI patient who was treated with AMP in a double-blind, placebo-controlled, crossover trial. They reported improved performance and consistency on a neuropsychological test battery when the patient received AMP.

Walker-Batson et al. treated 6 aphasic patients with AMP and speech therapy in an open label trial for 37 days. Five of the 6 showed accelerated language recovery compared with predicted scores. She also randomized 10 hemiplegic ischemic stroke survivors to receive AMP or placebo and found that the AMP group showed an increased rate and extent of recovery as judged by Fugl-Meyer scores.

24. What is the track record of MPH in the rehab setting?

MPH has been useful in treating poststroke depression. Since the prevalence of depression is as high as 30–60% in the first 2 years following stroke, recognition and proper treatment of this entity are critical. In a retrospective chart review, Lazarus et al. found equal efficacy of MPH (53%) as compared with nortriptyline (43%, a nonsignificant difference). However, the average response time for the MPH group was 2.4 days as compared with 27 days in the nortriptyline group. This is particularly meaningful for stroke survivors on inpatient rehabilitation units who often must demonstrate continuing gains every week or risk being discharged.

The record of MPH in TBI is mixed, with studies that both support and find little effect of MPH. Speech et al. subjected 12 "chronic" TBI patients (with an average time since injury of

4 years) to receive 1 week of MPH treatment or placebo using a double-blind, placebo-controlled, randomized crossover design. No significant differences were detected in the neuropsychologic testing. Although the authors claim no significant differences on the Katz Adjustment Scale, subjects on MPH scored higher on 9 of 11 subscales. In addition, 8 of 11 observers reported cognitive and personality improvement during the MPH treatment. Among the studies' weaknesses, none of the subjects was identified before enrollment as having deficits in attention that might be amenable to treatment; no washout period between treatments was provided (improvements due to MPH may have persisted for the placebo group); and no precautions were noted to prevent learning between the tests.

Kaelin, Cifu, and Matthies found MPH was associated with improvement in neuropsychological tests measuring attention and arousal and in function in 10 TBI patients using a multibaseline design.

Plenger et al., in a double-blind, placebo-controlled trial of 23 TBI patients found accelerated recovery as rated by the Disability Rating Score.

25. What is the locus ceruleus?
A nucleus of approximately 30,000 neurons located in the posterolateral tegmentum near the fourth ventricle. It is the major source of norepinephrine in the brain. Its axons extend throughout the cortex, subcortical centers, brainstem, cerebellum, and spinal cord. It plays a role in regulating arousal and mood and has been described as having an enabling effect on other brain systems and as enhancing signal-to-noise ratio.

26. What role does the locus ceruleus (LC) have in motor recovery following stroke?
Some LC neurons support axons that branch to both the sensorimotor cortex (SMCX) and to the contralateral cerebellum. Injury to one branch disrupts neurotransmission to the intact branches. Therefore, with SMCX damage, there is disruption of NE transmission to both the SMCX and the contralateral cerebellum. The projections of the LC to the cerebellum normally provide inhibition to the cerebellum's Purkinje cells. These Purkinje cells in turn provide inhibition to deep cerebellar nuclei. These nuclei project to the red nucleus from which the rubrospinal tract originates. It is hypothesized that the rubrocerebrospinal tract is active during well-known movements, while the corticospinal tract is involved in execution of new movements.

The sum of this line of reasoning is that damage to the SMCX causes a decrease in LC input to the Purkinje cells. This causes increased inhibition to the outflow of the deep cerebellar nuclei to the rubrospinal tract, causing a loss of well-known movements. This loss is somewhat reversible, as the LC projections to the cerebellum recover.

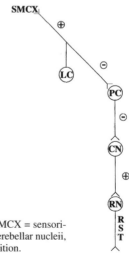

The normal influence of the locus ceruleus on the motor outflow. SMCX = sensorimotor cortex, LC = locus ceruleus, PC = Purkinje cells, CN = deep cerebellar nucleii, RN = red nucleus, RST = rubrospinal tract, + = facilitation, – = inhibition.

27. What other pharmacologic agents besides stimulants show potential to enhance cognitive recovery in the postacute stage?

The dopamine agonists levodopa/carbidopa, amantadine, bromocriptine, pergolide, and deprenyl (selegiline) have been used to improve arousal and motor activity.

Levodopa/carbidopa has been credited with promoting emergence from coma in case studies and small, uncontrolled trials of TBI patients.

Five unblinded trials of six or fewer patients have supported the use of **bromocriptine** to treat nonfluent aphasias.

Treatment with **tacrine** (Cognex), a potent, centrally active, reversible acetylcholinesterase inhibitor, provides a modest boost to memory function in early Alzheimer's disease.

Physostigmine, another acetylcholinesterase inhibitor, improved sustained attention of TBI patients in a double-blind trial involving 16 patients.

Various other agents have been employed to promote recovery and enhance cognition in the brain injured: tricyclic antidepressants, GM_1-ganglioside, carbaminol choline, CDP choline, phentermine, yohimbine, and apomorphine.

28. Are there any human data indicating that benzodiazepines inhibit recovery following stroke?

Goldstein et al., as part of a larger study on the effects of GM_1-ganglioside on stroke, prospectively studied the motor recovery of patients assigned to a control group who did not receive GM_1-ganglioside. This group was divided into those who were treated with any "detrimental drugs" ($n = 37$) during their hospital course versus those who were not ($n = 57$). Detrimental drugs were defined as implicated in animal trials as inhibitory to recovery following brain injury, specifically benzodiazepines, dopamine receptor antagonists (such as haloperidol), α_2-agonists, α_1-antagonists, phenytoin, and phenobarbital. Patients receiving detrimental drugs displayed significantly greater upper limb motor impairment and less recovery in activities of daily living.

Despite several weaknesses in its design, this prospective study should confirm the caution with which the detrimental drugs are used. Since benzodiazepines were the most commonly used detrimental drug in this study, they fall under the greatest suspicion.

29. What are the rationales for use and avoidance of haloperidol after traumatic brain injury?

Haloperidol is a butyrophenone neuroleptic that depresses the central dopaminergic/catecholaminergic neurotransmitter system, producing reduced restlessness and often sedation. It is often used to treat acute agitation and is widely used to treat confused or delirious individuals in danger of dislodging tubes or intravenous lines, extubating themselves or injuring staff. In this setting, haloperidol can be employed as a **chemical restraint**.

Haloperidol is causally associated with unpredictable development of tardive dyskinesia (automatic stereotyped movements) and has been shown to delay motor recovery in animal studies. Feeney's studies showing impaired motor recovery in brain-injured rats and cats after pharmacologic intervention with haloperidol are responsible, in part, for physiatrists' reluctance to use this agent. In addition, some believe that agitation is a normal stage in emergence from coma among the brain-injured and that unnecessary suppression of agitated behavior may impair recovery. A clinical trial by Rao et al., concluding good response and outcome after treatment of agitation with haloperidol, may partially explain the continued use of this agent by TBI rehabilitationists. Continued use, however, is difficult to support because of the significant methodologic limitations of the study. It was neither randomized nor blinded. The small sample size predisposed the study to type-II statistical error (i.e., the erroneous conclusion of no significant difference between study groups). Also, the outcome measures for determining severity of injury, cognitive recovery, and severity of agitation were insensitive. Although the only significant difference in the haloperidol-treated group was prolonged posttraumatic amnesia, there was also a trend suggesting a poorer recovery in the treated patients. The consensus among physiatrists specializing in TBI is that use of haloperidol should be avoided.

30. Is there any hope for multiple sclerosis (MS)?

While the exact pathophysiology of MS is unknown, several studies support an immune-mediated process as the prime culprit. The immunomodulatory agents interferon beta-1b and interferon beta-1a have decreased MS exacerbation rates. Low-dose methotrexate and interferon beta-1a have slowed disease progression; interferon beta-1b has shown a trend toward slowing disease progression.

31. Of what relevance is the mapping of the human genome?

Once the genetic defect for a disease is localized, the pathophysiology can be explored on a molecular level, treatments investigated, and genetic testing offered. Discovery of the defects underlying genetic diseases, many of which are treated by physiatrists, may ultimately lead to effective medical treatment.

Genetic Diseases of Relevance to Physiatry

DISEASE	CHROMOSOME
Huntington's chorea	4p
Duchenne-Becker muscular dystrophy	Xp
Myotonic dystrophy	19q
Facioscapulohumeral dystrophy	4q
Neurofibromatosis I	17q
Neurofibromatosis II	22q
Charcot-Marie-Tooth IA	17p
Friedrich's ataxia	91

32. Subarachnoid hemorrhage. Is it all dismal?

Prognosis of subarachnoid hemorrhage has improved because of early surgical intervention to prevent rehemorrhage. There also have been medical advances to salvage brain tissue and prevent further neuronal damage. Nimodipine, a calcium channel antagonist, is used to reduce vasospasm by inhibiting the contractile properties of smooth muscle cells and also results in vasodilatation of small arterioles, thereby increasing perfusion. It may also inhibit cell death by decreasing calcium influx into neurons. Triple H therapy (hypervolemia, hemodilution, hydration) is also used to prevent vasospasm.

33. Your patient with severe Parkinson's disease is noted to have a new lesion in the globus pallidus. Why is this good news?

Ablative neurosurgical procedures, such as pallidotomy and thalamotomy, can help to restore function in some neurologic diseases. The medial pallidum is believed to function normally as a motor control station. When it is diseased (as in Parkinson's), freezing of initiation and execution of movement results, which can be reversed with pallidotomy. **Pallidotomy** (placing selective lesions in the pallidum) was first used in the 1940s to decrease the rigidity, bradykinesia, and tremor of Parkinson's disease. It fell out of favor because of the difficulty in avoiding unwanted lesions in the internal capsule causing contralateral hemiplegia. The development of MRI stereotactic techniques has improved neurosurgical precision, reviving interest in pallidotomy.

Thalamotomy (lesions in selected portions of the thalamus) has also been tried to control tremor. Rarely, thalamotomy of the ventroposterior lateral nucleus is performed in hopes of controlling severe pain, as this is considered a prime central relay station.

34. What is apoptosis?

Apoptosis is the phenomenon of programmed cell death, first noted as a normal occurrence during embryogenesis. During embryogenesis and adult life, many cells die according to a predetermined genetic program triggered by environmental signals.

- Understanding the physiologic factors that trigger apoptotic cell death may be applied to help limit the secondary injury of neuronal tissue surrounding a primary CNS lesion.

• If apoptosis could be selectively activated in cancerous cells of CNS tumors, without threatening the viability of surrounding health tissue, great benefit could be gained.

35. What are neurotrophic factors? What are possible clinical applications?
Neurotrophic factors are secreted substances found in muscle and brain extracts that promote survival and maintenance of neurons both in vivo and in vitro. They are involved in regulation of structure, metabolism, and repair. During normal development of the CNS and PNS, approximately half of all neurons undergo programmed cell death (apoptosis). In mammalian studies, neurotrophic factors have been demonstrated to (1) promote survival of developing neurons and (2) prevent the death and atrophy of motor neurons that would be expected following peripheral axonotomy. Consideration is now being given for clinical trials of a glial-cell-line–derived neurotrophic factor (GDNF) to retard progression of motor neuron diseases.

BIBLIOGRAPHY
1. Bensimon G, Lacomblez L, Meininger V, the ALS/Riluzole Study Group: A controlled trial of riluzole in amyotrophic lateral sclerosis. N Engl J Med 330:585–591, 1994.
2. Boyeson MG, Harmon RL: Acute and postacute drug-induced effects on rate of behavioral recovery after brain injury. J Head Trauma Rehabil 9(3):78–90, 1994.
3. Challenor YB, Borkow RB: Central nervous system plasticity. In Downey JA, Myers SJ, Gonzalez EG, Lieberman JS (eds): The Physiological Basis of Rehabilitation, 2nd ed. Boston, Butterworth-Heinemann, 1994, pp 599–624.
4. Feeney DM, Baron JC: Diaschisis. Stroke 17:817–829, 1986.
5. Goldstein LB, Sygen in Acute Stroke Study Investigators: Common drugs may influence motor recovery after stroke. Neurology 45:865–871, 1995.
6. Lazarus LW, Moberg PJ, Langsley PR, Lingam VR: Methylphenidate and nortriptyline in the treatment of poststroke depression: A retrospective comparison. Arch Phys Med Rehabil 75:403–406, 1994.
7. Lipton SA, Rosenberg PA: Excitatory amino acids as a final common pathway for neurologic disorders. N Engl J Med 330:613–622, 1994.
8. Little KY: d-Amphetamine versus methylphenidate effects in depressed inpatients. J Clin Psychiatry 54:9:349–356, 1993.
9. Levy CE, Lis S: Dramatic recovery from herpes encephalitis via early administration of acyclovir, methylphenidate (Ritalin) and behavior modification. Presented at the American Congress of Rehabilitation Medicine–American Academy of Physical Medicine and Rehabilitation Annual Meeting, San Francisco, November 1992.
10. Meyer JS: Does diaschisis have clinical correlates? Mayo Clin Proc 66:430–432, 1991.
11. Wroblewski BA: Pharmacological treatment of arousal and cognitive deficits. J Head Trauma Rehabil 9(3):19–42, 1994.

42. MULTIPLE SCLEROSIS
Bertram Greenspun, D.O.

1. Who gets multiple sclerosis (MS)?
MS is the third most common cause of severe disability of people in their most productive years, affecting between 200,000–500,000 people in the United States. The prevalence is almost twice that of spinal cord injury. Women especially are prone to develop the disease. The number of women who become afflicted is double that of men. Twice as many white people as black people have MS.

2. What causes MS?
There are many hypotheses, but nothing has been proven. An early theory, proposed in the early 19th century, was that the disease was caused by the **suppression of sweat**. One of the

present-day theories concerns **genetic factors**, with the finding of HLA antigens being more frequent in patients with MS than in controls. Many feel that there is an **autoimmune mechanism**. Others feel that direct infection is the cause, with the most likely agent being a **slow virus**, possibly herpes simplex virus. There is the possibility that all of these factors may be at play.

3. What is peculiar about the geographic distribution of MS?
*   The prevalence rate is < 1/100,000 in equatorial areas as compared to 6–14/100,000 in southern Europe and the southern U.S. In Canada, northern Europe, and the northern U.S., the rate is 30–80 cases/100,000.
*   Interesting statistics indicate that there is a threefold increase in prevalence and a fivefold increase in mortality in New Orleans compared to Boston.
*   MS is associated with particular localities rather than an ethnic group in any locality. Individuals migrating prior to becoming 15 years of age assume the risk for MS of the new location, while those who migrate after 15 years of age retain the risk of their original birthplace.

4. Describe the mode of onset of MS.
It is a common misconception that MS starts in young people at a time when they are in perfect health. A careful history will often reveal a picture of easy fatigue, low energy, pain that is hard to localize or characterize involving muscles and joints, as well as a loss of weight. These symptoms may have been present for weeks to months prior to the onset of any neurologic symptoms. On the other hand, the onset of neurologic symptoms may start acutely, even within minutes or hours. This latter type of onset is seen in about 40% of patients, while approximately 30% have an onset over a period of 24–48 hours. Another 20% begin to be ill with neurologic symptoms over weeks to months. The final 10% have symptoms starting over months to years. The latter group is usually over 45 years of age.

5. What are some presenting signs and symptoms?

Weakness and/or fatigue (about 50% have this onset)	Limb tingling
	Girdle-like feeling (trunk, limbs)
Optic neuritis	Gait ataxia (often with nystagmus)
Double vision	Vertigo
Vomiting	Bladder dysfunction
Charcot's triad (scanning speech, intention tremor, nystagmus)	

6. What is optic neuritis?
Optic neuritis implies an inflammatory process. However, it now includes certain vascular diseases and degenerative diseases that interfere with optic nerve function:
Infection or inflammation: Inflammation spreading from orbit, sinuses, or eye; CNS infections spreading to eye; infections from distant sites (rarely)
Vascular diseases: Temporal arteritis, periarteritis nodosum, pulseless disease, atherosclerosis
Degenerative or systemic conditions: Toxic exposures (methyl alcohol, lead poisoning), sarcoidosis, collagen disease, hyperthyroidism, diabetes mellitus, blood disorders

7. Might there be a relationship between the sensory symptoms and the cause of MS?
Sensory signs and symptoms are second in frequency, while coordination deficits are the commonest finding. There is a hypothesis that the dorsal roots and cranial sensory ganglia might be the neuronal site in which a putative MS infectious agent lies concealed, but expensive and painstaking research would be required to prove this point. In addition, numerous autopsies would be needed, searching for an unknown agent or virus.

8. What is the pathologic process in MS?
No evidence of disease is noted by gross appearance. The surface of the spinal cord feels uneven on touch. Numerous scattered lesions are observed on sectioning. These appear pink-gray

in color due to the loss of myelin. It becomes obvious that the basic lesion in MS is **demyelination** with significant **lymphocyte invasion** into the plaques that are formed. The pathogenesis, while unknown, is thought by some to be the result of an interaction of genetic, infectious, and immune mechanisms.

9. Are there any diseases that might mimic or be confused with MS?

Transient ischemic attacks	Lacunar strokes	Tumors
Sarcoidosis	Vasculitides	Lupus
Lyme disease	Cerebral vasculitis	
Meningovascular syphilis	Behçet disease	

Vascular malformations of the brainstem and spinal cord with bleeds
Spinal cord compression due to tumor or cervical spondylosis
Tropical spastic paraparesis (HTLV-1 myelitis)

10. What signs and symptoms might be seen later in the course of MS?

These could include signs and symptoms related to involvement of the optic nerves, brainstem, cerebellum, and spinal cord. Between 30–40% show evidence of spastic ataxia and deep sensory changes in the extremities due to a spinal form of the disease. A small percentage (about 5%) show exclusive cerebellar or pontocerebellar findings, while a like number show an amaurotic form.

11. What is the story concerning cognition in MS? What accounts for the euphoria sometimes mentioned?

There is a wide range of estimates of cognitive changes in the population with MS. Numbers range from 43–72 percent, with the difference being due to the patient sample and/or method used to assess cognition. As for euphoria, its occurrence is overemphasized. When it does occur, it is most likely secondary to lesions located in the white matter of the frontal lobe, or it may be due to side effects of corticosteroids. Pathologic cheerfulness is seen almost always in association with other evidence of cerebral involvement. It may be part of the syndrome of pseudobulbar palsy.

12. Pseudobulbar palsy? What is it?

The "bulb," as you may or may not know, is the old name for the **medulla oblongata**. Pseudobulbar palsy consists of an inconsistency between the loss of voluntary movements of muscles innervated by the motor nuclei of the lower pons and medulla (inability to forcefully close the eyes, elevate and retract the corners of the mouth, open and close the mouth, chew, swallow, phonate, articulate, and move the tongue) and the preservation of movement of the same muscles in yawning, coughing, throat clearing, and spasmodic laughing or crying (i.e., in reflexive pontomedullary activities). In some cases, on the slightest provocation and sometimes for no apparent reason, the patient is thrown into hilarious laughter that may last for many minutes to the point of exhaustion. Or, far more often, the opposite happens—the mere mention of the patient's family or the sight of the doctor provokes an uncontrollable spasm that resembles crying.

13. How do you diagnose MS using clinical features?

There must be multiple neurologic signs that involve at least two areas of the CNS, but with predominant white matter pathology (long tract signs). There may be one of two time patterns. One pattern may include two or more episodes of worsening, each of which lasts > 24 hours and should be at least 1 month apart. Another pattern is a slow or stepwise progression extending over at least 6 months.

14. What diagnostic procedures can be used to help diagnose MS?

MRI is the most helpful tool to investigate abnormalities, especially in the posterior fossa and spinal canal, which can be common sites of MS involvement. Its sensitivity for detecting lesions approaches 90–95%. Single lesions in the spinal parenchyma are the most confusing since they appear similar to neoplasms.

In about one-third of patients, particularly those with an acute onset or exacerbation, there may be a slight to moderate mononuclear pleocytosis (usually < 50 cells/mm³) in the **cerebrospinal fluid** (CSF). In spinal fluid, the proportion of gamma globulin (in essence, IgG) is increased (above 10–13% of the total protein) in about two-thirds of patients.

About half of patients with definite MS will show an abnormal **brainstem auditory evoked response**. Somatosensory evoked auditory and tactile evoked responses are frequently utilized to help in the diagnosis. A perceptual delay on visual stimulation is seen in a positive test. There are no totally reliable markers of the activity of the disease—including MRI, altered blood-brain barrier, immunoglobulin synthesis, and myelin basic protein in CSF.

15. How serious a problem is fatigue in the individual with MS?

Fatigue is the most common complaint of MS patients. It can vary from quite mild to totally disabling—simply dressing may utterly exhaust the patient. It is not clear what causes the fatigue, but it is thought to be multifactorial and might include the immune system as so many patients have increased fatigue before and after an exacerbation of the disease. Fatigue frequently worsens with increased ambient temperature, and this may be due to conduction block in demyelinated fibers. Spasticity and weakness will contribute to fatigue, as might depression.

16. Any suggestions for dealing with fatigue in MS?

In most patients, **amantadine** will reduce fatigue somewhat. It can be used in a dosage of 100 mg twice a day for symptomatic benefit. It there is no improvement in the feeling of fatigue after 1 month, the drug should be discontinued. Those patients sensitive to heat should maintain the ambient temperature at a comfortable level. Dressing lightly will aid heat dispersion as well.

17. How important is bladder dysfunction in MS patients? What types of problems occur?

Most MS patients develop bladder symptoms at some time in the course of their disease. Because of the nature of the problem, major social difficulties can result.

The types of problems can be classified as obstructive or irritative. **Obstructive** symptoms include hesitancy and/or an interrupted and diminished force to the stream. Fullness after apparently emptying the bladder as well as urinary leakage, which can happen without warning, may occur. The flaccid neuropathic bladder is usually obstructive in nature. An **irritated bladder** can cause urgency, increased frequency, nocturia, as well as leakage. A urinary tract infection may complicate the irritative symptoms, and this will exacerbate the already existing problems. An uninhibited neuropathic bladder will cause mainly irritative symptoms.

There can be a great deal of overlap between the two types of neuropathic bladder described and a clinical history will usually not be enough to allow a diagnosis to be made and some testing will most likely be necessary.

18. What were the prognosis and treatment described by Charcot over 100 years ago?

"The **prognosis** has hitherto been of the gloomiest. . . . It is to be hoped that, when the disease has become better known, the physician will learn how to take advantage of that spontaneous tendency to remission which has been noticed in a great number of cases." Has much really changed since Charcot spoke these words? "After what precedes, need I detain you long over the question of **treatment**? The time has not yet come when such a subject can be seriously considered." He described the use of gold chloride and zinc phosphate, which seemed to worsen the symptoms. Strychnine sometimes resulted in tremor decreasing and helped the paresis of the limbs, but it did not last long. Arsenic, belladonna, ergot of rye, and potassium bromide were described as having no real benefit. Faradism and galvanism had no impact. What will be thought of our therapies 100 years from now?

19. What is the story concerning today's therapies?

They are controversial, and the response varies widely. There are no large controlled studies on the use of immunosuppressive therapy for acute exacerbations. **Methylprednisolone** gives superior results in one study, and **ACTH** does just as well in two others. The exact mechanism of improvement is not known. **Azathioprine** has reportedly also given mixed results in clinical trials. **Cyclosporine** has been shown to result in slight benefit with decreased progression of disease, relapse rate, and relapse severity. Unfortunately, there has been a twofold increase in side effects compared to azathioprine. Hypertension and nephropathy are the most serious. The use of **plasma exchange** offers no better results than azathioprine. **Interferons** have been proposed because of their immunomodulatory and antiviral properties. In a recent multicenter trial with interferon-β1b in relapsing/remitting MS, the rate of exacerbation was reduced by one-third compared with placebo.

20. Give some tips concerning exercise for the patient with MS.

It must be individualized
Weakness must be considered
Need to know patient's goals concerning exercise
Want to improve strength and endurance
Mild weakness: progressive resistive exercise/isokinetic exercise
Ataxia: Frenkel's exercises
Spasticity: reduce tone exercises
Best to exercise in the morning
Stress functional goals
Don't exercise to point of fatigue
Avoid a warm environment
Air-conditioning may be a medical necessity
If overheated, use cool baths and ice packs
Rest if acute exacerbation after exercise
Don't "push" patient toward inappropriate goals
Patient should "listen" to his/her body

21. What in the world are Frenkel's exercises?

These exercises were originally developed in 1889 to treat patients with problems of incoordination and cerebellar ataxia due to loss of proprioception from tabes dorsalis. The exercises are designed to substitute the use of vision and hearing for the loss of proprioceptive sensation and require a high degree of mental concentration and visual control of movement. They are not appropriate for all patients with MS, but in the patient with the ability to perform them, they can be effective in reducing ataxia and regaining some control of functional movement. Concentration and repetition are the keys to success with these exercises.

Techniques are available for both the upper extremities and lower extremities, although those for the latter are the common ones used. The exercises progress from postures of greatest stability (lying, sitting) to postures of greatest challenge (standing, walking). As voluntary control improves, the exercises progress to stopping and starting on command, increasing the range, and performing the same exercises with the eyes closed.

22. What outcome can be expected with inpatient rehabilitation for the MS patient with severe involvement or a recent exacerbation?

In one study from the early 1980s, 28 patients (with 33 admissions) were evaluated on admission, at discharge, and 3 months post-discharge. On admission, 18% were ambulating independently, while at discharge 76% could do so. There were 15 patients who went from dependence to independence in their ability to climb stairs. Improvement in ADLs was not as dramatic. In general, those who stayed in the center longer were initially more dependent and made greater relative gains. It is interesting to note that the average length of stay (ALOS) was 27 days for those individuals with a single admission, while those with more than one admission had an ALOS of 32 days. In today's era of managed care, though, it will be hard to justify such lengths of stay.

23. Tell me more about the use of interferons in the treatment of MS.

Interferon (IFN)-beta, administered intrathecally or systemically, significantly reduces MS exacerbations. The IFN-beta MS Study Group demonstrated a significant reduction in exacerbation rate following frequent subcutaneous injections of relatively high doses of IFN-beta over a 2-year period. The systemic study demonstrated decreased CNS lesion progression on serial MRIs of treated patients, the first clear evidence that IFN treatment can alter the basic pathologic course of the disease. These therapeutic trials had to be conducted in humans because of the species specificity of the IFNs.

24. What are some of the *sources* of psychosocial problems seen in the patient with MS?
- Difficulty in making the diagnosis with no pathognomonic test
- Major, unpredictable disruptions due to exacerbations
- Frequently given the wrong diagnosis, at least early in the course
- The patient may be told, "nothing can be done"
- A disease that is not curable
- Likelihood of financial problems, emotional depletion, interpersonal difficulties with a chronic illness
- Problems associated with aging and chronic illness

25. Describe the cognitive dysfunction seen in patients with MS.

In general, MS patients exhibit difficulty with recent memory, sustained attention, verbal fluency, conceptual reasoning, and visuospatial perception. Less frequently they show impaired language skills and difficulty with immediate and remote memory. There appears to be no correlation between cognitive impairment and duration of disease, depression, the course of the disease, or usage of medication. There is a weak correlation with physical disability.

26. How important a problem is depression in patients with MS?

Depression occurs in 27–54% of MS patients, and often at a moderately severe level. Patients are frequently angry, irritable, worried, and discouraged. As a general rule, they are not self-critical, withdrawn, or disinterested. Suicide does not appear to be a major problem. One reason for looking for depression in patients with MS is that it has a significant adverse effect on the functioning of the patient both at work and on the individual's family and social lives. It is felt that few patients with depression and MS receive adequate treatment.

BIBLIOGRAPHY

1. Adams RD, Victor M: Principles of Neurology, 5th ed. New York, McGraw-Hill, 1993, ch. 36.
2. Beatty WW, Goodkin DE: Screening for cognitive impairment in multiple sclerosis. Arch Neurol 47:297–301, 1990.
3. DeLisa J (ed): Rehabilitation Medicine: Principles and Practice. Philadelphia, J.B. Lippincott, 1993.
4. Greenspun B, Stineman M, Agri R: Multiple sclerosis and rehabilitation outcome. Arch Phys Med Rehabil 68:434–437, 1987.
5. Lee KH, Hashimoto MD, Hooge JP, et al: Magnetic resonance imaging of the head in the diagnosis of multiple sclerosis. Neurology 41:657–660, 1991.
6. Lublin FD, Whitaker JN, Eidelman BH, et al: Management of patients receiving interferon beta-1b for multiple sclerosis. Neurology 46:12–18, 1996.
7. Minden SL, Schiffer RB: Affective disorders in multiple sclerosis. Arch Neurol 47:98–104, 1990.
8. Sanders VJ, Waddell AE, Felisan SL, et al: Herpes simplex virus in postmortem multiple sclerosis brain tissue. Arch neurol 53:125–133, 1996.
9. Schapiro RT: Symptom management in multiple sclerosis. Ann Neurol 36(suppl):S123–S129, 1994.
10. Sullivan SB, Schmitz TJ: Multiple Sclerosis in Physical Rehabilitation, 3rd ed. Philadelphia, F.A. Davis, 1994.

43. TRAUMATIC BRAIN INJURY

Robert L. Harmon, M.D., M.S., and Lawrence J. Horn, M.D., M.R.M.

1. Why shouldn't I skip this chapter and simply read about stroke rehabilitation?

While stroke and traumatic brain injury (TBI) both may involve brain lesions due to is-chemia or hemorrhage, patients with TBI tend to have more diffuse impairments in brain function. These patients also classically tend to have more cognitive, personality, and behavioral impairments than persons following stroke. There is also a much larger proportion of younger patients with TBI than stroke. Understanding the issues surrounding TBI and its rehabilitation in addition can add to one's understanding about stroke and its rehabilitation, as well as other forms of brain injury such as encephalitis.

2. What are the common causes of TBI?

Over half of the TBI events that occur in the United States are related to **traffic accidents**. **Falls** are the next most common cause, most often occurring in those under 15 and over 70 years of age. **Assaults** and **failed suicide attempts** may also be significant causes in certain regions.

3. How does drug and alcohol use, use of motorcycle helmets, and use of seat belts impact the incidence of TBI?

Alcohol use is associated with the occurrence of motor vehicle accidents and may also contribute to the occurrence of intracranial hemorrhage following head trauma. Other **drugs**, both legal and illegal, can impair cognition or reaction time and may also increase the risk of a motor vehicle accident. Illicit drug use in some regions may also be associated with an increased risk of head injury from assaults.

The use of **seat belts** and **motorcycle helmets** has been shown to significantly decrease the number of head injuries for wearers. The presence of **air bags** in a vehicle may also be found to significantly decrease traumatic brain injury as more information becomes available. The occurrence of TBI, therefore, can be modified.

4. How often is TBI associated with spinal cord injury (SCI)?

It is difficult to know exactly how many patients have a combined TBI and SCI, as many relatively mild brain injuries go undetected. Because motor vehicle accidents cause both types of injury, these lesions may occur together in as many as 25–50% of cases. Cognitive deficits, or motor or sensory system abnormalities not explained by a single spinal cord lesion, in a patient with SCI should trigger an evaluation for a possible associated brain injury.

5. How often is TBI associated with extremity fractures?

For the reason given in question 4, this is difficult to determine. Also approximately 10–11% of patients admitted to a rehabilitation service following TBI have previously unrecognized skeletal trauma, including of the spine. This point is important because unrecognized fractures or joint dislocations may interfere with the functional restoration of these patients. Skeletal trauma may be associated with peripheral nerve injuries. Long bone fractures also may be associated with an increased risk of heterotopic ossification.

6. What are the principal types of primary injuries resulting from TBI?

Primary injuries to the brain occur as a direct result of the forces involved in the traumatic event upon the brain and are not preventable except by preventing the traumatic event itself. These primary injuries include:

Contusions and lacerations of the brain surface (typically occurring on the frontal and temporal lobes inferiorly where the brain contacts the base of the skull)

Diffuse axonal injury (related to shearing injury disrupting nerve axons in the brain white matter)

Diffuse vascular injury resulting in multiple petechial hemorrhages within the brain

Contusion or shearing of the cranial nerves (most commonly the olfactory nerve)

Tearing of the pituitary stalk.

7. What are secondary types of injury arising from brain trauma?

Secondary damage to the brain results from processes produced by the injuring event but tends to be delayed in its presentation, suggesting that it may be preventable (at least in theory). The principal types of secondary injuries include:

Intracranial hemorrhage (which may be extradural, subdural, subarachnoid, or intracerebral)

Brain swelling related to increased cerebral blood volume and/or cerebral edema

Increased intracranial pressure

Brain damage associated with hypoxia

Intracranial infection (particularly with penetrating injuries)

Hydrocephalus

The cascade of neurochemical events after brain injury that lead to neuronal death is also considered secondary injury.

8. Define diaschisis.

The term refers to one of several general theories that pertain to recovery of function following brain injury. Diaschisis includes the concept that damage to one region of the brain can produce altered function in regions adjacent to or distant from the site of damage as long as there is a connection between the two sites. Classically, this would appear as functional depression in intact areas of the brain that received inputs from a damaged area. The resolution of behavioral deficits would be expected to occur in conjunction with a return of activity in functionally depressed areas.

There are certainly other theories regarding the recovery of function, such as **vicariation** (where functions are taken over by brain areas not originally handling that function), **redundancy** (where recovery of function is based on the activity of uninjured brain regions that normally would contribute to that function), and **behavioral substitution** (where new strategies are learned to compensate for the behavioral deficit). Additionally, functional recovery would be dependent on the reversal of ischemia and edema in regions surrounding the areas of neuronal loss, changes in neurotransmitter levels and receptor number, and neuronal sprouting. Because areas involved by diaschisis are still intact, there have been attempts to modulate the rate of recovery from this process experimentally and in the clinical setting.

9. What happens neurochemically following brain injury?

Acutely after TBI, there is a release of large amounts of neurotransmitters, particularly excitatory neurotransmitters such as glutamate. These neurotransmitters bind to receptors in neuronal cell membranes, activating postsynaptic ion channels. Excess amounts of ionized calcium, in particular, are allowed to enter the cell this way, as well as through voltage-activated channels in the cell membrane, activating phospholipases within the cell. This results in increased arachidonic acid metabolism and the production of free radicals that may damage or destroy the neuronal membrane if levels exceed what cellular enzymes can remove. These processes may occur over the course of minutes to hours following brain injury. Postacute neurochemical changes relate to alterations in the level and turnover of various neurotransmitters and their receptors. These postacute changes may be responsible for diaschisis-like effects.

10. Can we intervene in this process to minimize the adverse effects?

In the acute brain injury period, experimental efforts have focused on using pharmacologic agents to **block neuronal calcium channels**, including receptor-activated channels (particularly the N-methyl-D-aspartate receptor) and voltage-activated channels. Because most calcium flow into neurons occurs within 30 minutes after injury, it is as yet unclear how clinically useful these agents might be. Other research has focused on using agents that inhibit the formation or increase the clearance of **free radicals**. Again, it is unclear how useful these agents might be, although some clinical trials are under way. In the postacute period, some limited clinical evidence suggests that various **dopamine agonists** may beneficially affect the rate of recovery of patients in low functioning states following TBI. While other medications have also been associated in case reports and small studies with improved behavioral recovery in the postacute period, in general, the clinical information available is quite limited with no large controlled trials of these medications.

11. What are the best prognostic indicators for patients following TBI?

Prognostic indicators related to the injury itself include the duration of **coma** (the shorter the better, but > 4 weeks is extremely bad), the duration of **post-traumatic amnesia** (again, the shorter the better, but > 11 weeks is inconsistent with independent living), and the motor response on the **Glasgow Coma Scale** (with active posturing, decorticate/decerebrate or worse represents a fairly clear demarcation prognostically from higher levels of motor function). Other clinical findings, including evidence for brainstem involvement such as dysconjugate gaze or altered pupillary responses, can add power to prognostication. Perhaps the most useful information that can be gleaned is the actual early recovery course that a patient demonstrates. Although site of lesion is not associated directly or very powerfully with outcome, knowing that the language areas, for example, have been damaged or that the patient has hemianopsia does have an impact on predicting ultimate outcome. Other useful prognostic indicators include a patient's age, with people under 20 years of age generally doing much better than those over 60 if they have sustained the same kind of injury. Between the third and sixth decades, there is not a great deal of variability decade by decade in terms of outcome. The exception to this rule of thumb is for very young children (under 2 years of age). Another variable unrelated to the injury itself is the patient's premorbid psychosocial status; an individual who has had considerable psychological impairment or social disruption can be anticipated to have a relatively poorer outcome from a brain injury than someone without these problems. This is particularly true in the case of significant substance abuse.

12. Which assessment scales are commonly used to measure function and outcome for TBI patients?

The most frequently used assessment scales include the Glasgow Outcome Scale and the Disability Rating Scale.

The **Glasgow Outcome Scale** is divided into 5 categories: dead, persistent vegetative state, severe disability, moderate disability, and good outcome. It has been criticized as being relatively insensitive, particularly given the span of the "severe disability" category from near-vegetative to complete independence with the exception of needing some assistance within a 24-hour period by a caregiver.

The **Disability Rating Scale** includes a reversed Glasgow Coma Scale and additional measurements of basic functional skills, employability, and total level of dependence. This scale has been correlated with evoked potential studies and has been demonstrated to be scientifically valid. It has also been proven to be far more sensitive than the Glasgow Outcome Scale.

The **Rancho Los Amigos Scale**, a descriptive scale with 8 categories, has been proved to be *not* scientifically valid. Its utility is essentially to expedite communication. Additional scales have been used to measure functional status, such as the **Functional Independence Measure** and **Functional Assessment Measure**, the latter being more specific for TBI injury as opposed to general disability. There are also scales that are used to assess patients in a vegetative state, such as the **Coma Near-Coma Scale** or the **Western Neuro Sensory Stimulation Profile**.

13. How should central dysautonomia, with its associated hypertension, tachycardia, and temperature elevation, be managed?

Central dysautonomia may present with any single symptom or sign alone or as a constellation which may also include periodic perspiration over the face and shoulders. The cardiovascular problems may involve a generalized increase in circulating catecholamines or may occur without this. In general, the hypertension and tachycardia have been proved to be effectively treated by β-blockers, although clonidine, calcium channel blockers, and even dopamine agonists have all been anecdotally reported to be effective. Central hyperthermia is typically managed with dopamine agonists. Again, there are anecdotal reports of response to β-blockers or clonidine. The utility of modalities for hyperthermia should not be underestimated; if necessary, iced saline lavage through a nasogastric tube can rapidly decrease the core temperature. The episodic perspiration may respond to β-blockers, but often transdermal scopolamine must be used. When the entire constellation presents as episodic severe dysregulation, it has been called **diencephalic fits**. In addition to the types of medications mentioned above, carbamazepine or valproic acid at times may be effective.

14. Are endocrine problems commonly associated with TBI?

Endocrine problems may accompany TBI and include central dysautonomia, disorders of temperature regulation, feeding/eating disorders (hyper/hypophagia), and disorders of the hypothalamic pituitary axis (including extrahypothalamic regulation). For hyperphagia, selective serotonin reuptake inhibitors may be helpful; for hypophagia, the use of mild psychostimulants may be effective. For disorders of the hypothalamic pituitary axis, treatment typically involves replacement of end-organ hormones (such as thyroid hormone, steroids, etc.). Correcting the actual hormone deficiency may be a bit complex, especially when dealing with fertility-related issues. Posterior pituitary problems include oversecretion or, less commonly, undersecretion of antidiuretic hormone and are often transient.

15. How do the occurrence and management of heterotopic ossification (HO) in TBI compare to that in SCI?

Admittedly, as in SCI, the exact etiology of HO is unknown. One main difference, however, is in the joint sites involved. HO involves the upper extremity and lower extremity equally following TBI, whereas the hip and knee are primarily affected following SCI. The incidence of HO following TBI ranges from 11–76%. It most commonly involves the shoulder, elbow, and hip, occurring infrequently at the thigh and knee. Patients at highest risk are those in coma for > 2 weeks, with spasticity, and with long-bone fractures.

While passive range of motion is advocated, as in SCI, to decrease the risk of HO, controversy exists as to whether these exercises may actually contribute to the ectopic bone formation. One small study of patients with TBI suggested that etidronate disodium may significantly decrease the risk of HO if given early after injury. The dose used was 20 mg/kg for 3 months, followed by 10 mg/kg for an additional 3 months, a longer period of treatment than has been suggested following SCI.

16. How does the management of spasticity associated with TBI compare to that in SCI?

Historically, there has not been much difference. The use of physical agents, splinting, neurolytic and motor point blocks, and surgical intervention usually follows the same line of decision-making regarding management in both patient populations. **Dantrolene sodium** has been considered the oral agent of choice in managing spasticity associated with various forms of brain injury; **baclofen** and **diazepam** tend not to be advocated as much as for spasticity of spinal origin because they have side effects that may include sedation and impairment of cognitive function. Recently, **clonidine**, as for spinal spasticity, has been shown to be effective in the treatment of spasticity from TBI. The use of clonidine in this patient population is complicated somewhat by the observation that baclofen reversed the beneficial effects of clonidine's action on spasticity in a stroke patient; this was not noted, however, when dantrolene sodium was added to clonidine treatment in a patient with TBI. More work in this area is required before any general recommendations can be made because these observations were limited to isolated cases.

17. Do TBI patients require anticonvulsants?

While some patients who have had brain injuries do require anticonvulsants, the general consensus currently is that anticonvulsant prophylaxis is overused. Approximately 5% of all head

injury patients develop seizures. This number may be higher, approaching 20%, in the more severely injured. Early seizures occur within the first week after brain injury, and early use of anticonvulsants suppresses the development of a seizure focus, but not beyond the first week.
While there is no cogent scientific data supporting this position, it would appear that treatment
prophylaxis is warranted when early seizures are present. Another case to treat prophylactically
and early is in missile or open injuries, which have an association with seizures of approximately 40%.

18. Which anticonvulsant medications are most appropriate for this patient population?

The choice of anticonvulsant agent continues to be controversial. **Phenytoin** and **phenobarbital** have an advantage in that they can be given parenterally. However, both have a considerable number of side effects. Although not entirely proven, it is recommended to convert
patients to **carbamazepine** or **valproic acid**, as these medications may be better tolerated in the
TBI population.

**19. What are some common intracranial complications that arise relatively late in the
course following TBI?**

Intracranial sequelae that occur in the weeks or months following TBI, sometimes overlapping with secondary injuries, may slow the functional recovery of a patient or actually lead to a
reversal of previous gains. One significant complication is **post-traumatic hydrocephalus**,
which should be differentiated from ventricular dilitation due to encephalomalacia or loss of
brain tissue associated with the brain trauma itself. **Cerebrospinal fluid fistulas** may also occur
as a consequence of head trauma, reaching an incidence as high as 5–11% in those patients with
basilar skull fractures. **Post-traumatic movement disorders**, such as tremor and parkinsonism,
may be significant sequelae of injury, impairing behavioral recovery. While **post-traumatic
seizures** have already been discussed, it is important to remember that post-traumatic epilepsy
may first occur relatively late (even several years) following injury.

20. What are some peripheral nervous system injuries commonly associated with TBI?

Plexopathies, particularly involving the upper extremity, may occur as a result of traction,
compression, or lacerations arising from the traumatic event itself. These may overlap **radiculopathies** resulting from nerve root avulsions or nerve root compression associated with spine
fractures. **Focal neuropathies** may occur as a result of heterotopic ossification (particularly involving the ulnar nerve at the elbow), spasticity producing extremity contractures (particularly
affecting the median nerve at the wrist and ulnar nerve at the elbow), and fractures and soft tissue
injury associated with the traumatic event. The **polyneuropathy** associated with prolonged alcohol use may be seen as well in that subgroup of patients who ultimately sustain brain injury.

21. What behavioral and personality changes are commonly seen following TBI?

Because the brain is the organ of consciousness and personality, virtually any change in behavior or intellectual function can be observed following injury. The most common problems
cognitively are deficits in **attention** (inability to concentrate, increased distractibility, or even
perseveration) and **memory**. As with stroke, specific cognitive disorders may emerge that include (but are not limited to) aphasias, agnosias, apraxias, temporal sequencing problems,
visual-perceptual and spatial dysfunctions, prosodic deficits, and, with frontal lesions, disorders
of judgment, planning, and other "metacognitive" skills.

Behaviorally, the most common problems have to do with **impulse control** or disinhibition
of the dampening system for an **emotional response** to a stimulus. This may present as anger and
violent behavior or as emotional lability, including crying or even laughing, which is out of proportion to a stimulus. Another problem may be "**agitation**," which in the early stages of recovery
is often related to confusion and post-traumatic amnesia; it is not necessarily related to any long-
term behavioral changes. More chronic problems include social impropriety, loss of pragmatic
skills, low frustration tolerance, and, less commonly, actual violence and aggression.

22. Discuss the recommended evaluation of behavioral and cognitive changes following TBI.

Most investigations relate to the environment and only require common sense. Does the patient have a normal sleep wake cycle? Is the patient in pain? Is the environment disorienting instead of orienting (e.g., intensive care unit settings)? Does the environment reinforce inappropriate behaviors? An organized approach should be followed to rule out correctable biologic etiologies for cognitive and behavioral problems. The patient should be evaluated for possible seizures, particularly partial complex seizures, and intracranial space-occupying lesions, such as hydrocephalus or subdural hematoma/hygroma. An endocrine evaluation, particularly of thyroid function, is important, as is ensuring electrolyte balance. All medications should be reviewed, including those prescribed and those used for recreational pursuits; pharmacologic agents are a common correctable etiology for cognitive or behavioral deficits. A search for toxins may also be important.

23. Describe some behaviorally and environmentally based strategies for managing TBI patients with disruptive or aggressive behavior.

It is important to remember that behaviors are defined by the context in which they occur. In some situations, it is tempting to consider sedation for those around the patient rather than treating the patient's "agitated" behavior. The first step in the approach to management should be to define the undesired behavior in a way in which all observers can agree. The behavior should then be observed in regard to its frequency of occurrence and associated environmental factors serving as its triggers. The environment should then be modified to remove triggers, if possible, and the behavior then monitored to see if its occurrence diminishes. Principles of operant conditioning may also be utilized to help extinguish the undesired behavior.

24. Which pharmacologic interventions are useful for TBI patients with disruptive or aggressive behavior?

A recent survey has suggested that even among practitioners experienced in the management of TBI patients, there is much discrepancy in the use of pharmacologic management. **Carbamazepine** and **amitriptyline** were some of the most commonly used medications. **Neuroleptics** were less commonly used by persons experienced in the management of these patients because of concerns related to cognitive impairment and potential slowing of behavioral recovery.

25. Getting back to the cognitive changes seen following TBI, does "cognitive remediation" therapy or pharmacotherapy really help improve these deficits?

Pharmacotherapy seems to have its clearest usefulness for problems of basic arousal and attention. Dopamine agonists and stimulating antidepressants improve attentional dysfunction, particularly distractibility and difficulty focusing, in higher level patients. There has been an indication that bromocriptine can be effective for motor aphasias and neglect in some patients. Evidence also suggests that cholinergic agonists, such as oral physostigmine, may specifically improve memory function in some patients. More work needs to be done in this area, however.

In general, **cognitive remediation** programs have not been shown to intrinsically improve the intellectual function of a patient for all situations. Their principal role is in teaching adaptive strategies and compensatory techniques. From this perspective, they are most effective when they are task-specific and site-specific, because one of the biggest problems people with brain injuries may have is generalizing performance from one site or one task to another. Indeed, there is increasing evidence to support "bringing therapy to the patient" (instead of the patient to a hospital or outpatient area), using job coaches or independent living counselor/therapists either at the job site or in the community to teach adaptive strategies to patients.

26. What evaluation should be done to rule out correctable causes for coma or vegetative state?

As with cognitive and behavioral changes, a search for possible seizures, space-occupying brain lesions, endocrine and electrolyte abnormalities, toxins, and potentially contributory pharmacologic agents is warranted.

27. What is the role of a "coma stimulation" program and of pharmacotherapy in the management of patients in low-functioning states following TBI?

An appropriate "coma stimulation" program would first of all need a different name—no one is trying to stimulate coma. At present, there is absolutely no cogent scientific evidence that any kind of therapy-based program will augment the cessation of coma or the vegetative state. However, an organized approach to a low-functioning patient permits a quantitative assessment of responses to stimuli and early recognition of changes or improvements in response to intervention or through spontaneous recovery.

There is a clear indication for preventative therapeutic interventions, particularly early on. These include basic rehabilitation strategies to manage bowel and bladder function, maintain appropriate nutrition, maintain skin integrity, control spasticity, and prevent contracture formation. The rationale is that if the patient comes out of the vegetative state or coma, this kind of "tertiary" prevention will permit more rapid participation in an active rehab program and a shorter total program length of stay. There is also some evidence that, for individuals who are "destined" to come out of a transient vegetative or akinetic mute state, or coma, this process may be hastened through the use of pharmacotherapy, particularly dopamine agonists such as combined levodopa/carbidopa, amantadine, or bromocriptine.

28. What is the prognosis for patients in low-functioning states following TBI?

In general, patients who are in a vegetative state or prolonged coma will remain significantly impaired upon "awakening." Prognosis for arousal and consciousness is largely dependent on the duration of time a person remains in a low-functioning state but also may be related to age. In general, it appears that children can sustain a more severe injury and cease being vegetative than can an older person, particularly those over 50 or 60 years of age. Other prognostic indicators relate to the pervasiveness of injury based on the Glasgow Coma Scale and include persistent posturing and ocular findings.

The time course of recovery suggests that most individuals with prolonged unconsciousness or post-traumatic unawareness will become conscious and cognizant within the first 3 months. There is a small number of low-functioning patients who then show improvement between 3–6 months and then a virtual trickle out to about 1 year post-injury. If a patient achieves consciousness after 1 year in a vegetative state, it is essentially a reportable case. Of those patients in a vegetative state at 1–3 months following injury, approximately 50–60% will die within the first year.

29. Which symptoms are commonly experienced by patients with mild TBI?

The symptoms largely parallel those of patients with more severe TBI. Physically, however, the most common complaint (and one fairly unique to the more mildly injured patient) is **headache**. **Vestibular** or **disequilibrium complaints** are also very common, as is a sense of **fatigue** and an assortment of complaints related to **weakness, numbness**, and **"tingling."** There may also be deficits with regard to **hearing**, complaints of blurred or "changed" **vision**, and dysfunction in **smell** and **taste**. With regard to cognitive function, the principal complaints relate to **attentional** and **memory problems**, although some of the other cognitive disorders described previously may also supervene. With regard to behavior, **irritability** and **disordered sleep** are the most common complaints, but mild TBI patients may also manifest aggression and other personality changes.

30. Explain the management strategies available to help patients following mild TBI.

Management of patients with mild TBI, as with other brain injuries, requires a coordinated team approach. The first management issue pertains to identification and possible verification of the organicity of the presenting signs and symptoms. While MRI and other imaging studies should be undertaken, much of this documentation occurs through a neuropsychologic assessment. It is important to distinguish individuals who have true organic changes from those with emotional or psychiatric problems and from those who have a combination of both. Of note, some of the physical and secondarily cognitive complaints may be related to injuries of the cranial nerves and craniocervical neurovascular systems. Also, a fair number of complaints can be attributed to musculoskeletal injury of the head and neck; this is particularly true in the case of post-traumatic headache, which nearly always has a musculoskeletal component. The incidence of overt malingering, while possible, is not felt to be very high. After a clear idea of a patient's cognitive, emotional, and intellectual state is established, along with some clarification as to organicity, evaluation and intervention should target those deficits that are brain injury-related. This may include the use of compensatory strategies and pharmacotherapy as already discussed. There is also a strong role for education and counseling of the patient and family members.

31. Given the wide range of cognitive and functional impairments associated with TBI, how does one decide what level of therapy intensity or what type of program is appropriate for a given patient?

Interventions by various therapeutic disciplines, including physical and occupational therapy, speech and language pathology, psychology, social work, therapeutic recreation, vocational counseling, and nursing, may be provided in a variety of settings depending on a patient's medical requirements, the patient's need for and potential benefit from specific therapeutic interventions (particularly those that require equipment that cannot be transported out of a facility), a patient's activity tolerance, and the unique skills of the health care providers involved. Often, a continuum of services is felt to be optimal to manage the evolving issues of a brain-injured patient throughout recovery.

As discussed under "coma stimulation" programs, the acute care hospital therapies focus on maintaining the body in readiness while waiting for neurologic recovery. Therapies may progress to include mobility training, self-care activities, and programs to facilitate communicative and cognitive functioning. Depending on a patient's needs, additional services may be provided in an extended-care facility with therapies, "subacute" rehab facility, intensive inpatient rehab program, as outpatient therapies either in a standard format or a more specialized community reentry program, or as home-based therapies (if services do not require extensive equipment). Socioeconomic and insurance coverage restrictions play a significant role in determining what options can be pursued.

32. How many patients with TBI subsequently return to work?

Reports vary widely, ranging from 12–100%. It is safe to say that most patients with TBI can return to work because about 80% of TBIs are of the mild type. However, for people who have sustained more moderate to severe brain injuries, the prospect of returning to work is considerably less optimistic. For severe injuries, the estimate is < 20%, perhaps even closer to 10%.

33. How much impact does TBI as a disorder really have on society?

A lot. It has been estimated that about 200 TBIs occur per 100,000 population annually in the U.S. (about 40 times the incidence of traumatic SCI), although study results vary depending on the methods used. Also, about 17–30 deaths occur annually due to brain injury per 100,000 population. The associated economic impact is more difficult to determine; a patient with severe brain injury may require $4.5 million in lifetime medical and care costs, excluding lost earnings and indirect costs to the patient or family. The costs, however, are not only economic but societal in terms of neurologic residua impacting a patient's ability to cope with life changes, have desired interpersonal relationships, and achieve a level of vocational performance that might have been anticipated prior to injury. It is worth mentioning again that TBI is a potentially preventable disorder. Ongoing efforts to minimize its occurrence should be encouraged and applauded.

ACKNOWLEDGMENT

The authors thank Pamela Harmon for her kind assistance in the preparation of this manuscript.

BIBLIOGRAPHY

1. Cooper PR (ed): Head Injury, 3rd ed. Baltimore, Williams & Wilkins, 1993.
2. Feeney DM: Pharmacologic modulation of recovery after brain injury: A reconsideration of diaschisis. J Neurol Rehabil 5:113–128, 1991.

3. Glenn MB: Anticonvulsants reconsidered. J Head Trauma Rehabil 6(3):85–88, 1991.
4. Hall KM, Hamilton BB, Gordon WA, Zasler ND: Characteristics and comparisons of functional assessment indices: Disability rating scale, functional independence measure, and functional assessment measure. J Head Trauma Rehabil 8(2):60–74, 1993.
5. Horn LJ, Cope DN (eds): Traumatic Brain Injury. Phys Med Rehabil State Art Rev 3:1–160, 1989.
6. Horn LJ, Glenn MB: Pharmacologic interventions in neuroendocrine disorders following traumatic brain injury: Pts1 and 2. J Head Trauma Rehabil 3(2):87–90, 1988 and 3(3):86–90, 1988.
7. Horn LJ, Zasler ND (eds): Medical Rehabilitation of Traumatic Brain Injury. Philadelphia, Hanley & Belfus, 1996.
8. Rosenthal M, Griffith ER, Bond MR, Miller JD (eds): Rehabilitation of the Adult and Child with Traumatic Brain Injury, 2nd ed. Philadelphia, F.A. Davis, 1990.
9. Stone LR (ed): Neurologic and Orthopaedic Sequelae of Traumatic Brain Injury. Phys Med Rehabil State Art Rev 7:441–670, 1993.
10. Whyte J: Neurologic disorders of attention and arousal: Assessment and treatment. Arch Phys Med Rehabil 73:1094–1103, 1992.

44. SPINAL CORD INJURIES

Steven Stiens, M.D., Barry Goldstein, M.D., Ph.D., Margaret Hammond, M.D., and James Little, M.D., Ph.D.

1. What is SCIWORA?

Spinal cord injury without radiologic abnormality. This condition is commonly seen in young children and older adults. Mechanisms of injury in children include traction in breech delivery, violent hyperextension, or flexion. Predisposing factors in children include their large head-to-neck size ratio, elasticity of the fibrocartilaginous spine, and the horizontal orientation of the planes of the cervical facet joints.

The typical presentation of SCIWORA in the elderly is an acute central cord syndrome after a fall forward and a blow on the head. The ligamentum flavum may bulge forward into the central canal and narrow the sagittal diameter as much as 50%.

Essential history in a person with head trauma or neck pain includes identifying any parathesias or other neurologic symptoms. Flexion and extension films should be done cautiously only after static neck films have been cleared by a radiologist and only if no neurologic symptoms or severe pains are present. Empiric use of a 24-hour cervical collar with repeat films at resolution of cervical spasm is warranted. Delayed onset of paralysis may occur due to vascular mechanisms or edema accumulation at the injury site, although this is uncommon.

2. What are the key muscles tested to define the SCI level clinically?

The American Spinal Cord Injury Association (ASIA) has developed guidelines that quantify impairment through objective recording of sensory and motor findings. Due to the multiple segmental innervation of muscles, antigravity ($\frac{3}{5}$) strength is considered enough to define a level if all muscles above have $\frac{4}{5}$ or greater strength. A patient is classified as **motor incomplete** if there is palpable contraction of the external anal sphincter on digital examination. The index muscles that define each motor level are:

C4—diaphragm
C5—biceps, brachialis
C6—extensor carpi radialis
 (longus and brevis)
C7—triceps brachii
C8—flexor digitorum profundus
 to middle finger

T1—abductor digiti minimi
L2—iliopsoas
L3—quadriceps
L4—tibialis anterior
L5—extensor hallucis longus
S1—gastrocnemius, soleus
S2—anal sphincter

3. How is sensory level defined and documented with bedside examination of persons with SCI?

It is most effective to work from areas of decreased or absent sensation toward areas of normal sensation. A **pinprick stimulus** (clean, unused safety pin) is presented lightly to the skin starting at S1 (lateral aspect of the 5th toe), then advanced by dermatome until normal perception is documented. Results are recorded as 0 = absent, 1 = present but abnormal, 2 = normal perception (as compared with areas above the lesion). The same process is repeated for **light touch** (brush or cotton). The **zone of partial preservation** is the area of partial sensation that separates areas without sensation from those with normal sensation. A patient is described as **sensory incomplete** if any anal canal sensation is present.

4. Why is sensation most likely to be spared in the perianal area?

Sacral sparing is due to spinal cord somatotopic organization. Sensory and motor fibers are laminated within the tracts of the spinal cord such that fibers that serve caudal regions are located laterally and closer to the surface. Contusions and spinal cord ischemia produce relatively more damage to centrally located spinal neurons and axons than those peripherally located within the spinal cord.

5. What are the most important long tracts in the spinal cord?

Long Tracts in the Spinal Cord

TRACT	LOCATION	FUNCTION
Gracile	Medial dorsal column	Proprioception from the leg
Cuneate	Lateral dorsal column	Proprioception from the arm
Spinocerebellar	Superficial lateral column	Muscular position and tone
Pyramidal	Deep lateral column	Upper motor neuron
Lateral spinothalamic	Ventrolateral column	Pain and thermal sensation

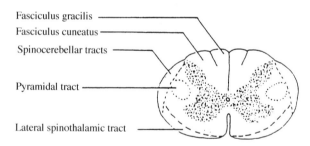

Fasciculus gracilis
Fasciculus cuneatus
Spinocerebellar tracts
Pyramidal tract
Lateral spinothalamic tract

(From Joynt R: Clinical Neurology. Philadelphia, J.B. Lippincott, 1992, with permission.)

6. Where in the cord is each of the major long tracts located?

The somatotopic organization of the major long tracts of the spinal cord. The dorsal columns have lower-extremity fibers (sacral and lumbar) lying medially, while the pyramidal and spinothalamic tracts have lower-extremity fibers lying laterally.

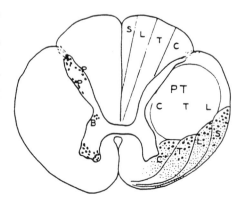

(C = cervical, T = thoracic, L = lumbar, S = sacral, PT = pyramidal tract.) (From Joynt R: Clinical Neurology. Philadelphia, J.B. Lippincott, 1992; with permission.)

7. What is the artery of Adamkiewicz?

The artery of Adamkiewicz is a major radicular branch that arises from the aorta and enters the cord between T10 and L3. Though radicular arteries supply each root, typically only this one large artery actually supplies the low thoracic and lumbar spinal cord via the **anterior spinal artery**. The anterior spinal artery supplies the anterior two-thirds of the spinal cord. It supplies the lumbar and lower thoracic segments, anastomosing with the anterior spinal artery in the lower thoracic region, which is thus the watershed area of the cord. The diagram shows the blood supply of the spinal cord. The **lumbar radicular artery** is commonly called the artery of Adamkiewicz. (From Joynt R: Clinical Neurology. Philadelphia, J.B. Lippincott, 1992, with permission.)

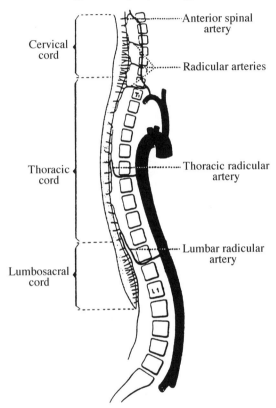

8. What is the arterial supply of the posterior third of the cord?

Paired dorsolateral **posterior spinal arteries** extend the length of the cord and supply the posterior third of the cord through circumflex and penetrating vessels. They arise from the vertebral or posterior inferior cerebellar arteries.

9. What is the difference between quadriplegia and tetraplegia?

It is a matter of medical etymology. *Quadra* is a Latin root meaning four. *Tetra* (four) and *plegia* (*plege*, meaning stroke or paralysis) are Greek roots. The compound word *tetraplegia* is more correct because it does not mix Greek and Latin roots.

10. Name the spinal cord injury syndromes. What are their lesions, clinical findings, and common causes?

Anterior cord syndrome. The clinical syndrome includes hyperreflexia, atrophy, variable motor loss, with preservation of position sensation but impaired pin prick (hypalgesia) and temperature sensation. Common causes for these findings are abdominal aortic aneurysm and aortic clamping for surgery which compromise segmental spinal cord circulation and thoracolumbar burst fracture.

Central cord syndrome. The clinical constellation includes weakness greater in the arms than legs, lower-extremity hyperreflexia, upper-extremity mixed upper motor neuron and lower motor neuron weakness, and preserved sacral sensation with the potential for preservation of bowel and bladder control. Common causes are spinal stenosis with extension injury, expanding intramedullary hematoma mass, or syrinx.

Brown-Sequard syndrome. This syndrome presents with hemi- or monoplegia or paresis with contralateral pain and temperature deficit. There is a good prognosis for motor recovery progressing from the proximal extensors to distal flexors, although spasticity may compromise total function. Causes include knife wounds to the back and asymmetrically oriented tumors.

Posterior cord syndrome. This uncommon presentation manifests with bilateral deficits in proprioception. The potential causes are vitamin B12 deficiency (subacute combined degeneration) and syphilis (tabes dorsalis).

11. Compare the Frankel classification and the ASIA Impairment Scale.

The **Frankel classification** was an attempt to separate SCI patients into various functional groups as follows:

Frankel A: motor and sensory function complete without any movement or sensation below the lesion

Frankel B: motor complete with some sensory sparing

Frankel C: motor and sensory incomplete without functional motor recovery

Frankel D: functionally useful movement below the lesion

Frankel E: motor and sensory recovery to normal function but residual clinical evidence of SCI may still be present

The **ASIA Impairment Scale** further refined distinctions between categories by specifying sensory dermatomes and muscle grades as follows:

ASIA A: complete (no motor or sensory S4 or S5 function)

ASIA B: incomplete sensory but no motor function preserved through S4–5

ASIA C: motor and sensory incomplete with the strength of most muscles below the lesion at grade 3 or less

ASIA D: motor and sensory incomplete (motor functional) with most muscles $\frac{3}{5}$ or greater in strength

ASIA E: normal motor and sensory function

12. What is the highest complete SCI level that is consistent with independent living without the aid of an attendant?

C6 complete tetraplegia. An occasional exceptionally motivated individual with C6 tetraplegia demonstrates the capability and chooses independent living in an accessible environment without the aid of an attendant. A review of outcomes from a subset of people with motor and sensory-complete C6 SCI revealed that the following percentage of patients were independent for key self-care tasks: feeding 16%, upper body dressing 13%, lower body dressing 3%, grooming 19%, bathing 9%, bowel care 3%, transfers 6%, wheelchair propulsion 88%. Feeding is accomplished with a universal cuff for utensils. Transfers require stabilization of elbow extension with forces transmitted from shoulder musculature through the limb as a closed kinetic chain. Bowel care is performed with a suppository insertion wand and Fickle finger for digital stimulation.

13. How much motor recovery is expected in a patient with a stable diagnosis of motor and sensory complete traumatic tetraplegia with central spinal cord edema and hematomyelia on MRI?

Recovery is greatest in muscles supplied within the zone of injury. Less than 30% of SCIs will go from C4 to C5 but > 66% of those at C5–8 gain one root level by 6–12 weeks. The ability to perceive pain from a pin stimulus over the lateral antecubital space (posterior brachial cutaneous nerve) is a good prognostic indicator for eventual recovery of the extensor carpi radialis to $\frac{3}{5}$. Eighty-five percent of patients' muscles that demonstrate $\frac{1}{5}$ strength initially within the zone of partial motor preservation (myotomes caudal to the neurologic level that remain partially innervated) will achieve > $\frac{3}{5}$ strength by 1 year. Below the injury zone, only 3% of patients initially (at 72 hours) Frankel A improved to grade D or E. Negative prognostic indicators on MRI include transection, hematomyelia, and edema, but MRI adds little to the clinical exam for prediction of prognosis.

14. What are the mechanisms of motor recovery after SCI?
    Motor recovery after SCI occurs rapidly during the first and second week; then recovery continues at a slower pace for the first 4 months and beyond. Initially, recovery could be mediated by central mechanisms (cortical reorganization) such as recruitment of latent pathways (unused until injury). At the injury site, edema and hematomyelia may resolve reducing secondary injury, neurapraxic block, and demyelination. Within the anterior horn, central synaptogenesis may occur in response to denervation hypersensitivity of the anterior horn cell. Root impingement may resolve with decompression, spinal alignment, and fixation as needed.

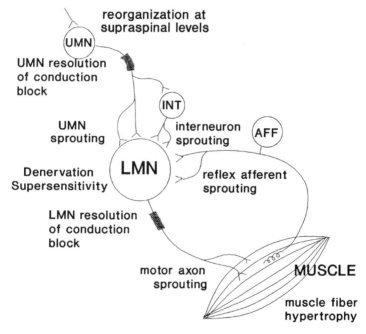

Mechanisms of recovery after SCI. (UMN = upper motor neuron; LMN = lower motor neuron; INT = interneuron; AFF = afferent.) (From Little JW, Stiens SA: Electrodiagnosis in spinal cord injury. Phys Med Rehabil Clin North Am 5:571–593, 1994; with permission.)

15. What are the most common and disabling contractures of the upper extremities after SCI?
    Adduction of shoulder, flexion of elbow, extension of the MCP, DIP, and MIP. Helpful contractures are mild flexion of the MCP, PIP, and DIP. They provide **tenodesis**, which is finger prehension (opposition of the thumb to the index finger) with active wrist extension. Even greater strength can come from a wrist-driven flexor hinge orthosis, which stabilizes the thumb, index, and middle fingers for a tight pincer grasp.

16. A T4 complete paraplegic complains of a pounding headache and was noted to have a blood pressure of 190/100 mmHg, gooseflesh of his trunk and legs, and a paradoxic brady-cardia at 50 bpm. What is the diagnosis, pathophysiology and treatment?

Autonomic dysreflexia is an acute hypertensive syndrome due to a hyperactive reflex sympathetic discharge often precipitated by viscus distention or noxious stimuli registered below the level of the SCI. The nerve cell bodies for sympathetic outflow are located in the **intermediolateral cell columns,** which run from T1 through L2 bilaterally in the spinal gray matter. Lesions above T6 cut off central modulation of sympathetic discharges. Hypertension often produced by excessive vasoconstriction is registered at the carotid baroreceptors, resulting in corrective parasympathetic outflow via the vagus nerve to reduce heart rate and contractility.

Treatment includes identification and elimination of the cause (commonly urologic obstruction/distention, bowel impaction, skin irritation, ingrown toenail, or intraabdominal processes). Sit the patient up and administer nifedipine orally or sublingually. Nitropaste can be placed for prevention in situations that may precipitate autonomic dysreflexia.

17. Why is deep vein thrombosis (DVT) a pervasive problem after SCI?

The primary risks were summarized in 1856 as Virchow's triad:

1. **Venous stasis** (paralysis, spinal shock)
2. **Hypercoagulability** (trauma, tumor as cause for increases in circulating thrombogenic factors)
3. **Vessel injury** (primary trauma or secondary injury due to sensory deficits after SCI)

The incidence of DVT after SCI ranges from 47–100% as revealed with various noninvasive surveillance techniques for subclinical disease. The risk is highest during the first 2 weeks to 3 months after SCI, and prevention of clot formation is essential.

18. How is DVT best prevented after SCI?

- Check a baseline activated partial thromboplastin time and platelet count.
- Immediate initiation of subcutaneous heparin, 5000 units every 12 hours, once emergency trauma management is complete and hemostasis has been achieved.
- Thigh-high Ted hose and heel protectors are placed and kept on all day to prevent edema and trauma.
- Stasis is reduced by sequential pneumatic compression, which should be continued for a minimum of 2 weeks.

Higher heparin doses have an increased effectiveness but also an increased incidence of hemorrhagic complications. Low-molecular-weight heparins do not bind thrombin or inhibit platelet function. Studies indicate that low-molecular-weight heparin given once daily is also effective.

19. What muscle function is typically required to allow community ambulation?

Walking ability is directly related to the proportion of lower-extremity joints that are animated with sufficient muscular force to overcome gravity. At least $\frac{3}{5}$ strength in hip flexion bilaterally with at least $\frac{3}{5}$ knee extension on one side is required for an effective reciprocal gait pattern to permit community ambulation. Bilateral bracing (ankle-foot orthosis or knee-ankle-foot orthosis) with forearm crutches or a walker maximizes efficiency. The calculation of the sum of bilateral lower-extremity strength measures produces the ASIA Lower Extremity Muscle Score (LEMS, normal 50). LEMS correlates with gait velocity, energy expenditure, and peak axial load by arms on crutches. Values above 30 are associated with community ambulation.

20. A chronic T2 ASIA B SCI patient presents to the clinic and mentions that he was unable to tell the difference between a cold and a warm beer by grasping the can with his hand at a recent party. What are your thoughts and actions?

This represents a change in temperature perception, which is carried by the superficially located lateral and ventral **spinothalamic tracts**. Afferent fibers enter through the dorsal root and *cross over* to the opposite side of the spinal cord via the anterior commissure just anterior to the central canal. A differential diagnosis might include progressive post-traumatic syringomyelia (an expanding intramedullary cyst that may originate at the injury site), tethered cord syndrome (progressive spinal cord dysfunction due to stretch or traction of the cord), myelopathy, radiculopathy, plexopathy, and peripheral neuropathy.

The patient should be questioned about shooting pain with sneeze or cough, history of Valsalva, or heavy-lifting, which may all increase subarachnoid pressures. The exam should include neck flexion to assess the presence of **Lhermitte's sign** (a sudden electric-like shock extending down the spine with head flexion), pinprick/touch sensation, reflexes, and strength. Further evaluation includes electrodiagnostic testing and MRI.

21. What is the treatment and outcome for progressive post-traumatic syringomyelia?

Conservative measures include avoidance of high-force isometric contractions, Valsalva, head elevation at night, and maintenance of the neck in a neutral position. Surgical shunting may be associated with shunt obstruction and syrinx reaccumulation.

22. How can an acute abdomen be diagnosed in a person with a spinal cord injury?

The diagnosis of abdominal emergencies requires a high index of suspicion, since it often produces subtle and minimal symptoms and poor localizing findings on examination. The most prominent objective finding may be just an elevated pulse rate!

Signs and symptoms depend on the level of injury and degree of completeness, thus dictating the responsiveness of the remaining intact nervous system. A person with an injury level above T6 may experience autonomic dysreflexia, vague nonlocalized abdominal discomfort, increased spasticity, and a rigid abdomen. A level between T6 and T10 may allow for some reflex responses and localization, depending on the specific organ involved. A level lower than T12 spares sympathetic splanchnic outflow and responses are normal.

Key symptoms, although not always present, include nausea, anorexia, restlessness, changes in spasticity, nonlocalized abdominal pain, and shoulder pain in the person with quadriplegia. Signs may include elevated pulse rate (although bradycardia may exist if autonomic dysreflexia is present), fever, and spasticity. Abdominal tenderness is not common in those individuals with a level above T5. Rapid diagnosis with laboratory studies (complete blood count, amylase) and imaging studies is warranted to improve on the all-too-common delays in diagnosis. There is a resultant 10–15% mortality rate in this population.

23. What is Charcot spine? Why would someone with SCI have it?

Jean M. Charcot was a French neurologist who treated many syphilitics. He described osteoarthropathy from trauma in people with **tabes dorsalis** (syphilitic posterior column deterioration) who lacked protective sensation.

Because of their spinal trauma and analgesia below the level of injury, those with SCI are particularly prone to this insensate joint destruction. After spinal fixation, the fusion mass acts as a lever, contributing to hypermobility at the joint just caudal to the fusion. The joints themselves can be a pain source that triggers autonomic dysreflexia or a nidus of infection after hematogenous spread.

24. A 17-year-old, newly SCI-injured, muscular, C6 incomplete tetraplegic complains of lethargy and abdominal cramping. What could it be?

Immobilization hypercalcemia should be considered. Symptoms of hypercalcemia can be remembered with the mnemonic **stones, bones, and abdominal groans**. Other symptoms include lethargy, nausea, and anorexia.

The diagnosis is made with measurement of the total serum calcium adjusted for the total protein. Serum ionized calcium is also elevated and is a more accurate test. The 24-hour calcium excretion normally should be < 250 mg. Treatment includes mobilization, rehydration with saline, and treatment with furosemide (which enhances Ca^{+2} secretion in the loop of Henle). Calcitonin can be used in resistant cases.

25. A 63-year-old man who has had T7 paraplegia for 37 years presents to your clinic with right shoulder pain of 2 years' duration. He describes the pain as insidious in onset (except for periods of bursitis), located in the posterolateral shoulder, and now interfering with reaching activities. Physical exam reveals significant atrophy of the involved supraspinatus and infraspinatus muscles and severe weakness of external rotation, abduction, and forward flexion. Radiographs reveal upward displacement of the humeral head against the coracoacromial arch. The patient has had approximately 6 steroid injections into the affected shoulder. He has a 75-pack-year smoking history. What is the differential diagnosis for shoulder pain in this individual with paraplegia?

The working diagnosis from his history and physical examination is a **rotator cuff tear** (RCT). However, there are other common causes of shoulder pain and/or weakness in this population, including rheumatologic diseases (glenohumeral osteoarthritis, acromioclavicular osteoarthritis), soft tissue disorders (subacromial bursitis, rotator cuff tendinitis, bicipital tendinitis), post-traumatic syringomyelia, cervical radiculopathy, heterotopic ossification, avascular necrosis, brachial neuritis, and various nerve palsies (long thoracic nerve, suprascapular nerve). Therefore, the physical examination and diagnostic evaluation should confirm the working diagnosis and rule out other etiologies. This is particularly important in individuals who have had paraplegia for many years because shoulder pain and RCTs are common findings. The diagnosis of RCT is supported by the upward displacement of the humeral head and could be confirmed by MRI, arthrography, arthroscopy, or surgery.

26. How is a rotator cuff tear treated in a paraplegic individual such as the 63-year-old man above?

Surgical treatment of RCT in persons with SCI is complex. At best, the surgery will be successful with full restoration of shoulder function. The individual will require many weeks of non-weight-bearing, placing great demands on the contralateral shoulder and great stresses on the vocational and home situation. The usual postoperative restrictions for an able-bodied person are much more difficult for the person with SCI to follow. Return to upper-extremity weight-bearing and extreme loading of the newly repaired cuff frequently occur more rapidly than the able-bodied population because anything less requires assistance from a family member or attendant. It is also important to remember that rotator cuff repairs commonly do not result in full restoration of function. Discouraging prognostic factors include an older age (> 65 years), insidious atraumatic onset, weakness > 6 months, a long smoking history, repeated steroid injections, previous cuff repair attempts, poor nutrition, severe weakness, and upward displacement of the humeral head. This patient has many negative prognostic factors.

Conservative treatment of RCT has not been well studied in the SCI population. However, nonoperative management of tears of the rotator cuff have been examined in the able-bodied population. In general, NSAIDs, stretching, and strengthening programs have been used. It is particularly important to strengthen the posterior shoulder musculature since individuals with paraplegia have relatively strong, shortened anterior muscles and weaker, lengthened posterior muscles. It is also important to identify and eliminate bad habits (e.g., poor transfer technique), to correct posture and optimize the wheelchair set-up, and to lose weight if obesity is a factor.

BIBLIOGRAPHY

1. Bayley JC, Cochran TP, Sledge CB: The weight-bearing shoulder: The impingement syndrome in paraplegics. J Bone Joint Surg 69A:676–678, 1987.
2. Charney KJ, Juler GL, Comarr AE: General surgery problems in patients with spinal cord injuries. Arch Surg 110:1083–1088, 1975.
3. Duchling P, Wilberger JE: Spinal cord injury without radiographic abnormalities in children. J Neurosurg 57:114–129, 1982.
4. Green D, et al: Prevention of thromboembolism in spinal cord injury: Role of low molecular weight heparin. Arch Phys Med Rehabil 75:290–292, 1994.
5. Hussey RW, Stauffer ES: Spinal cord injury: Requirements for ambulation. Arch Phys Med Rehabil 54:554–557, 1973.

6. Ingberg HO, Prust FW: The diagnosis of abdominal emergencies in patients with spinal cord lesions. Arch Phys Med Rehabil 49:343–348, 1968.
7. Sgouros S, Williams B: A critical appraisal of drainage in syringomyelia. J Neurosurg 82:1–10, 1995.
8. Stiens SA, Johnson MC, Lyman PJ: Cardiac rehabilitation in patients with spinal cord injuries. Phys Med Rehabil Clin North Am 6:263–296, 1995.
9. Waters RL, Adkins R, Yakura J, Virgil D: Prediction of ambulatory performance based on motor scores derived from standards of the American Spinal Injury Association. Arch Phys Med Rehabil 75:757–760, 1994.
10. Yarkony GM: Spinal Cord Injury: Medical Management and Rehabilitation. Gaithersburg, MD, Aspen, 1994.

45. STROKE

Elliot J. Roth, M.D.

1. How many people get stroke? Who are they?

Stroke is a very common clinical problem, occurring in approximately 500,000 people yearly in the U.S. About 150,000 die within 1 month after the stroke, making stroke the third leading cause of death in the U.S. About 3 million people are alive today who sustained a stroke at some time in the past, and a substantial proportion of these survivors have varying degrees and types of neurologic impairments and functional disabilities. Stroke is the second most frequent cause of disability (second only to arthritis), the leading cause of *severe* disability, and the most common diagnosis among patients on most rehabilitation units.

Men have a 30–80% higher incidence rate than do women, and African-Americans have a 50–130% greater incidence than do whites. The incidence is age-related, with the rate increasing 9-fold between the ages of 55 and 85. About two-thirds of all stroke patients are over age 65.

2. Name the risk factors for stroke.

Risk factors can be classified into three groups:

Risk Factors that are Modifiable with Behavior Change

Hypercholesterolemia	Cigarette smoking
Obesity	Alcohol abuse
Sedentary lifestyle	Cocaine use

Risk Factors that are Modifiable with Medical Care

Hypertension	Transient ischemic attack
Diabetes	Significant carotid artery stenosis
Heart disease	History of prior stroke

Unmodifiable Risk Factors

Age	Race
Gender	Family history

3. How can subsequent strokes be prevented in patients who have survived a first stroke?

Risk factor modification

Antiplatelet agents—aspirin and ticlopidine

Anticoagulation—warfarin

Carotid endarterectomy

Surgical procedure to correct cerebral aneurysm or arteriovenous malformation

4. What is a stroke?

A stroke is an acute neurologic dysfunction of vascular origin, with relatively rapid onset, causing focal or sometimes global signs of disturbed cerebral function lasting for > 24 hours.

5. What are the different types of strokes?

Stroke types are generally divided into two broad common etiologic categories, ischemic (65–80% of the total) and hemorrhagic (15–25% of the total). The cause of a few strokes (up to 10%) is either unknown or more unusual.

Type of Stroke	% of the Total
Ischemic strokes	
Thrombotic brain infarction	45–65%
Embolic brain infarction	10–20%
Hemorrhagic strokes	
Intracerebral (intraparenchymal) hemorrhage	5–15%
Subarachnoid hemorrhage	5–10%
Other strokes	0–10%

6. What are the common impairments caused by stroke and their relative frequencies?

Impairment	Acute	Chronic
Any motor weakness	90%	50%
Right hemiparesis	45	20
Left hemiparesis	35	25
Bilateral hemiparesis	10	5
Ataxia	20	10
Hemianopsia	25	10
Visuoperceptual deficits	30	30
Aphasia	35	20
Dysarthria	50	20
Sensory deficits	50	25
Cognitive deficits	35	30
Depression	30	30
Bladder incontinence	30	10
Dysphagia	30	10

7. Describe a lacunar stroke.

Accounting for about 15% of all strokes, lacunar strokes are caused by small deep infarctions located in the deeper portions of the brain and brainstem, resulting from occlusion of the deep penetrating cerebral arteries. Risk factors for lacunar stroke include hypertension and diabetes. Because the cerebral lesions are small, they usually do not cause severe impairment or disability. Because they are caused by deeper cerebral lesions, they usually do not impair higher cortical functions. The most common lacunar syndromes are:

Pure motor hemiplegia
Hemimotor-hemisensory syndrome
Pure sensory stroke
Dysarthria-clumsy hand syndrome
Hemiparesis-hemiataxia

8. What is locked-in syndrome?

It is a severely disabling condition, characterized by the combination of complete quadriplegia, facial paralysis, and anarthria. It is caused by interruption of the bilateral corticospinal and corticobulbar tracts that occurs with bilateral infarction of the ventral pons.

9. What is pseudobulbar palsy?

The combination of emotional lability, dysphagia, dysarthria, and hyperactive brainstem reflexes.

10. Describe the usual course of natural recovery after onset of hemiplegia.

Natural spontaneous recovery of motor function follows a relatively predictable sequence of stereotyped movement events for most patients who recover from stroke-induced hemiplegia. The pattern of recovery is most consistent in patients with cerebral infarction in the middle cerebral artery distribution. Lower-extremity function recovers earliest and most completely, followed by upper extremity and hand function. Tone usually returns before voluntary movement, volitional control over the proximal limb before the distal limb, and mass movement (synergy) patterns before specific isolated coordinated volitional motor functions. Most exceptions occur in patients with stroke types other than cerebral infarctions and with lesion locations other than middle cerebral artery distribution. The relative uniformity of these phases was first documented systematically by Twitchell in 1951 and later formalized into a series of stages by Brunnstrom in 1970.

11. Describe the features of the Brunnstrom stages of motor recovery in hemiplegic patients.

Stage I	Flaccidity
	Phasic stretch reflexes absent
	No volitional or reflex-induced active movement
Stage II	Spasticity, resistance to passive movement
	Basic limb synergy patterns
	Associated reactions
	Movement patterns stimulated reflexively
	Minimal voluntary movement
Stage III	Marked spasticity
	Semivoluntary
	Volitional initiated movement of involved limbs, resulting in synergy
	Usually flexion synergy in arm and extension synergy in leg
Stage IV	Spasticity reduced
	Synergy patterns still predominant
	Some complex movements deviating from synergy
Stage V	Spasticity declines more, but still present with rapid movements
	More difficult movement patterns deviating from synergy
	Voluntary isolated environmentally specific movements predominate
Stage VI	Spasticity disappearing
	Coordination improves to near-normal
	Individual joint movements possible
	Still some abnormal movement and faulty timing during complex actions
Stage VII	Restoration of normal variety of rapid complex movement patterns with normal timing, coordination, strength, and endurance

12. Name the components of the limb synergy patterns.

Synergy patterns are the stereotyped mass movement patterns that characterize limb activity after injury to the cerebral voluntary motor system. The affected upper and lower extremities each can assume a flexion or an extension synergy pattern. In the following list, the predominant movement in each pattern is marked with an asterisk.

Upper-extremity flexion synergy pattern

Scapular retraction	Forearm pronation
Scapular depression	Elbow flexion*
Shoulder internal rotation	Wrist flexion
Shoulder adduction	Finger flexion

Upper-extremity extension synergy pattern

Scapular protraction	Forearm pronation
Scapular depression	Elbow extension
Shoulder internal rotation	Wrist extension
Shoulder adduction*	Finger flexion

Lower-extremity flexion synergy pattern

Pelvic protraction	Knee flexion
Pelvic depression	Ankle dorsiflexion
Hip flexion*	Foot inversion
Hip abduction	Toe dorsiflexion
Hip external rotation	Great toe extension

Lower-extremity extension synergy pattern

Pelvic retraction	Knee extension*
Pelvic elevation	Ankle plantarflexion
Hip extension	Foot inversion
Hip adduction	Toe plantarflexion
Hip internal rotation	Great toe extension

13. What are the most common causes of death in stroke survivors?

In the first month following stroke, in order of descending frequency:

The stroke itself, with progressive cerebral edema and herniation

Pneumonia

Cardiac disease (myocardial infarction, sudden death arrhythmia, or heart failure)

Pulmonary embolism

After the first month, cardiac disease is the most common cause, and stroke is the second.

14. How common are venous thromboembolic phenomena in stroke patients?

Deep venous thrombosis (DVT) has been reported to occur in 22–73% of stroke survivors, with the best estimates of incidence of 40–50%. The incidence of pulmonary embolism (PE) in stroke is about 10–15%. Peak incidence is during the first week after stroke, but the risk of venous thromboembolism persists thereafter. Clinical features of DVT or PE are present in less than one-half of patients with these problems, making laboratory diagnosis necessary for most patients suspected of having these conditions.

15. What can be done to prevent venous thromboembolic complications?

Because of the high risk of venous thromboembolism, DVT prophylaxis is recommended for all patients with stroke who have muscle weakness and who undergo inpatient rehabilitation. Methods of prophylaxis include repeated doses of low-dose subcutaneous heparin or low-molecular-weight heparin compounds, external pneumatic calf compression boots, and other physical methods. The optimal duration of prophylaxis is not known, but persistence of severe muscle weakness and lack of ambulatory ability are considered indicators of increased DVT risk.

16. How common are dysphagia, aspiration, and pneumonia after stroke? What can be done about them?

The incidence of dysphagia in stroke patients is between one-third and one-half. Although dysphagia can be associated with cortical, subcortical, or brainstem lesions, the highest incidence is in patients with brainstem strokes.

One-third of stroke patients with dysphagia will have aspiration, defined as entrance of material into the airway below the level of the true vocal folds. Of those who aspirate, 40% will do so silently, without cough or other clinical manifestations of difficulty. To establish the dysphagia diagnosis and aspiration risk, a clinical evaluation of swallowing function and videofluoroscopic swallowing study can be done.

Complications of stroke-induced dysphagia include pneumonia, malnutrition, and dehydration. Pneumonia occurs in about one-third of all stroke patients, and the major cause of pneumonia is dysphagia with aspiration. Other factors that increase the risk of pneumonia are cognitive deficits, inadequate hydration and nutrition, impaired cough and gag reflexes, immobility, and decreased ability to cough resulting from expiratory muscle weakness, altered chest wall movement patterns, chest wall spasticity, and contracture.

Interventions to treat dysphagia include changes in posture and head position; oral motor exercises for the tongue and lips to increase strength, range of motion, velocity, and precision; use of thickened fluids and soft or pureed foods in smaller boluses; tactile-thermal application of cold stimuli; practice in proper eating techniques; and use of alternative feeding routes such as nasogastric, gastrostomy, or jejeunostomy tubes.

17. Describe the major bladder problems caused by stroke. What can be done to treat them?

The incidence of urinary incontinence is 50-70% during the first month after stroke and about 15% after 6 months, a figure comparable to that in the general population. Incontinence may be caused by the brain damage itself (resulting in an uninhibited spastic neurogenic bladder with a synergic sphincter), urinary tract infection, impaired ability to transfer to the toilet or remove clothing, aphasia, or cognitive-perceptual deficits that result in lack of awareness of bladder fullness. Bowel impaction and some medications may exert an adverse effect. Urinary incontinence can cause skin breakdown, social embarrassment, and depression, and it increases the risk of institutionalization and unfavorable rehabilitation outcomes.

The most important therapeutic approach to the neurogenic bladder that results from stroke is the implementation of a timed bladder-emptying schedule. Other important management strategies include treatment of urinary tract infection, regulation of fluid intake, transfer and dressing skill training, patient and family education, and, rarely, medications.

Urinary retention is less common but can occur in the presence of diabetic autonomic neuropathy or prostatic hypertrophy. Urinary retention may cause urinary tract infections requiring treatment with catheterization, medication, and attention to the primary genitourinary cause.

18. What is the incidence of bowel dysfunction in stroke? How can it be treated?

The incidence of bowel incontinence among stroke patients is 31%. While this problem usually resolves within the first 2 weeks after stroke, persistent bowel incontinence may reflect severe brain damage. Bowel continence may be adversely affected by infection resulting in diarrhea, inability to transfer to the toilet or to manage clothing, or inability to express toileting needs. The more common bowel complications are constipation and impaction, resulting from inactivity, inadequate fluid intake, and psychologic disturbances.

Management of bowel dysfunction emphasizes a timed toileting schedule; use of dietary fiber; adequate fluid intake; use of stool softeners, suppositories, or enemas; training in toilet transfers and communication skills; and judicious use of laxatives.

19. Explain the motor facilitation approaches frequently used in physical therapy with stroke patients.

Each of the neuromuscular facilitation exercise approaches has a neurophysiologic basis and a somewhat unique focus.

The **Neurodevelopmental treatment method**, developed by the Bobaths, is currently the most widely used approach for the treatment of hemiplegia resulting from stroke. This method emphasizes inhibition of abnormal tone, postures, and reflex patterns, while facilitating specific automatic motor responses that will eventually allow the performance of skilled voluntary movements.

The **Brunnstrom method** uses the reflex tensing and synergistic patterns of hemiplegia to improve motor control through central facilitation.

The **Rood method** relies on the peripheral input of cutaneous sensory stimulation, in the form of superficial brushing and tapping, to facilitate or inhibit motor activity.

Proprioceptive Neuromuscular Facilitation, introduced by Kabat and Knott, uses such mechanisms as maximum resistance, quick stretch, and spiral diagonal patterns to facilitate normal movement.

Only a few studies have investigated the relative effectiveness of these methods. Results are inconclusive, but no single method has been found to be more effective than any other to improve outcome after stroke. A common clinical practice is to incorporate elements of several methods.

20. What is the "forced use paradigm" of treatment after stroke?

In the forced use intervention, the nonhemiplegic limb is restrained in an attempt to force the individual to use the hemiplegic limb for functional activities. Based originally on favorable results derived from animal studies, this method was found in recent human studies to improve recovery of function among individuals with hemiplegia resulting from stroke. Although this form of treatment is not in common clinical use at this time, the potential and implications of this form of treatment are important.

21. Describe the common treatment approaches used for spasticity caused by stroke.

Hemispheric strokes affect motor activity in several ways, causing weakness and synergy patterns as well as spasticity. Typically causing more functional impairment in the upper extremity than in the lower limb, spasticity is usually (but not always) less severe in patients with cerebral lesions than in those with spinal cord lesions.

Treatment of spasticity relies most heavily on proper positioning, orthotics, and aggressive, consistent stretching exercises to maintain and improve range of motion. Other management strategies include casting, pharmacologic injection blocks of motor points or peripheral nerves (using phenol or botulinum toxin), therapeutic exercise other than stretching, casting, oral medications, and surgical release, the latter of which may be very effective in selected patients. The efficacy of medications remains controversial, but dantrolene sodium (Dantrium) is probably the drug of choice for patients with cerebral spasticity.

22. Describe common shoulder problems in stroke survivors. What can be done about them?

Approximately 70–80% of patients with stroke and hemiplegia have shoulder pain, contracture, or another form of dysfunction, making it one of the most common secondary complications of stroke. Causes of hemiplegic shoulder dysfunction are many and can include glenohumeral subluxation, adhesive capsulitis (frozen shoulder), impingement syndromes, rotator cuff tears, brachial plexus traction neuropathies, reflex sympathetic dystrophy syndrome ("shoulder-hand syndrome, present in up to 25% of patients), bursitis and tendinitis, and central pain. Often, there is either a history or radiographic evidence of a preexisting or long-standing shoulder problem, and it is likely that the abnormal mechanical forces resulting from the stroke either exacerbate or make manifest the chronic problem.

In some patients, pain and loss of range of motion are associated with improper positioning or handling, weakness of the shoulder girdle muscles, or spasticity. Shoulder dysfunction has been found to be present significantly more frequently in patients with spastic upper limbs than in those with flaccid upper limbs. Pain and glenohumeral subluxation may occur together or independently, and the extent to which there is a causal relationship between pain and subluxation is unclear.

Treatment of shoulder dysfunction is individualized and may consist of arm supports, shoulder slings, arm troughs, lap boards, medications, physical modalities, proper positioning and staff handling, and, most importantly, aggressive and consistently performed range-of-motion exercises. The use of shoulder slings is controversial, but if subluxation is the main cause of the shoulder dysfunction, then slings may be helpful. Ensuring consistent performance of stretching exercises is the major clinical task.

23. What is central post-stroke pain syndrome?

Previously known as **thalamic pain** or **Dejerine-Roussy syndrome**, central post-stroke pain syndrome is present in < 5% of stroke survivors. It causes severe and disabling pain sensations, which usually are described by patients as diffuse, persistent, and refractory to many treatment attempts. The most common descriptions of the pain are "burning and tingling," although many experience "sharp, shooting, stabbing, gnawing," and at times, "dull and achy." The dysesthesias are often associated with hyperpathia, which is an exaggerated pain reaction to mild external cutaneous stimulation. Only about 50% of the patients have thalamic strokes; the remainder have cerebrovascular lesions in a variety of locations. Treatment methods include:

Medical and nursing care
  Prevention and treatment of bladder, bowel, and skin problems
  Prevention and treatment of other medical problems such as infection
  Range-of-motion exercises
  Mobility exercises
Psychologic methods
  Relaxation, imagery
  Biofeedback
  Hypnosis
  Psychotherapy
  Preoccupation
Medications
  Analgesics
  Antidepressants
  Anticonvulsants
Surgical techniques (rarely used)

24. Describe the common types of aphasia that occur after stroke.

Global aphasia: loss of both expression and comprehension abilities. Patients have non-fluent or absent speech.

Broca's aphasia: reduction in expressive, and therefore repetition, abilities, but preservation of comprehension. Speech is nonfluent.

Wernicke's aphasia: reductions in comprehension and repetition, but with preservation of expression. Speech is fluent but often nonsensical.

Transcortical motor aphasia: expressive dysfunction with intact comprehension and repetition.

Transcortical sensory aphasia: loss of comprehension ability with intact expression and repetition.

Conduction aphasia (relatively rare): isolated loss of repetition, while expression and comprehension remain intact.

25. What is melodic intonation therapy, and how does it work?

It is a direct form of aphasia treatment that utilizes the patient's relatively unimpaired ability to sing, which can facilitate spontaneous speech in some patients. Therapy starts with the therapist and patient chanting simple phrases and sentences in unison to melodies that resemble natural intonation patterns. This progresses to a level at which the patient is able to chant answers to simple questions and, in some cases, the patient makes the transition off of intoned speech and into normal prosodic speech patterns. This method is most successful in patients with good auditory comprehension and limited verbal expression. It is thought that the effectiveness of this method derives from the reliance on the unimpaired musical functions of the right hemisphere to support the damaged motor speech function in the left hemisphere.

26. What is hemispatial neglect and how can it be treated?

Unilateral hemispatial inattention, or neglect, is lack of awareness of a specific body part or external environment. Neglect usually occurs in patients with right (nondominant) hemisphere cortical strokes; such patients ignore or have muted responses to visual, auditory, or tactile stimuli on the left side of the body or environment. Patients with severe hemi-inattention deny that they have an illness or that neglect is a problem, or they may not recognize their own body parts. Neglect can improve spontaneously but can impede performance of functional tasks and complicate rehab efforts.

Treatment methods emphasize retraining, substitution of intact abilities, and compensatory techniques. Specific treatment strategies include providing visuospatial cues, fostering awareness of deficits, and using computer-assisted training, visual scanning skill training, caloric stimulation, Fresnel prism glasses, eye patching, dynamic stimulation, and optokinetic stimulation.

27. What is Gerstmann's syndrome?

Gerstmann's syndrome occurs following damage to the left parietal region of the brain, which causes the four findings of dyscalculia, finger agnosia, right-left disorientation, and dysgraphia.

28. What are the apraxias?

The term *apraxia* is applied to a group of complex cognitive disorders that adversely affect motor function, usually characterized by difficulty in planning, organizing, sequencing, and executing learned voluntary movements, in the absence of weakness, ataxia, or extrapyramidal dysfunction. Several specific types of apraxias have been identified:

Motor or ideomotor apraxia: Can perform a particular movement automatically or spontaneously, but cannot repeat the movement when asked.

Ideational apraxia: Failure to hold on to ideas and plans necessary to perform an activity.

Constructional apraxia: Disturbance in the organization of individual spatial elements such that patient is unable to synthesize the elements into a whole. Inability to put together an object from separate parts or to draw a picture of an object.

Apraxia of speech: Deficit in motor programming of speech. Often associated with Broca's aphasia.

Dressing apraxia: Inability to dress self despite adequate motor ability.

Apraxia of gait: Difficulty in initiating and maintaining a normal walking pattern when sensory and motor functions are otherwise unimpaired. Usually associated with frontal lobe lesions.

29. How common is post-stroke depression? What can be done about it?

The incidence of depression after stroke ranges between 10% and 70%, with the best estimates at around 30%. Major depression is present in about one-third of all of those with depression. The depression may result from a biologic effect of the brain damage itself, a reaction to the losses caused by the stroke, effects of certain medications, manifestations of certain medical conditions, or a combination of these factors. Depression may adversely affect both participation in rehabilitation and functional outcomes

The choice of treatment depends on the cause and severity of the symptoms. Review of medications and treating intercurrent medical illnesses are important first steps. A rehab program that includes therapy for physical and cognitive disabilities, interaction with others, and attention and encouragement from family and staff is often extremely helpful. Many patients respond favorably to more intensive psychotherapy or to the use of antidepressant medications, which have been demonstrated in at least three randomized controlled clinical trials to be effective in treating post-stroke depression.

30. What are some of the typical functional outcomes after stroke?

It is estimated that only about 1 in 10 stroke patients is functionally independent immediately after stroke and that nearly one-half are independent at 6 months. Results of the Framingham Study provide estimates for the types and frequencies of long-term disabilities in stroke survivors:

Type of Disability	
Decreased vocational function	63%
Decreased socialization outside home	59
Limited household tasks	56
Decreased interests and hobbies	47
Decreased use of transportation	44
Decreased socialization at home	43
Dependent ADL	32
Dependent mobility	22
Living in institution	15

Estimates for disabilities in some of the specific activities after 6 months post-stroke are as follows:

Type of Disability	
Unable to walk	15%
Needs assistance to transfer	20
Needs assistance to bathe	50
Needs assistance to dress	30
Needs assistance to groom	10

31. Name some of the commonly cited predictors of unfavorable functional outcome after stroke.

Prior stroke	Unemployed
Urinary incontinence	Cardiac disease
Bowel incontinence	Coma at onset
Depression	Inability to perform ADL
Visuospatial perceptual deficits	(the most important)
Cognitive deficits	Poor sitting balance
Delayed acute medical care	Large cerebral lesions
Delayed rehabilitation	Dense hemiplegia
Low functional score on admission	(Homonymous hemianopsia)
to rehab program	(Aphasia)
Poor social supports	(Increased age)
Unmarried	(Medical comorbidity)

32. Describe some of the unique considerations in rehabilitation of older adults with stroke.

Because a substantial proportion of stroke survivors are over age 65 years, consideration of issues that tend to be more common among older adults assumes prominence in the care of stroke survivors. Some of the most important of these problems are the increased frequency of preexisting medical conditions and prior stroke, increased risk of secondary post-stroke medical complications, increased likelihood of recurrent stroke, and slower recovery from secondary intercurrent medical illnesses. Many of these problems result from reduced endurance and limited physiologic reserve among older adults. Older adults are at greater risk for falls with injuries, adverse drug reactions, and neurologic changes resulting in altered cognitive, sensory, and motor functioning.

For many older patients, the problem that is more significant than medical comorbidity is a relative lack of family, economic, and social resources. Spouses and other caregivers are often either not available or not able to provide post-rehab care for the older stroke survivor. Institutional discharges tend to be more common among older adults.

These problems may delay or inhibit participation in the therapeutic exercise program, complicate the rehabilitation course, and prolong hospitalization. It is important to note, however, that studies have shown that *older adults are able to make functional improvements in amounts that are similar to those of younger stroke patients.* Compared to younger individuals, older adults tend to have lower functional ratings on admission (and therefore at discharge), primarily because of the greater frequencies of comorbidities and prior strokes, and also because of greater stroke severities among older patients.

BIBLIOGRAPHY

1. Brandstater ME, Roth EJ, Siebens HC: Venous thromboembolism in stroke: Literature review and implications for clinical practice. Arch Phys Med Rehabil 73:S379–S391, 1992.
2. Davidoff G, Keren O, Ring H, Solzi P, Werner RA: Assessing candidates for inpatient stroke rehabilitation: Predictors of outcome. Phys Med Rehabil Clin North Am 2(3):501–516, 1991.

3. Gordon WA (ed): Advances in Stroke Rehabilitation. Boston, Andover Medical Publishers, 1993.
4. Gresham GE, Duncan PW, Stason WB, et al: Post-Stroke Rehabilitation: Guideline Report, No. 16. [AHCPR Publication No. 95-0662.] Rockville, MD, Agency for Health Care Policy and Research, 1995.
5. Hoogasian S, Walzak MP, Wurzel R: Urinary incontinence in the stroke patient: Etiology and rehabilitation. Phys Med Rehabil: State Art Rev 3(3):581–594, 1989.
6. Lorish TR, Sandin KJ, Roth EJ, Noll SF: Stroke rehabilitation: 3. Rehabilitation evaluation and management. Arch Phys Med Rehabil 75:S47–S51, 1994.
7. Roth EJ, Harvey RL: Rehabilitation of stroke syndromes. In Braddon RL (ed): Textbook of Physical Medicine and Rehabilitation. Philadelphia, W.B. Saunders, 1995.
8. Roth EJ, Noll SF: Stroke rehabilitation: 2. Comorbidities and complications. Arch Phys Med Rehabil 75: S42–S46, 1994.
9. Teasell RW, Gillen M: Upper extremity disorders and pain following stroke. Phys Med Rehabil: State Art Rev 7(1):133–146, 1993.
10. Wade DT, Langton Hewer R, Skilbeck CE, David RM: Stroke: A Critical Approach to Diagnosis, Treatment, and Management. Chicago: Year Book, 1985.

46. MOTOR NEURON DISEASE

James C. Agre, M.D., Ph.D., and Arthur A. Rodriquez, M.D.

1. What is a motor neuron disease?

A motor neuron disease produces dysfunction of the motor neurons, which results in weakness and muscle wasting. These diseases or conditions include those that affect the upper (corticobulbar and corticospinal) motor neurons and/or the bulbar and spinal lower motor neurons.

2. How are the motor neuron diseases classified?

In a number of different ways. One classification system is based on the location of the pathophysiologic involvement.

The Motor Neuron Diseases

Upper motor neuron disorders
  Primary lateral sclerosis
  Tropical spastic paraparesis
  Lathyrism
  Epidemic spastic paraparesis
  Familial (hereditary) spastic paraplegia

Combined upper and lower motor neuron disorders
  Amyotrophic lateral sclerosis (ALS)
  Familial ALS
  Western Pacific ALS—parkinsonism dementia complex
  Groote-Eylandt motor neuron disease
  Postencephalitic (encephalitis lethargica) ALS
  Juvenile inclusion body ALS

Disorders of the lower motor neuron
  Spinal (bulbospinal muscular) atrophies
  Monoclonal gammopathy and motor neuron disease
  Cancer and motor neuron disease
  Poliomyelitis and post-polio syndrome

Modified from Hudson AJ: The motor neuron diseases and related disorders. In Joynt RJ (ed): Clinical Neurology, vol 4. Philadelphia, J.B. Lippincott, 1991, pp 1–35.

3. Under the lower motor neuron disorders, how are the spinal (bulbospinal) muscular atrophies subclassified?

Spinal (Bulbospinal) Muscular Atrophies

Infantile
    Acute infantile spinal muscular atrophy (Werdnig-Hoffmann disease, type I spinal muscular atrophy, or acute proximal hereditary motor neuropathy)
    Chronic infantile spinal muscular atrophy (Werdnig-Hoffmann disease, type II spinal muscular atrophy, or chronic proximal hereditary motor neuropathy)

Juvenile/Adult
    Juvenile and adult proximal spinal muscular atrophy (Kugelberg-Welander disease, type III spinal muscular atrophy, or recessive proximal hereditary motor neuropathy; type IV spinal muscular atrophy or [juvenile] dominant proximal hereditary motor neuropathy; type V spinal muscular atrophy or [adult] dominant proximal hereditary motor neuropathy)
    Bulbar disease of childhood (Fazio-Londe disease and Brown-Vialettlo-van Laere syndrome)
    Distal spinal muscular atrophy (distal hereditary motor neuropathy)

Adult
    Scapuloperoneal (facioscapuloperoneal) muscular atrophy
    Chronic bulbospinal muscular atrophy of late onset
    Monomelic (segmental) spinal muscular atrophy

Modified from Hudson AJ: The motor neuron diseases and related disorders. In Joynt RJ (ed): Clinical Neurology, vol 4. Philadelphia, J.B. Lippincott, 1991, pp 1–35.

4. What is known about the pathophysiologic causes of the motor neuron diseases?

With few exceptions, the pathogenesis of the motor neuron diseases is unknown. One exception is **lathyrism**, which is an upper motor neuron disorder that is produced by an excessive consumption of the chickling pea (*Lathyrus sativus*). The toxic agent in the pea is thought to be β-N-oxalylamino-L-alanine (BOAA), which is an agonist of the excitatory neurotransmitter, glutamate. Lathyrism is endemic to the Indian subcontinent, where the chickling pea is used as an emergency food in times of drought or flooding.

The other exception is **poliomyelitis**. Poliomyelitis is caused by a viral infection.

5. Is it possible to get polio more than once?

Yes, it is possible, though improbable. The offending virus is a single-stranded RNA enterovirus (picornavirus), and there are three antigenically distinguishable viruses that cause poliomyelitis. Hence, the vaccine to prevent poliomyelitis is a trivalent vaccine. Following a poliomyelitis illness, the patient will have developed antibodies only to one specific virus and could possibly develop poliomyelitis upon exposure to either of the other two viral strains.

6. How is the poliomyelitis virus transmitted?

It usually enters via the oral route. Once in the body, the virus replicates in the lymphoid tissues of the pharynx and intestine and then spreads to the regional lymphoid tissues, resulting in a viremia and a nonspecific illness. Viremia is the most accepted mechanism for direct nervous system exposure to the virus. The reason for the selective vulnerability of certain cells, such as the motor neurons, to the poliomyelitis virus is unknown, but it may relate to specific receptors on their cell membranes.

7. It has been stated that most people who had polio in the past didn't even know they had the disease. Is that true?

The poliovirus is an extremely infectious agent, but only a fraction of those infected have any symptoms. The disease progresses to CNS involvement with paresis or paralysis in only 1–2% of cases. In 4-8%, only a nonspecific illness is noted by the individual, and in the others, the infection is inapparent.

8. How is it that polio caused weakness in the people who experienced paresis or paralysis?

The poliomyelitis viruses, for unknown reasons, appear to have an affinity for the anterior horn cells. In histologic studies of motor neurons of monkeys with acute paralytic poliomyelitis, nearly all (96–97%) of the motor neurons of severely paralyzed limbs were affected by the virus during the acute infection. About one-half of these motor neurons died during the early convalescent period, and the other half survived. A good correlation was found between the proportion of destroyed motor neurons and the severity of paralysis. With death of the motor neurons, wallerian degeneration occurs, and the muscle fibers associated with those neurons become "orphaned," resulting in motor weakness.

9. Why is it that polio patients often required several years to plateau in their functional recovery?

Survivors commonly recovered muscle strength gradually in muscles not completely paralyzed. Some lucky individuals ultimately recovered to a point of minimal or no residual dysfunction. Improvements in function often began in the first weeks but could continue for several years after the acute illness. The mechanisms of recovery include both resolution of dysfunction of partially damaged motor neurons as well as reinnervation of denervated muscle fibers by surviving motor units and muscle hypertrophy following reactivation.

10. Which motor neuron diseases are typically seen in a PM&R practice?

In the United States, amyotrophic lateral sclerosis (ALS) and poliomyelitis (post-polio syndrome).

11. Tell me about amyotrophic lateral sclerosis (ALS).

It is better known as Lou Gehrig's disease, since the Yankee first baseman died from this disorder. ALS encompasses two conditions: progressive bulbar palsy and progressive muscular atrophy, which differ only in their site of onset. Initially, progressive bulbar palsy affects the bulbar motor neurons, while progressive muscular atrophy initially affects the spinal motor neurons. These two diseases overlap the longer the patient survives. Death usually results from the bulbar involvement.

12. Who gets ALS?

The incidence of ALS is approximately 1.6–2.4 cases/100,000 population, but it may increase with age. For instance, in a study in southwestern Ontario, the incidence increased to 7.4 cases/100,000 population by the eighth decade, with an average age at diagnosis of 62 years. The average survival from time of diagnosis is approximately 2.5 years, though it is reported to be somewhat shorter for older patients than younger patients. The male-to-female ratio varies from 1.2 to 1.6:1.

13. Describe the typical clinical features of ALS.

The typical complaint is weakness. The most common findings at the time of initial examination include atrophy, weakness, and fasciculations (lower motor neuron signs). Additionally, muscle stretch reflexes can be depressed in regions where there is primarily lower motor neuron involvement or where atrophy is so advanced that upper motor neuron signs cannot be found. Otherwise, it is common to find brisk muscle stretch reflexes in areas of muscle atrophy. On occasion, the patient may present with only mild spasticity, suggesting a purely upper motor neuron disorder (e.g., spastic dysarthria or facies or both with no detectable lower motor neuron signs). Muscle cramping is also a frequent complaint.

In general, the most striking feature of ALS is the focal, often asymmetrical, onset of weakness, which then spreads to adjacent areas of the body. Spasticity can be disabling and make ambulation difficult. The bowel and bladder are spared in this disease, except for constipation related to inactivity or poor nutritional intake. Sensation is generally spared, although paresthesias and decreased vibratory sense can be found in up to 25% of patients.

14. What are some of the characteristic pathologic findings in this disorder?

Unlike poliomyelitis, where the pathogenesis is related to a viral infection, the pathogenesis of classic ALS is unknown. Some characteristic pathologic findings in classic ALS include degeneration and/or complete loss of motor neurons in the brainstem and spinal cord areas corresponding to the muscle atrophy and degeneration of the large pyramidal neurons in the primary motor cortex and the pyramidal tracts. The nucleus of Onuf (the nucleus controlling the striated muscles of the pelvic floor and the bowel and bladder sphincters) is preserved; hence, bowel and bladder function are preserved.

15. Are other motor neuron diseases found in children besides poliomyelitis?

Acute infantile spinal muscular atrophy (Werdnig-Hoffmann disease) is an autosomal recessive disorder with an estimated incidence of 1/15,000 to 1/25,000 livebirths. The disease is apparent at birth in one-third of the children and is usually diagnosed by age 3 months. Survival averages 6–9 months from diagnosis and does not exceed 3 years. The clinical picture is dominated by severe hypotonia and weakness and resultant delays in motor milestones. The infants characteristically lie motionless with the lower limbs abducted in the frog-leg position. Fasciculations of the tongue are almost pathognomonic for the disease. Death usually results from respiratory failure.

Chronic infantile spinal muscular atrophy (chronic Werdnig-Hoffmann disease) is much more slowly progressive than the acute form of this disease. Clinical signs are usually present by age 3 years, but occasionally as early as age 3 months. This disease has variable progression, with the average age of death being over 10 years. It also has an autosomal recessive inheritance.

Juvenile proximal spinal muscular atrophy (Kugelberg-Welander disease) is characterized by slowly progressive weakness and atrophy of the proximal limb and girdle musculature. It is usually transmitted as an autosomal recessive disorder (type III proximal hereditary motor neuropathy) but also has an autosomal dominant form (type IV juvenile proximal hereditary motor neuropathy). The clinical onset of the disease can occur anytime between childhood and the seventh decade of life (in the adult form, type V proximal hereditary motor neuropathy) but usually occurs between ages 2–17 years. Both the juvenile and adult forms of this disease begin with symmetrical atrophy and weakness of the pelvic girdle and proximal lower limbs, then progress to involvement of the shoulder girdles and upper arms.

Progressive bulbar paralysis of childhood has two forms, Fazio-Londe disease and Brown-Vialettlo-Laere syndrome. Both cause a slowly progressive weakness of the muscles of the face, tongue, and pharynx. Fazio-Londe disease, which has been described rarely since 1925, produces bilateral deafness as the first symptom. This occurs between the ages of 18 months and 31 years (average onset, 12 years). Cranial nerve palsies usually appear about 4–5 years later. Survival may exceed 2 decades. Inheritance is apparently autosomal recessive.

Distal spinal muscular atrophy (spinal form of Charcot-Marie-Tooth disease) has several forms with different inheritance patterns: (1) autosomal recessive juvenile mild (onset, 2–10 years of age) and juvenile severe (onset, 4 months–20 years), and (2) autosomal dominant in the juvenile (onset, 2–20 years) and in the adult (onset, 20–40 years). Life expectancy is normal except in some severe juvenile cases. Clinical features include weakness and atrophy, which usually start distally in the legs.

16. Can cancer cause motor neuron disease?

This possibility has been raised, as some individuals with cancer become extremely weak and appear as having a motor neuron disorder. However, this observation has not yet been substantiated, and there are many other explanations for these neurologic findings, such as metastases to the nervous system and meninges, cachexia, neuropathy, myopathy, mixed neuropathy/myopathy, and other factors.

17. What is post-polio syndrome?

Post-polio syndrome is essentially a diagnosis made by exclusion in polio survivors. A good definition of post-polio syndrome has been given by Halstead and Rossi (1987) and is based on five criteria:

1. A confirmed history of paralytic poliomyelitis
2. Partial to fairly complete neurologic and functional recovery
3. A period of neurologic and functional stability of at least 15 years' duration
4. Onset of 2 or more of the following health problems since achieving a period of stability: unaccustomed fatigue, muscle and/or joint pain, new weakness in muscles previously affected and/or unaffected, functional loss, cold intolerance, new atrophy
5. No other medical diagnosis to explain these health problems

18. What are the most frequent complaints of patients with post-polio syndrome?
In general, new musculoskeletal and neuromuscular symptoms. The table lists the most frequent new health and ADL problems of post-polio individuals, whether they were seen in a post-polio clinic or had responded to a national survey. The most prevalent new health-related complaints were fatigue, muscle or joint pain, and weakness. The most prevalent new ADL complaints were difficulties with walking and stair-climbing.

New Health and ADL Problems in Post-Polio Patients

	PERCENT WITH COMPLAINT		
SYMPTOM	HALSTEAD[1] (n = 539)	HALSTEAD[2] (n = 132)	AGRE[3] (n = 79)
New health problems			
Fatigue	87	89	86
Muscle pain	80	71	86
Joint pain	79	71	77
Weakness			
Previously affected muscles	87	69	80
Previously unaffected muscles	77	50	53
Cold intolerance	—	29	56
Atrophy	—	28	39
New ADL problems			
Walking	85	64	—
Stair-climbing	83	61	67
Dressing	62	17	16

1. Halstead LS, Rossi CD: Orthopedics 8:845–850, 1985.
2. Halstead LS, Rossi CD: In Halstead LS, Wiechers DO (eds): Research and Clinical Aspects of the Late Effects of Poliomyelitis. White Plains, NY, March of Dimes Birth Defects Foundation, 1987, pp 13–26.
3. Agre JC, Rodriquez AA, Sperling KB: Arch Phys Med Rehabil 70:367–370, 1989.

19. How many polio survivors have post-polio syndrome?
The answer is not precisely known. One study reported that 41% of respondents to their questionnaire had new complaints compatible with post-polio syndrome, another study reported approximately 25%, and a third study reported 28.5%. One might estimate from these reports that somewhere between 25–40% of polio survivors may be experiencing post-polio syndrome at present. As these individuals age, this proportion may well increase significantly.

20. What evidence is there for progressive loss of strength in polio survivors?
Although the development of late-onset weakness in polio survivors was first reported well over a century ago, at present there is little objective evidence in the literature to indicate that the rate of loss in strength is greater than that expected as a result of the normal aging process. Several reports have simply relied on the patient's complaint to determine a progressive loss in strength. Preliminary analyses from our research laboratory show that both stable and unstable post-polio individuals lost strength in the quadriceps femoris musculature, but not from the biceps humerus musculature, over a 5-year follow-up. The rate of loss of strength in the quadriceps, however, was not greater than that found in control (non-polio) subjects. Despite the present lack of objective

evidence, it is most probable that polio survivors are losing strength at a greater rate. Further research on this and the possible causes of strength loss is needed.

21. Why are these post-polio individuals losing strength as they age?

A number of plausible reasons have been suggested to explain a more rapid decline in strength in polio survivors. However, to date, there is no empirical evidence that the loss of strength is directly related to poliomyelitis. Instead, it may be a reflection of the aging process in individuals with impaired function. A number of possible pathophysiologic and functional etiologies have been suggested, including premature aging of motor neurons damaged by the poliovirus, premature aging of the motor neurons due to the increased metabolic demand, loss of muscle fibers within the surviving motor units, death of motor neurons due to the normal aging process, disuse weakness, overuse weakness, or weight gain. It may be that different polio survivors have differing combinations of the above factors related to their complaints.

22. Outline the evaluation of a patient with a possible motor neuron disease?

As with all diseases, the initial assessment to determine the diagnosis includes obtaining a detailed history, performing a good physical examination, and obtaining appropriate laboratory values.

• **History**
   1. Major complaints of the patient (and/or parents)
   2. Pattern of weakness (in general, motor neuron diseases produce proximal weakness, while neuropathic disorders cause distal weakness, often accompanied by sensory abnormalities)
   3. Age of onset of difficulties and rate of progression
   4. Family history

• **Physical examination**
   1. Visual inspection for areas of muscular atrophy, muscular hypertrophy, and fasciculations
   2. Sensory examination (Sensory loss is very rare in motor neuron diseases, but common in neuropathic disorders.)
   3. Muscle stretch reflexes (increased in upper motor neuron disorders, increased or decreased in the combined upper and lower motor neuron disorders, and decreased in the lower motor neuron disorders)
   4. Manual muscle testing to show the level of residual muscle function and distribution of the weakness (proximal, distal, or asymmetrical)
   5. Range of motion testing to detect contractures (including passive ROM)
   6. Functional assessment (to determine the patient's level of functional abilities for assistive devices)

• **Laboratory studies**
   1. Muscle biopsy
   2. Nerve conduction studies (to check for peripheral neuropathy)
   3. Electromyography (to differentiate neuropathy and myopathy and to determine loss of motor neurons, amount of denervation, and presence of collateral reinnervation)
   4. Other evaluations, depending on the clinical presentation of the patient (to look for specific disorders, e.g., rare disorders, diabetes mellitus, thyrotoxicosis)
   5. Urinalysis (to check for heavy metal intoxication, such as lead or mercury)

23. What are the general principles of rehabilitation management of a patient with a motor neuron disorder?

The management should be divided into prospective care and expectant care. **Prospective care** includes all the usual health measures provided to any individual regardless of their health status and includes such things as appropriate vaccinations and health screening tests. **Expectant care** is focused on the individual's specific situation and disease. It includes anticipation of complications that might occur during the course of the patient's motor neuron disease. Aggressive measures can be made to prevent or minimize complications and maximize function and independence for as long as possible. The expected complications could include pain, muscle tightness, deformities of bones and joints, weakness, impaired ventilation, and impaired functional abilities.

24. Is pain a common problem in patients with motor neuron diseases?

Pain is not usually a major problem, except in patients with acute poliomyelitis, who may have severe muscle pain. In them, control of pain can usually be accomplished by both physical and pharmacologic treatments. The use of hot packs, especially the Kenny hot packs (made from woolen blankets), applied at 5-minute intervals for 20 minutes, can be helpful. The heat treatments along with stretching are useful in the acute stages to control pain and maintain range of motion. NSAIDs may also be used. Many patients, however, may have mechanical pain related to weakness, contracture, or deformity.

25. How does one treat muscle contractures?

Muscle contracture is a common problem in patients with motor neuron diseases. The best treatment is **prevention**. Contractures usually first occur at muscles that span two joints with the joints in the flexed position. Common sites include the shoulder adductors, elbow flexors, forearm pronators, finger adductors, hip flexors or internal rotators, knee flexors, ankle plantar flexors, and foot invertors.

The physical treatment includes passive, active assistive and active range of motion, depending on the condition of the patient, usually after the application of superficial heat. Prolonged stretching is required to correct contracture. When using orthotics to help prevent contractures, one must carefully assess the kinesiologic factors. When preventing or correcting shortening of a muscle that spans two joints, it is important to ensure that the muscles are stretched at both joints that they cross. Also, splinting and casting can be used to treat contracture. Surgery is only rarely needed. Appropriate positioning can aid in the prevention of deformity.

26. How is spasticity treated in patients having motor neuron disorders?

Considerable spasticity can occur in some motor neuron diseases. Their treatment is no different than the treatment in spinal cord injury or other upper motor neuron disorder.

27. How does one treat deformity in patients with motor neuron disorder?

Malalignment of body segments leads to contracture and deformity; therefore, appropriate **prospective treatment** is needed to prevent or minimize the development of contracture or deformity. Appropriate stretching, bracing, and positioning can help prevent contractures. For instance, in a child sitting in a large wheelchair with a sling-type seat, frequently one hip will be higher than the other, with the hips internally rotated and adducted, and the child leaning on one elbow for support. This position will lead to contracture and subsequent scoliotic deformity. The minimal wheelchair prescription should include a firm seat, with adequate lumbar, truncal, and arm support. Also, thoracolumbosacral orthotic devices can help to prevent progressive scoliotic deformity in patients with significant weakness of the trunk.

Some patients with post-polio syndrome place significant stress upon the knee while ambulating. This can cause either genu valgus and/or genu recurvatum deformity to develop, which is usually treated with a knee-ankle-foot orthosis.

28. How is scoliosis managed?

Prevention and management of scoliosis comprise one of the major goals in the management of neuromuscular disease. Scoliosis occurs with increasing age and with advancing disability. Most children with motor neuron disease develop a collapsing, paralytic type of scoliosis. Usually, the paraspinal muscular weakness is symmetrical, and while the child is ambulatory, the development of scoliosis is uncommon; however, once the child becomes nonambulatory, scoliosis develops rapidly.

The initial approach to managing scoliosis is to order the most appropriate wheelchair, which must be measured for each child. The child must maintain a symmetrical sitting posture with adequate upper and lower extremity support; the sling seat should be avoided because it permits asymmetrical pelvic rotation. A solid foam-padded seat cushion can be used to level the pelvis during sitting in the early stages. Children tolerate sitting-support orthoses until the curve reaches > 40°. At that point, a relatively rapid progression continues that generally cannot be managed orthotically, and surgery may be indicated.

29. Can weakness be treated in patients with motor neuron disease?

Yes, with strengthening exercises, if prescribed judiciously and followed carefully. Although not well studied, vigorous, fatiguing, progressive resistive exercise appears to be contraindicated in most motor neuron diseases, because such exercise can lead to overuse weakness. Low-intensity, nonfatiguing exercise may be beneficial for maintenance or improvement in muscle strength and cardiorespiratory fitness. Weakness is also treated with appropriate orthotic devices for support.

30. How does one treat the patient with respiratory difficulty?

When weakness and/or deformity sufficiently limits the patient's ability to ventilate, mechanical ventilatory assistance is needed. Early signs and symptoms of hypoxia include difficulty with sleeping, nighttime dyspnea, nightmares, and daytime somnolence. As these signs appear, appropriately prescribed ventilatory aids (such as cuirass or plastic wrap) enhance ventilation in the recumbent position. In the later stages of motor neuron disease, oral positive-pressure ventilation, pneumobelt, or cuirass ventilators can be used throughout the day, energized by the wheelchair battery. Tracheostomy is rarely needed, and its use is somewhat controversial.

31. What is the primary goal in the treatment plan?

The primary goal in treating patients with motor neuron diseases is to assist the patient in the maintenance of function, independence, and quality of life for as long as possible. This requires a coordinated effort by the entire rehabilitation team in prospective and expectant care of the patient. Appropriate preventive and therapeutic interventions for the treatment of pain, soft-tissue tightness, deformity, scoliosis, weakness, and respiratory dysfunction can minimize complications and maximize the patient's ability to function. Functional training for locomotion, dressing, eating, and other ADLs is also recommended. Assistive devices and selective surgical procedures (such as tendon transfers, releases, and arthrodeses) represent management techniques that can be judiciously applied to improve the patient's ability to function.

BIBLIOGRAPHY

1. Agre JC, Rodriquez AA, Tafel JA: Late effects of polio: Critical review of the literature on neuromuscular function. Arch Phys Med Rehabil 72:923–931, 1991.
2. Agre JC: The role of exercise in the patient with post-polio syndrome. Ann NY Acad Sci 753:321–334, 1995.
3. Dumitru D: Electrodiagnostic Medicine. Philadelphia, Hanley & Belfus, 1995.
4. Grimby G, Einarsson G: Post-polio management. CRC Crit Rev Phys Med Rehabil 2:189–200, 1991.
5. Halstead LS, Grimby G (eds): Post-Polio Syndrome. Philadelphia, Hanley & Belfus, 1995.
6. Hudson AJ: The motor neuron diseases and related disorders. In Joynt RJ (ed): Clinical Neurology, vol 4. Philadelphia, J.B. Lippincott, 1991, pp 1–35.
7. Kottke FJ: Therapeutic exercise to maintain mobility. In Kottke FJ, Lehmann JF (eds): Krusen's Handbook of Physical Medicine and Rehabilitation, 4th ed. Philadelphia, W.B. Saunders, 1990, pp 436–451.
8. Matthews DJ, Stempien LM: Orthopedic management of the disabled child. In Sinaki M (ed): Basic Clinical Rehabilitation Medicine. St. Louis, Mosby, 1993, pp 399–411.
9. Sinaki M: Exercise and rehabilitation measures in amyotrophic lateral sclerosis. In Tsubaki T, Yase Y (eds): Amyotrophic Lateral Sclerosis [Excerpta Medica International Congress series 769]. Amsterdam, Elsevier Science Publ., 1988, pp 343–368.
10. Taylor RG, Lieberman JS: Rehabilitation of the patient with diseases affecting the motor unit. In DeLisa JA (ed): Rehabilitation Medicine: Principles and Practice. Philadelphia, J.B. Lippincott, 1988, pp 811–820.

47. MOVEMENT DISORDERS

Kenneth Silver, M.D., and Paul Fishman, M.D., Ph.D.

1. How do movement disorders differ from other motor impairments commonly encountered in rehabilitation medicine, such as with stroke or spinal cord injury?

1. Typically, primary movement disorders are not associated with weakness or sensory loss, as are the other diagnoses.

2. Degenerative diseases are commonly the cause of movement disorders, but infarct, trauma, or pharmacologic agents may also result in characteristic symptoms of insufficient or excessive movements.

3. The predominant area of the brain affected in movement disorders is the basal ganglia, but other pathways or structures may be involved (e.g., the cerebellum).

2. How are the involuntary movement disorders categorized?

By either too little (hypokinetic) or too much movement (hyperkinetic):

Hypokinetic	Hyperkinetic
Parkinson's disease	Tremors
Parkinson-like conditions	Tics
Progressive supranuclear palsy	Gilles de la Tourette syndrome
Drug-induced	Dystonia
Olivopontine-cerebellar degeneration	Dyskinesias (incl. tardive dyskinesias)
Multisystem atrophy, Shy-Drager	Hemifacial spasm
syndrome	Athetosis
Nigrastriatal degeneration	Chorea (incl. Huntington's disease)
	Hemiballismus
	Myoclonus

3. What are the major clinical features of Parkinson's disease?

Resting tremor
Bradykinesia (slowness of movement)
Rigidity (increased muscular tone)
Masked facies
Stooped posture
Hypometria (reduction of the amplitude of movements)
Hypophonia (soft monotone speech)
Micrographia (small, less legible handwriting)
Slowed walking
Reduced stride length
Turning "en bloc" (pivoting is replaced with a series of small steps)

4. Who gets Parkinson's disease?

Older people. Its frequency is 20/100,000 in the general population and 1% in those over age 65. Although the cause of Parkinson's disease is unknown, people with a history of exposure to pesticides and herbicides (as in farmers) appear to be at increased risk.

5. How does Parkinson's usually begin?

The most common initial symptom is **tremor**, typically of the hand, which goes away when the limb is in motion. Activities that involve other limbs, such as walking, usually increase the tremor. Patients may feel clumsy or weak as well as slow and stiff. Certain normal activities, such as dressing (particularly buttoning), shaving, cutting food, and writing, become more difficult. Family members may notice the patient's appearance and feel that he or she is "depressed."

6. What other conditions can look like Parkinson's disease?
1. **Drug-induced parkinsonism:** symptoms identical to Parkinson's disease, with prominent tremor
2. **Shy-Drager syndrome:** autonomic failure with prominent postural hypotension
3. **Progressive supranuclear palsy** (PSP): reduction in vertical gaze and slowing of eye movements
4. **Vascular parkinsonism:** early dementia with brisk tendon reflexes
5. **Multiple head trauma—"parkinsonism pugilistica":** early dementia with brisk tendon reflexes
6. **Olivopontocerebellar degeneration** (OPCA): prominent intention tremor and ataxia

7. What drugs are associated with drug-induced parkinsonism?
Antipsychotics, such as haloperidol (Haldol) and thioridazine (Mellaril), and **antinausea drugs**, such as metoclopramide (Reglan) and prochlorperazine (Compazine). Symptoms are related to the dose of medication. They develop within days to weeks after starting the medication and resolve within days to weeks after its discontinuation.

8. Which medications are used to treat Parkinson's disease?
L-**Dopa** in combination with **carbidopa (Sinemet)** is the most effective treatment but is usually not the first medication given. Patients develop loss of L-dopa efficacy, usually within 3–5 years, so an effort is made to manage early disease with other medications. Anticholinergic drugs such as **trihexyphenidyl** (Artane) and **amantadine** (Symmetrel) are useful medications in early disease. Although its effect in early disease is controversial, the monoamine oxidase inhibitor **deprenyl** (selegiline, Eldepryl) is widely given to newly diagnosed patients.

Within 1–2 years, most patients will have sufficient difficulties with movement and ADLs to require L-dopa. A common starting dose is 25/100 bid (25 mg carbidopa, 100 mg L-dopa). As the disease progresses, the improvement seen with each dose seems to "wear off" before the next dose. Gradually, the frequency of dosing as well as the total dose needed will increase, along with the need for other adjunctive medications (e.g., the dopamine agonists bromocriptine and pergolide).

9. What are the common side effects of drug treatment in Parkinson's disease?
The commonest side effects of L-dopa are **nausea, abdominal cramping**, and **diarrhea**. These side effects are significantly reduced when L-dopa is given in combination with carbidopa, a peripheral decarboxylase inhibitor that prevents the peripheral conversion of the levodopa to dopamine. Pergolide and bromocriptine can cause nausea more frequently than the L-dopa/carbidopa combination. All anti-Parkinson drugs cause **postural hypotension**, which can reach symptomatic levels. Virtually all antiparkinson drugs can cause **confusion**, hallucinations, and even psychosis.

10. Describe the usual course of Parkinson's disease.
Parkinson's disease usually begins in one limb, but all eventually become affected. Most patients have increasing disability, despite medical treatment, within 3–5 years of diagnosis. In moderately affected patients, gait and postural stability become impaired. Patients with more advanced disease can also have sudden loss of action of L-dopa (**freezing**) at times not simply related to end-of-dose (**on-off syndrome**). Involuntary jerking and twisting movements (dyskinesias) can result from medication dose increases. Advanced patients move frequently from periods of relative immobility ("off" or akinesia) to normal mobility ("on"). Stooped posture and permanent kyphosis can occur after years of disease. Freezing, loss of postural stability (with falling), stooping with kyphosis, and dementia respond poorly to drug therapy. Depression, commonly seen in Parkinson's patients, improves with standard antidepressants such as the tricyclics or the serotonin re-uptake inhibitors, though not usually with L-dopa.

11. What are the causes of disability in Parkinson's disease?

Even mildly affected patients require additional effort to perform many physical activities, leading to declining efficiency at work and abandonment of leisure activities. Manual dexterity is invariably impaired as Parkinson's worsens, affecting many ADLs. Social isolation, often due to changes in physical appearance, is common.

Walking becomes impaired as the disease progresses. Postural alterations include increased neck, trunk, and hip flexion, which, coupled with a decrease in righting and equilibrium reactions, lead to balance deficits and an increased risk of falling. Slowing of gait is typically seen, with difficulty turning and a tendency toward short, shuffling steps. Worsening proximal muscle rigidity significantly reduces trunk rotation and arm swing. Affected persons tend to stagger backwards (retropulsion) when pushed from the front; when pushed from the back, they stumble forward (propulsion) and similarly with lateral forces. The risk of falls is exacerbated by the tendency of the feet to "freeze" when confronted with a complex spatial task. Attempts to increase speed of walking result in more rapid stepping, but not in increased stride length.

12. What characteristics of the person with Parkinson's disease should be emphasized in the rehab evaluation?

1. Assess the degree of rigidity and bradykinesia and how these symptoms interfere with ADLs. Established scales for Parkinson's disease, such as the Unified Parkinson's Disease Rating Scale (UPDRS), can be used. Note not only which tasks can be performed, but how long is required.

2. Gauge the general pattern of gait, including walking speed and distance. Forward and backward stepping as well as the ability to navigate obstacles need to be checked.

3. Periodically assess fine motor tasks such as writing.

4. Measure and record restrictions in joint mobility, particularly hips, knees, shoulders and trunk.

5. Analyze equilibrium, including tandem walking.

6. Evaluate ability to perform simultaneous and sequential tasks (Parkinson's patients have difficulty in performing complex movements).

7. Test cognitive function and swallowing if clinically indicated.

13. Which occupational therapy strategies can help the person with Parkinson's?

OT can provide vital input for maintaining the home, vocational, leisure, and transportation capabilities of the patient. **Adaptive equipment** is provided when deficits in upper-extremity control limit efficient and safe function. For instance, plate-guards or specialized dishes, weighted or large-handled cups and utensils, and swivel forks and spoons can help with feeding. Buttons on clothing can be replaced with Velcro or zipper closures.

Environmental aids can help keep the person productive at work. Workplace adaptations to accommodate for Parkinson's-related impairments and disabilities may include equipment to support writing (built-up pens and forearm supports) and typing skills (electronic keyboards and computerized scanning and pointing devices), as well as power mobility devices (scooters or wheelchairs).

The slowing of motor responses as the disease worsens may place these patients at risk when driving. OTs can help assess and retrain patients in driving skills, particularly extremity reaction timing and visual field scanning. Families should be counseled to have the patient undergo driver's testing and training early when mobility and ADL performance first begin to suffer.

14. What are the nonparkinsonian tremors? How are they classified?

Tremor, the most common form of involuntary movement disorder, is characterized by rhythmic oscillations of a body part. Tremors that are worst at **rest** are exclusively associated with Parkinson's disease or other parkinsonian states. The **movement** tremors can be classified as to the situation in which they are most prominent:

1. **Postural or static tremor** occurs with maintained posture; it is tested by holding the arms out in front. Examples include physiologic tremor, essential (familial or senile) tremor, tremor of basal ganglia disease, tremor of peripheral neuropathy, and alcoholic tremor.

2. **Kinetic or intentional tremor** occurs with movement from point to point; it is tested by the finger-to-nose maneuver. Examples include cerebellar tremor and rubral tremor.

3. **Task-specific tremor** occurs only with a specific type of movement. Examples include writing tremor, vocal tremor, or orthostatic tremor.

15. Are physiologic tremors worrisome?

No, they are usually of no clinical significance. Often they increase or are precipitated by emotional stress, are aggravated by fatigue, hypoglycemia, thyrotoxicosis, exercise, alcohol withdrawal, and fever, and can be drug-induced (caffeine, theophylline, lithium). They can be treated by educating the patient to avoid precipitating conditions.

16. How are other tremors treated?

The most useful medications are **propranolol,** the anticonvulsant **primidone,** and the benzodiazepine **clonazepam.** Measures to reduce or alleviate anxiety are useful, as are strategies to dampen oscillation excursion with weights or other mechanical compensations.

17. What is the physiologic basis for tics?

This is largely unknown. They are sustained nonrhythmic muscle contractions that are rapid and stereotyped, often occurring in the same extremity or body part during times of stress. Usually, the muscles of the face and neck are involved, with a rotational movement away from the body's midline. They are often seen in otherwise normal children, predominantly males, between ages 5 and 10 and usually disappear by the end of adolescence. Tics result in minimal physical impairment and disability but may cause social consequences and handicaps. Tics can be seen as representing a spectrum of disease from transient to chronic disorder, with Tourette's syndrome lying somewhere on that spectrum.

18. Describe some of the aspects of Gilles de la Tourette syndrome.

The most notable aspect is the involuntary use of obscenities (**coprolalia**) and obscene gestures (**coproraxia**), yet this may be mild and transient and occurs only in a minority of afflicted persons. Other features include vocal and motor tics, echolalia, loud cries, and yips. The tics can begin with the eyes or as a facial grimace, but can involve the head, neck, trunk or legs. Some affected individuals have few symptoms, while others can be quite handicapped. The tics may not always be present, having a waxing and waning quality, and the patient may be able to voluntarily suppress them.

19. How are the dystonias distinguished from other movement disorders?

Dystonias are slow, sustained contractions of muscles that frequently cause twisting movements or abnormal postures. The disorder resembles athetosis but shows a more sustained isometric contraction. When rapid movements are involved, they are usually repetitive and continuous. The movements are a result of simultaneous co-contraction of agonists and antagonists. Dystonia often increases with emotional or physical stress, anxiety, pain, or fatigue and disappears with sleep. Therefore, symptom severity can vary through the day. Patients often develop methods to self-inhibit or diminish the dystonic movements by changing posture or touching the affected body part.

20. How are the dystonias classified?

Usually by the distribution of affected muscles. **Focal** dystonias include torticollis (neck), blepharospasm (periorbital), oromandibular (mouth/jaw), and writer's or occupational cramp (arm/leg). **Segmental** dystonias begin in one body part and spread to another. These are often subdivided into cranial, axial, brachial (arm), or crural (leg) distributions. **Multifocal** dystonias occur in more than one body part (e.g., torticollis plus leg dystonia) or may be generalized, such as dystonia musculorum deformans.

21. Describe spasmodic torticollis.

Spasmodic torticollis is the most common focal dystonia, affecting predominantly women in their fourth or fifth decade. It most frequently involves the sternocleidomastoid, trapezius, scalenes, and posterior neck muscles in an asymmetric pattern. The movement can be tonic or intermittent with head rotation, or it can assume a predominantly forward (antecolic) or backward (retrocolic) position. Symptoms can be lessened with certain gestures of the hands to the head (e.g., lightly touching the chin with a finger) and are worsened by prolonged standing and walking or with stress or fatigue. Associated pain is common. Complete or partial remissions can occur.

Social stigmatization is a major concern, as is functional disability which can include driving, reading, or activities that involve looking down and using the hands. Primary treatment remains pharmacologic, especially intramuscular injection of botulinum toxin. Rehabilitation management includes pain control, stretching tight musculature, and trigger point injections. Exercises to strengthen contralateral, uninvolved muscles and reciprocally inhibit involved ones have been used, but some feel this worsens symptoms. Biofeedback has been used but is not routinely effective.

22. Describe some of the other common dystonias.

Blepharospasm is characterized by intermittent contractions of the orbicularis oculi. Early presentation may be as uncontrolled, excessive blinking from presumed eye irritation, but the condition progresses to irregular and more forceful and sustained closure of the lids.

Writer's or **occupational cramp** involves the dominant hand and wrist and appears during certain activities, such as writing, typing, or playing a musical instrument. It presents with onset of a specific activity as an uncontrollably tight grip, accompanied by flexion of the wrist. Jerking or sustained movements are often associated.

Oromandibular dystonia involves muscles of the tongue, mouth, and jaw, causing the mouth to pull open or forcibly shut. The mentalis and platysma muscles may also be involved.

Dystonia musculorum deformans is a rare hereditary disorder, appearing between ages 5–15, with symptoms of sustained movements with torsional spasms of the pelvis and legs resulting in abnormal gait. Upper extremity, neck, and facial muscles become involved later in the course, and in the more severe forms, progression to death within 5–10 years occurs.

23. What agents are used to treat dystonias?

Detection and correction of an underlying abnormality (drug-induced, structural cause) are the first steps. Among children, a small group (10–20%) may improve with **L-dopa**. Anticholinergics such as **trihexyphenidyl** and **benztropine** are the most effective oral agents for both generalized and focal dystonias. **Baclofen, carbamazepine,** and **clonazepam** are sometimes helpful. Focal dystonias are now commonly treated with **botulinum toxin.**

24. What is hemifacial spasm?

Hemifacial spasm is the most frequent form of the facial hyperkinetic movement disorders. The etiology is generally unknown (vascular compression?), but it usually involves a region of abnormal electrical impulse generation and transmission in the peripheral facial nerve (cranial nerve VII). The spasms, which are tonic, usually begin in the orbicularis oculi and later involve other muscles innervated by CN VII. They are aggravated by stress and fatigue. They are more often seen in women in middle age and can interfere with vision and be socially and psychologically handicapping. Treatment options usually boil down to either surgery for facial nerve decompression (very often successful) or botulinum toxin injection.

25. What causes tardive dyskinesia (TD)?

TD is characterized by involuntary, choreiform movements of the face and tongue associated with chronic use of neuroleptic medication. Common movements include chewing, sucking, mouthing, licking, "fly-catching movements," puckering, or smacking (buccal-lingual-masticatory syndrome). Choreiform movements of the trunk and extremities can also occur along with dystonic movements of the neck and trunk. TD is seen in up to 20% of patients treated chronically with neuroleptics (dopamine antagonists) and probably represents hypersensitivity of dopamine receptors and overactivity of the dopamine system due to long-term dopamine receptor blockade. Duration of treatment, dose, and patient age are risk factors for the development of TD. Resolution of TD after withdrawal of neuroleptic drugs is slow and incomplete, with half of TD patients still symptomatic a year after drug discontinuation.

26. Define akathisia and rabbit syndrome.

Akathisia is the state of motor restlessness accompanied by a sensation of unpleasant, dysphoric inner tension or anxiety (unable to sit still, shifting in their seats, rocking, shaking legs, or pacing) induced by antipsychotic medications. It is felt to be an extrapyramidal reaction to dopamine blockade and can occur in 20–40% of patients on antipsychotic drugs.

Rabbit syndrome also can develop after long-term use of antipsychotics in 2–5% of users. It is characterized by fine, rhythmic lip movements that resemble a rabbit's chewing. It usually resolves with the use of anticholinergic medication.

27. What causes ataxia? How can it be treated?

The cerebellum plays an important role in monitoring movement and modulating motor control. When cerebellar disease occurs, a spectrum of symptoms may result, including disequilibrium, tremor during voluntary movement, reflex changes, and disturbances in timing and coordination (**ataxia**). Common causes include stroke, multiple sclerosis, and toxicity (alcohol). Slowly progressive ataxia may represent a group of hereditary disorders.

The response to drug therapy has been poor. The mainstay of treatment is **occupational therapy** to develop compensatory techniques for performing basic self-care and occupational activities. Weighted bracelets or similar devices can dampen limb oscillations by increasing mass. Gait training and education in the use of assistive devices for walking can prevent falls and enhance mobility.

28. How do athetosis, chorea, and hemiballismus differ?

Athetosis: Involuntary, slow, writhing, and repetitious movements; slower than choreiform movements and less sustained than dystonia; usually involves the face and distal upper extremities. Onset may be idiopathic, but often secondary to another neurologic disease, such as stroke, tumor, or Wilson's disease.

Chorea: Nonstereotyped, complex, unpredictable, and jerky movements that interfere with purposeful motion; can affect any or all body parts, but usually the oral structures, causing abnormal speech and respiratory patterns; may occur in almost any disease affecting the CNS or be secondary to anti-Parkinson's medication. The most familiar, generalized form is **Huntington's disease**.

Hemiballismus: An uncommon disorder consisting of extremely violent flinging of the arms and legs on one side of the body; usually secondary to hemorrhage or infarction of the contralateral subthalamic nucleus.

29. What is Huntington's chorea?

Chorea means *to dance*, and the gait in these patients takes on an ataxic, dancing appearance. Huntington's disease unfortunately is a terminal disorder involving involuntary, choreiform movements that are abrupt and purposeless and associated with progressive dementia. It is an autosomal dominant disorder affecting 4–6 persons/100,000 population and reached the public's attention as afflicting Woody Guthrie, the well-known American folksinger. Symptom onset can range from childhood to the eighth decade, but most individuals become affected after age 30. The abnormal movements begin in the fingers, toes, and facial regions, often with dysarthria, teeth grinding, and facial grimacing. With time, movements become less choreiform and more parkinsonian and dystonic (i.e., restricted motions, immobility and unsteadiness of gait). Dementia and psychosis invariably occur and progress rapidly to become the most disabling features. The rate of suicide among these patients is 2,000 times the national average. Symptoms progress over a 10–25-year period and death is usually by aspiration pneumonia.

30. What is myoclonus?

Myoclonus is one of the most common involuntary movement disorders of CNS origin. It is characterized by sudden, jerky, irregular, or periodic contractions of a muscle or group of muscles. It can be subdivided into **reflex myoclonus** that is stimulus-sensitive, appearing with volitional movement, muscle stretch, or superficial stimuli like touch; or **nonspontaneous myoclonus**, which is non-stimulus-sensitive and occurs at rest.

31. What are the different types of myoclonus?

Etiologically, myoclonus can be classified as one of four types:

Physiologic—occurring in normals while falling asleep, walking, or with anxiety (e.g., sleep jerks and hiccups)

Essential—increasing with activity; sometimes disabling but without neurologic deficit

Epileptic—associated with generalized seizures, as in juvenile myoclonic epilepsy

Symptomatic—part of a more widespread neurologic disorder, such as encephalopathy or stroke. For example, **spinal myoclonus** involves a group of muscles innervated by a certain spinal segment (segmental myoclonus) and can be associated with spinal cord disease, such as trauma, multiple sclerosis, and tumors.

BIBLIOGRAPHY

1. Duvaisin R: Parkinson's Disease: A Guide for Patients and Families. New York, Raven Press, 1991.
2. Elbe R, Koller W: Tremor. Baltimore, Johns Hopkins Press, 1990.
3. Hallett M: Classification and treatment of tumor. JAMA 266:1115, 1991.
4. Jankovic J, Hallett M: Therapy with Botulinum Toxin. New York, Marcel Dekker, 1994.
5. Johnson R, Griffen J (eds): Current Therapy in Neurologic Disease. St. Louis, Mosby, 1993.
6. Melnick M: Basal ganglial disorders. In Umphred DA (ed): Neurological Rehabilitation. St. Louis, Mosby, 1995, pp 606–640.
7. Pentland B: Parkinsonism and dystonia. In Greenwood R, Barnes M, McMillan T, Ward C (eds): Neurological Rehabilitation. London, Churchill Livingstone, 1993, pp 474–485.
8. Weiner W, Lang A: Movement Disorders. New York, Futura, 1989.

---

48. THE SHOULDER

Rene Cailliet, M.D.

---

1. What are the two most common categories of shoulder injury?
External trauma (impact injury) and overuse syndromes (repetitive injuries).

2. What are the key structures of the shoulder complex that are susceptible to pain and injury?
The glenohumeral, acromioclavicular, scapulocostal, and claviculosternal joints and the bicipital tendon are commonly the source of pain and impairment. (The term *shoulder complex* is considered more descriptive than *shoulder joint*.)

3. Identify the most frequent causes of shoulder pain.
The **impingement syndrome** (entrapment syndrome) is probably the most common. As the arm is abducted, the head of the humerus glides down the glenoid fossa, and by concurrent external rotation (with abduction), the greater tuberosity passes behind the overhanging acromium. Repeated overhead arm elevation causes the greater tuberosity to impinge on the acromium and undergo deterioration.

In **acute tendinitis**, the arm can abduct to 60° without significant pain. There is pain from 60–120° of abduction. As the humerus has externally rotated (placing the greater tuberosity behind the acromium), the remaining elevation to 180° is pain-free if there is no capsular contraction.

Within the glenohumeral joint are numerous other tissues that are nociceptive.

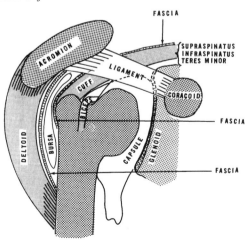

Contents of glenohumeral joint. (From Cailliet R: Shoulder Pain, 3rd ed. Philadelphia, F.A. Davis, 1991, with permission.)

4. How can you differentiate clinically between a completely torn supraspinatus tendon and one that is partially torn or frayed?

When the tendon is frayed and/or irritated, the arm does not abduct or forward flex past the horizontal range, but it can be held there once achieved. When the tendon is completely torn, the arm does not abduct or forward flex and, when placed in that position, cannot be held for more than a brief period of time.

5. Name the individual muscles comprising the rotator cuff.

S—Supraspinatus

I—Infraspinatus

T—Teres minor

S—Subscapularis

6. What role does each of the rotator cuff muscles play during shoulder abduction?

Supraspinatus—helps to pull the humeral head into the glenoid cavity and slightly rotates the humerus into abduction.

Infraspinatus—rotates the humeral head and pulls it down slightly.

Subscapularis—acts to internally rotate the humerus around its longitudinal axis and to pull the head of the humerus into the glenoid.

Teres minor—exerts a pull in a downward fashion.

7. What is the drop arm test?

With a complete tear of the rotator cuff, the arm, when passively abducted, can be held momentarily and weakly by the deltoid muscles. Since there is no stabilization of the humerus within the glenoid fossa by the cuff muscles, the arm gradually drops. This clinical sign is indicative of a complete cuff tear.

8. Aside from faulty shoulder abduction, is there another test to determine the presence of a complete rotator cuff tear?

Yes. Since a portion of the rotator cuff is represented by the tendinous insertion into the tuberosity of the supraspinatus and infraspinatus muscles, in a complete tear, active external rotation of the arm is not possible.

9. Are diagnostic tests always necessary to determine rotator cuff disease?

No. Rotator cuff tears can often be detected clinically, although MRI or arthrographic studies will help to confirm the extent of the tear.

10. A patient presents to your office with a painful arc in abduction. Is the diagnosis tendinitis or bursitis?

To fully understand the answer to this question, consult your local anatomy book! Since the inner sheath of the supraspinatus bursa is the same as the outer sheath of the tendon, either tendinitis *or* bursitis or *both* may be the culprit!

11. Besides rotator cuff disease, what other differential diagnostic possibilities must be considered in evaluating shoulder pain?

Suprascapular nerve entrapment	Thoracic outlet syndrome
Shoulder instability	Cervical radiculitis
Acromioclavicular degenerative joint disease	Bicipital tendinitis

12. Can other painful joints of the shoulder be clinically diagnosed?

Yes! When the acromioclavicular joint is injured, it becomes tender to palpation and undergoes painful crepitation in scapular elevation and circumduction. An analgesic injection into the joint is diagnostic as well as therapeutic.

13. How should acute glenohumeral joint limitation be treated in order to prevent undesirable sequela?

Early elimination of pain through ice application, oral anti-inflammatory medication, intra-articular analgesic injection, and possibly, steroid injection are helpful measures. The most important strategy, however, is to begin active-passive joint movement to prevent a frozen shoulder.

14. Suggest a convenient way of initiating active-passive shoulder movement.

Pendulum (Codman's) exercises are a simple way of instituting active-passive motion of the glenohumeral joint. This is best achieved with the patient bent forward, with the arm in the dependent (pendular) position and the body "actively" moving to "passively" move the pendular arm.

15. What is meant by the term *frozen shoulder*?

Inflammation of the tissues within the glenohumeral joint can result in adhesive capsulitis or adhesive bursitis. The term *adhesive* implies that the synovial tissue of the capsule and the bursa become adherent, which results in a *frozen* ability to move the glenohumeral joint.

16. In evaluating the sequela of a painful shoulder and/or adhesive capsulitis, why is it important for the examiner to inspect the rest of the arm and hand carefully?

The shoulder-hand syndrome is one of the most serious manifestations of reflex sympathetic dystrophy. Often, swelling of the hand, albeit minimal soft tissue edema, is an early indication of this syndrome.

17. In the advent of a frozen shoulder, must surgery be immediately advocated?

Not immediately, as many frozen shoulders respond to intensive conservative treatment. Manual mobilization and manipulation are effective in treating this condition.

18. Is posture a factor in the painful shoulder?

Most assuredly. A rounded upper back (kyphosis) causes the overhanging acromium to move downward and cause a greater incidence of impingement of the cuff tendon.

19. Is shoulder pain ever a site of referred pain?

Cervical radiculitis refers to the shoulder area and must be ruled out.

20. In the setting of a complete brachial plexus disruption, what is the ideal (most functional) way of performing a shoulder fusion procedure?

Generally, it is agreed that fixation of the shoulder in flexion, abduction, and internal rotation will facilitate function, although the precise degree is debated.

21. Why does shoulder dislocation occur?

The shoulder dislocates because of its unusual anatomy, including lax ligaments, shallow glenoid cavity, and redundant capsule. Anterior dislocation is more common than posterior dislocation. The coracoclavicular ligament is usually torn in forcible dislocation of the shoulder.

22. What is the scapulohumeral rhythm?

Well, it certainly is not a new pop song! Scapulohumeral rhythm refers to the balanced contribution of glenohumeral and scapulothoracic joint movement during arm abduction. During abduction, scapulothoracic movement contributes 69° and glenohumeral motion contributes 120° to abduction of the arm by the shoulder complex. This 2:1 rhythm is important because scapulothoracic migration is required to rotate the position of the glenoid to permit glenohumeral abduction *without acromial impingement*. The normal shoulder capsule is redundant (has slack), permitting the humeral head to drop into interiorly on the glenoid labrum (lip).

23. What is shoulder subluxation? Why does it occur in the hemiplegic patient?

Shoulder subluxation is characterized by the presence of a palpable gap between the acromion and humeral head. Although there are few objective standardized radiologic or clinical criteria for diagnosing subluxation, the examiner often measures severity in terms of fingerbreadths.

Changes in the mechanical integrity of the glenohumeral joint may cause subluxation. While the exact cause of subluxation is not known, several factors are thought to play a role in compromising glenohumeral stability, including the angulation of the glenoid fossa, the influence of the supraspinatus muscle on humeral head seating, the support of the scapula on the rib cage, and contraction of the deltoid and rotator cuff muscles on the abducted humerus.

24. How do you treat shoulder subluxation?

While a variety of slings are touted for subluxation treatment, their use is frequently controversial. An ill-fitting sling or one that fails to mechanically realign the humeral head into the glenoid fossa can exacerbate flexion synergy patterns, placing the patient at risk for contracture. A sling can be used for protection of the flaccid hemiplegic arm during ambulation but can also interfere with balance and standing activities. Shoulder subluxation can often be managed through optimal arm positioning on the wheelchair armrest, lapboard, or forearm trough.

25. What are the other sources of shoulder pain in the hemiplegic?

Shoulder pain, while uncommonly associated with subluxation, may originate from unrelated pathology including rotator cuff tear, prior musculoskeletal injury, bicipital tendinitis, adhesive capsulitis, arthritis, and subdeltoid bursitis. Other causes of shoulder pain in the stroke patient include shoulder capsule stretching secondary to disuse, shoulder-hand syndrome, and thalamic syndrome.

26. Describe the three stages of the shoulder-hand syndrome.

During the **acute stage**, the shoulder-hand syndrome is variably known as sympathetically maintained pain syndrome, causalgia, and reflex sympathetic dystrophy. The patient presents with shoulder and/or wrist pain, periarticular edema, and vasomotor changes (i.e., skin temperature changes, color changes, sweating).

This can progress to a **dystrophic stage** highlighted by intensification of pain, decreased nail growth, brawny edema, loss of range of motion, atrophy, and osteopenia.

The end stage, or atrophic stage, is manifested by less pain; joint contracture; cool, pale, cyanotic, glassy skin; muscle wasting; bone demineralization; tapering digits; and alteration in edema.

27. How is shoulder-hand syndrome prevented and treated?

Prevention can be achieved through proper alignment and mobilization of the plegic upper extremity, prevention of shoulder subluxation, hand splinting, and ranging of the upper extremity. Once edema develops, arm elevation, retrograde massage, and compression devices can be implemented. The goal is to avoid the onset of pain

When shoulder-hand syndrome has progressed to its maximal state, aggressive management including the addition of modality intervention (heat, cold, contrast baths, TENS, and ultrasound), pharmacologic intervention (NSAIDs, oral prednisone, calcitonin), and anesthetic and steroid injections into the painful shoulder may be of benefit. For more severe pain, sympathetic blockade may be needed. The use of psychologic counseling should be used early on in refractory cases.

"It is easier not to allow the seed of pain to be planted than to uproot the entire tree."

BIBLIOGRAPHY

1. Andren L, Lundberg BJ: Treatment of rigid shoulders by joint distention during arthrography. Acta Orthop Scand 36:45, 1965.
2. Cailliet R: Shoulder Pain, 3rd ed. Philadelphia, F.A. Davis, 1991.
3. Grey RG: The natural history of "idiopathic" frozen shoulder. J Bone Joint Surg 60A:564, 1978.
4. MacNab I: Rotator cuff tendinitis. Ann R Coll Surg 53:271, 1973.

5. Neer CS: Impingement lesions. Clin Orthop 173:70, 1983.
6. Stiens SA, Goldstein BA: Rehabilitation after overuse injuries of the shoulder. In Gordon S (ed): Overuse Injury of the Upper Extremity. American Academy of Orthopedic Surgeons NIH Symposium Series, Repetitive Motion Disorders of the Upper Extremity, 1995, pp 517–537.
7. Stiens SA, Haselkorn JK, Peters DJ, Goldstein B: Rehabilitation intervention for patients with upper extremity dysfunction: Challenges of outcome evaluation. Am J Ind Med 29:590–601, 1996.

49. THE ELBOW

Ramon Vallarino, Jr., M.D., and Francisco H. Santiago, M.D.

1. Name the articulations comprising the elbow joint.
Humeroulnar joint, humeroradial joint, and proximal radioulnar joint.

2. Describe the functions of the elbow.
• Positions the hand in space for functional activities.
• Effectively lengthens and shortens the upper extremity.
• Helps stabilize the upper extremity for power and detailed work activities.
• Provides power to the arm for lifting.

3. What is the carrying angle of the elbow?
The carrying angle refers to the normal anatomic valgus angulation between the upper arm and forearm when the elbow is fully extended. Normally, the angle is 5–10% in males and 10–15% in females. A carrying angle of > 20% is considered abnormal.

4. What is a gunstock deformity of the arm?
This refers to a cubitus varus deformity of the elbow, usually secondary to fractures or epiphyseal injury to the distal humerus.

5. Which muscles originate at the medial epicondyle?

Flexor carpi radialis	Flexor digitorum superficialis
Flexor carpi ulnaris	Flexor digitorum profundus
Palmaris longus	Pronator teres

6. Which muscles originate at the lateral epicondyle?

Extensor carpi radialis	Extensor digitorum communis
Extensor carpi radialis longus	Supinator
Extensor carpi ulnaris	Anconeus

7. Describe the ligamentous support of the elbow.
• Medially by the ulnar collateral ligament.
• Laterally by the radial collateral ligament.
• Annular ligament, which holds the head of the radius in proper position in relation to the ulna and humerus.

8. Is there a normal functional position of the elbow?
Yes. The elbow is in 90° of flexion with the forearm midway between supination and pronation. In this position, the olecranon process of the ulna and the medial and lateral epicondyles of the humerus normally form an isosceles triangle when viewed posteriorly—this is known as the **triangle sign**. If there is a fracture or dislocation or a degeneration leading to loss of bone and/or cartilage, the distance between the apex and base decreases, and the isosceles triangle no longer exists.

9. What is the most common congenital anomaly around the elbow?
Congenital radial head dislocation.

10. Describe Panner disease.
Panner disease is a condition of unclear etiology in which there is osteochondrosis of the capitellum. It is seen most often in young boys who complain of tenderness and swelling over the lateral aspect of the elbow with limited extension. Radiographs show patchy areas of sclerosis and lucency, which may appear to be fragmented. Treatment includes immobilization with a long-arm cast followed by protected motion. Patients may be left with an elbow flexion contracture.

11. What is osteochondritis dissecans of the elbow?
This is an idiopathic condition affecting the capitellum of the humerus, with ensuing avascular necrosis. It is usually seen in the dominant arm of teenage boys, especially ones involved in throwing sports. It is characterized by poorly localized elbow pain, and the radial head is sometimes involved. Treatment includes immobilization followed by gentle range of motion. Rapid, forceful movements are to be avoided.

12. Describe tennis elbow.
This term has traditionally been used to describe numerous symptoms around the elbow. Presently, it is most commonly used in reference to **lateral epicondylitis**, in which the extensor carpi radialis brevis is affected by repetitive strain injury.

13. What is Cozen's test?
This test is used in the physical examination to confirm the presence of lateral epicondylitis. The examiner stabilizes the elbow with a thumb over the lateral epicondyle. The patient is asked to make a fist, pronate the forearm, and radially deviate and extend the wrist against resistance. This causes pain in the lateral epicondyle.

14. What is the radial tunnel syndrome?
This condition is associated with a resistant tennis elbow in which the posterior interosseous nerve is entrapped in the lateral aspect of the proximal forearm. There is pain in the lateral elbow and weakness in the extensors.

15. What is usually responsible for golfer's elbow?
Repetitive strain injury of the flexor-pronator musculature at or near its insertion on the medial epicondyle, causing medial epicondylitis.

16. How do you test for golfer's elbow?
The examiner resists wrist flexion and forearm pronation, causing medial epicondyle pain.

17. Is there a boxer's elbow? What causes it?
Yes. This condition, otherwise known as hyperextension overload syndrome or olecranon impingement syndrome, is caused by repetitive valgus extension of the elbow in the boxer's jab or in sports that involve throwing.

18. What is little leaguer's elbow?
An injury occurring in children and adolescents in which the medial epicondyle is inflamed and there is partial separation of the apophysis. Radiographs are important in the diagnostic evaluation to rule out an avulsion fracture of the medial epicondyle, which must be corrected surgically.

19. Where does ulnar nerve entrapment at the elbow typically occur?
The cubital tunnel, which is a passageway formed by the two heads of the ulnar collateral ligament and the tendon of the flexor carpi ulnaris. The patient complains of tingling or paresthesias

in the ulnar nerve distribution of the forearm and hand. These symptoms may be exacerbated when the elbow is held in a flexed position for 5 minutes (elbow flexion test).

20. What is draftsman's elbow?

Inflammation of the olecranon bursa, which may be secondary to a number of conditions, including repetitive or acute trauma, rheumatoid arthritis, gout, and pseudogout. It is also known as student's elbow and miner's elbow. There is pain posteriorly around the olecranon and swelling when compared to the opposite elbow. A septic bursa must be ruled out by aspiration of its fluid, followed by Gram stain and culture. Radiographs are useful for finding bone spurs and to rule out osteomyelitis. Treatment of nonseptic olecranon bursitis includes protective padding, NSAIDs, maintenance of functional range of motion, and occasional drainage.

21. What is a "pushed" elbow? "Pulled" elbow?

A pushed elbow describes subluxation of the radial head in a proximal direction, which is often seen after a person falls on an outstretched hand. The radial head impinges on the capitellum. It is occasionally associated with Colles' fracture. Treatment consists of traction and repetitive stretching.

A pulled elbow is subluxation of the radial head in a distal direction, which may follow a forceful traction to the forearm. Common in children, this condition produces limited supination and elbow pain.

22. When is the balanced forearm orthosis used?

To assist both elbow and shoulder function in the presence of profound weakness and/or pain of the upper extremity. It consists of a trough in which the proximal portion of the forearm rests. A pivot and linkage system underneath the trough can be adjusted and preset so that the patient can learn to use the upper extremity functionally.

23. What is unique about the brachioradialis muscle?

It is the only muscle producing flexion of the elbow that is not supplied by the musculocutaneous nerve. Rather, it is supplied by the radial nerve.

BIBLIOGRAPHY

1. Andrews JR, Whiteside JA, Wilke KE: Rehabilitation of throwing and racquet sport injuries. In Buschbacher RJ, Braddom RL (eds): Sports Medicine and Rehabilitation: A Sports-Specific Approach. Philadelphia, Hanley & Belfus, 1994, pp 47–65.
2. Braddom RL (ed): Physical Medicine & Rehabilitation. Philadelphia, W.B. Saunders, 1995, pp 771–781.
3. Hoppenfeld S: Physical Exam of the Spine and Extremities. Norwalk, CT, Appleton & Lange, 1976.
4. Kottke F, Lehmann J: Krusen's Handbook of Physical Medicine & Rehabilitation, 4th ed. Philadelphia, W.B. Saunders, 1990.
5. Magee DJ: Orthopedic Physical Assessment, 2nd ed. Philadelphia, W.B. Saunders, 1992, pp 143–167.
6. Weinstein S, Buckwalter J: Turek's Orthopaedics, 5th ed. Philadelphia, J.B. Lippincott, 1994, pp 401–416.

50. THE HAND

Francisco H. Santiago, M.D., and Jaywant J. P. Patil, M.B.B.S., F.R.C.P.C.

1. Name the eight carpal bones.

As they say, "scared lovers try positions that they cannot handle." Which translated means:

S = Scaphoid   T = The anticonvulsant
L = Lunate   T = Trapezoid
T = Triquetrum   C = Capitate
P = Pisiform   H = Hamate

2. Describe the contents of the 6 dorsal compartments of the hand.

The 6 dorsal compartments contain extensor tendons to the hand. From radial to ulnar, they are as follows:

1. Abductor pollicis longus, extensor hallucis brevis
2. Extensor carpi radialis longus, extensor carpi radialis brevis
3. Extensor pollicis longus
4. Extensor digitorum communis, extensor indices proprius
5. Extensor digiti minimi
6. Extensor carpi ulnaris

3. What are the key actions of the interossei muscles?

Remember *dab* and *pad:*

Dab = Dorsal interossei—Abduct and assist in metacarpophalangeal (MCP) flexion.
Pad = Palmar interossei—Adduct and assist in MCP flexion.

4. What structures make up the borders of the anatomic snuff box?

Floor: scaphoid bone
Radial border: abductor pollicis longus and extensor pollicis brevis muscles
Ulnar border: extensor pollicis longus

5. How is the function of the lumbrical muscles related to its anatomy?

Since the lumbrical muscles originate from the tendons of the flexor digitorum profundus and insert into the extensor hood tendons, their main action is flexion of the MCP joints and extension at the interphalangeal joints.

6. Where is "no man's land" in the hand?

It is the area of the hand where the flexor tendons (i.e., the flexor profundus and sublimis) are tightly enclosed within the tenosynovium. It is located in the palm between the distal palmar crease and the crease of the proximal interphalangeal (PIP) joints. Generally, primary repair of the tendons in this region is contraindicated. (See also Chapter 60).

7. Define deQuervain's disease.

Tenosynovitis of the extensor pollicis brevis and abductor pollicis longus tendons can result from direct injury or repetitive activity and may be associated with arthritis. Thickening of the tendon sheath often results in stenosis of the tenosynovium and inflammation. Pinching, gripping, and wrist and thumb movements are associated with pain, and there is tenderness over the tendon on the radial side of the wrist. The patient's symptoms often can be reproduced by the Finkelstein's test (see question 23). There may also be swelling over the involved tendon on the radial side of the wrist.

8. What is a trigger finger?

Trigger finger occurs secondary to tenosynovitis involving the flexor tendon sheaths. The usual presentation is a fusiform swelling around the area of the flexor sublimis tendon in the vicinity of the metacarpal head. A constriction of the tendon sheath results in locking or obstruction of finger flexion.

Finger locking often occurs in the morning. At times, there is a popping sensation perceived when the fingers go from the flexed to the extended position. This type of trigger finger could be associated with trauma, osteoarthritis, or inflammatory arthritis, such as rheumatoid arthritis.

9. Name the three common deformities associated with rheumatoid arthritis in the hands. Describe the mechanism of the deformities.

Boutonniere deformity. There is hyperextension at the MCP joint, flexion at the PIP joint, and extension at the DIP joint. Often in the rheumatoid process, there is weakness and tearing of the terminal portion of the extensor's hood, which tends to hold the lateral band in place. In this deformity, the lateral bands tend to slip down and flex the PIP joint and exert tension to hyperextend the DIP joint.

Swan-neck deformity. This often occurs as a result of contractures and shortening of the intrinsic muscles causing flexion at the MCP joint, hyperextension at the PIP joint, and flexion at the DIP joint. Contractures and spasm of the intrinsic muscles cause dorsal subluxation of the tendons, resulting in hyperextension of the PIP joint. This hyperextension is further aggravated by synovitis that causes laxity of that joint. Flexion and tension on the long flexor result in flexion of the DIP joint.

Ulnar deviation of the fingers. This deformity is often associated with ulnar deviation of the wrist. Basically, the flexor tendons enter the tunnel of the flexor pulley. In rheumatoid arthritis, the mouth of the tunnel becomes more relaxed, and this results in the flexor tendons' deviating more toward the ulnar side.

10. Where are Herberden's nodes usually found?

These discrete but palpable bony nodules are found on the dorsal and lateral surfaces of the DIP joint and may be features of osteoarthritis. The nodules found in the PIP joint are called Bouchard's nodes.

11. What happens to the flexor pollicis longus in rheumatoid arthritis?

The flexor tendon most commonly ruptures as it rubs over an osteophyte on the volar aspect of the scaphoid trapezial joint.

12. How does a mallet finger occur?

This injury, also called baseball finger or cricket finger, occurs when a sudden unexpected passive flexion of the DIP joint, with the extensor tendon under tension, avulses a fragment of the bone from the base of the distal phalanx into which the tendon is inserted. Alternatively, the extensor tendon may rupture just proximal to its insertion. In either case, the DIP joint remains flexed and can no longer be actively extended. Treatment usually involves splinting the finger with the DIP extended.

13. What is a boxer's fracture?

This injury is more appropriately considered a street fighter's fracture, since it results from an unskillful blow with a clenched fist. It fractures the neck of the fifth metacarpal bone.

14. Describe a Bennett's fracture.

In adults, a longitudinal force along the axis of the first metacarpal in the flexed thumb may produce a serious intra-articular fracture-dislocation of the carpometacarpal joint. A small triangular-shaped fragment at the base of the metacarpal remains in proper relationship to the trapezium, but the remainder of the metacarpal, which carries with it the major portion of the joint surface, is dislocated and assumes a position of flexion.

15. Who usually gets a scaphoid fracture?
Fracture of the carpal scaphoid is relatively common in young adults, particularly males. The responsible injury is usually a fall on the open hand, with the wrist dorsiflexed and radially deviated. This fracture is frequently overlooked at the time of injury and is usually dismissed as a sprain. Scaphoid fracture can be associated with serious complications, including avascular necrosis, delayed union, nonunion, and post-traumatic degenerative joint disease.

16. Who gets Keinbock's disease?
Osteochondrosis or avascular necrosis of the lunate occurs most frequently in young adults and may be secondary to trauma. Workers such as carpenters and riveters are often affected.

17. How could a gamekeeper and a skier possibly develop the same sort of thumb injury?
Both gamekeeper's thumb and skier's thumb are caused by forcible abduction of the thumb associated with injury to the ulnar collateral ligament of the first MCP. Gamekeeper's thumb earned its name from British gamekeepers who sustained this injury when killing rabbits (with a ski pole?). A skier who falls is at risk for an injury via a similar mechanism.

18. What is bowler's thumb?
Traumatic neuropathy of the thumb's digital nerve can be caused by repeated friction or compression by the edge of the thumb-hole in the bowling ball. The digital nerve can also be compressed in racquet sports or by direct injury from playing handball.

19. How do you test the flexor digitorum profundus muscle?
Ask the patient to bend the DIP joint while you stabilize the PIP joint in extension.

20. How do you test the integrity of the flexor digitorum superficialis tendon?
With the superficialis test. The flexor digitorum superficialis flexes the PIP joint. While the examiner holds the adjacent fingers in full extension, the patient flexes the finger. If there is no injury or tear in the flexor digitorum superficialis tendon, the patient is able to flex the PIP joint, but the DIP joint remains in extension or neutral.

21. How can you test the integrity of the flexor digitorum profundus tendon to one particular finger?
By the **profundus test**. The MCP and PIP joints are held in extension by the examiner, and the patient flexes the DIP joints. If the patient can do this, then the long flexor, or the profundus tendon, to that finger is intact.

22. What does the absence of an okay sign mean?
Absence of flexion of the interphalangeal joint of the thumb as well as the DIP joint of the index finger, and therefore inability to make an okay sign, may signal a deficit in the anterior interosseous innervated muscles of the median nerve.

23. How is the Finkelstein's test done?
With the patient's thumb flexed into the palm of the hand while the fingers are "fisted" over the thumb, the examiner twists the wrist inward (ulnar deviation). This maneuver maximizes tension on the abductor pollicis longus and extensor pollicis brevis tendon. In deQuervain's disease (stenosing tenosynovitis), pain is reproduced over the radial wrist.

24. What is the Froment's sign?
Although the adductor pollicis is paralyzed in ulnar nerve lesions, the movements of palmar and ulnar adduction can still be performed. When the patient attempts to grasp an object such as a piece of paper between the thumb and the edge of the palm, the purpose is accomplished by flexing the thumb at the interphalyngeal joint by means of the flexor pollicis longus, supplied by the median nerve. This is described as a positive Froment's sign.

25. Name the two different types of grips in the hand.
  • Prehension, which includes pinch, tip, as well as lateral grip.
  • Power, which includes hook, grasp, and palmar grip.

26. Describe the Bunnell-Littler test.
  This test evaluates the tightness of the intrinsic muscles of the hand (lumbricals and the interossei). To test the tightness of the intrinsic muscles, hold the MCP joint in a few degrees of extension and try to move the PIP joint into flexion. If in this position the PIP can be flexed, then the intrinsics are not tight. If the PIP joint cannot be flexed, either the intrinsics are tight or there are joint capsule contractures.

BIBLIOGRAPHY

1. American Society for Surgery of the Hand: The Hand Examination and Diagnosis, 3rd ed. New York, Churchill Livingstone, 1990.
2. Ariyan S: The Hand Book. New York, McGraw Hill, 1989.
3. Browner B, Jupiter J, Levine A, Trafton P: Skeletal Trauma: Fractures, Dislocations, Ligamentous Injuries. Philadelphia, W.B. Saunders, 1992, pp 925–1024.
4. Cailliet R: Neck and Arm Pain, 3rd ed. Philadelphia, F.A. Davis, 1991.
5. Cailliet R: Hand Pain and Impairment. Philadelphia, F.A. Davis, 1995.
6. Hoppenfeld S: Physical Exam of the Spine and Extremities. Norwalk, CT, Appleton & Lange, 1976.
7. Hunter JM, Mackin EJ, Callahan AD: Rehabilitation of the Hand: Surgery and Therapy, 3rd ed. St. Louis, Mosby, 1994.
8. Skinner H: Current Diagnosis and Treatment in Orthopedics. Norwalk, CT, Appleton & Lange, 1995, pp 453–511.
9. Weinstein S, Buckwalter J: Turek's Orthopaedics, 5th ed. Philadelphia, J.B. Lippincott, 1994, pp 417–446.

51. THE HIP

Neil Spiegel, D.O.

1. What is the normal angle of inclination between the neck and shaft of the femur for males and females?
  125° in male adults and 115–120° in females, giving females a wider pelvis. The angle between the neck and shaft of the femur influences where the gravitational line of force falls in relation to the hip and knee.

2. Name the deformities caused by an increased and decreased angle of inclination.
  A decreased angle is known as **coxa vara**, which tends to shorten the leg and limit hip abduction. This abnormality forces the knee into valgus. **Coxa valgus** is caused by an increased angle, which tends to lengthen the leg and cause a lateral displacement of the hip on the knee, a varus deformity.

3. What are the chief ligaments of the capsule of the hip joint?
  The iliofemoral (which is considered the strongest ligament in the body), the ischiofemoral, and the pubofemoral ligaments.

4. What is the normal range of all the hip motion?

Flexion	0–120°	Extension	0–15°
Abduction	0–45°	Adduction	0–30°
Internal rotation		External rotation	
With hip flexed	0–45°	With hip flexed	0–45°
With hip extended	0–35°	With hip extended	0–45°

5. What is the maximal force across the hip joint? At what stage of gait cycle does it occur?

The maximal force across the hip joint reaches approximately three times the body weight. It occurs during the early and late periods of stance phase of the gait cycle and the force increases to 4.3 times the body weight upon jogging.

6. Why and how is the Thomas test performed?

The Thomas test is performed to assess for flexion contracture of the hip. The patient lies supine on the examining table. To test the right hip, the left hip and knee are maximally flexed. A positive result or a flexion contracture is present if the right thigh elevates above the table passively.

7. Why and how is the Ober test performed?

The Ober test is done to evaluate for a contracture of the tensor fascia lata (TFL). The patient lies on his or her side with the lower leg flexed at the hip and knee for stability. The examiner then passively abducts and extends the patient's upper leg with the knee flexed to 90°. The examiner then releases the upper limb; if contracture is present, the upper leg will remain abducted and will not fall to the table.

8. What are the predisposing factors for bursitis of the hip?

Low back pain	Rheumatologic conditions
Herniated lumbar disk	Hip trauma
Leg-length discrepancy	Previous surgery
Hip disease	Hemiparesis

9. What is a hip pointer? In which sports do they most commonly occur?

A hip pointer is caused by a fall directly on the iliac crest, contusing the soft tissue (a hematoma forms at the point of contact). It occurs commonly in football, basketball, gymnastics, and volleyball.

10. What is myositis ossificans? How is it treated?

Myositis ossificans is essentially the formation of heterotopic ossification (HO) within the muscle after a direct blow to the hip or thigh. X-rays will show a soft tissue mass. Calcific flocculations can develop within 7–10 days and progress to HO between the second and third week.

The initial injury may be aggravated by the early use of heat, ultrasound, or massage or by repeated unprotected thigh contusions. Gentle active range of motion exercise can be done to prevent contractures. Progressive strengthening is encouraged, and protective padding prior to return to contact sport is recommended. If surgery becomes necessary, it must be delayed 9–12 months or until the lesion matures.

11. Name the common factors associated with hamstring and quadriceps muscle strains. How are they graded?

Poor flexibility, inadequate warm-up, exercise fatigue, poor conditioning, and muscle imbalance. A rehab program needs to assess and modify these risk factors (the normal strength ratio for hamstrings to quadriceps is 3:5). The injury occurs during the eccentric phase of muscle contraction and ranges in severity from grade I (strength injury) to grade III (a complete tear).

12. What common causes of femoral compressive neuropathy are likely to be seen on the rehabilitation ward?

There are many different causes of femoral neuropathy, but in a patient on a rehab ward who has a rapid onset of pain in the groin and thigh, one must rule out a hemorrhage secondary to anticoagulant therapy in the retroperitoneal space. Femoral neuropathy can also occur from heat that is produced by the cement used in total hip replacement surgery.

13. What is meralgia paresthetica and how does it present?

Injury of the lateral femoral cutaneous nerve is commonly called meralgia paresthetica. Patients complain of numbness, burning pain, ache, or tingling sensation over the anterolateral thigh. Common causes include pressure from tight clothing, seatbelt injury, and diabetes.

14. When referring to Travell's trigger points, what muscle in the hip can cause a sciatic like syndrome?

The referred pain pattern of the anterior portion of the gluteus minimus extends over the lower lateral buttock and the lateral aspect of the thigh, knee, and leg to the ankle. The posterior part gives a pattern that is more down the back of the thigh into the calf.

15. What is the referred pain pattern from a Travell trigger point in the piriformis muscle?

Pain from a trigger point in the piriformis refers into the sacroiliac region, laterally across the buttock, and over the hip region posteriorly into the proximal two-thirds of the posterior thigh. Primary dysfunction of the sacroiliac joint may present in a similar fashion.

16. Which athletes are prone to stress fracture of the proximal femur?

Endurance athletes, such as runners.

17. How do stress fractures usually present? What two types of stress fractures occur?

The patient usually presents with groin pain or hip tenderness with decreased range of internal rotation on examination. The two types of stress fractures are:

1. Transverse type—The fracture line goes across the superior portion of the femoral neck. This type is more prone to a complete break, and therefore internal fixation may be necessary.

2. Compression type—This more common type of stress fracture usually occurs along the inferior neck of the femur. It is more stable and therefore is treated more conservatively.

18. What is the most common neurologic cause of referred pain into the hip?

Lumbar radiculopathies, either by a dermatologic pattern L1–3 or a myotomal pattern L4–S3.

19. How many patients after hip fracture return to their prefracture level of function? How many die?

Of those who survive, 25–50% regain their premorbid level of function. The mortality rate is 20–29% after 1 year and 40% at 2 years.

20. List the common risk factors associated with osteoporotic hip fracture.

- Fixed risk factors
  Advanced age—two-thirds after age 75 yrs
  White race—2–3:1 white-to-black ratio among females
  Female sex
- Modifiable risk factors
  Smoking—decreases bioavailability of exogenous estrogens
  Alcohol use > 2.5 gm/day—increases bone loss
  Caffeine—increases urinary calcium excretion
  Slim body habitus
  < 90% of ideal body weight
  Certain medications—e.g., tricyclic antidepressants, benzodiazepines, antipsychotics

21. How common is venous thromboembolism following hip surgery?

It occurs in at least 50% of unprotected patients.

22. When does the period of the maximum risk for pulmonary embolism occur after total hip replacement surgery?

During the second and third week, when 70% of pulmonary emboli occur.

23. Which diagnostic test is the most sensitive and has the highest specificity in detecting venous thrombosis for the postoperative hip patient?

Venography

24. What is the most common complication after total hip replacement?
Heterotopic ossification, with an incidence of about 50%. But, only about 7% of patients will experience a loss of motion.

25. Which methods are commonly used as prophylaxis for heterotopic ossification?
Radiation and NSAIDs

26. How long is the average length of stay on a rehab ward after a total hip replacement?
7–10 days. There is a current trend to reduce the length of stay.

27. How does loosening of the hip prosthesis present? How is it usually detected?
Loosening at the cement–bone or cement–prosthesis interface presents with new onset of thigh or groin pain, worse during transfers and early ambulation. Plain x-rays may pick up a bone cement lucency > 2 mm wide.

28. Name the common complications of anterior and posterior hip dislocations.
Anterior dislocations may be associated with an injury to the femoral nerve. Posterior dislocation, which is more common, is associated with an injury to the sciatic nerve, and avascular necrosis can occur in 10–20% of patients.

29. What are the most common known causes of avascular necrosis of the hip?
Alcohol abuse and systemic steroid use.

30. Name the most common cause of a painful hip in children under 10 years of age.
Acute transient synovitis, which is usually nonspecific and self-limiting.

31. What is Legg-Calvé-Perthes disease?
Avascular necrosis of the femoral head. It usually occurs in children aged 5–12 years and may be due to interruption of the vascular supply of the hip leading to ischemic necrosis.

32. What is the most common pediatric tumor involving the hip?
Osteogenic sarcoma.

33. What sources can cause metastatic disease in the femur?
Prostate, breast, lung, kidney, and colon cancers.

34. What is the primary etiology of hip deformities and instability in children with cerebral palsy?
Spasticity.

BIBLIOGRAPHY

1. Bonica JJ: The Management of Pain. Philadelphia, Lea & Febiger, 1990.
2. Brown DE, Neumann: Orthopedic Secrets. Philadelphia, Hanley & Belfus, 1995.
3. Dumitru D: Electrodiagnostic Medicine. Philadelphia, Hanley & Belfus, 1995.
4. Johnson RJ, Lombardo J: Current Review of Sports Medicine. Philadelphia, Current Medicine, 1994.
5. Nicholas JA, Hershman EB: The Lower Extremity and Spine in Sports Medicine. St. Louis, Mosby, 1986.
6. Travell JG, Simons DG: Myofascial Pain and Dysfunction: The Trigger Point Manual. Baltimore, Williams & Wilkins, 1992.

52. THE KNEE

Warren Slaten, M.D.

1. How do meniscal injuries occur?
In traumatic injuries, twisting is usually described by the patient. This may be accompanied by a valgus force or a varus force with rotation in medial meniscal injuries and a varus force or a valgus force with rotation in lateral meniscal injuries. Swelling may occur, though in isolated meniscal injuries, this occurs more gradually (several hours to 2 days) than in anterior cruciate ligament (ACL) injuries. With a valgus force to a flexed and rotated knee, the medial meniscus, medial collateral ligament, and ACL may all be injured. This is **O'Donoghue's triad**.

2. What tests can be used to diagnose a meniscal tear?
The most sensitive signs on physical exam are joint line tenderness and positive hyperflexion test (pain toward the end range of flexion when passively flexing the knee). McMurray's test and Apley's compression test can also be used.

3. Describe McMurray's test.
The patient is supine with the knee fully flexed. To evaluate the lateral meniscus, the tibia is medially rotated, which will cause a click often accompanied by pain. As the degree of knee flexion is changed, the maneuver tests different parts of the meniscus, with the more anterior parts of the meniscus tested as the knee is extended. Laterally rotating the tibia stresses the medial compartment for testing the medial meniscus.

4. Describe Apley's compression test.
Apley's test can be used to diagnose a meniscal tear. The patient lies prone with the knee flexed to 90° and the thigh immobilized by the examiner's knee. While the tibia is rotated medially and laterally, the leg is compressed into the knee, which may result in pain if a meniscal tear is present. Pain when the leg is distracted rather than compressed suggests ligamentous injury.

5. Can meniscal injuries be treated without surgery?
Yes. Initially, the **PRICE** (**P**rotect, **R**elative rest, **I**ce, **C**ompression, and **E**levation) acronym is used until the effusion is reduced. During the first days after injury, range-of-motion (ROM) exercises are started, especially if restrictions are present. Strengthening exercises for the hamstrings and quadriceps can provide support for and stabilize the knee. Proprioceptive exercises can facilitate return to functional exercises, which may begin as the patient tolerates. A neoprene sleeve can be used to improve proprioception and provide some relief of symptoms caused by a coexisting Baker's cyst.

6. When is surgical treatment indicated for meniscal tear?
- Locking, or inability to fully extend the knee because of mechanical blockage
- Motion restricted despite a trial of physical therapy
- Instability, which may predispose to further intra-articular damage
- Baker's cyst resulting from a meniscal tear
- Refractory pain not improving with physical therapy and symptomatic management

7. What tests are used to diagnose an ACL tear?
The ACL helps prevent anterior displacement of the tibia relative to the femur and provides rotatory stability, so tests to stress the tibia anteriorly will test ACL function. These tests include Lachman's test, anterior drawer test, and pivot shift test.

8. Describe Lachman's test.

This is a test of anterior knee stability. With the patient supine, the knee is held between 15–30° of flexion. The femur is stabilized by the examiner, while the proximal tibia is pulled forward. With the ACL disrupted, there will be no clear end point to the tibia's motion. Placing a rolled towel under the femur may help relax the patient to facilitate testing.

9. Describe the anterior drawer test.

The patient's knee is placed in 90° flexion, and the patient's foot is stabilized by the examiner's body. Place your hands around the proximal tibia and draw the tibia forward on the femur. A positive test is > 6 mm of movement of the tibia. The test is not very sensitive because hemarthrosis, hamstring spasm, and other structures (such as the posterior capsule) can limit forward movement of the tibia.

10. What does the pivot shift test add to this?

It assesses the anterolateral rotatory stability of the knee.

11. Describe the rehabilitation of the patient with an ACL injury.

Again, the **PRICE** acronym is used until the effusion is reduced. ROM exercises should begin in the first few days after injury. Strengthening exercises should emphasize the hamstrings to help stabilize the tibia in the absence of ACL function. The quadriceps should be strengthened with terminal range squats to prevent patellofemoral pain, a common sequela of ACL injury. Proprioceptive exercises and agility training will prepare the patient for functional activities. Functional bracing with a brace that limits terminal extension and rotation will provide further control and should be fitted when thigh girth of the injured limb is near-normal.

12. How does a patient with a tear of the medial collateral ligament (MCL) typically present?

An MCL injury typically occurs after a valgus blow to the knee, often when the knee is slightly flexed. Patients often describe weakness with or without pain. On examination, there may be tenderness medially along the ligament and tenderness anteromedially. Knee stability is tested at 0° and 30° flexion. With the knee in 30° of flexion, valgus stressing causes the knee to "open," often with a vague end-feel.

13. What is the classification of MCL injuries?

Grade I—partial fiber disruption. Valgus stressing results in pain, but valgus stability is intact.

Grade II—nearly complete rupture of the ligament with the capsule intact. Swelling and hemorrhage with the valgus instability are evident on examination. An endpoint is appreciated.

Grade III—rupture of the superficial and deep portions of the ligament and rupture of the surrounding capsular structures. With valgus stressing, there is no end point.

14. How is a grade I MCL injury treated?

Ice, NSAIDs, and early (as soon as tolerated, usually within the first week) ROM and strengthening exercises, with the functional goal of returning to activities within 1–3 weeks post-injury. Functional bracing may be used for several weeks to protect the ligament from further injury.

15. How is grade II MCL injury treated?

Treatment differs from that for grade I injuries in that mobilization begins more gradually to allow for ligament healing. Applying a functional rehabilitation brace that allows for progressive ROM has been advocated. ROM exercises between 30° and full flexion can be done within the first week, gradually progressing to full extension within a few weeks. Resistive exercises can begin as tolerated within the cast brace, progressing as tolerated to functional exercises. By 4–5 weeks, functional activities can begin, with use of a double upright functional knee brace continuing for 2–3 months post-injury.

16. How are grade III MCL injuries treated?

Treatment is similar to that for grade II injuries, though ROM exercises should be delayed until the second week. After 2 weeks, strengthening exercises can begin, including bicycle ergometry but with extension limited to 30°. When strength is near-normal and the valgus instability is improved, functional activities can begin, again with use of a functional knee brace.

17. What is osteochrondritis dissecans?

This condition is characterized by fragmentation of the articular cartilage with subchondral bone, most commonly the medial femoral condyle or the patella. The cause is usually acute or repetitive trauma in predisposed individuals, predominantly adolescent males.

The usual presentation is stiffness and aching with an effusion. If a loose body is present, the knee may lock. Examination reveals tenderness over the affected area and possibly an effusion or limited ROM. X-rays with tunnel views may reveal the defect.

18. What are some common causes of patellofemoral pain?

Biomechanical factors—e.g., weak quadriceps, weak hamstrings, increased Q angle, patella alta, vastus lateralis muscle hypertrophy, vastus medialis oblique muscle dysplasia, and femoral trochlea dysplasia.

Overuse with repetitive activities stressful to the patellofemoral joint—e.g., jumping, changing directions, and decelerating.

19. What is the Q angle?

Also known as the quadriceps angle or patellofemoral angle, this is the angle formed between a line drawn from the anterior superior iliac spine to the midpoint of the patella and a line drawn from the tibial tubercle to the midpoint of the patella. This angle is measured with the hip and foot in neutral position. Normally, the angle is 13–18° (though if the quadricep is contracted the angle is normally 8–10°), and it is lower in males.

20. Describe the typical signs and symptoms of patellofemoral pain.

Anterior knee pain with gradual onset, which worsens with repetitive knee flexion
Pain with prolonged sitting or upon arising after sitting (positive **theater sign**)
Pain with squatting or with descending stairs

21. What are the rehabilitation principles for treating patellofemoral pain?

Because lateral tracking is often implicated as a cause of patellofemoral pain, treatment is aimed at correcting this. Correcting muscle imbalances that predispose to lateral tracking may include strengthening the vastus medialis obliquus and stretching the iliotibial band. Quadricep strengthening should be done between 0–30° flexion because angles greater than this cause patellar compression. Also, closed-chain kinetic exercises with co-contraction of the quadriceps, hamstrings, and gastrocnemius reduce excessive forces across the patella and provide functional strengthening. Tightness of the lateral retinaculum may be corrected with manual stretching with medial patellar glide stretches. McConnell taping of the patella may improve tracking during functional activities, while the strengthening phase of rehabilitation is in progress. Correcting pronation with orthotics and controlling tibial alignment with wedging may also be necessary.

22. What is jumper's knee?

This is patellar tendinitis caused by overuse of the patellofemoral extensor mechanism characterized by microtearing of tendon fibrils. The site of involvement is most commonly the inferior pole of the patella, though the superior pole of the patella or the insertion site at the tibial tubercle can also be involved. A typical presentation is pain at the onset of the activity, with improvement during the activity followed by recurrence after completion of the activity.

23. How is jumper's knee treated?

Rest by avoiding activities that stress the patellar mechanism, ice to the knee, NSAIDs, and exercises that include isometric quadricep exercises and inferior patellar glides to mobilize the patella, progressing to isotonic quadricep exercises and hamstring stretching, and then eccentric quadricep strengthening. Also, proper athletic shoes are essential, which may include orthotics to correct for hyperpronation.

24. What is Osgood-Schlatter disease?

Apophysitis at the insertion of the patellar tendon into the tibial tubercle. It may start as tendinitis at the tubercle and progress to avulsion of a fragment of the tubercle or a tear of the tendon. Extension is limited with quadriceps weakness developing. Also, the patella may ride higher on the affected side. Palpation reveals localized tenderness over the tibial tuberosity.

25. What is Sinding-Larson-Johannson disease?

This is apophysitis at the insertion site of the patellar tendon into the distal pole of the patella. It is caused by overuse with repetitive trauma to the patellar tendon.

26. What is the iliotibial band (ITB) syndrome?

The ITB, which is the fascial and tendinous continuation of the tensor fascia lata muscle, can become inflamed with overuse activities. It is commonly described in runners who increase their training level quickly or run excessively on hills.

Patients often describe lateral knee pain, and on exam, there is tenderness over the ITB as it crosses the knee over the lateral femoral condyle. Tightness of the ITB can be shown by a positive Ober's test.

27. Define plica.

This is a fold of synovium and has been implicated as a source of pain in the knee. It has been described in the infrapatellar, suprapatellar, and mediopatellar aspects, with the mediopatellar most commonly implicated as a source of pain. With direct knee trauma, hemarthrosis, or ACL injury, the plica can thicken and become inflamed. It commonly accompanies patellofemoral pathology and can accompany other conditions that cause pain, such as ACL tears and meniscal tears. Thus, it is unclear whether it is a cause of pain or a sequela of other pathologies.

28. Which bursae around the knee are frequent sources of pain?

The prepatellar, superficial and deep infrapatellar, tibial collateral ligament, and pes anserine bursae.

29. List the common causes of bursitis.

Acute trauma such as with a direct blow, chronic overuse, infection, and underlying degenerative knee disease.

30. What is prepatellar bursitis?

The prepatellar bursa between the patella and skin may become inflamed with direct trauma, such as falling on the bent knee or kneeling (known as **housemaid's knee**). When inflamed, the bursa is tender and the skin becomes tight, limiting knee flexion. Treatment is with ice, compression, and rest, and, if necessary, needle aspiration followed by application of direct pressure.

31. What is vicar's knee?

Superficial infrapatellar bursitis, which is inflammation of the bursa that lies between the patellar tendon and the overlying skin. It is associated with kneeling in the upright position, hence its name. It usually responds to compression and ice without drainage.

32. If vicar's knee is caused by kneeling in prayer and housemaid's knee is caused by housework, what causes a Baker's cyst?

I bet you were going to say baking. But this is a synovial cyst that may communicate with the joint capsule. The etiology is not certain, though trauma and joint effusion have been implicated. Often, there is underlying pathology (most commonly a meniscus tear) which should be sought, and treatment includes addressing the underlying pathology.

ACKNOWLEDGMENT

The author thanks Dr. Gerard Malenga for his feedback and assistance.

BIBLIOGRAPHY

1. Dillingham MF, King WD, Gamburd RS: Rehabilitation of the knee following anterior cruciate ligament and medial collateral ligament injuries. Phys Med Rehabil Clin North Am 5(1):175–194, 1994.
2. Buschbacher RJ, Braddom RL (eds): Sports Medicine and Rehabilitation: A Sports-Specific Approach. Philadelphia, Hanley & Belfus, 1994.
3. Magee DJ: Knee. In Orthopedic Physical Assessment, 2nd ed. Philadelphia, W.B. Saunders, 1992, pp 372–447.
4. Nisonson B: Anterior cruciate ligament injuries: Conservative vs. surgical treatment. Physician Sportsmed 19(5):82–89, 1991.
5. Rowland GC, Beagley MJ, Cawley PW: Conservative treatment of inflamed knee bursae. Physician Sportsmed 20(2):67–77, 1992.
6. Smith AD, Tao SS: Knee injuries in young athletes. Clin Sports Med 14(3):629–647, 1995.
7. Tindel NL, Nisonson B: The plica syndrome. Orthop Clin North Am 23(4):613–618, 1992.

53. THE ANKLE AND FOOT

Lew C. Schon, M.D., Stuart D. Miller, M.D., and Steven B. Weinfeld, M.D.

1. What does the foot do during the four phases of gait?

Phase I—from heel-strike to foot flat. The ankle moves from dorsiflexion to neutral, the anterior tibialis muscle helps to decelerate the forefoot, the heel moves from initial supination to pronation, and the tibia rotates internally.

Phase II—foot flat to heel-off. The ankle moves from initial neutral to 15° of dorsiflexion at heel-off, the posterior tibialis muscles and the intrinsic muscles help to raise the heel, the heel moves from pronation to supination, and the tibia continues to rotate internally.

Phase III—heel-off to toe-off. The ankle plantarflexes, the posterior tibialis and intrinsic muscles help to launch the foot, the heel remains supinated, and the tibia rotates externally.

Phase IV—swing phase. The posterior tibialis muscle is relaxed, and the anterior tibialis muscle contracts to help clear the forefoot from the ground.

2. What are the common problems in foot alignment?

Pes planus (flatfoot) may be flexible or rigid. A flexible flatfoot may be due to posterior tibial tendon rupture, ruptured plantar fascia, or instability of the medial column joints (especially the first metatarsocuneiform [MTC] and talonavicular joints) of the foot. A rigid flatfoot may be caused by arthritis, tarsal coalition, or late-stage flexible flatfoot.

Pes cavus, or a high-arched foot, can be secondary to Charcot-Marie-Tooth disease, neurologic problems, or physiologic factors (such as a familial pes cavus). Pes cavus also can be flexible or rigid. In the patient with subtalar fusion or coalition, there is an increase in stresses on the adjacent joints, such as the ankle, talonavicular, and calcaneocuboid joints. When a cavus or planus foot is symptomatic, it is important to identify the underlying etiology.

3. Define a hammertoe.

A hammertoe is a flexion contracture of the proximal interphalangeal (PIP) joint, usually associated with flexion contracture of the distal interphalangeal (DIP) joint. Conservative treatment includes added-depth shoes or a pad over the PIP joint. Surgical treatment includes removal of bone or fusion of the PIP joint with tendon transfer, lengthening, or release.

4. Clawtoe.

A clawtoe is a flexion contracture of the PIP joint, and often the DIP joint, with hyperextension of the MTP joint. Treatment is similar to that for hammertoe.

5. Mallet toe.

A mallet toe is a flexion deformity at the DIP joint, often with a painful callus at the tip of the toe or dorsally over the joint. If conservative treatment is not adequate, surgical release of the flexor digitorum longus, with or without resection of a portion of the middle phalanx, may be necessary.

6. What is meant by splaying of the toes?

This condition occurs when there is weakening of the adjacent collateral ligaments with progressive spreading of the toes at the MTP joints. The splaying usually occurs with neuritis of the involved webspace and clawing of the toes. Early treatment includes strapping of the toes and wider, higher toebox shoes. Surgical treatment includes tendon transfers and bone resection to realign the toes.

7. How do calluses, corns, warts, and bunions differ?

Callus is a protective hypertrophy of the keratinized layer of the skin in places of increased friction or pressure. Typically, there is an underlying bony prominence. A **corn** is a more localized hypertrophy of the tissues that occurs only on the toes. A soft corn develops between toes, and a hard corn is a callus on a dorsal or plantar surface. **Warts** are hard white growths caused by papovavirus infection. Unlike a callus, a wart exhibits punctate bleeding when scraped. A wart also interrupts normal skin whirls and creases, whereas a callus does not. A **bunion** refers to the medial protuberance of the first metatarsal (with hallux valgus being the angular malalignment of the first MTP joint).

8. What is sesamoiditis?

Sesamoiditis is pain on or around the sesamoid bones, which are located underneath the first MTP joint. Sesamoiditis may be caused by acute fracture, stress fracture, and/or osteonecrosis. Overuse injuries can also result in insertional flexor hallucis brevis tendinitis (where the tendon joins the sesamoid or the proximal phalanx).

A congenital bipartite sesamoid, which is a normal variant, may be injured and become as symptomatic as an acute or chronic sesamoid fracture. In this case, the two halves that were joined by fibrocartilage may acutely separate.

9. What causes the painful heel syndrome?

The most common cause is an attritional tearing of the plantar fascia near or at its origin in the medial plantar tubercle of the calcaneus. This condition, which results in acute and chronic inflammation, is termed **plantar fasciitis**.

10. How significant are heel spurs in the etiology of plantar fasciitis?

Many patients (nearly 80%) with plantar fasciitis demonstrate a plantar heel spur. Although the heel spur is often thought to be the cause of the heel pain, most clinicians deem it an incidental finding without significance to prognosis or treatment. Although 30% of patients with plantar fasciitis have heel spurs, approximately 16% of the general population have asymptomatic heel spurs. Most patients with a "painful heel spur syndrome" actually have plantar fasciitis.

11. What are other causes of plantar heel pain?

Irritation of the first branch of the lateral plantar nerve or the nerve to the abductor digiti quinti (Baxter's nerve), irritation or entrapment of the calcaneal branch of the tarsal tunnel, proximal irritation of the tibial or sciatic nerve, plantar heel bursitis, plantar medial venous plexus thrombosis, insufficient fat pad, post-traumatic fat pad incompetency (often after calcaneal fracture), and calcaneal stress fracture.

12. How is plantar fasciitis treated?
  • **First-line treatment**
  1. Heel cup or heel pad to cushion and lift the heel
  2. Stretching program (dorsiflexion of the ankle)
  3. Anti-inflammatories
  • **Second-line treatment**
  1. Lidocaine, bupivicaine, or corticosteroid injection at the origin of the plantar fascia
  2. Custom-molded foot orthoses, soft supportive shoes, foot strapping, and physical therapy with stretching modalities
  3. Night ankle/foot orthotic (AFO) or short-leg walking cast or brace
  • **Third-line treatment**
  1. Surgery (consider only if all nonoperative modalities fail after 1 year)

13. How does an acute rupture of the Achilles tendon present?

The patient complains of sudden calf pain, which may be severe, followed by weakness. Typically, there is weakness of plantarflexion, and there may be a palpable defect, usually 2–6 cm proximal to the insertion of the Achilles tendon on the calcaneus. The Thompson test is positive—squeezing the gastrocnemius-soleus proximally does not plantarflex the ankle because the connection has been disrupted.

14. For conservative treatment, how is the patient casted or braced?

A cast is applied in the equinus position to oppose the tendon ends. Then, the dorsiflexion is increased gradually to neutral, so that by 8–10 weeks, the patient's foot is in neutral position (the foot is at a right angle to the leg). Casting is continued for a total of 12 weeks. For 3–6 months thereafter, the patient uses a heel lift. The patient is instructed to increase his or her activity level gradually and to avoid going uphill, sudden dorsiflexion of the foot, or lunge movements that may suddenly stretch the healing tendon.

15. For a patient who is athletically active, is operative or nonoperative treatment recommended?

Direct repair is recommended for acute ruptures in an active or athletic individual. These individuals generally do not tolerate the prolonged casting, bracing, and inactivity and are better served with a technique that will have lower risk of re-rupture and ultimately better function and power.

16. How are patients with chronic Achilles tendon rupture treated?

These patients may be placed in an AFO to stabilize the foot and ankle, or surgery may be recommended to reconnect the Achilles tendon. At surgery, it is often necessary to span a persistent gap by grafting the defect with a local tendon. It is critical surgery to reestablish normal tension of the ankle against passive dorsiflexion.

17. What is Achilles tendinosis?

Achilles tendinosis, which is inflammation and degeneration of the tendon, is an overuse condition seen often in athletes such as runners and participants in racket sports. Typically, there is tenderness and thickening of the tendon 2–6 cm above the insertion point. There may also be crepitus, edema, and mild erythema.

18. What can happen to the posterior tibial tendon?

The posterior tibial tendon may rupture acutely during trauma. Typically, it can be inflamed from systemic disease, arthritic conditions, or chronic overuse. The tendon may also become degenerative and gradually attenuate and even rupture in a subacute fashion without an precipitating trauma.

19. What are the disorders affecting the peroneal tendons?

The peroneal tendons can sustain acute rupture (rarely), develop tenosynovitis and/or stenosis, and subluxate or dislocate.

20. When does tenosynovitis of the peroneal tendons occur?

Peroneal tenosynovitis occurs in persons participating in running and field sports and in dance. It is associated with ankle and subtalar sprains (inversion injuries), but may also be associated with connective tissue disease, especially seronegative arthritis, and stenosing lesions after calcaneal or fibular fracture.

It is treated first by evaluating for any underlying mechanical etiology. Then, anti-inflammatories and relative rest, followed by an ankle stirrup brace, cast, or AFO, may be helpful. Physical therapy with modalities using gentle strengthening and conditioning exercises are often beneficial.

21. How does stenosing tenosynovitis of the flexor hallucis longus (FHL) present?

FHL stenosing tenosynovitis occurs in dancers who perform *en pointe* or in any plantarflexed position of the foot. It may also be seen in runners or soccer players. Patients complain of tightness of the first MTP joint, with pain somewhere along the course of the FHL tendon between the posterior aspect of the ankle and under the arch toward the big toe. With dorsiflexion of the hallux, there is a locking or clicking of the FHL.

22. How does progressive degeneration of the anterior tibial tendon present?

The degenerating anterior tibial tendon often develops an asymptomatic or mildly symptomatic nodule on the dorsal aspect of the anterior tibial ankle. With time, this thickening becomes more symptomatic, and the patient develops dorsiflexion weakness. As the disease progresses, the tendon may attenuate or rupture. These patients present with foot-drop but a normal neurologic examination.

23. How is the rupture of the anterior tibial tendon treated?

Rupture of the anterior tibial tendon is treated with aggressive Achilles stretching combined with a dorsiflexion-assist AFO, such as a spring-leaf design. Patients who do not respond to this treatment may be candidates for surgical treatment.

24. Which ligaments are involved in ankle sprain?

In the nonmedical sense, an ankle sprain is any twisting of the ankle. It typically refers to an inversion and most commonly involves the anterior talofibular (ATF) ligament. But all the lateral ligaments are vulnerable to stresses with an inversion injury. From anterior to posterior, these are the ATF ligament, the calcaneal fibular (CF) ligament, and the posterior talofibular (PTF) ligament.

25. Can the medial ligaments be involved in ankle sprain?

Yes, the medial ligaments, including the different portions of the deltoid ligament that connect the medial malleolus to the talus, calcaneus, and naviculum, may be involved in an eversion injury. They may also be injured in an ankle fracture when the fibula fractures laterally, and the forces continue to cause medial ligament damage instead of fracture of the medial malleolus.

26. How long does it take to recover from a sprain?

Depending on whether the tear is a partial tear, minor tear, partial intersubstance tear, or complete tear, an ankle sprain may take between 2–3 months for nearly complete recovery and comfort. A severe ankle sprain, which may be associated with a syndesmotic injury, may take 6 months or longer to heal.

27. If a grade 3 ankle injury is treated properly, what percentage progress to chronic instability?

Depending on the magnitude of the injury and the mode of treatment, approximately 5–20% will have chronic instability.

28. How is chronic instability of the ankle assessed?

An **anterior drawer maneuver**—performed by grabbing the heel, pushing it anteriorly while the other hand stabilizes the tibia, pushing it posteriorly—will demonstrate ATF ligament incompetence. An **inversion stress test**, in which one hand is used to tilt the heel into inversion and the other to stabilize the tibia and palpate the ankle joint, may demonstrate an opening up of the ankle joint. To avoid aggravating the initial injury, the inversion tilt test should not be done forcefully until 10–12 weeks post-injury. The anterior draw test can be done at 6 weeks, but an extremely rigorous test should also be postponed until 10–12 weeks. A radiographic stress test during performance of these maneuvers may also be helpful.

29. If a patient has persistent critical instability at 3 months, is an operation indicated?

If the patient is a high-performance athlete, surgery may be indicated at this point. Otherwise, the patient should progress with his or her activities. If the patient at any time after 3 months experiences functional instability, surgical reconstruction of the torn ligaments may be considered.

30. Discuss the principles of treating ankle fractures.

The most important goals in treating ankle fractures are to restore the mortise (the tibiofibular relationship) and to recreate a symmetrical joint space. Stabilizing structures of the ankle include the lateral malleolus and its associated ligaments, the medial malleolus and its associated ligaments, and the anterior and posterior syndesmosis. Depending on the amount of displacement and instability, the fracture may be treated by closed or open means. A nondisplaced stable fracture is usually treated in a cast, brace, or AFO. Displaced unstable fractures are treated with open reduction and internal fixation (ORIF).

31. How can the heel bone be injured? How is it treated?

Calcaneal fractures, usually high-energy injuries associated with multiple other injuries (including spinal trauma), are characterized by widening of the heel and disruption of the subtalar joint. A CT scan is excellent for assessing joint displacement. Anatomic restoration of the posterior facet of the subtalar joint is the most important goal of treatment. Most displaced calcaneal fractures that are not extremely comminuted may be treated with ORIF and early motion. This procedure is not universally performed, and some consider it a high-risk procedure with a fair prognosis. Nondisplaced fractures can be treated with early motion, a compression bandage to decrease swelling and soft-tissue damage, and non-weight-bearing for 2–3 months. Relatively comminuted calcaneal fractures may require primary or delayed fusion of the subtalar joint.

32. What is the most common joint involved in gout?

Half of all initial gout attacks involve the first MTP joint of the toe, and this joint is involved at some point in > 90% of all patients with gout. However, gout may affect any other joint or tendon in the foot or ankle. Tophus formation (large collections of crystals adjacent to prominent joints) are a hallmark of the disease in its chronic state.

33. What are the signs of hallux rigidus?

Hallux rigidus describes the loss of motion in the first MTP joint (literally, a stiff big toe), usually caused by arthritis. The signs are:

1. A large, often tender, dorsal osteophyte at the head of the first MTP joint and/or the base of the proximal phalanx;
2. Limited ROM at the first MTP joint (normal range, 60–90° dorsiflexion);

3. Pain with extreme passive dorsiflexion and plantarflexion;
4. Mild erythema and swelling at the dorsal aspect of first MTP joint;
5. Lateral transfer of weight-bearing during the toe-off stage of the gait cycle.

34. Where are the common sites for degenerative or post-traumatic arthritis?

In the foot and ankle, degenerative arthritis may occur spontaneously in any joint(s), and post-traumatic arthritis can develop in any injured or surgically treated joint(s).

35. How is arthritis of the foot treated?

For midfoot joint arthritis without deformity, shoe modifications and orthotic devices (even an AFO) are useful. Intra-articular steroids can provide temporary relief. Cases resistant to conservative modalities or associated with severe deformity may require midfoot fusion with or without osteotomy.

In hindfoot arthritis, if an AFO or foot orthotic does not control the pain or deformity, a triple arthrodesis (including the talonavicular, calcaneocuboid, and talocalcaneal joints) should be performed. In patients with loss of bone stock in addition to the arthritis, a fusion with iliac bone graft may be required.

36. What can be done for ankle arthritis?

If medications, intra-articular injections, and an AFO with or without a rocker-bottom shoe cannot control the pain, a resection of the arthritic portions of the joint (cheilectomy) may be useful in select cases. Most patients require ankle fusion to manage the persistent pain and deformity.

37. What is the most common seronegative arthropathy to affect the foot?

Reiter's syndrome.

38. Describe the typical foot changes secondary to rheumatoid arthritis.

Rheumatoid arthritis of the hindfoot typically produces a valgus deformity with a flattening over the longitudinal arch. In the forefoot, involvement of the MTP joints is characteristic. In the first MTP joint, this leads to a hallux valgus deformity. Disease of the MTP joint of the lesser toes often results in lateral deviation of the toes, subluxation and dislocation of the MTPs, and clawing of the toes. Classically, there will be tender plantar prominences.

39. What are the nonoperative treatment options for rheumatoid arthritis involving the mid- or hindfoot?

Shoes must have enough depth to accommodate a soft orthotic device. This pads the plantar surface of the foot and reduces the metatarsalgia. A high, wide toebox shoe is needed to provide room for the hallux valgus and the clawtoes. A Velcro strap on the shoes will help patients with hand involvement put on and remove the shoes. Bracing with an AFO may also help diminish some symptoms. Corticosteroid injections into isolated joints can reduce synovitis, but injection of tendons should be avoided, as it may increase the risk of tendon rupture.

40. What are the surgical treatment options for rheumatoid arthritis involving the foot?

In the forefoot, typically the dorsal subluxation/dislocation of the lesser MTP joints and clawtoe deformities are treated with resection arthroplasty of the metatarsal heads. Removal of the metatarsal heads eliminates the problem of arthritic grinding at the joint and reduces the metatarsalgia from the painful, prominent metatarsal heads. The first MTP joint often needs to be fused to correct the deformity and provide stability to the forefoot.

Instability of the midfoot joints that results in persistent pain, a dropped arch, or separation of the metatarsals can be addressed with a midfoot fusion. Hindfoot joints with chronic pain, valgus, or (rarely) varus deformity may be improved with a hindfoot fusion. Occasionally, an osteotomy of the hindfoot or midfoot bones can correct the deformity.

41. What about the rheumatoid ankle?

Rheumatoid arthritis of the ankle can often be managed with an AFO and intra-articular injections of steroids. A joint that remains painful or becomes progressively more deformed is treated with an ankle fusion. In some cases, an ankle joint replacement may be indicated.

BIBLIOGRAPHY

1. Clanton TO, Schon LC: Athletic injuries to the soft tissues of the foot and ankle. In Mann RA, Coughlin MJ (eds): Surgery of the Foot and Ankle, 6th ed. St. Louis, Mosby-Year Book, 1993, pp 1095–1224.
2. Lutter LD, Mizel MS, Pfeffer GB: Foot and ankle. In Orthopaedic Knowledge Update. Rosemont, IL, American Academy of Orthopaedic Surgeons, 1994.
3. Moore TJ: Acquired neurologic disorders of the adult foot. In Mann RA, Coughlin MJ (eds): Surgery of the Foot and Ankle, 6th ed. St. Louis, Mosby-Year Book, 1992, pp 603–612.
4. Papa J, Myerson M, Girard P: Salvage, with arthrodesis, in intractable diabetic neuropathic arthropathy of the foot and ankle. J Bone Joint Surg 75A:1056–1066, 1993.
5. Pfeiffer WH, Cracchiolo A, III: Clinical results after tarsal tunnel decompression. J Bone Joint Surg 76A:1222–1230, 1994.
6. Schon LC: Plantar fascia and Baxter's nerve release. In Myerson M (ed): Current Therapy in Foot and Ankle Surgery. St. Louis, Mosby-Year Book, 1993, pp 177–182.
7. Schon LC, Marks RM: The management of neuroarthropathic fracture-dislocations in the diabetic patient. Orthop Clin North Am 26:375–392, 1995.
8. Wapner KL, Sharkey PF: The use of night splints for treatment of recalcitrant plantar fasciitis. Foot Ankle 12:135–137, 1991.

V. Rehabilitation of System-Based Disorders
D. The Spine

54. NECK PAIN

Rene Cailliet, M.D.

1. Discuss the basic architecture of the cervical spine.

The spine is composed of a super-imposed assemblage of vertebrae lined one atop another. The cervical spine has a total of 7 vertebrae, the upper 2 of which are architecturally unique and the lower 5 of which are similar in structure.

The upper spine includes the occiput, atlas (C1), axis (C2), and the lower cervical segments. The structures below the axis consist of a posterior gliding section and an anterior shock-absorbing, weight-bearing section. The upper segment has no intervertebral discs, foramina, or facets, as do the lower elements.

(Figure from Calliet R: Neck and Arm Pain, 3rd ed. Philadelphia, F.A. Davis, 1991, with permission.)

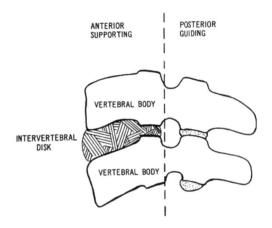

2. What are the common sites of pain production in the neck?

Since the neck has many pain-sensitive tissues compactly concentrated in a small area, nociceptive input can result from injury, irritation, inflammation, and infection. Common sites of pain production include the anterior and posterior longitudinal ligaments, facet articulation, muscle, nerve root, dura, and facet capsule.

3. Is the cervical disc itself pain-sensitive or -insensitive?

Although traditionally the disc was thought to be a pain-insensitive tissue, recent literature reports unmyelinated nerves in the outer annular rings of the disc that probably are transmitters of pain.

4. What are the two components of the disc? What is their composition?

The shock-absorbing disc is composed of two parts, the mucopolysaccharide **nucleus pulposus**, which is an avascular tissue that receives its nutrition by imbibition, and the **annulus**, which is a fibroelastic mesh.

5. What factors may amplify pain intensity?

Abnormal posture is a major one, since the foramina open on neck flexion and narrow on neck extension. Lateral bending and head turning cause the foramina to close on the side toward which the head bends and turns. Whiplash injury is obviously a major mechanism of neck injury resulting in pain.

6. In a clinical evaluation from history, what are the major factors to be determined?

History and physical must determine the precise **movements** and **positions** that cause or aggravate the pain. Position (posture), duration of this position, and the precise position reproducing the symptoms should be elicited.

7. Where does most of the movement come from in the cervical spine?

The most significant contribution to cervical spine movement occurs in the upper spine between the atlas and axis. As much as 90° of rotation from right to left is achievable. Flexion and extension in an anterior-posterior plane occurs between the occiput and atlas to produce head nodding. Flexion is typically 10° and extension is 25°. Most lower cervical movement occurs at the C4–5 and C5–6 levels.

8. Is the cervical musculature a significant basis for pain and disability?

Most assuredly. The cervical muscles are replete with numerous unmyelinated nerve endings that transmit nociceptive afferent impulses. The cervical muscles are also significantly innervated with spindle cells that modulate muscular activity.

9. In the evaluation of cervical pain, is the routine x-ray of significant value?

No. Although x-rays can help to rule out fractures and major subluxations, in addition to revealing "reversal" of normal lordosis, they are not useful routinely.

10. How are the first two cervical vertebrae different from one another?

The **atlas** (C1) lacks a body but has an anterior arch instead. The upper surface is occupied by two large concave facets which provide support to the occipital condyles. On the **axis** (C2), there is a large odontoid process that projects up from the body and articulates with the anterior arch of the atlas.

11. Where does the movement of the head and neck take place?

Nodding, i.e., flexion and extension of the head and neck, takes place at the **atlanto-occipital joint**, while rotation happens at the **atlantoaxial joint**. The atlas and the skull move as a unit. Movement also occurs at the lower segments C3–7.

12. How does the shape and orientation of spinal elements affect movement patterns?

The posterior C3–7 facet joints are virtually perpendicular to the sagittal plane, allowing horizontal rotation and lateral bending. The most mobile segments of the cervical spine are C4–6. Movement also occurs at the lower segments C3–7.

13. Why is the cervical spine less susceptible to damage induced by posterior disc displacement and herniation?

Since the nucleus pulposus is more anterior in the cervical spine, the posterior portion of the annulus is thickest. The anterior dimension of the disc is twice the posterior height, and the joints of Luschka decrease the vulnerability of the cervical cord to damage from posterior disc displacement.

14. What is the most common ailment involving the cervical spine?

External forces, such as auto and football injuries, are common modes of cervical spine injury. Cervical sprain and strain often result.

15. What is the stinger?

The stinger is widely recognized as an acute cervical compression occurring in football which causes transient (and occasionally permanent) nerve root irritation.

16. How do a strain and a sprain differ?

A **sprain** is a tearing or excessive stretching with microscopic contusion or hemorrhage or both. A **strain** is a pulling of the ligamentous, capsular, or tendinous structures without tearing.

17. What are some of the common signs and symptoms of cervical strain/sprain?

The patient often presents with headache, limitation of cervical movement, occipital pain, cervical pain, and shoulder, arm, and hand pain, with occasional paresthesia. The physical exam shows decreased ROM, spinous process tenderness, and shoulder and neck muscle spasm. On exam, there is no nerve root involvement and no localizing neurologic findings. X-rays may rule out fracture, trauma, or subluxation.

18. How does a herniated disc of the cervical spine present?

The onset of symptoms in a patient with a herniated disc is often dated to a specific event, typically a traumatic one. Herniation may occur because of high pressure in the nucleus or weakening of the annulus. Headache may be a symptom, and radicular pain and numbness may also occur. Acute herniation can cause compression of the spine. Myelopathy is not uncommon with chronic disc herniation. The secretion of phospholipid A_2 in response to matrix degeneration is a factor irritating the posterior longitudinal ligament and the root dura. Pressure on a noninflamed nerve does not cause pain.

19. Are there any other common pathologies of the cervical spine?

Cervical spondylosis occurs at the vertebral endplate as a result of disc degeneration. Degeneration and inflammation lead to changes in surrounding structures, especially the bones and meninges. Osteoarthritis in the cervical spine, including the joints of Luschka, is secondary to the intervertebral disc disease.

20. What is the most common disease of the spine during middle age or later?

Cervical spondylosis and facet pain.

21. Can osteoarthritic spurs affect vascular structures?

Yes, the vertebral and basilar arteries can be compressed by osteoarthritic spurs and can produce signs and symptoms including drop attacks and vertigo, especially when the neck is extended or rotated. It is often difficult to differentiate these from labyrinth disorders. Vertebral angiography can reveal arterial osteophytic compression by the joints of Luschka.

BIBLIOGRAPHY

1. Bogduk N: Innervation and pain patterns in the cervical spine. Clin Phys Ther 17:1–13, 1988.
2. Cailliet R: Neck and Arm Pain, 3rd ed. Philadelphia, F.A. Davis, 1991.
3. Cailliet R: Soft Tissue Pain and Disability, 3rd ed. Philadelphia, F.A. Davis, 1996.
4. Maigne R: Diagnosis and Treatment of Pain of Vertebral Origin. Baltimore, Williams & Wilkins, 1996.
5. Teasell RW, Shapiro AP (eds): Cervical Flexion-Extension/Whiplash Injuries. Spine: State Art Rev 7(3):329–578, 1993.

55. LOW BACK PAIN: CLINICAL EVALUATION AND TREATMENT

James W. Leonard, D.O., P.T.

1. How frequently does low back pain occur?

Each year, 10–17% of adults have an episode of back pain. Low back pain (LBP) results in approximately 10% of all chronic health conditions and is the second most common reason for office visits. Low back injuries account for approximately 20% of workers' compensation claims.

2. What are the key aspects to elicit when taking a history in a patient with LBP?

Onset of pain (sudden or gradual), its duration, and location

Any specific event that caused the pain

Initial course of symptoms, any changes over time

Any numbness, weakness, or change in bowel or bladder control

Course of pain over a 24-hour period (sleep disturbance, morning stiffness or pain, increase or decrease of symptoms during the day)

Aggravating or relieving factors

Previous episodes of pain and duration of symptoms

Previous tests and results

Previous treatment and results

Current medications and amount used

Medical history (especially any past tumors or infections)

Educational level

Stress level

3. What should the physical examination include?

The key components of the exam include:

Gait	Neurologic tests
Range of motion (including spine and extremities)	Special tests (straight leg raise, etc.)
	Palpatory findings

Neurologic Exam

NERVE ROOT	REFLEX	SENSATION	MOTOR	MOST COMMON LEVEL OF DISC HERNIATION AFFECTING NERVE
L4	Patellar	Medial calf	Quadriceps	L3–4
L5	None	Lateral calf	Extensor hallucis	L4–5
S1	Achilles	Lateral foot	Gastroc-soleus	L5–S1
S2–4 (cauda equina)	None	Perirectal	External anal sphincter	Multiple levels

4. What are Waddell's tests?

If three out of five of the following tests are positive, then a nonorganic psychologic cause is likely:

Tenderness, superficial or nonanatomic

Pain on simulated stressing tests

Inconsistent findings when testing the patient while he or she is distracted

Nonanatomic regional disturbances

Over-reaction

5. Describe the straight leg raise test.

This is a nerve tension sign. It is usually done with the patient supine, with the hip in a neutral position and the knee extended. One leg at a time is passively raised, and the angle at which the patient has pain is noted. True stretch on the nerve occurs between 30–60° of hip flexion. When recording the result of the test, note at what degree of flexion the patient had pain and where the pain was located. Also note if the crossed straight leg raise test is positive. This occurs when the straight leg raise test brings on pain on the opposite side.

6. Which lab tests should be done?

A complete blood count, ESR, and urinalysis are good screening tests. More specific tests depend on any specific entity you are attempting to define.

7. When should you order an electromyograph and nerve conduction study?

These tests may be ordered in a patient with radicular symptoms approximately 3 weeks after onset of the problem.

8. Which radiologic studies should be done?

Plain films should include anteroposterior and lateral views. A cone-down view of L5–S1 may be needed for better visualization. Oblique views are required to rule out a pars interarticularis fracture, which is seen in spondylolysis. An anteroposterior view of the pelvis may be adequate to evaluate the sacroiliac joints. If not, then specific sacroiliac joint views should be done.

9. When should you get an MRI or CT scan of the lumbar spine?

These studies are not routinely required to make a diagnosis or plan a conservative treatment program. They should be reserved for the patient who is not improving despite having undergone appropriate treatment, or for those in whom there is suspicion of more serious pathology.

Generally, MRI appears to be used more than CT. Both can adequately visualize the lumbar area and identify disc herniations. MRI is superior in imaging the conus medullaris portion of the spinal cord and at evaluating discs for dehydration. After lumbar disc surgery, MRI with contrast is preferred to differentiate recurrent disc herniation versus scar formation. CT is generally superior in evaluating bony structures.

While myelograms and discograms are also options, they are rarely needed for nonoperative evaluation and treatment planning.

10. What other imaging modalities may be helpful? When?

Bone scans, particularly SPECT scans, are very helpful in defining subtle abnormalities, such as spondylolysis or evidence of bone trauma, that may not be evident on other studies.

11. What are the most common diagnoses seen in a spine clinic?

About only 15% of patients presenting with acute low back problems can be given a specific diagnosis. So while it is important to try to be as specific as possible in giving a diagnosis, also realize that the lack of objective findings in many patients will allow only a general impression of the problem. If the following list of common diagnoses is considered when you see a patient, then you are less likely to miss a major problem.

Myofascial pain	Stenosis
Herniated disc	Fibromyalgia
Spondylolysis/spondylolisthesis	Infection
Fracture	Spondyloarthropathy
Facet syndrome	Tumor

12. What are the most common causes of lumbar pain by age group?

While soft tissue strains are the most common, several other conditions are also commonly seen in specific age groups. In teenagers, it is spondylolysis, especially in the athletic population. For those aged 20–60, a herniated disc would be a high suspicion. For those over age 60, spinal stenosis or fracture is frequent.

13. List the possible treatments to consider in a patient with LBP.

Rest	Manipulation
Medications (analgesics, anti-inflammatories, antispasmodics)	Injections
	Bracing
Modalities (heat, ultrasound, hydrotherapy, etc.)	Education
	Psychological intervention
Aerobic exercise	Ergonomic modifications
Specific spinal exercises (flexion, extension, stabilization	Surgery
	Vocational counseling

14. When is surgery indicated?
Absolute indications
    Cauda equina syndrome (loss of bowel/bladder control)
    Progressive neurologic deficit
Relative indications
    Intolerable pain
    Persistent pain that markedly compromises a patient's functional abilities

15. When are flexion, extension, or stabilization approaches used?
When planning any program, remember the three-joint complex of the vertebra, and the effect of any degenerative process on this (e.g., disc space narrowing resulting in increased facet loading and abnormal mechanical forces). The types of exercises and the aggressiveness of any program will depend on where a patient is in the degenerative cascade.
- For discogenic pain, the McKenzie approach, with emphasis on passive extension initially, is usually preferred.
- For posterior element pain, such as facet dysfunction or spondylolysis, flexion approaches are preferred, as there is less stress placed on these structures. William's flexion exercises would fall in this group.
- For patients with a very "irritable" back that flares with any activity, gentle isometric approaches may be preferred. Then, as they can tolerate more activity, functional stabilization exercises are very effective. These could range from simple balance exercise, frequently using a gym ball, to higher-level functional training with pulleys and other athletic or functional activities. Their role is not only strengthening but also coordination training (neuromuscular re-education).

Once the patient is beyond the acute stage, progressing them to as near of normal strength and range of motion of the spine as possible is the goal.

Exercise Approaches and General Indications for Their Use

DIAGNOSIS	AEROBICS	FLEXION	EXTENSION	STABILIZATION
Myofascial pain	+	+	+	+
Herniated disc (not a free fragment)	+	±	±	+
Spondylolysis	+	+	Not acutely	+
Fracture (stable)	+	Not acutely	Not acutely	+
Facet syndrome	+	+	–	+
Spinal stenosis	+	+	–	+
Fibromyalgia	+	+	+	+
Infection	Mild	±	±	±
Spondyloarthropathy	+	±	±	+
Tumor	Varies	±	±	±

16. What general exercise approaches should be recommended?
Almost all patients need to be involved in some type of aerobic exercise. Most choose walking, with swimming, biking (regular or stationary), stair-steppers, ski machines, and running as alternatives. With discogenic pain, sitting intolerance may preclude use of the exercise bike.

An individual who has been limited due to pain for 1–2 months should start at a low level of activity, such as walking for 10–15 minutes, one to two times per day. This can be gradually increased by 3–5 minutes per session every week until the patient is up to 30–45 minutes of sustained activity every day. If a patient is having so much pain with activity that he or she cannot sleep at night or has severe pain that persists into the next day, then the patient is progressing too quickly.

17. How long should a patient be on bedrest?

Most patients do not require bedrest but would benefit from an alteration in their activity until the pain subsides. More than 4 days of bedrest is not recommended for most acute conditions. It is becoming rarer for patients with acute back pain to undergo hospitalization for bedrest.

18. Describe the natural history of LBP.

Eighty to 90% of episodes of LBP resolve within 1 month. Practitioners will spend most of their time with the 10–20% of cases that do not improve rapidly. Kirkaldy-Willis eloquently addressed the natural history of spinal degeneration: dysfunction leads to instability, with the body attempting to stabilize itself eventually. As patients age, their LBP will probably subside, but they will be stiffer in this area, which is the price paid for stabilization.

19. What are some common "red flags" that identify the 10–20% of cases less likely to improve well?

Poor educational level (less than a high school degree)
Tobacco/alcohol use
Presence of significant emotional stressors
Pending medical-legal issues

20. When should the patient be sent to a psychologist?

- Obvious emotional distress (anxiety, apathy, decreased motivation, suicidal comments)
- Failure to comply with medical recommendations
- Behavioral problems on the job (decreased performance, tardiness, lack of follow-through)
- Any evidence of alcohol/drug abuse
- Any traumatic injury requiring significant adaptation (back/hand injuries, etc.)
- "Too good" of adaptation (overcompensating that may prove stressful in the long run)
- Failure to cope with stressors outside the job

21. What are the most important points to impress on the patient?

- A severe medical or surgical condition has either been addressed or ruled out.
- Back pain is usually a lifestyle issue, and unless there is an alteration of risk factors, there is a high rate of recurrence.

22. When has a patient reached the point of maximal medical improvement (end of healing)?

When the treatment goals have been achieved, or when it is obvious that the goals are unachievable and the patient is not making significant progress. The amount of time it takes to reach this point varies greatly among patients.

23. What are the real keys to successful treatment?

Defining the problem for the patient
Having a motivated patient
Correctly structuring the treatment program
Knowing the patient and his or her problem well enough to set realistic expectations for final outcome in an appropriate time frame

BIBLIOGRAPHY

1. Bigos S, Bowyer O, Braen G, et al: Acute Low Back Problems in Adults: Clinical Practice Guideline No. 14. (ACHR Publication No. 95-0642.) Rockville, MD, Agency for Health Care Policy and Research, 1994.
2. Kirkaldy-Willis WH: Managing Low Back Pain, 2nd ed. New York, Churchill-Livingstone, 1988.
3. McKenzie R: The Lumbar Spine: Mechanical Diagnosis and Therapy. Upper Hut, New Zealand, Spine Publications, 1981.
4. Pope MH, Andersson GBJ, Frymoyer JW, Chaffin DB: Occupational Low Back Pain: Assessment, Treatment, and Prevention. St. Louis, Mosby, 1991.

5. Spengler DW, Bigos SJ, Martin NA, et al: Back injuries in industry: A retrospective study: 1. Overview and cost analysis. Spine 4(2):129–134, 1986.
6. Spitzer WO, et al: Scientific approach to the assessment and management of activity-related spinal disorders: A monograph for clinicians: Report of the Quebec Task Force on Spinal Disorders. Spine 12(suppl 7):S1–S59, 1987.
7. Twomey L, Taylor J: Physical Therapy of the Low Back, 2nd ed. (Clinics in Physical Therapy.) New York, Churchill-Livingstone, 1994.
8. White AA, Panjabi MM: Clinical Biomechanics of the Spine, 2nd ed. Philadelphia, J.B. Lippincott, 1990.

56. DIAGNOSTIC IMAGING IN LOW BACK PAIN

Maury Ellenberg, M.D., and Michael Schwartz, M.D.

1. Why are radiologic techniques important in managing patients with low back pain (LBP)?

They can detect cancer, infection, disc disease, fracture, and other conditions, such as synovial cysts or tethered cord. They can direct treatment and help the physician follow the response to treatment in specific disorders. Negative x-rays can also be useful guides.

2. Does every patient with LBP need to be x-rayed?

No! The history and physical examination are still the most effective screening tools for diagnoses. Imaging is required to confirm or rule out a condition suggested by the clinical picture. In today's cost-conscious environment, cost/benefit ratios must always be considered. You must ask yourself how the intervention will be used to change the management of the case. Also, these techniques are not completely innocuous. There is some radiation exposure and studies requiring contrast also carry a small but definite risk of anaphylaxis.

3. Which imaging techniques are used in patients with LBP?

Plain x-ray	CT
Myelography	MRI
Radionuclide studies	Discography

4. How do you decide which patients need to be imaged?

In **acute** problems, if there is trauma, image—something could be broken and may place the contents of the spinal canal at risk. If there is no trauma, imaging is generally not helpful or necessary, unless there is suspicion on a clinical basis that a disease process such as infection, compression fracture (as in a postmenopausal female with acute localized pain), or malignancy (history of prostate or other cancer) is present. Then immediate imaging is indicated. If the pain does not improve or if it worsens in 3–4 weeks, imaging is indicated. If there is progressive weakness or if the patient develops bilateral signs and symptoms or bowel and bladder symptoms, immediate imaging is needed based on these new acute symptoms or findings.

For long-standing complaints of back pain (> 8 wks), first check the clinical scenario carefully. A young person with no risk factors with an aching back could be treated first. If anything seems suspicious or if the patient is an older individual, imaging may be indicated.

The general rule is don't image unless it will make a real difference in the treatment. There are times, however, when imaging can provide information independent of treatment. A negative study can be reassuring to both clinician and patient and permits more active treatment. A positive study that demonstrates a herniated disc as the cause of the problem can reassure the patient and explain pathogenesis and prognosis.

5. Which imaging technique should be used first?

That depends on the situation. Despite the advanced technology of CT and MRI, plain films are still the foundation of imaging.

6. What imaging technique would be used in a trauma patient?

The main concerns are fracture as well as alignment and stability of the spine, since these can affect the cord or cauda equina or be the source of pain. Traumatic hematomas compressing the cord or nerve root must also be considered. In a patient who was involved in a car accident or a short fall and has localized pain and tenderness with a negative neurologic examination, get plain spine films that adequately image the affected areas. These will usually suffice to rule out fractures and dislocations.

7. What imaging techniques would you use on a young person who presents with lumbar radiculopathy without preceding trauma?

That depends on the precise situation and the timing. If you have a young person presenting within a week or two of the onset of the radiculopathy, no imaging is necessary. If the patient has undergone treatment for a 3-week period and has had less than expected improvement, plain x-rays and subsequent close clinical follow-up will suffice. The decision for further imaging should depend on continued clinical progress, response to nonsurgical treatment, discussion with the patient regarding the need for surgical intervention, and the degree of functional limitation the current problem imposes. It is possible, at this point, that cross-sectional imaging (CT or MR) is indicated.

8. Compare the advantages of CT and MRI.

Each technique has its advantages and disadvantages, but which you order depends on the circumstance and patient.

CT	MRI
Lower cost	No ionizing radiation
Better information on calcifications and cortical bone detail	Better information on soft tissue anatomy
Images less sensitive to patient motion	Multiplanar images possible (saggital, coronal, and axial)

With MRI, metal can cause problems. Larger, well-fixed metal implants such as hip prostheses or Harrington Rods may cause artifact. Some metal implants such as cerebral aneurysm clips, cardiac pacemakers, and metal in the eye are absolute contraindications. However, almost all patients with prosthetic heart valves can be imaged.

9. When should contrast (gadolinium) be used with MRI?

First, it's not just an MRI with contrast, because it should always be done without and with to allow comparison. Gadolinium, the contrast medium used for MRI, works by breaching the blood-brain barrier when this barrier is disrupted by infection, inflammation, or malignancy, thereby increasing the contrast between the lesion and the surrounding normal tissue. As such, gadolinium is the most effective way of visualizing spinal tumors. MRI with contrast is also the best way to distinguish scar from recurrent or persistent disc herniation in the postoperative back, although in the early postop period (at least the first 6 months), even this technique is unreliable.

10. Why are the invasive procedures—myelography or discography—not used much anymore?

The biggest problem with **myelography** was not the procedure as much as the side effects of the contrast media. Pantopaque, an oil-based medium, could produce arachnoiditis, and more recently, Metrizamide, a water-soluble medium, caused a high incidence of headaches, nausea and vomiting, and seizures. The current medium is a water-soluble, non-ionic product that results in considerably fewer side effects. As MRI use increased, the need for CT-myelography (myelography is almost never performed without a followup CT scan) has diminished. Its role today is almost exclusively for unusual problem-solving cases.

Discography is the injection of contrast material into the disc under fluoroscopic guidance, often followed by CT imaging. This procedure allows observation of the internal architecture of the disc and pain response of the patient. Discography's value in diagnosis and predicting treatment outcome is very controversial. Most physicians feel it adds little to the other diagnostic methods.

11. What is the role for bone scanning?

Bone scanning is often nonspecific, but under the right circumstance, it can be helpful. It can help distinguish an acute from a long-standing process in conditions such as compression fractures or pars defects. It will be positive in small fractures invisible to plain x-rays and can detect stress fractures and avascular necrosis before x-ray. One of its most important uses is to detect disseminated disease.

12. Does an MRI or CT scan showing disc herniation mean the patient has radiculopathy?

Definitely not. Large numbers of asymptomatic patients (21–37.5%) can have disc herniation (asymmetric extrusion of disc material at a weak spot in the annulus fibrosis), spinal stenosis, or facet degenerative joint disease without radiculopathy. Disc bulges (symmetric prominence) are present in 53–80% of individuals, with the incidence increasing with age. A bulge should therefore be considered a normal finding.

13. In patients with disc herniation who have lumbar radiculopathy, do these herniated discs have to be removed?

No, 75–90% of patients with proven radiculopathy can improve with nonsurgical treatment.

14. What happens to the disc if you don't operate?

Multiple studies have found that in about 50–70% of patients, the herniation disappears or is visible to only a very small extent on follow-up imaging after nonsurgical treatment.

15. So when the disc herniation resolves, the patient is better?

No, not at all! There is not always a correlation between the follow-up imaging findings and clinical symptoms. Some patients who have persistent large herniations can be totally asymptomatic. Also, these patients are better long before the disc herniation is no longer present, since symptoms may go away in a matter of weeks and the disc herniation may persist on imaging studies for much longer. In addition, appearance of the disc—whether it is large or small, lateral or central, extruded or not—on initial scans does not predict recovery or the need for surgery. Therefore, don't decide on surgery based on the imaging study; that decision remains clinical.

16. In a patient with back and leg pain, if the imaging scan is normal, does that mean the patient does not have radiculopathy?

Definitely not. Disc herniation does not equate with radiculopathy and, in fact, can be present with no symptoms whatever. And the converse is also true: radiculopathy does not equate with disc herniation. That is, you can have a radiculopathy without a disc herniation or other anatomic abnormality. Remember, we do not treat imaging studies; we treat patients.

17. Will electrodiagnostic studies be abnormal in these cases?

Yes, they may. An electrodiagnostic study is an assessment of the pathophysiology and complements the history and physical examination. Electromyography (EMG) identifies motor axon damage, the H-reflex assesses the sensory motor reflex arc, and compound motor action potentials reflect the amount of motor axon loss. Therefore, if there is an abnormality of the nerve root, there will likely also be an abnormality in the EMG.

18. Which is more accurate in radiculopathy diagnosis, EMG or imaging?

These are clearly not mutually exclusive techniques, but complementary techniques to help the clinician focus the intervention. EMG defines the pathophysiology and helps to determine whether radiculopathy is present and something about its extent, but gives no information regarding the cause. Imaging, although it cannot diagnose radiculopathy, certainly can help determine the etiology and confirm anatomic localization once the clinician has determined there is a radiculopathy (i.e., discs, spinal stenosis, infection, trauma, tumor, etc.).

BIBLIOGRAPHY

1. Deyo RA, Bigos SJ, Maravilla KR: Diagnostic imaging procedures for the lumbar spine [editorial]. Ann Intern Med 111:865–867, 1989.
2. Ellenberg MR, Ross ML, Honet JC, et al: Prospective evaluation of the course of disc herniations in patients with proven radiculopathy. Arch Phys Med Rehabil 74:3–8, 1993.
3. Gehweiler JA Jr, Daffner RH: Low back pain: The controversy of radiologic evaluation. AJR 140: 109–112, 1983.
4. Jensen MC, Brant-Zawadzki MN, Obuchowski N, et al: Magnetic resonance imaging of the lumbar spine in people without back pain. N Engl J Med 331:69–73, 1994.
5. Kaye JJ: Imaging of disorders of the spine. Curr Opin Radiol 3:719–726, 1991.
6. Liang M, Komaroff L: Roentgenograms in primary care patients with acute low back pain: A cost-effectiveness analysis. Arch Intern Med 142:1108–1112, 1982.
7. Saal JA, Saal JS, Herzog J: The natural history of lumbar intervertebral disc extrusions treated nonoperatively. Spine 7:683–686, 1990.
8. Taveras JM: Radiologic aspects of low back pain and sciatic syndromes [editorial]. AJNR 10:451–452, 1989.
9. Thornbury JR, Fryback DG, Turski PA, et al: Disk-caused nerve compression in patients with acute low-back pain: Diagnosis with MR, CT, myelography, and plain CT. Radiology 186:731–738, 1993.
10. Weber H: The natural history of disc herniation and the influence of intervention. Spine 19:2234–2238, 1994.

57. SCOLIOSIS

Mark A. Thomas, M.D.

1. What is scoliosis?

Curvature of the spine. The deformity in the spine's postural curve (lateral spinal curvature) is commonly associated with a rotational deformity. As the spine bends laterally, the vertebral body may rotate toward the convex side of the curve. Lateral curvature may lead to abnormal height of a hemipelvis or shoulder, while the rotational deformity leads to "humping" of the right or left paraspinal surface.

2. What are the common types of scoliosis? What causes the deformity?

Scoliosis can be considered either structural or functional. **Functional** scoliosis is due to malpositioning or unilateral paraspinal muscle pull. This may be associated with back pain and muscle spasm ("bowstring sign of Forestier"). In this type of curve, there is no significant vertebral body rotation, and the scoliosis is reversible.

Structural forms of scoliosis are not reducible and may be idiopathic, congenital, or acquired. Congenital malformation or loss of structural integrity may affect the vertebral body, disc, or supporting structures. Curvature may also result from weakness and chronic malpositioning of the spine, as with spinal muscular atrophy or muscular dystrophy. Scoliosis is a frequent finding in patients with neurofibromatosis, presumably due to the mechanical obstruction to normal alignment presented by the neurofibroma. There is no defined etiology for idiopathic adolescent scoliosis, although spinal cord or brainstem pathology are possible factors.

Classifying Scoliosis

FUNCTIONAL	STRUCTURAL
Muscle spasm	Congenital
Paraspinal strain	Bar
Herniated disc (unilateral)	Block
Postural	Hermivertebra or other body anomaly
	Idiopathic
	Adolescent (spinal cord or brainstem disease?)
	Juvenile
	Associated with congenital heart disease
	Acquired
	Degenerative
	Post-traumatic (fracture)
	Overuse (repetitive microtrauma)
	Senile
	Secondary (disease-related)
	"Paralytic" neuromuscular disease (spinal muscular atrophy, muscular dystrophy, myelomeningocele, etc.)
	Connective tissue disease (Ehlers-Danlos, chondrodysplasia, Marfan's, etc.)

3. How is scoliosis evaluated?

Patient height, leg lengths, and angle of back inclination (as a reflection of the degree of spinal rotation) are measured serially, generally every 6 months to 1 year. Vital capacity may be measured, and back extensor and abdominal strength, flexibility of the back, and flexibility of the musculature around the hip should be assessed. In many instances, x-ray evaluation is important to assess the curve as well as estimate bone age (e.g., Risser's sign, which assesses the development of iliac apophyses in grades 0, immature, to 5, mature.

4. How is the type of curve described?

Scoliosis is named by the location and direction of curvature, i.e., by the location of the **apex** of curve (the convex side, right or left) and the **segment** of spine (thoracic or lumbar).

Curves may be further characterized by other findings that also have prognostic value:

Pattern of curve (C or single major, S or double major, multiple or serpentine, compensatory primary)

Degree of rotation (1–4, judged by x-ray position of the pedicles on an AP view)

Risser score (bone age, 0–5)

Degenerative or congenital, depending on associated x-ray findings

Cosmetic spinal score, or angle of inclination of the back

5. What is PLEAD?

This is a useful way to remember the factors considered in naming the scoliotic curve:

P—Pattern (S, C, serpentine, primary, secondary)

L—Location (thoracic, thoracolumbar, lumbar)

E—Etiology (idiopathic, congenital, degenerative, disease-related)

A—Apex (thoracic, lumbar)

D—Direction (right, left)

6. How are x-rays used in the evaluation of scoliosis?

The parameters most commonly assessed by plain radiographs include the Cobb angle, spinal rotation, pelvic and spinal growth centers, and the rib-vertebral angle difference. X-ray evaluation is important in decision-making when treating scoliosis. The films should be done with the patient standing. Low-dose AP films, with shielding of radiosensitive tissue (e.g., genitalia) are preferred to PA views for more accurate depiction of the spine. Serial evaluation is necessary for anticipating the course of disease and determining treatment or for assessing effectiveness and modifying treatment.

X-ray allows measurement of the curve by the Cobb angle, which has been demonstrated to have a reasonable inter-rater reliability. The most likely source of error in x-ray evaluation is related to the way in which the radiograph is produced (i.e., PA vs. AP view). X-rays also offer the possibility of identifying other pathology, such as spondylolisthesis or spondylolysis.

7. How is the Cobb angle measured? Rotation?

The **Cobb angle** is measured by dropping lines perpendicular to the endplates of the most severely tilted vertebral bodies in the curve. The angle at which these perpendicular lines intersect is the Cobb angle, which is the most common definition of the severity of the lateral deformity in scoliosis.

Rotation is assessed by viewing the films with attention to symmetry of pedicle position and position of the spinous process (normally midline). Rotation is graded 0 (no rotation) to 4 (one pedicle rotated entirely out of view.).

8. Which growth centers are assessed on x-ray films in scoliosis?

In the adolescent, the film routinely incorporates the **iliac** (Risser's sign) and **ischial apophyses**, which may be open, capping, consolidating, or closed (graded 0–5). The film may also incorporate the proximal **humeral growth plate**, which is helpful to see since closure of growth centers proceeds in a caudal to cephalad manner. The **ring apophyses** (spinal growth centers) may or may not be clearly defined on plain films. The timing and window of nonsurgical intervention for adolescent idiopathic scoliosis can be estimated by evaluating these growth centers.

9. When does scoliosis require treatment?

While the primary factor in the decision to treat scoliosis is the **degree of lateral curvature**, several other variables help anticipate the natural course of the deformity. These may weight the decision whether to observe, brace, or operate. The type of scoliosis, pattern of the curve, cosmesis, severity of rotation and location of the curve, patient age, effects of deformity (pain, neurologic, pulmonary, or cardiac compromise), patient compliance, and available resources all help dictate what treatment should be offered to a patient.

10. What are the available options?

In general, treatment most often provided for the different types of scoliosis includes:
Congenital scoliosis: surgery; bracing
Paralytic scoliosis: wheelchair seating systems, bracing, surgery
Idiopathic scoliosis:
    < 20°: observation
    20–40°: bracing
    > 40°: surgery
Marked rotation/humping (nonsurgical curve): bracing
Degenerative scoliosis:
    < 60°: posture, exercise, supportive (corset, NSAIDs, etc.)
    > 60°: surgery

Alternative treatments (exercise, electric stimulation, biofeedback, traction, manipulation) have been recommended at various times on an anecdotal basis. These treatments have not been shown to effectively alter the natural progression of deformity, although they might be useful as treatment for any associated mechanical back pain.

11. Why treat scoliosis?

Curvature of the spine, particularly during growth or when > 20°, is likely to be progressive. Complications of deformity, such as pain, psychosocial consequences of poor cosmesis, and even possible respiratory failure (with curves > 110°) are compelling reasons to intervene when there is a reasonable prospect of controlling (or correcting) scoliosis.

12. Which prognostic factors predict the likelihood that deformity will progress in the scoliotic patient?

Determining the Likelihood that Scoliosis Will Progress

PROGNOSTIC VARIABLE	UNFAVORABLE	FAVORABLE
Type of scoliosis	Congenital, juvenile, "paralytic"	Other
Degree of curvature	> 20–40°	< 20°
Location of curve	Thoracic	Lumbar
Pattern of curve	Single, short	Serpentine, compensatory, long
Degree of rotation	2–4	0–1
Risser sign/growth	0/immature	5/mature
Change on serial evaluation	Rapid increase in curve size	Minimal change in curve size
Gender	Female	Male
Menarchal status	Premenarchal	Regular menses
Osteoporosis	Present	Normal bone mineral density
Prior spinal surgery	Discectomy or laminectomy	None

13. What surgical options are available for treatment of scoliosis?
Surgical strategies aim to either stabilize the spine or to correct deformity and then stabilize the spine. The goal is to limit the progression of spinal deformity.

Surgery in general addresses lateral and rotational deformity by distraction or derotation, and instability by either compression or bony fusion. Instrumentation that requires bony fusion of the spine is used for distraction procedures (i.e., Harrington rods); these procedures may or may not include rib resection in an attempt to improve appearance. Postoperatively, these patients are placed in a cast or body jacket to immobilize the operated segment. Cotrel-Dubousset instrumentation and the various modifications that work to derotate the spine do not require either fusion or immobilization with a body jacket nor rib resection. Other procedures such as osteotomy, laminectomy, and fusion are done as appropriate.

14. What are the potential complications of surgery?
Complications include slipping of anchoring hooks, fracture of the rod, failure of bony fusion, wire pull-out, progressive pelvic obliquity, rod bending, pseudarthrosis, and migration of hardware. Progression of the curve is possible. For the adolescent in whom spinal growth continues, the "crankshaft phenomenon" (progressive deformity resulting from continued growth of the anterior spine after posterior arthrodesis) may occur. This may result in some increase in scoliosis, rotation, rib-vertebral angle difference, and, less likely, kyphosis, but is usually not problematic. The patient with degenerative scoliosis who has undergone successful surgery may experience persistent pain or restricted mobility.

15. How do braces work for scoliosis?
When bracing is used optimally, the probability that surgical intervention will be required decreases by up to a factor of 4. Braces provide force acting in a direction opposite to the deformity. Most work by providing an anteriorly directed force against a posteriorly rotating segment, using a rib or transverse process as a lever to transmit corrective forces to the spine. This, in effect, "de-rotates" the spine and ideally either stops or slows curve progression. With scoliosis in a growing patient, some correction may actually occur. In order to apply force effectively, the brace must anchor firmly against the bony pelvis.

Patients with significant weakness may be assisted by an orthotic to help correct posture and stabilize the trunk, and patients with significant spondylosis may experience some relief of pain with orthotic support.

16. What are the orthotic (brace) options available for use?

Orthotics Used in the Treatment of Scoliosis

Bracing to control spinal curvature
  Body jacket type: Boston, Denver, Risser localizer cast, etc. (TLSO or LSO)
  Milwaukee: CTLSO or TLSO
  Shoe lift (with leg-length discrepancy)
Bracing to improve stability and comfort
  Soft Boston
  Corset-type TLSO or LSO
  Adaptive seating

TLSO, thoracolumbosacral; LSO, lumbosacral, CTLSO, cervicothoracolumbosacral.

17. Are there potential complications from the orthotics used to treat scoliosis?

Complications of bracing include skin breakdown, excessive sweating, and allergic skin reactions. Bracing may result in a decrease in rib cage and abdominal wall movement. Increased gastric pressure and gastroesophageal reflux due to body jacket braces have also been reported, as has spontaneous fracture of the sternum (one case). Discomfort and rejection of the brace due to poor appearance are probably the most common complications seen.

18. Describe a typical patient with degenerative scoliosis.

Degenerative scoliosis affects between 3–30% of the geriatric population, with the incidence increasing with age and female gender. The typical patient is a female over age 50 years with a history of low back pain. The curve is located between T12 and L5, there is a history of spondylosis, and on diagnosis, the curve is frequently as high as 50° or 60° (Cobb angle). In general, the curve will increase about 3° per year. There may be a history of osteoporosis.

These patients have spondylosis, degenerative disc disease, facet arthritis, and possibly stenosis (of the lateral recess or neural foramen due to related arthritic change, or of the spinal canal as a result of listhesis and/or scoliotic deformity). Degenerative scoliosis is a lumbar curve without any compensatory thoracic curve.

19. When is surgery indicated in degenerative scoliosis? What are the potential complications?

Indications for surgery include severe pain that does not adequately respond to conservative care, progressive deformity, and/or loss of sagittal plane balance. Surgery also prevents such secondary morbidity as the loss of rib cage movement, decrease in vital capacity, and cardiopulmonary impairment due to scoliosis. Unsuccessful surgery with persistent pain is usually related to failure of fusion (associated with smoking), failure to restore lumbar lordosis, or late problems distal to the site of fusion.

20. Does exercise have a role in the treatment of scoliosis?

No clear value of exercise in correcting the curve has been demonstrated in a well-done study. Nonetheless, it is generally agreed that exercise is useful in maintaining strength, flexibility, and conditioning. This may be particularly important in the elderly patient with degenerative scoliosis, in whom exercise may have a positive impact on gait and balance as well as general well-being.

BIBLIOGRAPHY

1. Edelman P: Brace treatment in idiopathic scoliosis. Acta Orthop Belg 58(suppl 1):85–90, 1992.
2. Goldberg CJ, Dowling FE, et al: A statistical comparison between natural history of idiopathic scoliosis and brace treatment in skeletally immature adolescent girls. Spine 18:902–909, 1993.

3. Kennedy JD, et al: Effect of bracing on respiratory mechanics in mild idiopathic scoliosis. Thorax 44:548–553, 1989.
4. Korovessis P, et al: Adult idiopathic lumbar scoliosis: A formula for prediction of progression and review of the literature. Spine 19:1926–1932, 1994.
5. Lonstein JE, Winter RB: The Milwaukee brace for the treatment of adolescent idiopathic scoliosis: A review of one thousand and twenty patients. J Bone Joint Surg 76A:1207–1221, 1994.
6. Mehta MH: The conservative management of juvenile idiopathic scoliosis. Acta Orthop Belg 58(suppl 1): 91–97, 1992.
7. Montgomery F, Willner S: Screening for idiopathic scoliosis: Comparison of 90 cases shows less surgery by early diagnosis. Acta Orthop Scand 64(4):456–458, 1993.
8. Perennou D, et al: Adult lumbar scoliosis: Epidemiologic aspects in a low-back pain population. Spine 19:123–128, 1994.
9. Weiss HR: Characteristics of physical therapy of scoliosis patients in adulthood. Rehabilitation 31(1): 38–42, 1992.
10. Winter RB: The pendulum has swung too far: Bracing for adolescent idiopathic scoliosis in the 1990s. Orthop Clin North Am 25(2):195–204, 1994.

VI. *Rehabilitation of the Orthopedic Patient*

58. SHOULDER REHABILITATION AFTER SURGERY

Brian M. Torpey, M.D., and Edward G. McFarland, M.D.

1. When is a shoulder arthroplasty indicated?

Common indications for shoulder replacement surgery are pain due to joint incongruity, decreased range of motion, and diminished function. Shoulder replacements are performed for severe arthritis, avascular necrosis, acute fracture, or neoplasm.

2. How does total shoulder arthroplasty differ from hemiarthroplasty?

Total shoulder arthroplasty (TSA) involves surgical replacement of both the humeral and glenoid side of the joint, while **hemiarthroplasty** involves the humeral side of the joint. Most surgeons recommend TSA for patients with an intact rotator cuff, and hemiarthroplasties for arthritic patients with massive rotator cuff tears or patients with complex fractures of the proximal humerus.

3. When is shoulder arthroplasty not indicated?

Contraindications include severe osteoporosis, neuropathic joint, paralysis, and recent joint infection.

4. What are the most frequent complications after TSA?

Humeral fracture, axillary or suprascapular nerve injury, instability/dislocation, infection, perioperative rotator cuff tear, reflex sympathetic dystrophy, and loosening. Shoulder infection, although infrequent (< 1%), can be caused by *Staphylococcus aureus* and may require debridement and intravenous antibiotics or, in more severe cases, prosthetic removal and revision. Chronic instability may be caused by a malpositioned prosthesis or an impaired rotator cuff mechanism. The rehabilitationist needs to adhere strictly to ROM precautions.

Loosening of the shoulder prosthetic presents with pain, instability, and progressive dysfunction of the arm. Loosening is often identified on x-rays as radiolucent lines.

5. What ROM precautions need to be followed after TSA?

No extension past neutral
No external rotation past 15°
No active abduction or flexion until 4–6 weeks postop

6. What's the outcome after TSA? Does the shoulder still hurt?

Although pain relief is anticipated, a significant improvement in ROM is less consistently predictable.

7. Discuss the role of surgery in treating rheumatoid arthritis of the shoulder.

Many areas of the shoulder complex can result in pain. In the arthritic patient, pain commonly originates from the glenohumeral joint, acromioclavicular joint, or subacromial joint space. Most rheumatoid shoulder surgery is aimed at the glenohumeral joint. The acromioclavicular joint can be treated by excision of the clavicular end along with anterior acromioplasty and subacromial decompression. Arthritis-associated rotator cuff tears are often not repairable because of size and poor tendon quality. If articular surfaces are smooth and congruent, a synovectomy may be performed for shoulder synovitis unresponsive to medical management.

8. After TSA is performed, how is the patient rehabilitated?

As with the replacement of other joints, rehab after shoulder arthroplasties should be tailored to the individual patient. Goals include pain relief, restoration of musculoskeletal function, and joint protection strategies.

Rehabilitation After Shoulder Arthroplasty

DURATION	PRECAUTIONS	TREATMENT
Phase 1		
0–3 wks postop	Non-weight-bearing Sling worn at all times except exercise Avoid active abduction, extension > 0°, external rotation > 15°	Gentle passive and active ROM; flexion to 90°, abduction to 90°, internal rotation to 45°, external rotation to 15° Pendulum exercises Isometric strengthening as tolerated by pain in flexion, extension, and rotation One-handed ADL
3–6 wks postop	Continue sling and non-weight-bearing May begin active abduction	Vigorous isometrics as tolerated Active-assisted progressing to active ROM exercise "Wall-walking" with hand used as stabilizing assist
Phase 2		
6–12 wks postop	May lift objects up to 2 lb Discontinue sling Continue ROM precautions	Vigorous isometrics Progressive isotonics (e.g., elastic tubing exercises) as tolerated Active-assisted ROM and active AROM past 90° Two-handed ADL encouraged
Phase 3		
> 12 wks postop	Discontinue ROM precautions	Active ROM exercises, progressive resistance, strengthening Stretching in flexion, abduction, and rotation

Adapted from Brander VA, Hinderer SR, Alpiner N, Oh TH: Limb disorders in rehabilitation in joint and connective tissue diseases. Arch Phys Med Rehabil 76(suppl):S-52, 1995.

9. What is the best way to rehabilitate a patient with a humeral neck fracture?

It depends. If the patient is **elderly**, an impacted humeral neck fracture is commonly treated conservatively with a sling. Gentle passive ROM exercises and active-assisted ROM during the first week are advisable. Pendulum exercises should be initiated as soon as tolerable. Adhesive capsulitis must be prevented. With improvement in pain, isometric strengthening exercises are performed. As ROM gradually improves, isotonic exercise can be implemented. Wall-walking and arm raises are particularly helpful. To preserve shoulder function, the elderly patient should acquire about 90° of abduction and flexion, 45° of internal rotation, and 15° of external rotation. With enhanced shoulder function, use of a sling can be tapered and one-handed techniques can be adopted. Full weight-bearing of the shoulder as well as aggressive stretching and strengthening exercises can begin once callus formation occurs. (Note that in acute fractures of the surgical neck of the humerus, the proximal segment is often abducted because of the action of the supraspinatus muscle.)

If the patient is **young**, there is a heightened risk for malunion, although less of a risk for adhesive capsulitis. Immobilization of stable fractures for 6–12 weeks is important until healing occurs. Isometric strengthening exercises along with gentle active-assistive ROM exercises can be implemented 2–3 weeks after the fracture. This can be upgraded to isotonic exercises at 6 weeks. At 12 weeks, progressive resistive and stretching exercises can be instituted.

10. What is impingement syndrome?

Shoulder impingement, also called rotator cuff tendinitis or subacromial bursitis, refers to compression of the rotator cuff by the acromion, coracoid process, coracoacromial ligament, and/or the acromioclavicular joint. This compression occurs as the glenohumeral joint is put through its ROM, specifically forward flexion and internal rotation. The supraspinatus tendon is most frequently involved, and the patient typically complains of pain into the deltoid region of the shoulder and arm or pain radiating to the forearm.

11. Describe the staging system for shoulder impingement.

Neer has outlined three stages of shoulder impingement:

Stage I   age < 25 yrs reversible edema, hemorrhage
Stage II   age 25–40 yrs, fibrosis, tendinitis
Stage III   age > 40 yrs, bone spurs on acromion, tendon rupture

12. How is impingement treated?

Acute impingement syndrome usually responds well to conservative therapy, including rest, ice massage, and NSAIDs. With resolution of the acute tendinitis, a shoulder rehab program emphasizing shoulder motion maintenance, modification of work or sport, and rotator cuff strengthening should be initiated.

Patients with persistent pain (often at night) following a course of rest, medication, and therapy may benefit from a corticosteroid injection into the subacromial space. If no relief in symptoms occurs after 6 months of treatment, evaluation for a rotator cuff tear is performed with shoulder arthrography, MRI, or ultrasound.

13. When are the various imaging tools used for shoulder assessment?

Plain films can be used to assess gross bony abnormalities of the shoulder complex. An AP view highlights the relationship of the humerus to the glenoid cavity, the relationship of the clavicle to the acromion, and the presence or absence of focal calcification in the tendons, particularly the supraspinatus and infraspinatus. An AP "stress view" can demonstrate third-degree sprain or glenohumeral inferior laxity. An axial lateral view of the shoulder highlights the relationship between the clavicle, scapula, humerus, and glenoid cavity. The sternoclavicular joint is optimally assessed in this view.

MRI is valuable for evaluating shoulder abnormalities including impingement syndromes, rotator cuff disruption, instability syndromes, bicipital tendon abnormalities, arthritic changes, occult fractures, ischemic necrosis, and intra-articular bodies.

Ultrasound is sometimes used as a "poor man's" imaging tool to identify rotator cuff tears.

Arthrography can be used to look at soft-tissue structures and recesses around the glenohumeral joint. Alone, arthrograms are frequently used to evaluate rotator cuff tears. When used in conjunction with CT scanning, arthrograms allow for excellent visualization of the glenoid labrum and for the diagnosis of glenohumeral instability.

14. When is shoulder surgery advisable?

Imaging-proven rotator cuff tendon tears, associated with persistent pain and shoulder dysfunction, may require surgical intervention. An acromioplasty can be done for patients with tendinitis or partial rotator cuff tears. Full-thickness rotator cuff tears are usually repaired unless they are chronic and/or too large to repair.

15. What causes a frozen shoulder?

A frozen shoulder (adhesive capsulitis) is diagnosed when pain associated with severe restriction of active and passive ROM of the glenohumeral joint occurs in all planes. Idiopathic frozen shoulder happens without any history of injury or primary precipitating event. Onset is insidious. Atrophy of the shoulder girdle muscles is often noted. Plain films are often normal but may show humeral head osteopenia. Arthrography frequently demonstrates a small retracted capsule with reduced dimension of the recesses. Patients with idiopathic frozen shoulder may experience a subsequent contralateral frozen shoulder in up to 20% of cases.

16. What are the stages of frozen shoulder?

Patients with idiopathic frozen shoulder typically experience three stages of symptoms and gradual improvement:

Painful stage: Complaints of vague global shoulder pain without history of a precipitating event. Pain is progressive in onset, lasting 2–9 months.

Stiffening stage: Progressive loss of shoulder motion in external and internal rotation and abduction. This stage may last from 4 months to 1 year.

Thawing stage: Progressive increase in shoulder motion. Although most patients re-develop functional motion, complete restoration of motion is not assured. Pain typically resolves. Secondary frozen shoulder may develop as a result of associated trauma to the shoulder, shoulder tendinitis, shoulder immobilization, disuse or paralysis.

17. How are frozen shoulders treated?

Stretching programs, in conjunction with analgesics, may offer relief in early frozen shoulder. Exercises should include Codman's, home pulley use, and active-assistive ROM using a cane or dowel rod. Stretching exercises should preferably be performed for short periods of time, several times a day. After pain control is established, physical therapy should be directed toward promoting stretching (internal and external rotation, and forward nexion) and eventually strengthening exercises. This nonoperative program may take up to 9–12 months before improvement of motion in the frozen shoulder is evident.

Corticosteroids injection in conjunction with exercise programs can be done. Subacromial injections especially may be useful in patients with concomitant impingement syndrome. Brisemont (distension arthrography) and manipulation under anesthesia, although controversial (because of the potential risk of fractures or brachial plexus injury) can be utilized when all other methods of treatment fail.

18. What causes glenohumeral instability?

Anterior glenohumeral instability can develop secondary to traumatic or atraumatic causes. Damage to the anterior glenolabral complex (glenoid labrum and inferior glenohumeral ligament) can occur during anterior shoulder dislocations. Detachment of the glenoid labrum (Bankart lesion), as a result of a traumatic anterior shoulder dislocation, may predispose to recurrent anterior shoulder instability, especially in the patient under age 20 (up top 80–90% have recurrent dislocation).

Atraumatic anterior instability of the humeral head is seen most commonly in overhead-throwing athletes. In this phenomenon, the anterior shoulder structures stretch and become lax because of the stresses placed on the shoulder during repetitive throwing motions. The humeral head subluxes partially over the anterior glenoid lip, causing discomfort and instability (dead arm syndrome), but a frank anterior dislocation does not occur.

Atraumatic anterior shoulder instability is also seen in patients with soft tissue laxity (Ehlers-Danlos syndrome). Some patients may be able to voluntarily subluxate their shoulder(s). These individuals often experience multidirectional instability, where the humeral head subluxes anteriorly, posteriorly, and inferiorly.

19. What are the treatment options for anterior glenohumeral instability?

Young athletes who experience traumatic anterior shoulder dislocation often benefit from a shoulder rehabilitation program. A brief period of shoulder immobilization, followed by ROM therapy, should be prescribed prior to the initiation of an exercise program. Exercises in this program should include strengthening of the anterior shoulder girdle muscles, the scapular stabilizer muscles, and the rotator cuff musculature. If these individuals experience recurrent anterior instability despite an aggressive shoulder stabilization/rehab program, then surgical reconstruction should be considered.

Some professional competitive athletes may benefit from early surgical reconstruction. Nonathletic individuals and older patients (> 40 years old) may not require surgery after an initial anterior dislocation. Physical therapy and return to restrictive activities may suffice to prevent anterior instability. Overhead throwing athletes who experience anterior shoulder subluxation should be started on a shoulder stabilization program which includes anterior shoulder girdle muscular development. Continued instability in athletes who have undergone a prolonged shoulder rehab program may require surgery. Patients who experience episodes of atraumatic instability due to hyperlaxity should be treated nonoperatively. Extensive physical therapy, as well as psychosocial evaluations, may be necessary to treat these patients. Surgery is rarely indicated for patients with voluntary dislocating shoulders.

20. Describe the biomechanics of throwing a baseball.
Six phases have been identified:

Wind-up	Acceleration
Early cocking	Deceleration
Late cocking	Follow through

The throw begins with a wind-up. By drawing back on one leg and turning sideways, a pitcher is able to elevate the center of gravity as high as possible. The arm is then cocked back as the pitcher's foot touches the ground (early cocking), which allows the arm to cock back to its furthest limit (late cocking). The ball is accelerated by the concentric contraction of the anterior shoulder and scapular muscles, trunk rotation, and ground reaction force. After the ball is released, deceleration occurs and includes eccentric contractions of posterior shoulder stabilizers to slow the extremity. In follow through, energy is dissipated as the pitcher's arm comes to a resting position. A balanced strengthening of the shoulder stabilizers prevents injury.

BIBLIOGRAPHY

1. Brander VA, Hinderer SR, Alpiner N, Oh TH: Limb disorders in rehabilitation in joint and connective tissue diseases. Arch Phys Med Rehabil 76:S-52, 1995.
2. Kircher MT, Cappuccino A, Torpey BM: Muscular violence as a cause of humeral fractures. Contemp Orthop 6:475–480, 1993.
3. Lundberg BJ: The frozen shoulder. Acta Orthop Scan (Suppl) 119:1–59, 1969.
4. Neer CS: Involuntary inferior and multidirectional instability of the shoulder: Etiology, recognition, and treatment. In AAOS Instructional Course Lectures, vol 34. Ruby Ridge, IL, American Academy of Orthopaedic Surgeons, 1985, pp 232–238.
5. O'Sullivan SB, Schmitz TJ: Physical Rehabilitation: Assessment and Treatment. Philadelphia, F.A. Davis, 1988.
6. Rizk TE, et al: Adhesive capsulitis (frozen shoulder): A new approach to its management. Arch Phys Med Rehabil 64:29–33, 1983.
7. Rockwood CA, Matsen FA: The Shoulder. Philadelphia, W.B. Saunders, 1990.
8. Simonet WT, Cofield RH: Prognosis in anterior shoulder dislocation. Am J Sports Med 12(1):19–24, 1984.
9. Sullivan PE, et al: An Integrated Approach to Therapeutic Exercise Theory and Clinical Application. Reston, VA, Reston Publ. Co., 1982.

59. ELBOW REHABILITATION AFTER SURGERY

Jason Rudolph, M.D., Brian M. Torpey, M.D., and Edward G. McFarland, M.D.

1. What are the indications for performing elbow replacement surgery?

Three groups of patients commonly benefit from elbow arthroplasty:

1. Patients with rheumatoid arthritis that causes elbow pain and loss of motion, with or without instability. Elbow x-rays that show loss of cartilage or significant resorptive arthropathy are important indicators for elbow arthroplasty.

2. Patients with post-traumatic arthritis, who have destroyed elbow joint surfaces, limited motion, and severe pain. Surgery is usually performed only in patients older than 60 years.

3. Patients with malunion or nonunion of distal humerus fractures.

2. Are there any contraindications to elbow arthroplasty?

Absolute contraindications
    Previous open wounds about the elbow associated with trauma
    Previous infection of the elbow joint
    Arthrodesis of the elbow joint
Relative contraindications
    Paralysis of biceps or triceps (unless muscle transfer can be done as substitute motor power)
    Severe joint capsule contractions
    Young active patients

3. How do the different types of elbow replacement prostheses work?

There are two basic types of elbow replacement prostheses. **Constrained** elbow prostheses were the original, custom-designed, hinged implants that provided immediate stability; however, loosening at bone-cement interface was common. **Semiconstrained** prostheses provide a similar degree of stability but they allow 8–10° of varus-valgus and axial toggle, allowing the capsule and ligaments to transmit some of the force and thereby reducing the risk of mechanical loosening.

4. Describe the postoperative management required after elbow replacement surgery.

After implantation of a semiconstrained prosthesis, the arm is elevated for 2–3 days, the compression dressing is removed after 4–5 days, and a collar and cuff are applied. Patients are started on active elbow flexion and extension in conjunction with occupational therapy for ADLs. Strength exercises are avoided; no lifting greater than 1 lb with the affected elbow is allowed for 3 months. Even then, patients are advised to never use their affected arm to lift objects weighing > 5 lbs. If a flexion contracture of 45° was present prior to surgery, an extension splint is used at night for 4–12 weeks.

5. What causes elbow contractures?

Elbow contractures may be classified by origin (intra-articular versus extra-articular), position (flexion or extension), or most commonly, etiology (traumatic, congenital, or acquired). Traumatic contracture may be extra-articular (due to soft tissue injury, pain, and subsequent hemarthrosis) or intra-articular (due to direct injury to joint surface). Congenital contractures are usually due to primary muscle or nerve deficiency. Acquired elbow contractures are usually caused by primary inflammatory processes (osteoarthritis, hemophilia, Still's disease, and septic arthritis).

6. How are elbow contractures treated nonoperatively?

Conservative treatment is preferred in contractures < 1 year old: local heat, active gentle assisted stretch, ultrasound, dynamic splinting, and occupational modulation. It is important to recognize the need for slow, static stretching or dynamic assistive stretching in elbow contractures, in contrast to the shoulder which responds more to aggressive manipulation.

7. What types of surgery are used to treat elbow contractures?

Operative intervention is indicated only when conservative treatment has failed. There are three types of operative intervention:

1. Excision, release of contracture, and early joint motion (recommended for most extra-articular contractures).
2. Release of contracture and muscle transfer (used in arthrogryposis and cerebral palsy)
3. Arthroplasty and distraction of joint (used with some types of intra-articular contractures)

8. Who is at increased risk for developing heterotopic ossification (HO) about the elbow?

Four groups of patients are at risk for developing HO: those with elbow trauma, traumatic brain or spinal cord injury, burn injury, and genetic conditions. The incidence of HO after simple elbow dislocation is approximately 3%, whereas patients with elbow dislocations and radial head fractures have a 20% incidence. Elbow dislocations associated with other fractures cause HO in approximately 16% of individuals.

9. In what direction do elbow dislocations most commonly occur?

Because a fall onto an outstretched arm is the most common mechanism of elbow dislocations, dislocations are most often posterior followed by anterior (seen in children) or, rarely, divergent (after high energy trauma). Associated injuries include fractures (radial head or condyles), arterial injury (beware of Volkmann's ischemic contracture), or associated nerve injury (median, ulnar).

10. Do elbow dislocations require surgery?

Typically, no. Management consists of emergent closed reduction and splint application with the elbow in a flexed and pronated position. Open reduction may be necessary if dislocation has been neglected, if soft tissue is interposed in the joint, or if concomitant intra-articular fractures are present. The elbow is placed into a padded posterior splint initially in full pronation and flexed at 90° (after assessment for instability has been made). The splint is removed 3–10 days later, and active unprotected flexion/extension exercises are encouraged. If the elbow remains unstable, a cast brace is applied, gradually increasing extension weekly. No immobilization is used beyond 3 weeks. Muscle strengthening is then encouraged. If full motion has not been attained by 6–8 weeks, static flexion and extension splints are advocated.

11. What are the treatment options and potential complications of fractures and dislocations about the elbow in adults?

Elbow Fractures and Dislocations (Adults)

INJURY	TREATMENT	COMPLICATIONS
Supracondylar	Undisplaced: Immobilize 1–2 wks Displaced: ORIF with bone grafting Early ROM exercises	Neurovascular injury, nonunion, malunion, contracture, pain, decreased ROM
Transcondylar	ORIF if displaced	Decreased ROM
Condylar		
Lateral	Undisplaced: Immobilize in supination Displaced: ORIF	Cubitus valgus
Medial	Undisplaced: immobilize in pronation Displaced: ORIF	Cubitus varus (gunstock deformity)
Capitellar	Undisplaced: Splint 2–3 wks Displaced: ORIF Comminuted: Excise fragment	—

(Table continued on following page.)

Elbow Fractures and Dislocations (Adults) (Cont.)

INJURY	TREATMENT	COMPLICATIONS
Olecranon	Undisplaced: Immobilize in 45–90° of flexion for 3 weeks	Decreased ROM, post-traumatic arthritis, ulnar nerve
Neurapraxia	Displaced: ORIF with tension band wiring Comminuted: Excision, reattachment of triceps Fracture-dislocation: ORIF with intramedullary device Rehab started once postoperative pain has subsided (usually after 3–7 days) Extremes of motion should be avoided Strengthening exercises delayed until union achieved (usually 8 wks)	Instability
Coronoid process	If fragment < 50%, excision with early ROM If fragment > 50%, ORIF	Instability and post-traumatic arthritis
Radial head	Undisplaced: Early motion Displaced: Use "Rule of 3's"—> 30° angulation, 3 mm of displacement, or $\frac{1}{3}$ of radial head involved → ORIF Comminuted: Excision	Posterior interosseous nerve injury
Elbow dislocation	Usually posterior dislocation: closed reduction, stabilize in a splint for 2–7 days, then gentle active ROM If irreducible: may require open reduction	Median, ulnar nerve injury Brachial artery injury Flexion contracture Heterotopic ossification

ORIF—open reduction and internal fixation.

12. What are the indications for fusing the elbow (arthrodesis)?

Chronic osteomyelitis, residual traumatic arthritis, tuberculosis (occasionally), and failed total elbow arthroplasty.

13. What is the most appropriate position to fuse the elbow joint?

For unilateral fusions, the elbow should be placed at 90° of flexion. For bilateral fusions, one elbow is placed at 110° flexion (to reach the mouth) and one at 65° (for personal body hygiene).

14. What preoperative considerations are important in patients requiring elbow disarticulation/amputation?

Amputations about the elbow result primarily from trauma or neoplasm. If disarticulation is performed, then an external prosthetic hinge is typically required. This hinge design is required to preserve cosmetic symmetrical bilateral arm length. Amputation at levels above the elbow commonly allows for an internally located elbow hinge because the prosthesis can be stabilized without having to comprise joint location. On the other hand, pronation and supination motion is much easier to control in patients with elbow disarticulation surgery. The preserved humeral condyles allow for better rotational control than the cylindrical distal humeral shaft in patients with above-elbow amputations.

The basic principle of all upper-extremity amputations is preservation of maximal length consistent with satisfactory wound management. One should also strive to maintain function of muscles, nerves, and arteries. The scar should be nontender, not adherent to bone, and healthy enough to withstand force transfer. Underlying bone should be contoured and smooth. Major nerves should be ligated and sharply sectioned (to prevent neuroma formation).

15. How soon after an elbow-level amputation can a patient be fit with a prosthesis?

A terminal device may be fitted the day after surgery. A body-powered prosthesis with a conventional shoulder girdle harness allows rapid return to bimanual activities. If a myoelectrical device is planned for the prosthesis, surface electrodes are placed on appropriate muscle signal areas in the inner wall of the cast. Shoulder and shoulder girdle exercises are started immediately after the amputation. Young, active patients may gain effective control of the temporary prosthesis within a few days after amputation. A permanent prosthesis is usually allowed after 5–6 weeks (to allow for adequate soft-tissue healing).

16. When is surgery indicated for median entrapment neuropathies at the elbow?

The median nerve is vulnerable to compression mainly between a supracondylar process and the ligament beneath the bicipital aponeurosis (the ligament of Struthers), deep to the arch of origin of the pronator teres, and under the origin of the flexor digitorum superficialis. The principal symptoms are numbness in the radial $3\frac{1}{2}$ digits and thenar muscle weakness (similar to carpal tunnel syndrome). Compression of the anterior interosseous nerve results in a loss of motor function (patient unable to end pinch index finger and thumb) without sensory involvement.

Few patients require surgery. However, when conservative management fails, surgical decompression of all possible impinging sites is required. Active ROM is commenced as tolerated after 4–5 days.

17. Ulnar entrapment neuropathies?

Ulner nerve compression occurs at the cubital tunnel. Sites of compression which must be explored at surgery include the arcade of Struthers, the medial intermuscular septum, medial epicondyle, soft-tissue structures within the cubital tunnel, and the deep flexor pronator aponeurosis.

Mild cases of ulnar nerve compression may be treated conservatively including use of nighttime extension splinting and avoidance of resting the elbow on a table during the day. Simple decompression achieved by releasing the arch of the flexor carpi ulnaris tendon may be appropriate if there is only localized nerve percussion signs. Anterior ulnar nerve transposition is preferred for cases with bony deformity, subluxation, or dislocation of the nerve or severe cases with motor deficits in younger patients. All previously mentioned sites of compression must also be explored. Some surgeons also routinely perform a medial epicondylectomy. However, the best indication for this procedure is nonunion of an epicondylar fracture with concomitant ulnar neuritis symptoms.

18. And radial nerve entrapment?

Radial nerve entrapment occurs at the elbow rarely, usually after strenuous muscular activity. Compression of the posterior interosseous nerve causes weakness (ECRB, supinator, ECU, EDC, EIP, EDQ, APL, EPL, EPB) but no sensory disorders. Possible anatomic sites of compression include the fascial tissue superficial to the radiocapitellar joint, a leash of vessels from the recurrent radial artery (the leash of Henry), the proximal edge of the supinator (arcade of Frohse), and the distal edge of the supinator.

Conservative therapy that includes rest, restriction of repetitive strenuous forearm motion, and NSAIDs may cause resolution of symptoms. Surgical intervention may be required to release all actual and potential sites of nerve compression. Recovery may continue for up to 18 months after surgery.

19. Describe the biomechanical considerations in sports injuries of the elbow.

The pitching motion is analogous to many other overhead motions in sports. The six phases of throwing include windup, early cocking, late cocking, arm acceleration, arm deceleration, and follow-through. Analysis has shown that the elbow is flexed to about 85° and maintained in this position during windup and cocking. The elbow is then rapidly extended during early acceleration at a velocity of 2300 m/sec to 20° of flexion at the time of ball release. Various forces on the elbow during throwing include varus torque, tensioning the medial structures (cocking), extension torque (during elbow extension), compression (maximum at ball release), and flexion/valgus torque.

20. How are elbow injuries related to sports classified?
Understanding the various forces acting about the elbow has assisted in classifying the injuries.
Medial elbow injuries—due to tension overload
 Medial epicondylitis
 Flexor-pronator tendinitis
 Ulnar collateral ligament tears
 Spur formation
 Ulnar neuritis
Lateral elbow injuries—due to compression overload
 Osteochondral fractures
 Osteochondritis dissecans
Posterior elbow injuries—due to a combination of compression, traction, and torsion
 Olecranon tip avulsions
 Olecranon stress fractures
 Olecranon fossa hyperostoses

BIBLIOGRAPHY

1. Donatelli RA, Wooden MJ: Orthopaedic Physical Therapy. New York, Churchill Livingstone, 1994.
2. Gould JA, Davies GJ (eds): Orthopaedic and Sports Physical Therapy. St. Louis, Mosby, 1985.
3. Jobe FW, Kvitne RS: Elbow instability in the athlete. In AAOS Instructional Course Lectures, vol 40. Park Ridge, IL, American Academy of Orthopaedic Surgeons, 1991, p 17.
4. Jobe FW, Nuber G: Throwing injuries of the elbow. Clin Sports Med 5:621, 1986.

60. HAND REHABILITATION AFTER SURGERY
Richard A. Rogachefsky, M.D.

1. What is synergy? How is this concept important in the rehabilitation of tendon transfers?
Synergy is the active complementary contraction of two muscle groups occurring simultaneously. For example, active wrist extension places the hand in a position to augment active finger flexion.

Why is it important? Transferring a muscle that normally acts in concert with the desired motion requires minimal transfer retraining. For example, in a high median nerve palsy, one of the necessary functions that must be obtained from a tendon transfer is finger flexion. Since the extensor carpi radialis longus normally contracts during digital flexion, the transfer of this muscle to the flexor digitorum profundus requires minimal functional retraining.

2. What is tenodesis with regard to hand motion?
Tenodesis is the passive motion of a joint or series of joints caused by the active contraction of the synergistic muscle related to that motion. For example, active wrist extension increases the passive tension in the finger flexor tendons. This increased tension pulls the digits and thumb passively into flexion.

3. How is tenodesis important in hand rehabilitation?
Tenodesis is used in rehabilitation after surgery or trauma, when patients have difficulty gaining active digital motion due to pain and swelling. By actively moving the wrist, the passive motion of the digits assists active finger motion.

4. What is quadregia and what is its significance?

The flexor digitorum profundus (FDP) tendons of the long, ring, and small fingers are linked by a common muscle origin. Quadregia is the balance of tension in these flexor tendons. The analogy is the chariot with four horses linked by a common rein. If the tension in one of the FDP tendons is altered, the motion of the other fingers is inhibited. For example, when the FDP tendon to the ring finger is repaired with excessive tension, the excursion of the FDP tendons to the long and ring fingers is reduced. This decreases the active flexion of those digits. This phenomenon is seen in flexor tendon repairs, metacarpophalangeal (MCP) joint fusions, amputation revisions, and infections.

5. What is the normal resting cascade of the fingers?

When the hand is in the relaxed position, the wrist is in neutral and the fingers maintain a position of increasing flexion from the index to the small finger, respectively. For example, the order of flexion is index<long<ring<small. If this normal position of the fingers at rest is altered, this may indicate an injury such as a tendon laceration, fracture, or contracture.

6. What are the techniques to control hand edema?

Ice	Controlled active motion
Elevation	Compressive garments
Bulky dressing	

7. Name the three stages of wound healing.

1. Inflammation—influx of edema fluid, leukocytes, and macrophages into a wound to debride devitalized tissue
2. Fibroplasia—invasion of the wound by capillaries and fibroblasts which form granulation tissue
3. Maturation—remodeling, softening, and strengthening of the wound scar

8. What are the post-treatment rehabilitation goals for the upper extremity after a distal radius fracture that has been treated by casting or open reduction and internal fixation?

1. Edema control
2. Improvement of active and passive ROM
3. Strengthening

9. What is functional fracture bracing? When is it used?

Functional fracture bracing uses prefabricated braces applied to the limb, providing external compression to the soft tissue to maintain fracture reduction. It can be used in long bone shaft fractures, such as humerus or ulna, that have minimal displacement and are inherently stable. This treatment is not effective for intra-articular fractures or unstable fractures that are severely displaced. Fracture bracing stabilizes the fracture while leaving the adjacent joints free. This allows early joint mobilization, decreasing swelling and stiffness.

10. Discuss the advantages of open reduction and internal fixation (ORIF) of fractures in the upper extremity with regards to rehabilitation.

ORIF provides early skeletal stabilization. This allows the discontinuation of external casts and other immobilization devices and allows the therapist to institute early joint mobilization. This enhances tendon gliding, improves joint motion, and controls edema. As a result, complications such as joint stiffness, contracture, and dystrophy may be avoided.

11. What is the intrinsic mechanism for tendon healing?

Multipotential cells from the epitendinous layer of the flexor tendon invade the repair site and actively synthesize collagen that matures and strengthens along lines of stress. This mechanism of healing is stimulated by the early controlled mobilization of the tendon.

12. When is a tendon repair the weakest?
At approximately 10–12 days, the tendon repair is the weakest and most susceptible to rupture.

13. What is dynamic range of motion?
Dynamic ROM occurs by passively pulling a single joint or multiple joints through a desired motion without active muscle contraction. For example, after a repair of a flexor tendon, a volar splint is fabricated with rubber bands that attach to the fingernails and pull the fingers into flexion. This provides tendon gliding while placing minimal force on the repair site.

14. Explain the concept of early controlled passive mobilization.
After tendons are repaired, active muscle contraction causes the greatest force on the tendon repair and the greatest chance for rupture. Pulling the joints dynamically or pushing the joints passively in the plane of musculotendinous contraction (alternating with active motion in the opposite direction) provides tendon excursion, which improves tendon healing and decreases adhesion formation. For example, after extensor tendon repair, a dorsal forearm splint with outriggers, rubber bands, and finger loops dynamically pull the fingers into extension. The digits are then allowed to actively flex to maximize tendon gliding.

15. What is early active short arc motion for extensor tendon repairs at the central slip?
This is a rehab program for extensor tendons that are repaired at the central tendon insertion at the proximal interphalangeal (PIP) joints of the digits. A volar splint template is made with a 30° bend at the level of the PIP joint. Under supervision, the splint is applied to the finger, and the patient is allowed to actively flex the PIP joint to 30°, to the limit of the splint, and then completely extend the PIP joint actively to 0°. When the patient is not exercising, a volar splint that keeps the PIP joint in neutral is used. This regimen is used for 2 weeks, and then the bend in the splint is increased to allow PIP active flexion to increase 10° each week. Then, at 4 to 5 weeks, full PIP joint active flexion is instituted. This regimen demonstrates improved total motion at the PIP joint on long-term follow-up.

16. What is the deformity in low ulnar nerve palsy?
The intrinsic muscles to the hand are the main flexors to the MCP joints and extensors to the PIP and distal interphalangeal (DIP) joints of the digits. When these muscles are nonfunctional due to a low ulnar nerve palsy, the ring and small fingers assume a claw deformity. This results from the unopposed active hyperextension of the MCP joints by the extensor digitorum communis tendons and the unopposed active flexion deformity of the PIP and DIP joints by the flexor digitorum profundus tendons.

17. Which splint is used to counteract this deformity?
An ulnar nerve palsy (anti-claw) splint attaches to the hand with a dorsal hood that extends over the MCP joints and blocks the MCP joints from hyperextending during active digital extension. This prevents the claw deformity in the ring and small fingers until permanent correction is obtained through nerve regeneration or tendon transfer.

18. What is the deformity in radial nerve palsy?
The radial nerve innervates the extensors of the forearm and hand. When the radial nerve is nonfunctional, the patient is unable to actively extend the wrist, fingers, or thumb due to the paralysis of the extensor carpi radialis longus and brevis, extensor digitorum communis, and extensor pollicis longus and brevis.

19. Which splint is used to correct this deformity?
A static volar or dorsal wrist control splint is applied to support the wrist in 30° of extension to correct the wrist flexion deformity and to facilitate active digital flexion. No supportive splint

is necessary for the digits because the intrinsic muscles will provide enough extension to clear the palm for grasp function and prevent permanent contracture until correction of the deformity is obtained through nerve regeneration or tendon transfer.

20. What are the clinical signs of early reflex sympathetic dystrophy?
1. Severe pain
2. Swelling
3. Excessive sweating
4. Stiffness
5. Discoloration

21. Describe the open-palm (McCash) technique for excision of Dupuytren's disease.
This technique utilizes transverse incisions to excise the Dupuytren's fasciitis. These incisions are left open to heal by secondary intention. This technique allows easier ROM by the patient during rehabilitation by decreasing postoperative hematoma formation, swelling, and pain.

22. What is the most important factor to determine use of an upper-extremity prosthesis?
Early fitting and use of a prosthesis, within 30 days of the amputation, greatly increases the probability of long-term prosthetic function and return to work. Patients who start to use a prosthesis later have poor compliance because they learn to adapt by using only the normal upper extremity.

BIBLIOGRAPHY

1. Amadio P: Current concepts review: Pain dysfunction syndromes. J Bone Joint Surg 70A:944–949, 1988.
2. Evans R: Early active short arc motion for repaired central slip. J Hand Surg 19A:991–997, 1994.
3. Freeland AE, Jabaley ME, Hughes JL (eds): Stable Fixation of the Hand and Wrist. New York, Springer Verlag, 1986, pp 28–35.
4. Gelberman RH (ed): Operative Nerve Repair and Reconstruction. Philadelphia, J.B. Lippincott, 1991, pp 813–826.
5. Gelberman RH, Vande Berg JS, Lundborg GN, Akeson WH: Flexor tendon healing and reconstruction of the sliding surface. J Bone Joint Surg 65A:70–80, 1983.
6. Green DP, Hotchkiss RN (eds): Operative Hand Surgery, 3rd ed. New York, Churchill Livingstone, 1993.
7. Hunter JH, Mackin EJ, Callahan AD (eds): Rehabilitation of the Hand: Surgery and Therapy, 4th ed. St. Louis, Mosby, 1994.
8. Malerich MM, Baird RA, McMaster W, Erickson JM: Permissible limits of flexor digitorum tendon advancement: An anatomic study. J Hand Surg 12A:30–33, 1987.
9. Pinzur MS, Angelat J, Light TR, et al: Functional outcome following traumatic upper limb amputation and prosthetic limb fitting. J Bone Joint Surg 19A:836–839, 1994.

61. HIP REHABILITATION AFTER SURGERY

Michael A. Mont, M.D., W. Stephen Tankersley, M.D., and David S. Hungerford, M.D.

1. What is a hip arthroplasty?
A hip arthroplasty is a replacement of damaged or arthritic surfaces of the hip joint with materials to restore the integrity of the joint. Most often materials are made of metals and plastics.

2. How do total arthroplasty and hemiarthroplasty differ?
A total hip replacement resurfaces both the femoral head and acetabulum. A hemiarthroplasty only resurfaces the femoral head. It is often used for displaced femoral neck fractures.

3. What are the indications for these procedures?

The main indications are to relieve pain caused by arthritis, correct deformity, and restore range of motion (ROM) and function. More specifically, candidates for hip replacements have severe degenerative changes on their hip x-rays and the failure of nonoperative treatment to relieve their pain. Nonoperative methods include anti-inflammatory medications, the use of a cane, loss of weight when indicated, and decreased activity. These methods should be used for 3–6 months before considering a hip arthroplasty.

Occasionally, after certain types of hip fractures, the procedure of choice may be hip replacement. This option is chosen when the fracture cannot be repaired or repair has little chance for clinical success, such as in an 80-year-old with a severely displaced femoral neck fracture.

4. What are the causes of osteoarthritis in the hip that progresses to a total hip replacement?

Idiopathic primary osteoarthritis (approximately 70%)
Slipped capital femoral epiphysis
History of trauma leading to joint incongruity
Rheumatoid arthritis
Developmental dysplasia of the hip
Avascular necrosis
Other inflammatory arthritides

There is no proof that factors such as obesity, occupational hazards, or a long history of jogging are risk factors for progression to a hip replacement.

5. How many hip arthroplasty procedures are performed in the United States annually?

Approximately 150,000.

6. How successful are these operations?

At 1 year, approximately 95% of patients can expect a good to excellent clinical result, with minimal to no pain, the ability to walk > 1 mile, increased ROM, as well as patient satisfaction with the procedure. These results are generally maintained at 6 to 10 years after the procedure. There is about a 1% failure rate per year, yielding about a 90% success rate at 10 years.

7. Can patients develop allergies to the materials used to construct hip replacement components?

Allergic reactions to these metal and plastic components are essentially nonexistent.

8. How are the components fixed to bone?

The components can be cemented with polymethylmethacrylate or affixed with noncemented methods such as press-fit and biological ingrowth prostheses. For a press-fit prosthesis, the component is placed in direct contact with bone, and the bone is finely machined to ensure an exact fit. In biologic ingrowth prostheses, components have a porous or meshed surface that allows bone to grow into the interstices, achieving true biologic fixation.

9. Does the mode of fixation affect rehabilitation?

Most patients after hip surgery are kept on partial weight-bearing for 6 weeks. In theory, patients with cemented prostheses are capable of bearing full weight immediately after surgery. The cement has reached 90% of its strength 10–15 minutes after mixing. Patients who have a porous ingrowth prosthesis should be on protected weight-bearing for up to 12 weeks, as this allows time for the bone to grow into the pores of the component.

10. Should the physiatrist be aware of the surgical approach used in a hip arthroplasty?

Yes and yes. The **lateral approach** involves splitting the abductors with repair back to the greater trochanter or trochanteric osteotomy with repair of the osteotomy. In either case, the repair needs 6–8 weeks to heal. The abductors (gluteus medius and minimis) are most commonly weakened and should be a target of strengthening.

The **posterior approach** involves splitting the gluteus maximus and releasing the short external rotators, which are repaired. The hip extenders and the short external rotators are affected and should be targeted. Concentric strengthening can be started earlier. The rehabilitation specialist should be wary of the higher incidence of posterior dislocation with this approach. In addition, the hip flexors, quadriceps, and hamstrings should all be strengthened after hip replacement.

11. How long will patients have significant pain after hip surgery?

Most patients recognize within 1 or 2 days after surgery that their pain is markedly different than preoperatively. The arthritis pain is typically eliminated immediately. The surgical pain can last for 2–3 weeks but progressively gets better after the first 1–2 days.

Persistent pain, especially after activities and ambulation, can persist for several months or more depending on various factors, such as the preoperative deformity or degree of muscle atrophy. It may take many months to rebuild the required muscle mass and strength to reduce this activity-related pain.

12. Can patients return to playing sports after hip replacement surgery?

Most patients can return to playing low-impact sports, such as golf, doubles tennis, and bowling, walking, and using exercise machines such as a stationary cycles and cross-country ski simulators. High-impact exercises such as running, singles tennis, basketball, volleyball, and football should be avoided, as this may lead to excessive wear of the prosthesis (unless you are Bo Jackson).

13. How long will a total hip replacement last?

Although this will vary from patient to patient, many large series show continued good to excellent results in > 90% of patients at 10 years. Hopefully, future hip replacements will last even longer.

14. What is the most common cause for failure in a patient with total hip arthroplasty?

Loosening. The young, very active, and obese people are at high risk. Evidence of loosening can be detected radiographically in 5–30% of cases at 10 years.

15. When will the patient receive full benefit after hip arthroplasty?

Typically, by 3 months, the patients have regained most of their strength across the joint as well as ROM. They continue to improve throughout the first year after surgery. Usually, by 1 year, the patient has achieved full benefit from the operation.

16. Describe a general management approach in a patient with total hip arthroplasty.

Day of surgery	Deep breathing exercises, incentive spirometry
	Active ankle ROM exercises
Postop day 1	Quadriceps isometric exercises
	Gluteus muscle isometrics depending on surgical approach
	Maintain hips in abduction
	Active assisted and knee flexion exercises as tolerated
Postop day 2–6	Begin ambulation with a walker or crutches; initiate progressive gait training
Cemented total hip replacement	Weight-bearing as tolerated
Bony ingrowth total hip replacement	Toe-touch weight-bearing for 6 wks, then advance to weight-bearing as tolerated
Trochanteric osteotomy	If secure reattachment, start weight-bearing as tolerated; if tenuous, partial weight-bearing
	Instruct hip precautions
	Instruct energy conservation and work simplification techniques
	Active assisted exercise, progress to active ROM motion and strengthening exercises
	Teach adaptive ADLs without violating hip precautions

Postop day 7–3 mos	Progressive strengthening and ranging of the trunk, hip, and knee
	Closed kinetic chain exercises
	Improving endurance and gait pattern
	Eliminating the use of assistive devices
	Pool therapy, bicycling, long-distance walking, progressive stair climbing, and isotonic exercises with weights are encouraged
Postop 3 mos	Follow-up visit
	Focus on level and location of pain, daily walking distance, sitting or standing duration, use of assistive devices, method of stair climbing, use of analgesics, and community reintegration

17. How long should a patient maintain total hip precautions?

For 12 weeks after the procedure. This allows for a pseudocapsule to reform. The incidence of dislocation is reduced by > 95% after 12 weeks.

18. How should a patient ambulate stairs after hip surgery?

"Up with the good and down with the bad." When going up stairs, the patient leads with the nonoperative extremity and then follows with the crutches and operative extremity, taking one step at a time. When descending, the patient leads with crutches and the operative extremity and then follows with the nonoperative extremity.

19. What are the most common causes of falls after hip surgery?

Most falls are caused by decreased visual acuity and a decreased balance sensation that occurs in the elderly population. With this in mind, accident prevention tips should be stressed while the patient is on a rehabilitation service, and in-home visit for safety should be considered. Fall prevention should include measures such as ensuring that rooms are well lit in the patient's home; avoiding throw rugs on floors; and avoiding thick carpets, which may cause stumbling. Finally, the patient should have a well-lit and easy path from the bed to the bathroom, as many falls occur when patients get up at night to visit the bathroom.

20. Do patients need prophylaxis for deep venous thrombosis after hip replacement?

The incidence of deep venous thrombosis measured by Doppler studies or venograms after hip surgery is > 50% in most reported series. It is therefore considered the standard of care to give some form of prophylaxis for deep venous thrombosis after hip surgery. This prophylaxis can include mechanical adjuncts, such as support hose and pneumatic compression devices, which should be continued throughout the course of the hospitalization. In addition, many surgeons give some form of pharmacologic prophylaxis, such as warfarin.

21. Define weight-bearing.

Body weight supported through the affected limb is measured by placing the limb on a weight scale and applying force on the scale.

None	0% of body weight
Toe-touch weight-bearing	Up to 20% of body weight
Partial weight-bearing	20–50% of body weight
Weight-bearing as tolerated	50–100% of body weight
Full weight-bearing	100% of body weight

22. When can patients bear full weight after hip surgery?

Patients are typically kept on partial weight-bearing for 6–12 weeks. Most patients will walk with crutches or a walker with foot-flat weight-bearing on the operative side for the first 6 weeks. Foot-flat weight-bearing allows 50–60 lbs to be placed across the hip joint during this time. Patients are rapidly progressed from a walker or crutch ambulation to cane ambulation for an additional 4–6 weeks and then to weight-bearing without an ambulatory assistive device usually after 3 months.

This period of partial weight-bearing is necessary to accomplish three goals:
1. It allows the soft tissues to heal adequately.
2. It allows for the muscles to reattach firmly to bone or for the trochanteric osteotomy to heal.
3. It allows adequate time for bone ingrowth to be achieved if the patient received bone-ingrowth prosthesis.

23. What are the dangerous positions to move the hip after hip arthroplasty?

There are four basic positions to be avoided after hip arthroplasty, particularly for the first 3 months:
1. No flexion of the hip past 90° with respect to the axis of the body
2. No adduction of the leg past the midline of the body
3. No combined extension of the hip joint with external rotation of the lower extremity
4. No flexion with internal rotation

24. Why should abduction pillows be utilized? When? For how long?

Use of the abduction pillow prevents the patient from getting into positions that could cause dislocation of the hip prosthesis (adduction, internal rotation). The pillows should be used after all total hip arthroplasties while the patient is sleeping or resting in bed.

Abduction pillows are typically worn for 6–12 weeks. At the end of that time, a pseudocapsule has formed around the hip joint, and the musculature is usually sufficiently strengthened to allow proprioceptive control and stability of the joint itself. Patients who have had previous hip surgery are at higher risk for dislocation and frequently require abduction bracing.

25. What ranges of motion of the hip are allowed after hip arthroplasty?

Typically patients are allowed to flex the leg to 80–90° and to extend it fully. They are allowed gentle (20–30°) internal and external rotation of the lower extremity. They are also allowed passive abduction as tolerated. Active abduction should be avoided for the first 6 weeks in patients who have undergone a lateral approach.

26. What is the sequence of ambulatory aids usually given to patients after total hip replacement?

For the first day or two, the patient usually works in physical therapy on the parallel bars. He or she is then progressed to crutches or a walker for the first 6 weeks. The patient is then advanced to one crutch or cane, which is continued for an additional 6 weeks. Greater than 70% of patients are ambulatory without an assistive device at the end of 3 months.

27. Give four goals of occupational therapy after total hip replacement.

1. To reestablish basic activities of daily living (ADL) with modifications that keep the patient's ROM within restricted limits
2. To teach joint protection
3. To review fall risks
4. To provide equipment with training

28. What special devices are used to achieve modified independence in ADL?

Elevated toilet seats, shower seats, shoe horns, elastic shoe laces, reachers that allow socks to be pulled on, and other devices.

29. Are resisted concentric exercises important after hip or knee surgery?

Concentric exercises against resistance should be avoided for the first 6–8 weeks. During that time, the patient can perform isometrics and active ROM exercises against gravity. After the first 6–8 weeks, resisted open kinetic chain strengthening can start in the place of joint motion with 1–10 lbs. Exercises performed with heavy weights against resistance cause undue wear on the prosthetic components.

30. What about sex after joint replacement?
Absolutely. Many people express a concern about a dislocation or damage to the prosthesis while having intercourse after a hip replacement. After 10–12 weeks, the pseudocapsule has re-formed around the hip joint, and the muscles typically have been rehabilitated so that the risk of a dislocation or damage to the prosthesis is negligible. Certainly, for patients who have had to cease coitus because of pain or a loss of ROM prior to hip surgery, the return of sexual activity should be one goal postoperatively.

31. Where are the most frequent sites of hip fracture in the elderly?
Femoral neck and the intertrochanteric and subtrochanteric areas.

32. What are the surgical indications and rehabilitations for the various hip fracture types?

Surgical Procedures and Rehabilitations for Hip Fractures

FRACTURES AND TYPE	SURGICAL PROCEDURE	WEIGHT-BEARING STATUS
Femoral neck		
Displaced fracture (Garden III and IV)	Hemiarthroplasty	Weight-bearing as tolerated
Undisplaced and impacted fractures (Garden I and II)	ORIF	Depends on the stability of surgical fixation
Intertrochanteric		
Undisplaced, displaced two-part fractures, or unstable three-part fractures	Treated operatively with multiple pins or screws and side-plate devices	Depends on degree of fracture stabilization, bone stock, patient's frailty, and risks of immobility
Subtrochanteric		
Simple, fragmented, or comminuted	ORIF with a blade plate and screws or an intramedullary nail	Delayed until fracture demonstrates evidence of healing

ORIF = open reduction and internal fixation.

33. Are there negative predictors of ambulation after hip fracture?
Lack of social support   Lower-limb contractures
Age > 85 years   Poor prefracture functional status

34. What factors are associated with institutionalization after fractures?
Inability to transfer or ambulate, incontinence, dementia, fewer hours of physical therapy, and lack of family involvement.

35. Name two major risk factors for hip fracture.
Osteoporosis and falls.

36. How can osteoporosis be prevented?
More than 50% of hip fractures are thought to occur without a precipitating trauma or fall and are presumably secondary to osteoporosis. Proper calcium intake, weight-bearing exercise, and hormonal replacement at menopause are beneficial in preventing osteoporosis. Reducing the risk factors for osteoporosis, such as smoking, alcohol use, and caffeine intake, are also helpful. For more progressive osteoporosis, one might consider calcitonin, calcitriol, and/or biphosphonates therapy. (See also the chapter on osteoporosis).

37. What factors are associated with an increased risk of falls?
Prevention of falls cannot be overemphasized in the elderly. Factors that increase the incidence of falls include lower-limb impairment such as weakness and ankle/foot problems, gait abnormalities, use of multiple medications, balance disorders, dementia, visual impairment, previous history of falls, Parkinson's disease, and palmomental reflex.

38. How commonly does avascular necrosis occur?

This hip disease annually afflicts about 5,000–10,000 young adults under age 45 years old and causes bone in the femoral head to die. Untreated, it leads to disabling hip arthritis and accounts for approximately 10% of the hip replacements that are performed in the United States each year.

39. What are the causes or associated factors for avascular necrosis?

In many cases in the population over age 60 years, femoral neck fractures will impair the blood supply of the femoral head and lead to avascular necrosis of the femoral head, necessitating hip replacement. In other cases, there is no recognized direct cause-and-effect relationship, but the disease is associated with various factors. These factors include steroid use and alcohol use, which account for about 90% of the known causes of avascular necrosis in the patient population under age 45 years.

Clinical Conditions Associated with Avascular Necrosis

Corticosteroids use	Gaucher disease
For systemic lupus erythematosus	Myeloproliferative disorders
For rheumatoid arthritis	Coagulation deficiencies
After renal transplantation	Trauma
For asthma	Chronic pancreatitis
Alcohol use	Caisson disease
Sickle-cell and other anemias	Radiation

Adapted from Mont MA, Hungerford DS: Non-traumatic avascular necrosis of the femoral head. J Bone Joint Surg 77A:459–474, 1995.

40. Describe a rehabilitation program for a patient with avascular necrosis.

The rehabilitation program includes exercise, pain control, and joint-protection techniques. Isotonic exercises, such as straight-leg raising, that distribute the stress through the hip joint must be avoided. Gravity-eliminated active assistive exercise, such as pool therapy and isometric exercises, can improve hip ROM and strength.

41. What is the prognosis for patients with avascular necrosis treated with nonoperative modalities that restrict weight-bearing?

Most studies have reported > 90% progression of collapse and the need for total hip replacement within 4 years.

BIBLIOGRAPHY

1. Anderson FA Jr, Wheeler HB: Natural history and epidemiology of venous thromboembolism. Orthop Rev 23:5–9, 1994.
2. Bowman AJ Jr, Walker MW, Kilfoyle RM, et al: Experience with bipolar prosthesis in hip arthroplasty: A clinical study. Orthopedics 8:460–467, 1985.
3. Brander VA, Hinderer SR, Alpiner N, Oh TH: Rehabilitation in joint and connective tissue diseases: Limb disorders. Arch Phys Med Rehabil 76 (Suppl 5):S-47–S-56.
4. Dall DM, Grobbelaar CJ, Learmonth ID, Dall G: Charnley low-friction arthroplasty of the hip: Long-term results in South Africa. Clin Orthop 211:85–90, 1986.
5. Engh CA, Bobyn JD, Glassman AH: Porous-coated hip replacement: The factors governing bone ingrowth, stress shielding, and clinical results. J Bone Joint Surg 69B:45–55, 1987.
6. Grady-Benson JC: High-risk factors and diagnostic challenges associated with venous thromboembolic disease. Orthop Rev 23:10–16, 1994.
7. Harris WH: Factors controlling optimal bone ingrowth of total hip replacement components. In AAOS Instructional Course Lectures, vol 35. Park Ridge, IL, American Academy of Orthopaedic Surgeons, 1986, pp 184–187.
8. Kavanagh BF, Ilstrup DM, Fitzgerald RH Jr: Revision total hip arthroplasty. J Bone Joint Surg 67A:517–526, 1985.
9. Krackow KA, Mont MA, Maar DC: A new neck preserving total hip arthroplasty for the young patient. Orthopaedics 17:253–259, 1993.

10. Lachiewicz PF, Rosenstein BD: Long-term results of Harris total hip replacement. J Arthroplasty 1:229–236, 1986.
11. Lausten GS, Vedel P, Nielsen PM: Fractures of the femoral neck treated with a bipolar endoprosthesis. Clin Orthop 218:63–67, 1987.
12. Levy RL, Capozzi J, Mont MA: Intertrochanteric hip fractures. In Browner BD (ed): Skeletal Trauma. Philadelphia, W.B. Saunders, 1991.
13. Mont MA, Hungerford DS: Non-traumatic avascular necrosis of the femoral head. J Bone Joint Surg 77A:459–474, 1995.
14. National Institutes of Health Consensus Conference: Prevention of venous thrombosis and pulmonary embolism. JAMA 256:744–749, 1986.

62. KNEE REHABILITATION AFTER SURGERY

W. Stephen Tankersley, M.D., Michael A. Mont, M.D., and David S. Hungerford, M.D.

1. Define knee arthroplasty.

A knee arthroplasty is a replacement of damaged or arthritic surfaces of the distal femur and proximal tibia and the rest of the knee joint with metal and plastic materials to restore the integrity of the joint.

2. What are the indications for this procedure?

The main indication is to relieve pain caused by arthritis. Secondary goals are to correct deformity and restore function. More specifically, candidates for knee replacements have severe degenerative changes of their knee joint seen on radiographs and have failed multiple methods of nonoperative treatment to relieve their pain. These methods include anti-inflammatory medications, the use of a cane, loss of weight when indicated, decreased activity, as well as interarticular corticosteroid injections. These methods should be tried for 3–6 months before considering a knee arthroplasty.

3. How many knee arthroplasty procedures are performed in the United States annually?

Approximately 150,000.

4. What are the goals of knee arthroplasty?

1. To restore a painfree joint
2. To restore range of motion (ROM)
3. To allow function that approaches normal for the patient

5. How successful are these operations?

About 95–97% of patients can expect a good to excellent clinical result. This clinical result encompasses minimal to no pain, the ability to walk > 1 mile, increased ROM, and patient satisfaction with the procedure. These results generally hold up at 5- and 10-year follow-ups, with about a 1% failure rate per year. Thus, one can expect about 90% success with these procedures at 10 years.

6. How long does significant pain last after knee surgery?

Most patients know within 1 or 2 days after surgery that their pain is markedly different than preoperatively. The arthritis pain is typically eliminated immediately. The surgical pain lasts for 2–3 weeks but progressively gets better after the first 1–2 days.

7. When should a knee manipulation be seriously considered?

If you have only 70° flexion by 14 days postoperatively.

8. Since the continuous passive motion machine does not appear to affect long-term ROM, why should one use it in a patient with total knee replacement?
It may be cost effective. It improves knee flexion and may reduce the number of hospital days and frequency of manipulations.

9. Can patients return to playing sports after knee surgery?
Most patients can return to low-impact sports, such as golf, doubles tennis, and bowling, walking, and use such exercise machines as a stationary cycle and cross-country ski simulators. High-impact exercises such as running, singles tennis, basketball, volleyball, and football should be avoided as these may lead to undo wear and tear on the prosthesis.

10. Describe a general rehabilitation program in a patient with total knee arthroplasty (TKA).

Day of surgery	Deep breathing exercises
	Active ankle ROM
Postop day 1	Lower-limb isometrics including quadriceps, hamstrings, and gluteal sets
	Wearing a knee immobilizer until the development of active knee extension and demonstration of good leg control during ambulation
	Weight-bearing after TKA may be partial or full, depending on the surgeon's discretion
Postop day 2	Standing at the bedside with knee immobilizer and partial weight-bearing on the operated limb
	Active assisted ROM
Postop day 4	Progressive isotonic and isometric knee and hip muscle strengthening
	Concentrate on terminal knee extension through active knee extension exercises

11. How long will a total knee replacement last?
Although this will vary from patient to patient, many large series in orthopedic literature show continued good to excellent results in > 90% of patients at 10 years.

12. When will the patient receive full benefit after knee arthroplasty?
Typically, by 3 months, the patients are doing quite well. Usually, by that time, they have regained most of their strength across the joint as well as ROM. They continue to improve throughout the first year after surgery, and by 1 year, the patient has achieved full benefit from the operation.

13. How should a patient ambulate stairs after knee surgery?
When going up stairs, the patient leads with the nonoperative extremity and then follows with the crutches and operative extremity, taking one step at a time. When descending, the patient leads with crutches and the operative extremity, following with the nonoperative extremity.

14. Is prophylaxis for deep venous thrombosis needed after knee surgery?
Yes.

15. List the usual sequence of ambulatory aids given to patients after total knee replacement.
- For the first day or two, the patient usually works in physical therapy on the parallel bars.
- He or she is then progressed to crutches or a walker for the first 6 weeks.
- The patient is then advanced to one crutch or cane, which is continued for an additional 6 weeks.
- Most patients (70%) are ambulatory without an assistive device by 3 months

16. What are four goals of occupational therapy after total knee replacement?

1. To reestablish basic activities of daily living (ADL), with modifications that keep the patient's ROM within restrictions
2. To teach joint protection
3. To review for falls risk
4. To provide equipment with training

17. Is sex possible after knee replacement?

Provided it does not involve chasing your partner around the room (or other obstacle-laden course) at high speeds.

18. When can patients bear full weight after knee surgery?

Most patients are kept on partial weight-bearing (50%) for 6–8 weeks, with progression to full weight-bearing usually at the end of 6 weeks. For biologic fixed components, full weight-bearing may not be allowed until 12 weeks to ensure bone ingrowth.

19. Which muscles should be targeted after knee surgery?

The muscles most affected by surgery are the **quadriceps** muscles (vastus lateralis, vastus medialis, vastus intermedius, and rectus femoris). Isometric strengthening and active ROM should begin immediately after surgery. For the first 6 weeks, the quadriceps should be strengthened with isometric exercises. Then, progressively resisted isokinetic or isotonic strengthening should be added. Other muscles that act at the knee through the open and closed kinetic chains should be strengthened: hamstrings, gastrocsoleus, and ankle dorsiflexors.

20. How should knee range of motion be measured and recorded?

ROM should be measured from the lateral side of the patient's leg with a goniometer. Full extension—i.e., an angle between the femur and tibial shaft of 0°—should be recorded as 0. The knee is then brought to full flexion and measured again from the lateral side of the patient's knee, and this is recorded as a positive number, somewhere between 0–135°. If the patient's leg cannot be fully extended, i.e., lacks 10° of complete extension, this should be recorded as +10 extension and the flexion recorded as whatever the patient is able to flex past that number. For example, the patient flexing to 100° but lacking complete extension of 10° should be recorded as having an ROM +10–105°. If the patient's knee comes to hyperextension, then the amount past 0° should be recorded as a negative number. For example, if the subject hyperextended approximately 5° and flexed to 100°, the ROM is recorded as -5–100°.

21. After total knee replacement, what should be the expected range of motion for the patient's knee? What are the preliminary goals?

The biggest predictor of postoperative ROM is preoperative ROM. The average postoperative ROM is 105–110° for most patients At least 90° of ROM is desirable for a good functional outcome. It is hoped that at least 90° of motion will be obtained within the first 7–10 days after surgery.

22. What is meant by the term "extensor lag"?

With an extensor lag, the patient cannot actively extend to a completely straight position (angle of 0° measured between the femur and tibia). Passive extension is not limited however. This condition occurs because of a lengthening or weakening of the quadriceps after surgery or because of prosthetic component positioning.

23. What is meant by the term "flexion contracture"?

This term is applied to patients who cannot fully extend the leg either actively or passively. This condition is usually caused by a mechanical block, such as a retained osteophyte, scarring of the posterior capsule or posterior structures, extremely tight hamstrings, or malposition of the prosthetic components. A flexion contracture significantly increases the energy required for ambulation.

24. How do you check the stability of the knee after a knee replacement?

Medial/lateral testing (varus or valgus): The knee is checked throughout the ROM starting at full extension and proceeding to 30°, 60°, and 90°. At each position, the patient's leg should be stressed medially and laterally. Any opening or closing of > 5° should be considered excessive.

Anterior/posterior testing: Again, the knee is checked throughout the ROM with a **Lachman's** or **anterior drawer** test, and the position of the greatest instability is recorded. This displacement is normally 5–8 mm of anterior translation, as the anterior cruciate ligament has been sacrificed in all total knee replacements.

25. Should the physiatrist be made aware of any particular circumstances after knee surgery?

The physiatrist should be aware if the patient has had any surgical procedure performed in addition to the routine surgical exposure. These adjuncts may include a **quadriceps muscle turn-down**, performed by splitting this muscle in an oblique fashion to allow the patella to be retracted distally, for better exposure of the joint. In addition, a **tibial tubercle osteotomy** sometimes is performed to allow exposure of the joint; it is performed by reflecting a portion of the bone underneath the tibial tubercle with the attached patella tendon laterally and then repairing this with some form of internal fixation. In either case, the ROM may be altered after surgery, and the strengthening part of rehabilitation may be delayed to allow the tendon or bone to heal.

26. Are resisted concentric exercises important after knee replacement surgery?

Concentric exercises against resistance should be avoided for the first 6–8 weeks. During that time, the patient can perform isometric and active ROM exercises against gravity. After the first 6–8 weeks, resisted open kinetic chain strengthening can start in the place of joint motion with 1–10 lbs. Exercises performed with heavy weights against resistance cause undue wear and tear on the prosthetic components.

BIBLIOGRAPHY

1. Brander VA, Hinderer SR, Alpiner N, Oh TH: Rehabilitation in joint and connective tissue disease: 3. Limb disorders. Arch Phys Med Rehabil 76(Suppl 5):S-47–S-56, 1995.
2. Fu FH (ed): Surgery of the Knee. Baltimore, Williams & Wilkins, 1994.
3. Insall JN, Kelly M: The total condylar prosthesis. Clin Orthop 205:43–48, 1986.
4. Insall JN, Windsor RE, Scott WN, et al (eds): Surgery of the Knee, 2nd ed. New York, Churchill Livingstone, 1993.
5. Krackow KA (ed): The Technique of Total Knee Arthroplasty. St. Louis, Mosby, 1990.
6. Lombardi AV Jr, Mallory TH, Eberle RW: Constrained knee arthroplasty. In Scott WN (ed): The Knee. St. Louis, Mosby, 1993, pp 1305–1323.
7. Mont MA, Antonaides S, Krackow KA, Hungerford DS: Total knee replacement following high tibial osteotomy. Clin Orthop 299:125–130, 1993.
8. Mont MA, Alexander N, Krackow KA, Hungerford DS: Total knee arthroplasty after failed high tibial osteotomy. Orthop Clin North Am 23(3):515–525, 1994.
9. Mont MA, Mathur SK, Krackow KA, et al: Cementless total knee arthroplasty in obese patients: A comparison to a matched control group. J Arthroplasty 1996 (in press).
10. Rand JA (ed): Total Knee Arthroplasty. New York, Raven Press, 1993.
11. Serna F, Mont MA, Krackow KA, Hungerford DS: Total knee arthroplasty in diabetic patients—A comparison to a matched control group. J Arthroplasty 9:375–380, 1994.

63. REHABILITATION AFTER FRACTURES

Arun J. Mehta, M.B., F.R.C.P.C.

1. How common are musculoskeletal injuries?

The National Health Interview Survey reported 32 million musculoskeletal injuries, including 6.1 million fractures, in 1 year in the U.S. (1988). Nearly 1 million patients required hospitalization for treatment, and two-thirds of the patients with fractures had to restrict some of their activities. The total cost, both direct and indirect, was estimated at $20 billion.

2. Why does a patient with a fracture need rehabilitation?

It takes a lot of force to break a bone. The same force damages soft tissues around the bone. Treatment of fractures usually involves prolonged immobilization which may lead to secondary impairments such as stiffness of joints, weakness of muscles, loss of function of the involved extremity or part of the body. Restoration of joint movements, muscle strength, and function requires rehabilitation. Even if the fracture does not require manipulation or operation, restoration to the premorbid condition makes rehab an essential component of fracture management.

3. Describe the mechanisms of injury that lead to fracture.

Direct injury—A direct blow to a bone fractures it at the site of impact.

Indirect injury—Force is applied at one point and fracture occurs at a site remote from the impact

Transverse or oblique fracture—The force tends to bend a long bone.

Spiral fracture—A result of twisting force.

Compression fracture—Compressive forces crush a soft spongy bone (e.g., vertebral body).

4. Name some of the factors that predispose a patient to fractures.

Age—The incidence of fractures increases with advancing age because of increasing occurrence of osteoporosis and falls in the elderly. Children usually break bones because they are more active and take more risks than adults.

Osteoporosis—Bone loss is a major contributing factor in fractures of the neck of femur and compression fractures of the spine. It is seen 10–15 years earlier in females than in males.

Falls—An elderly person is more likely to fall and break a bone because of neurologic disorders, such as peripheral neuropathy secondary to diabetes, cerebrovascular accidents, visual impairment, Parkinson's disease, or dementia.

5. What is an open fracture? Why is it important to treat it differently than a closed fracture?

The skin overlying the fracture is intact in a **closed** fracture. A laceration or even a puncture wound near the fracture site makes it an **open** fracture. This breakdown of skin cover makes the injured tissues very vulnerable to later infection. Also, in an open fracture, external bleeding may lead to blood loss. Infection and blood loss may delay fracture healing.

6. What systemic complications can occur after a fracture?

1. Urinary tract infection due to indwelling catheter
2. Constipation due to pain killers containing codeine
3. Pressure ulcers due to localized pressure of the cast or bedrest without change in position
4. Anemia resulting from blood loss at the time of injury or surgery
5. Fat embolism
6. Deep vein thrombosis
7. Pneumonia

7. How does a fracture heal?

Blood vessels are torn at the time of injury, and blood accumulates in tissues. The hematoma is replaced by new blood vessels and fibroblasts. Later, osteoblasts from periosteum and endosteum proliferate. These cells form the intercellular matrix in which calcium salts are deposited to form callus. The **callus** is gradually replaced by mature bone tissue. Bone is a living tissue and changes according to stress applied to it. New bone is deposited along lines of increased stress (**Wolff's law**) or fracture, and bone tissue is removed from the site where there is less stress. On x-rays, this is seen as thickening of cortical bone and more prominent trabeculae in cancellous bone. Mechanical loading of bone generates electrical potentials. This is known as the **piezoelectric** property of the bone. These very small negative electrical potentials are recognized by osteoblasts and guide new bone formation. This is the basis for the clinical use of electromagnetic devices in promoting bone healing. Increasing compression forces or stresses at the fracture site signal formation and orientation of collagen fibers, deposition of minerals, and strengthening of callus. Some prostaglandins participate in the formation of new bone, and therefore anti-inflammatory NSAIDs can potentially reduce ectopic bone formation and callus at the fracture site.

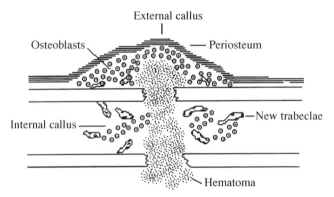

Fracture repair.

8. What do you look for on plain x-rays?

Where is the fracture?

Does it involve diaphysis, metaphysis, epiphysis, or articular surface?

Fracture line (transverse, oblique, or spiral)

Deformity (alignment, angulation, rotation, displacement of bony fragments, direction and distance from normal position)

Number of fragments and distance between fragments

Condition of the bone (other bone pathology like osteoporosis)

Adjacent joints (rule out dislocation or effusion)

Soft tissue swelling in the involved extremity (amount of blood loss)

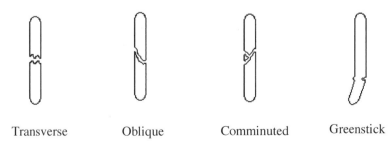

Transverse   Oblique   Comminuted   Greenstick

Types of fractures.

9. When do you suspect pathologic fracture?

A pathologic fracture occurs after a minor trauma that ordinarily would not break a bone. Sometimes, the patient may have had pain (especially night pain) in the region before the fracture. If a patient already has a malignant tumor and later develops a fracture, that fracture may likely be due to metastatic disease.

10. Which malignant tumors commonly metastasize to bone?

Malignant tumors of the breast, lung, prostate, colon, rectum, kidney, thyroid, and bladder are common primaries that metastasize to bones. The vertebrae, pelvis, ribs, and long bones are the common bones involved.

11. When should you order a bone scan?

If the initial x-rays do not show a fracture but there is a strong clinical suspicion (especially in suspected stress fractures), a radionuclide bone scan may be very useful. Fracture of the scaphoid is another example of a fracture that may not be visible on initial x-rays, and increased uptake on bone scan may help in diagnosis and management.

12. Is CT useful in the diagnosis and management of fractures?

CT scans may help reveal important characteristics of fractures of the skull, pelvis, and spine. A loose fragment of bone in a joint (joint mouse) can also be visualized better on CT.

13. How about getting an MRI done?

Partial and complete tears of ligaments and hematomas within ligaments are seen well on MRI. This may help in deciding on open or closed treatment of ligament injuries. Bone and muscle hematomas can also be visualized with MRI.

14. What are the goals of treatment after a musculoskeletal injury?

Control pain

Correct any deformity—If there is significant deformity, it needs to be corrected by closed reduction, traction, or open reduction.

Protect injured tissue—Movement at the fracture site is usually prevented by a cast, but internal fixation devices (intramedullary rod, screw, or plate and screws) or external fixation devices may be used.

Prevent complications, secondary impairment

Regain function

15. What are the different methods of immobilization?

The fracture fragments are immobilized and protected to help the natural process of healing. A limited amount of movement between fracture fragments promotes callus formation, whereas excessive movement leads to formation of cartilage and nonunion. Following methods are used to immobilize fractures:

Traction—Prolonged continuous force is applied to align and maintain fracture fragments.
  Skin traction
  Skeletal traction
External fixation
  Plaster cast
  External fixator
Internal fixation—Pins, plates, screws, and intramedullary rods are used to immobilize fracture fragments.

16. What are some of the local complications of a fracture?

Nerve and **blood vessels** can be damaged at the time of initial injury, during manipulation of a fracture, or during a change of cast or any other orthopedic procedure. It is very important to examine and document arterial pulsations, sensation, and muscle power of the involved extremity after the initial injury and before and after each orthopedic procedure.

Compartment syndrome should be suspected when the patient complains of very severe pain, numbness of toes or fingers, inability to move toes or fingers, poor capillary circulation under the nails.

Delayed union occurs if a fracture is not healed after a reasonable time. The site and type of fracture, age of the patient, and presence of any bone pathology are considered in determining a reasonable time for healing of any fracture since there is no absolute time limit to healing.

Nonunion is considered to occur when the bone ends look sclerotic and smooth on x-rays.

Malunion occurs when a fracture unites in an altered alignment.

Stiffness of joints and **atrophy** of muscles adjacent to the fracture site are very common because of immobilization necessary for fracture healing.

Early **degenerative joint disease** may result from incongruous and rough joint surfaces. When fracture involves articular cartilage, all efforts should be made to achieve perfect healing.

17. What is cast disease?

Cast disease includes the following constellation of signs: muscle atrophy, weakness, osteoporosis, and joint stiffness.

18. Which patients require a systematic, holistic approach to fracture rehabilitation?

Any patient who is at risk for significant functional impairment or complications:

Geriatric patients at risk for falls and with multiple medical problems. Deconditioning secondary to prolonged bedrest or inactivity makes it difficult to achieve independent ambulation.

Multitrauma patients with more than one fracture and/or injury to other systems. A careful review for occult injuries overlooked during triage is essential.

Special fractures (e.g, fractures of the scaphoid) are notorious for a high incidence of nonunion.

Preexisting medical conditions. Osteoporosis or osteogenesis imperfecta need special precautions during rehabilitation. Prescription of exercises for patients with cardiorespiratory diseases has to be modified to avoid new complications or aggravating existing ones.

19. Which factors should be considered in planning a rehab program for a patient with a fracture?

Age of patient—The bones (like any other tissue) of elderly patients heal slowly.

Quality of bone—Advanced osteoporosis or metastatic disease slows the healing process or interferes with bony union and may require consultation with an endocrinologist or oncologist.

Fracture site—Some fractures, such as the femoral neck or distal one-third of the tibia, are known to heal slowly or result in a nonunion.

Fixation—If the bone fragments are securely immobilized by internal or external fixation, then the patient has greater freedom to load the fracture site to facilitate healing.

Extent of soft tissue injury, neurovascular complications, or injury to other organs may slow down the progress of the patient in rehabilitation therapies.

20. Weight-bearing is a very important function of the lower extremity. How do you determine when the patient is ready for weight-bearing?

No specific timetable can be offered for any particular fracture. Decisions are made after considering following five factors:

1. **Type of fracture**—Weight-bearing can be tolerated earlier on a transverse fracture in normal alignment than an oblique, spiral, or communited fracture or a fracture with displaced fragments.

2. **Method and quality of fixation**—Intramedullary rods or plate and screws immobilize the fracture fragments much better than a cast, though rods and screws are not strong enough to support the weight of the body during ambulation.

3. **Condition of the bone**—Fracture through a metastasis does not heal well.

4. **Patient's ability to control weight-bearing**—Elderly patients with dementia or stroke may not be able to follow orders of partial weight-bearing. Similar difficulties may be encountered in persons with head trauma or multiple fractures.

5. **Bony union**—Union of bone fragments is determined by clinical and radiologic examination. A gentle bending force is applied to stress the fracture site. If there is no pain and no movement, then the fracture is said to be clinically united. Radiologic union occurs a few weeks after the clinical union.

21. What are some of the problem fractures in children?

Supracondylar fracture of the humerus is notorious because of the complication of Volkman's ischemic contracture.

Dislocation of the head of radius may be missed initially or may recur after reduction and immobilization in a cast in Monteggia fracture-dislocation (fracture of the shaft of ulna with dislocation of the head of radius). All movements (flexion, extension, and rotations) at the elbow are limited.

Metaphyseal and epiphyseal fractures, since they involve the growth plate, can lead to premature closure of the epiphysis and a shorter extremity.

22. Which signs increase the suspicion of child abuse?

1. When the type and distribution of bruises and fractures do not fit with the history of injury.

2. When the history of injury is not consistent from one day to the next or when father and mother give different stories.

3. When there is a delay in seeking medical attention.

4. The abused child may not cry because of fear.

5. When there are other types of injuries, such as burns, scars of previous trauma, or bruises of different colors suggesting multiple, separate incidents.

6. X-rays reveal multiple fractures at various stages of healing.

23. How are fractures in children different from those in adults?

• All tissues heal well and more rapidly in children.
• Joints do not become stiff as easily as in adults.
• Remodeling process corrects deformity to a much greater extent in younger children.
• "Greenstick" fractures, in which the cortex buckles on only one side of the shaft of a long bone, are seen only in children.
• Epiphyseal injuries may affect the growth plate and growth of a long bone in children.

24. What are some of the common fractures seen in the elderly?

Compression fracture of the spine—This fracture is due to flexion injury and is common in the osteoporotic spine. Metastatic disease and infection should always be ruled out.

Fracture of the femoral neck—Approximately 250,000 patients per year are hospitalized for treatment of fractures of the neck of femur. They usually require internal fixation or replacement arthroplasty and a rehabilitation program to get them back on their feet. A high rate of complications and mortality is associated with this fracture.

Fracture of distal radius—Colles' fracture is often associated with osteoporosis and a fall onto an outstretched arm.

Fracture of the neck of humerus—This injury may lead to marked limitation of movements in the shoulder joint.

25. Where do stress fractures commonly occur?

Ordinary fractures occur as a result of single injury; stress fractures occur as a result of cumulative effect of small, repeated stresses, resulting in a hairline crack in a bone. Stress fracture of the 2nd, 3rd, or 4th metatarsal is called "march fracture" because it was described in poorly conditioned soldiers after long marches. Long distance running and ballet dancing are other activities that may cause this injury. The proximal tibia, fibula, neck of femur, and pubic ramus are other frequent sites for stress fractures. The history includes a complaint of pain on weight-bearing after a few weeks of large amount of activity. There is localized tenderness over the fracture site.

26. Which fractures are missed (more often than others) on initial evaluation?

Hairline fractures of the scaphoid may not show on initial x-rays. A patient with a history of a fall on an outstretched hand, with pain and tenderness over the anatomical snuff box (radial side of wrist), should be treated empirically as having a scaphoid fracture (splinting or casting) for 10 to 15 days and then x-rayed again. If a fracture is not evident at that time and fracture of scaphoid is still suspected on clinical grounds, a bone scan is warranted.

A patient may be able to walk despite a fracture of the neck of femur if the bone fragments are impacted. The fracture line may be difficult to visualize on initial x-rays. Management of this problem is similar to that of suspected fracture of the scaphoid.

27. What is the difference between dislocation and subluxation?

In **dislocation**, the articular surfaces are totally separated from each other; there is no contact at all. In **subluxation**, there is partial contact between articular surfaces. A good example of subluxation is seen in the shoulder joint after a stroke. The head of the humerus slides downward because of gravity and the inability of weak muscles to maintain it in normal position. Fracture-dislocation is more severe and occurs when bone forming the joint is fractured. This type of injury may need open reduction and internal fixation to restore stability of the joint. Fracture-dislocations occur in the shoulder, ankle, elbow, and hip.

28. What goals do you want to achieve for your patient during rehabilitation?

1. **Prevent complications**, such as joint stiffness, disuse atrophy, contractures, pressure sores, and re-displacement of fracture fragments. Premature weight-bearing or very vigorous exercises can re-displace the bone fragments.

2. **Restore** range of movement, muscle strength by isometric or resistive exercises, function of the extremity, vocational and avocational activities.

BIBLIOGRAPHY

 1. Adams JC: Outline of Fractures, 9th ed. Edinburgh, Churchill Livingstone, 1987.
 2. Browner BD, Jupiter JB, Levine AM, Trafton PG (eds): Skeletal Trauma. Philadelphia, W.B. Saunders, 1992.
 3. McRae R: Practical Fracture Treatment, 2nd ed. Edinburgh, Churchill Livingstone, 1989.
 4. Mehta AJ (ed): Rehabilitation of Fractures. Phys Med Rehabil State Art Rev 9:1–283, 1995.
 5. Mehta AJ (ed): Common Musculoskeletal Problems. Philadelphia, Hanley & Belfus, 1996.
 6. Mehta AJ, Nastasi AE: Rehabilitation of fractures in the elderly. Geriatric Clin North Am 9:717–730, 1993.
 7. Philip AP, Traisman ES, Philip M: Musculoskeletal injuries in child abuse. Phys Med Rehabil State Art Rev 9:251–268, 1995.
 8. Praemer A, Furner S, Rice DP: Musculoskeletal Conditions in the United States. Park Ridge, IL, American Academy of Orthopedic Surgeons, 1992.
 9. Rockwood CA, Green DP, Bucholz RW (ed): Rockwood and Green's Fractures in Adults, 3rd ed. Philadelphia, J.B. Lippincott, 1991.
10. Salter RB: Textbook of Disorders and Injuries of the Musculoskeletal System, 2nd ed. Baltimore, Williams & Wilkins, 1983.

64. REHABILITATION OF WHIPLASH AND MUSCULOSKELETAL INJURIES FOLLOWING VEHICULAR TRAUMA

Howard Hoffberg, M.D.

1. What is the leading cause of musculoskeletal trauma?

Motor vehicle accidents are the most common mechanism of trauma and are frequently associated with musculoskeletal injury. In the United States, trauma is a major cause of death in people < 40 years of age and accounts for approximately 150,000 deaths annually. As a leading cause of disability in America, trauma causes 400,000 cases of permanent disability with an economic cost of $50 billion annually.

2. What types of musculoskeletal problems result from motor vehicle accidents?

Orthopedic and visceral damage includes chest trauma, abdominal trauma, brain injury, hematomas, long-bone fractures, spine fractures, traumatic nerve entrapments, and discogenic radiculopathies. **Soft tissue injuries** include strains, sprains, contusions, abrasions, and lacerations.

3. List some important historical questions you should ask the accident victim.

1. What was the nature of the accident (rollover, head-on collision, speed of impact, etc.?)
2. Was a seatbelt and/or shoulder harness worn?
3. Was the steering wheel or windshield broken?
4. Was there any body damage to the vehicle?
5. Was there any loss of consciousness?

4. How is the cervical spine of a trauma victim assessed radiologically?

X-rays of the cervical spine provide important structural information. A **lateral** view reveals vertebral bodies, intervertebral spaces, facet joint alignment, and prevertebral soft-tissue structures. Lateral views with flexion and extension can highlight alignment problems. **Anteroposterior** views (frontal) show the lower vertebral endplates and the joints of Luschka. An **open-mouth** view reveals lateral atlantoaxial malalignment, while a lateral projection shows anteroposterior subluxation. **Oblique** views help identify osteophytic encroachment of the intervertebral foramina.

5. What pain syndromes, other than neck pain, are seen with motor vehicle accidents?

Intervertebral disc tears and anterior longitudinal ligamentous disruption can trigger neck pain as well as scapular, shoulder, and upper extremity pain. Nerve root impingement may be attributed to disc herniation. Patients with a structurally compromised spine, with cervical spondylosis, or with osteophytic or thickened ligamentum flava (diagnosed or unknown) can develop central cord syndrome. With this syndrome, upper extremity strength is weaker than lower extremity strength, and sensory changes below the lesion may be present. Other injuries include "dashboard" knee contusions, which usually result in patellofemoral dysfunction and plica syndrome.

6. Describe the five types of fractures-dislocations of the spine.

1. **Jefferson** fracture is a burst fracture of the ring of the atlas (C1 vertebra) secondary to axial compression. It is often unassociated with neurologic deficits. Jefferson fractures are divided into 6 subtypes.

2. **Hangman's** fracture involves the neural arch and is induced by flexion, extension, or both, and axial compression. An abrasion on the forehead or chin is usually seen.

3. **Odontoid** fracture is a fracture in which shearing occurs. Only a small percentage of cases (5%) is associated with spinal cord injury due to the fracture's relatively small size. An open-mouth x-ray of the cervical spine can identify it.

4. **Chance** fracture is a common fracture of the thoracolumbar spine with associated abdominal injuries due to seatbelt wear. It is caused by a pure distraction force. Typically, it extends through the vertebral body, pedicle, and posterior spinal structures.

5. **Clay-shoveler's** fracture is an avulsion fracture of the spinous process. It can occur at any level of the spine and is associated with vigorous paraspinal muscle activity.

7. What is "whiplash"?

According to the Quebec Task Force, whiplash is defined as: "an acceleration–deceleration mechanism of energy transfer to the neck. It may result from rear-end or side-impact motor vehicle collisions, but can occur during diving or other mishaps. The impact may result in bony or soft tissue injuries (whiplash injuries) which may in turn lead to other clinical manifestations." An impact of 6–8-km/h (4–5 mph) is sufficient to produce enough force to induce cervical spine sprain. The Quebec Task Force, an international consortium of health professionals including physiatrists, neurosurgeons, orthopedists, physical therapists, and others, has recently proposed a classification system to categorize injury severity.

Quebec Classification of Whiplash-associated Disorders*

GRADE	CLINICAL PRESENTATION
0	No complaint about the neck No physical sign(s)
1	Neck complaint of pain, stiffness, or tenderness only No physical sign(s)
2	Neck complaint *and* Musculoskeletal sign(s)[†]
3	Neck complaint *and* Neurologic sign(s)[‡]
4	Neck complaint *and* Fracture or dislocation

* Dotted lines indicate limits of terms of reference of Task Force. Symptoms and disorders that can be manifest in all grades include deafness, dizziness, tinnitus, headache, memory loss, dysphagia, and temporomandibular joint pain.
[†] Musculoskeletal signs include decreased range of motion and point tenderness.
[‡] Neurologic signs include decreased or absent deep tendon reflexes, weakness, and sensory deficits.
From Spitzer WO, et al: Scientific monograph of the Quebec Task Force on Whiplash-associated Disorders. Spine 20(8s): 1995, with permission.

8. How do front-end collisions differ from rear-end collisions?

Rear-end collisions may commonly lead to hyperextension injuries and, depending on severity, may induce stretching injury to the sternocleidomastoid, longus, colli, and scalene muscle groups. Pain, muscle spasm, and range-of-motion limitation can ensue.

Front-end collisions are associated with hyperflexion stretch injury to the trapezius, levator scapula, and cervical paraspinal muscles. In frontal deceleration accidents, chest wall injuries, pulmonary contusion, myocardial contusion, and aortic rupture may occur.

9. What is the most common x-ray finding following cervical strain?

Reversal (straightening or flattening) of the cervical lordosis is often seen and indicates cervical paraspinal muscle spasm.

10. What is the difference between a strain and a sprain?

Strain: a stretch injury to a tissue unassociated with any tearing. Severity is described as mild, moderate, or severe.

Sprain: a stretch or tension injury associated with tissue tearing and bleeding. Its classification is first, second, or third degree depending on severity.

11. What other types of disability may result from traumatic impact to the thoracic, lumbosacral, and pelvic regions?

Pelvic girdle dysfunction, including quadratus lumborum, glutei, piriformis, and iliopsoas muscle dysfunction, may occur with pelvic trauma. As a result of pain and muscular imbalance, a functional leg-length discrepancy and scoliosis may occur. Lumbar strains are usually associated with lumbar paraspinal and quadratus lumborum involvement. Thoracic strain usually affects the thoracic paraspinal muscles, rhomboids, trapezium, levator, and shoulder girdle muscles. Rib injuries are more common in the elderly and may be associated with underlying osteoporosis.

12. List the types of headaches seen in accident victims.

Headaches, or cephalalgia, can occur as a referral pattern from cervical muscle strain, craniofacial pain, upper cervical facet pain, upper cervical radiculopathy, or postconcussive syndrome. Vascular (migrainous) headaches, stress and muscle tension headache, and mixed or combination headaches may be seen.

13. Do auto accidents really cause craniofacial dysfunction?

Strain of the temporomandibular joint can cause neck pain. A head-forward posture, frequently seen following cervical strain, alters the position of the jaw which can contribute to symptoms. If a patient has preexisting jaw problems, including poor bite alignment and bruxism (teeth grinding), symptoms can be significantly worsened following a motor vehicle accident. Jaw pain is frequently associated with masseter, pterygoid, sternocleidomastoid, temporalis, and submental trigger points.

14. What is injured when the patient "pulls his head over to the side" after an auto accident?

Shoulder strains may occur as a result of the torquing of the shoulder by the shoulder harness, which can affect the acromioclavicular, sternoclavicular, glenohumeral, or scapulothoracic joints, or due to direct trauma. The physical findings usually involve trigger points in the rotator cuff muscles, pectoralis, bicipital groove, and coracoid process. The most frequent findings following shoulder strain are restrictions of internal rotation and horizontal extension with myofascial pain.

15. What is reflex sympathetic dystrophy?

Sympathetically maintained pain syndromes affecting the extremities are occasionally associated with traumatic sprains, contusions, fractures, and crush or peripheral nerve injuries following an auto accident. The typical presentation is a swollen, cool (sometimes hot), discolored, sweating limb with exquisite sensitivity to light touch. Pain is often out of proportion to the objective findings.

16. Do cervical collars work?

Although cervical collars provide no stability to the cervical spine, they do serve to remind the patient to avoid extremes of motion. Debatedly, they may be helpful in those patients with guarded motions immediately following an accident. On the other hand, they can contribute to cervical muscular weakness and a head-forward posture.

BIBLIOGRAPHY

1. Allen ME, et al: Acceleration perturbations of daily living—A comparison to whiplash. Spine 19:1285–1290, 1994.
2. Cailliet R: Soft Tissue Pain and Disability. Philadelphia, F.A. Davis, 1977.

3. Junsson H, et al: Findings and outcome in whiplash-type neck distortions. Spine 19:733–743, 1994.
4. Merli GJ: Medical consultation in the patient with multiple trauma. Med Clin North Am 77:493–507, 1993.
5. Newman PK: Whiplash injury. BMJ 301:395–396, 1990.
6. Schofferman J, Wasserman S: Successful treatment of low back pain and neck pain after motor vehicle accident despite litigation. Spine 19:1007–1010, 1994.
7. Teasell RW, Shapiro AP (eds): Cervical Flexion-Extension Whiplash Injuries. Spine State Art Rev 7(3):329–578, 1993.
8. Travell J, Simons D: Myofascial Pain and Dysfunction: The Trigger Point Manual. Baltimore, Williams & Wilkins, 1992.
9. Waylonis GW, Perkins RH: Post-traumatic fibromyalgia: A long term follow up. Am J Phys Med Rehabil 7:403–409, 1994.
10. Young MA, Hillis A, Lenz FA: Sensory sequela and thalamic pain. In Outcome After Head, Neck, and Spinal Trauma: A Medicolegal Guide. Oxford, Butterworth-Heinemann.
11. Young MA, O'Young BO, McFarland EG: Rehabilitation of the orthopedic trauma patient. General principles. Phys Med Rehabil State Art Rev 8(1):185–201, 1995.

65. CHRONIC PAIN (BENIGN) SYNDROMES

Jaywant J. P. Patil, M.B.B.S., F.R.C.P.C.

1. What is the internationally recognized definition of pain?

The International Association for the Study of Pain defines pain as "an unpleasant sensory and emotional experience associated with actual or potential tissue damage or described in terms of such damage." Pain is always a subjective experience. The application of the word is learned in childhood by experiences related to injury or trauma; how one reacts to pain may be influenced greatly by the individual's personality, mood, ethnic background, and past experiences of pain. Pain indeed is unpleasant and therefore frequently an emotional experience.

Pain was recognized may centuries ago by Aristotle, who considered it to be an emotion. He described pain to be the opposite of pleasantness and considered it a quality of the soul.

2. What are the dimensions of the pain experience?

Pain can be a multidimensional experience. Melzack and Casey have suggested three distinct dimensions of pain:

1. The **sensory-discriminative** dimension is the physical, sensory component of pain. Transmission of the sensory component of pain is well explained in basic neurophysiology. This dimension can be mapped in terms of time (e.g., intermittent vs constant, acute vs chronic) and space (location).

2. The **cognitive-evaluative** dimension is an on-going perception and appraisal of the meaning of the sensation. This dimension can be mapped in time (present, past, or future). This is the coping dimension of pain or "why should this happen to me, oh Lord?" dimension of pain.

3. The **affective-motivational** dimension is the mood dimension of pain. It can be mapped in time within the social network.

All three dimensions can be seen in varying degrees in most pain experiences, be it acute or chronic pain. They can be remembered by the mnemonic "SAC," which stands for the **s**ensory, **a**ffective, and **c**ognitive dimensions of pain.

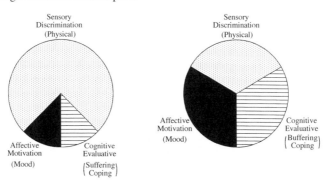

The three dimensions of pain. (Adapted from Chaplin ER: Chronic pain: A sociobiological problem. Phys Med Rehabil State Art Rev 5(1):1–48, 1991.)

3. How do chronic pain and the so-called chronic pain syndrome differ?

Acute pain can persist and eventually become subacute and, with the passage of time, chronic in nature. **Chronic pain** is generally considered a pain that continues to persist long after the expected healing time. Persons who suffer from pain make both physiologic and behavioral adaptations with time. Pain sufferers learn to cope and adapt to their pain in different ways. The persons who suffer from **chronic pain syndrome** exhibit maladaptive patterns of behavior for dealing with their persistent pain.

4. Name the five D's of the chronic pain syndrome.

1. Drug abuse or misuse
2. Dysfunction or decreased function in life
3. Disuse resulting in loss of flexibility, strength, and endurance
4. Depression or depressed mood
5. Disability resulting in inability to perform activities of daily living (ADL) or pursue gainful employment

To these five D's previously described by Brena, one could add a sixth D—disturbed sleep pattern, where stage 4 sleep is significantly adversely affected.

5. What common pain behaviors does one observe in clinical practice?

In acute pain, one sees automatic-type behaviors that may or may not be helpful to the patient. **Respondent behaviors** are spontaneous responses to painful stimuli, such as holding one's foot after dropping a heavy object on it. With the passage of time, the pain does become subacute, and many **volitional behaviors**, such as walking slowly or using a cane, emerge in an attempt to decrease the pain. **Chronic pain behaviors** as those behaviors that have been positively encouraged or enforced so that the frequency of that behavior is much greater than one would expect. For instance, rubbing a painful area of the body may be respondent behavior in the initial stages of pain, but if the pain sufferer gets the desired sympathy and TLC (tender loving care), the frequency of the behavior may increase, and then that behavior transforms itself into an **operant pain behavior**. This type of behavior may eventually control and limit the patient's mobility and function as the pain becomes chronic.

6. How does the DSM-IV 1994 classify chronic pain?

The *Diagnostic and Statistical Manual-IV* (DSM-IV) puts pain disorders under the general category of **somatoform disorders**. Pain disorders are further subclassified into:
- Pain disorder associated with psychological factors (judged to have a major role in the onset, severity, exacerbation, and maintenance of pain)
- Pain disorder associated with psychological factors and general medication conditions (judged to have an important role in the onset, severity, exacerbation, and maintenance of pain), and
- Pain disorder associated with general medical conditions

Many of the patients who fall under the category of chronic pain syndrome could indeed come under the category of pain disorder associated with both psychological factors and general medical conditions according to DSM-IV.

Under the general category of somatoform disorder, in addition to pain disorder, there are also other psychiatric conditions that include somatization disorder, undifferentiated somatoform disorder, conversion disorder, hypochondriasis, body dysmorphic disorder, and somatoform disorder not otherwise specified. It appears that the DSM-IV has tried to define the processes that are involved in pain disorders in general. This approach seems to be a more practical and logical one. Why not call a spade a spade and not something else to confuse the issue? Other diagnostic labeling, such as fibromyalgia or myofascial pain syndrome, do not fully describe the pain process.

7. How is operant conditioning therapy used in a pain program?

Behavior or operant conditioning therapy is a vital part of any good chronic pain program. It is assumed that the physiologic disorder represents a combination of learned factors as well as biological determinants. The dysfunctional behavior in chronic pain is a product of faulty or inadequate learning to cope with the pain and may be alleviated by applying the techniques and principles of learning new behaviors.

The team treating the patient would have to reinforce positive behavior and discourage negative maladaptive behavior. The patient's family should become involved so that the family can also reinforce positive behaviors. In other words, operant conditioning or behavior modification programs reinforce positive behavior and ignore negative maladaptive behavior. Similar techniques of behavior modification are used to train children and pets with behavior problems.

8. Outline a good 10-step approach to managing a patient with chronic benign pain.

1. As a physician, one must **accept that the patient's pain is real**. Find out why the patient experiences so much discomfort. Try and analyze to what degree the different dimensions of pain are contributing to the patient's total pain experience.

2. **Avoid excessive, unnecessary invasive procedures** and tests that do not help in the management of the patient's pain and only fuel the fires of the chronic pain process.

3. **Set realistic goals.** Make it clear to the patient that you are not trying to cure the pain, but rather to manage it and help the patient to be as functional as possible, despite the pain.

4. **Evaluate the patient's level of function.** Make realistic goals to increase his or her function gradually in terms of different physical tolerances such as walking, sitting, standing, etc. The patient should be taught how to pace himself or herself and how to organize work activities so that he or she can carry out the needed or wanted tasks despite the pain. In other words, the patient has to learn to work his or her life around the obstacle of pain, rather than letting pain restrict the quality of life.

5. If the patient is on medication for pain, this **medication should be taken on a time-contingency basis** rather than on an as-needed basis. Taking the medication as needed may reinforce pain behavior and may not be the best way to approach chronic pain. Also, very gradually reduce the amount of narcotic pain killers that the patient is taking.

6. **Prescribe an exercise program** for the patient, including a physical activity program, that should be very gradually increased over time. Many chronic pain patients are deconditioned because of lack of activity due to the fear of pain in the past. These patients need a reconditioning exercise program.

7. **Educate the patient and family** regarding the chronic pain process. If the patient and family understand the problem well, it then becomes easy to deal with it. The patient's focus should be directed not toward the pain but toward becoming more functional and active in society despite the discomfort and pain.

8. **Help the patient to get involved in recreational and pleasurable activities** to keep themselves physically as well as mentally busy. People who have something better to do don't hurt as much.

9. If the patient has a nonrestorative sleep pattern, take action to **restore a normal sleep pattern** so he or she gets adequate amounts of stage 4 sleep at night. Adequate sleep may help muscles relax completely, make patients psychologically less irritable during the day, and help them to cope better with pain.

10. **Treat depression.** If the patient suffers from some degree of depressed mood, a small dose of tricyclic antidepressants could help. It may also help stage 4 sleep.

9. What 10 factors may predispose a person with chronic pain to develop "chronic pain syndrome"?

1. A past history of anxiety, depression, panic attacks, or child abuse
2. Poor working conditions or no job to return to
3. Substance abuse
4. Multiple medical problems
5. Limited education with poor command of the local language (English)
6. Tendency to miss medical appointments

7. Inconsistent physical findings
8. Preexisting medical conditions
9. No response to different modalities of treatment
10. Previous injury claims with difficult rehabilitation

As a physician dealing with chronic benign musculoskeletal pain, one must be cognizant of the above predisposing factors. In addition, your evaluation should consider other factors, such as stress, coping difficulties with the trials and tribulations of life including pain, disturbed sleep pattern, depressed mood, major psychosocial upheavals (such as marriage separation), divorce, and ongoing litigation.

10. Describe the neurophysiologic process in the posterior horn of the spinal cord that contributes to chronic persistent pain.

Recent research has looked at the contribution of the dorsal horn cells in the production of chronic persistent pain. The **polymodal wide dynamic range neurons** (WDR) have many surface receptors, including the N-methyl D-aspartate (NMDA) receptors and neurokinin (NK) receptors. Excitatory amino acids released from sensory fibers, such as the A-delta fibers, act on the NMDA receptors, while **substance P**, which is released by the afferent C fibers, acts on both the NMDA and NK receptors. The action of substance P on the NK receptors results in decreased magnesium-dependent block on the NMDA receptors, which in turn results in influx of calcium ions into the WDR neurons. This results in increased depolarization of the NMDA receptors.

If painful sensations keep bombarding the WDR neurons with substance P transmitted via the C fibers, the WDR neurons undergo a **hyperpolarization state** or "wind-up." This wind-up phenomenon results in long-lasting cellular changes within the WDR neurons. There is loss of inhibitory mechanisms in the WDR neurons, which in turn results in continual pathologic persistent pain. One can prevent this pathologic state of hyperpolarization of WDR neurons by blocking the C fibers which release substance P with opiates or nerve blocks. It is now recognized that vigorous management of acute pain, postoperative pain, and preemptive analgesia (analgesia just prior to surgery) can prevent central sensitization and the process of "wind-up" that results in chronic persistent pain.

11. What is the role of tricyclic antidepressants in the management of noncancer chronic pain?

Tricyclic antidepressants are used extensively in the management of chronic benign pain. In addition to having an analgesic effect on certain types of chronic pain, they also have a positive effect on the affective dimension of chronic pain. The normally used dosage of this medication is generally much smaller than that used in psychiatric practice. Often, 10–75 mg of amitriptyline or doxepin is effective in managing chronic pain. The medication can be given in one dose at nighttime, which also helps improve the quality of sleep. New tricyclic antidepressants which act on the serotonin pathway are available in the market, but their efficacy in the management of chronic pain is not yet well established. The efficacy of older tricyclic antidepressants, such as imipramine, amitriptyline, and doxepin, has been well established.

12. Is there a connection between fibromyalgia syndrome, myofascial pain syndrome, and chronic pain syndrome?

Fibromyalgia syndrome is a form of nonarticular rheumatism characterized by widespread musculoskeletal aching and stiffness associated with tenderness on palpation at characteristic sites called **tender points.**

Myofascial pain syndrome can present as localized muscle pain or a more generalized form of muscle pain. It is associated with stiffness, aching, gelling, tightness, numbness, tingling, weakness, or coolness in a localized area of the body, along with taut bands found in the involved muscles. There is tenderness in the muscle bands and **trigger points** that give rise to pain in sites remote from the trigger point. A localized muscle twitch response may be elicited by snapping or needling of the taut bands.

Both syndromes, when chronic, can be associated with deconditioning, psychosocial dysfunction, symptoms of depression, and disturbed stage 4 sleep or nonrestorative sleep pattern. It is possible that people who suffer from a generalized form of myofascial pain syndrome may fulfill the criteria for fibromyalgia. It is also possible that people who have tender points in fibromyalgia may also have trigger points in the same location.

In **chronic pain syndrome**, a patient suffers from chronic pain and has associated psychological abnormalities such as depression or anxiety. They also exhibit the typical five D's of the syndrome (*see* Question 4). This patient may also present with tender points as found in fibromyalgia or trigger points as found in myofascial pain syndrome. It is possible that a patient who starts with regional myofascial pain syndrome may eventually develop a spread of their pain over their body and fulfill the criteria for fibromyalgia syndrome. It is also possible that both groups of patients may later go on to fulfill the criteria for chronic pain syndrome. This makes one wonder whether we are looking at the same condition which tends to progress over time and which tends to get labeled by different physicians at different points in time. Unfortunately, this type of change in diagnostic labeling results in confusion for the patient and more anxiety, which in turns feeds into the chronic pain process or chronic pain syndrome.

BIBLIOGRAPHY

1. Beitel RE, Dubner R: Response of unmyelinated (C) polymodal nociceptors to thermal stimuli applied to monkey's face. J Neurophysiol 39:1160–1175, 1976.
2. Bennett RM: Myofascial pain syndrome and fibromyalgia syndrome: A comparative analysis. Adv Pain Res Ther 17:43–65, 1990.
3. Brena SF: Chronic Pain: America's Hidden Epidemic. New York, Atheneum/SM1, 1978.
4. Chaplin ER: Chronic pain: A sociobiological problem. Phys Med Rehabil State Art Rev 5(1):1–48, 1991.
5. Coderre TJ, Katz J, Vaccarino KL, Melzack R: Contributions of central neuroplasticity to pathologic pain: Review of clinical and experimental evidence. Pain 52:259–285, 1993.
6. Diagnostic Criteria from DSM-IV. Washington, DC, American Psychiatric Association, 1994.
7. Fordyce WE, Fowler RS, Lehmann JF, et al: Ten steps to help patients with chronic pain. Pat Care 12:263, 1978.
8. King JC, Kelleher WJ: The chronic pain syndrome: The inpatient interdisciplinary rehabilitative behavior modification approach. Phys Med Rehabil State Art Rev 5(1):165–175, 1991.
9. Melzack R, Casey KL: Sensory motivational and central control determinants of pain: A new conceptual model. In Densholo D (ed): The Skin Senses. Springfield, IL, Charles C Thomas, 1968, p 427.
10. Merskey H: Classification of chronic pain: Description of chronic pain syndrome and definition of pain terms. Pain 26(suppl 3):S215–S221, 1986.
11. Patil JJP: Prevention and principles of treatment of chronic pain syndrome in soft tissue injury. Nova Scotia Med J 142(Aug):141–143, 1993.
12. Wolfe F, Smythe HA, Yunus MB, et al: American College of Rheumatology 1990 criteria for classification of fibromyalgia: Report of multicentre criteria committee. Arthritis Rheum 33:160–172, 1990.

66. FIBROMYALGIA AND THE MYOFASCIAL PAIN SYNDROMES

Norman B. Rosen, M.D.

1. Why is there so much confusion regarding the diagnosis and treatment of both these syndromes?

Because both syndromes lack true objective findings and laboratory markers. The few objective findings characteristic of these syndromes—tenderness, pain, characteristic distribution, fatigue, poor sleep, stiffness, weakness, and palpable taut bands (or nodules)—have been challenged as being subjective descriptions depending on the patient and evaluator. In addition, emotional and interpersonal factors often affect these presentations, as does the possibility of secondary gain.

2. What are the myofascial pain syndromes?

In 1952, Drs. Janet Travell and Seymour Rinzler coined the phrase *myofascial pain*. They define myofascial pain syndromes as involving an area of

(1) **local tenderness** ("trigger points") within

(2) a palpable **taut band** which,

(3) on **compression** or **needling**, results in a variety of

(4) **local** or

(5) **referred** manifestations to more remote areas. Trigger points cause **local** dysfunction by perpetuating the local tightness and weakness and **remote** dysfunction in the referral area(s). Every muscle in the body has the capacity to develop a myofascial pain syndrome.

3. Why do myofascial pain syndromes develop?

The major cause is muscle overload or overuse. Trigger points can develop due to a variety of factors, including direct or indirect trauma, tight compressive dressings, cold temperature, overuse, overwork, stress, or other factors that cause reflex muscle spasm. Any factor that causes an increase in muscle tension can cause **focal hypoxia** in that muscle, which then causes and perpetuates the reflex muscle spasm—possibly as a result of hyperactivity of the spindle. The result is that a localized band of tightness develops (the **taut band**), in which a trigger point then develops.

4. Are the fibromyalgia and myofascial pain syndromes two distinct conditions or different manifestations of the same condition?

They are two separate conditions that differ in diagnostic criteria and in expected outcome. Although classically they are differentiated by many authors only by their extent of involvement (regional or focal distribution for the myofascial pain syndromes and more generalized for fibromyalgia), it should be kept in mind that the myofascial pain syndromes may often be multifocal in nature and can mimic the more generalized fibromyalgia picture. The perpetuation of both of these conditions may be due to central events, which maintain muscle spasm in response to peripheral events including trigger points.

5. What are the criteria for the diagnosis of fibromyalgia?

The American College of Rheumatology (ACR) in 1990 set forward two criteria:

1. **Widespread pain and tenderness** present for at least 3 months involving the upper *and* lower and the right *and* left halves of the body.

2. Presence of tenderness at **11 or more of 18 predetermined tender points** on palpation (elicited by exerting a 4 kg/cm pressure, enough to cause blanching of the thumbnail) at the point. These 18 palpation points include specific areas present bilaterally:

- Suboccipital
- Lower anterior cervical (at the intertransverse spaces at C5–7)
- Trapezius (midpoint of the upper border)
- Supraspinatus (at the origin, near the medial scapular border)
- Second rib (at the second costochrondral junction)
- Lateral epicondyle (2 cm distal to the epicondyles)
- Gluteal (upper outer gluteus maximus)
- Greater trochanter (posterior to the trochanteric prominence)
- Knee (at the medial fat pads just proximal to the joint line)

6. What is fibrositis? How does this differ from fibromyalgia?

Fibrositis was first defined in 1904 by Gowers and probably referred to a **localized myofascial** pain syndrome involving the low back. Over the next 60–70 years, the term fibrositis was misapplied to any enigmatic condition involving muscle, including the myofascial pain syndromes, fibromyalgia, psychogenic rheumatism, nonarticulant rheumatism, and mechanical musculoskeletal dysfunction. In fact, the term fribrositis is a misnomer since there is no itis or inflammation involved in these conditions. In the late 1970s, Hench suggested the current term, **fibromyalgia**.

7. What other conditions fulfill the ACR criteria for the diagnosis of fibromyalgia?
1. Sleep deprivation (described as the rheumatic sleep modulation disorder)
2. Chronic fatigue syndrome
3. Multifocal pain syndromes that coincidentally coexist in different parts of the body
4. Psychophysiologic musculoskeletal dysfunctions (psychosomatic, psychogenic, or stress-related disorders)
5. Generalized myalgias of other etiologies

8. Is there a difference between a tender point and a trigger point?
Tender points and trigger points have in common focal point tenderness. However, they are differentiated by the fact that the **trigger point** is an area of firmness (or tautness) which, on compression or needling, can cause a variety of local or remote (referred) manifestations. Palpation or needling of a **tender point** reveals only local discomfort and softness to the needle tip and no referred manifestations. Furthermore, needling a trigger point results in a local twitch response, whereas needling a tender point does not.

9. What referred phenomena can occur from trigger points?
Although the most well-known of these are sensory in nature (**pain, tenderness**) other referred phenomena include **motor effects**, which may be inhibitory or excitatory in nature, and referred **autonomic dysfunctions** (lacrimation, coryza, vasodilatation, or vasoconstriction in the referral zone).

10. Are there any peripheral dysfunctions noted in the fibromyalgia population?
Yes, many.
1. Widespread reproducible tenderness in discrete points throughout the body
2. Weakness and fatigue of muscles, both on static and dynamic loading
3. Abnormalities of phosphate metabolism in muscle biopsies (low-energy disease, controversial)
4. Morning stiffness and "gelling," the etiology of which is not clear
5. Dermatographia in 15–25% of patients
6. Aggravation of symptoms in the cold and symptoms of Raynaud's phenomenon
7. Subjective swelling of the distal extremities (idiopathic edema?)

11. Are there fibromyalgia subsets?
There probably are several fibromyalgia subsets. First, fibromyalgia is currently defined by ACR criteria as not one disease, but probably encompassing *multiple* subsets and conditions within the fibromyalgia population. These subsets, in fact, may not even be related except for sharing a common set of diagnostic criteria. These subsets can be listed as:
1. Peripheral fibromyalgia [true(?) primary fibromyalgia]
2. Cold-induced fibromyalgia
3. Histamine-sensitive fibromyalgia
4. Sympathetic nervous system-mediated fibromyalgia
5. Centrally-mediated fibromyalgia
6. Affective-spectrum disorders and other psychologically mediated disorders
7. Sleep deprivation
8. Abnormalities of hypothalamic-pituitary-adrenal axis
9. Multifocal myofascial pain syndromes
10. Chronic fatigue syndrome
11. Other conditions (infectious [Lyme disease, HIV, etc.], rheumatologic, toxic, allergic, neuromuscular, etc.), generalized muscle pain and tenderness as a result of other conditions.

12. What is "myofascial dysfunction"?

Myofascial dysfunction is the clinical expression of the impairment due to muscular tightness or weakness. Myofascial dysfunction is often manifested by the presence of an imbalance between the agonistic and antagonistic muscle groups. In addition, dysfunction of the proximal stabilizers of the dysfunctional unit may also be present. Myofascial dysfunction has also been called **somatic dysfunction** by the osteopathic community.

13. Is there a difference between myofascial pain and dysfunction and the myofascial pain syndromes?

Yes. Myofascial pain refers to pain and tenderness in the muscles and their fascial components, whereas the myofascial pain syndromes are a unique group of syndromes that satisfy the criteria promulgated by Travell and Rinzler. The criteria include the physical findings of trigger points, taut bands, localized twitch responses, subtle shortening and weakness of involved muscle groups, referred pain upon compression or needling of the trigger points, and immediate reversal of weakness and restricted joint range of motion following successful inactivation of the trigger point.

14. What is unique about the development of the myofascial pain syndromes?

The most unique aspect is that they all develop **secondary** to some other factor, but they then develop the unique ability to become **independent** and **autonomous** pain generators (i.e., they cause pain and dysfunction both locally and elsewhere) and tend to **persist** long after the initial cause of the trigger point is no longer active.

15. What are the common "perpetuating factors" of the myofascial pain syndromes?

1. Postural abnormalities with resultant overload of tissues and development of localized muscle spasm (most common)
2. Underlying metabolic or endocrine dysfunction (particularly of thyroid metabolism)
3. Nutritional deficiencies (e.g., ascorbic acid, B vitamins, etc.)
4. Anemia (including low ferritin level)
5. Electrolyte imbalance (e.g., calcium, magnesium, etc.)
6. Medications (including narcotics)
7. Possible allergy
8. Environmental stessors
9. Temperature
10. External compression interfering with the innervation or circulation to the muscle
11. Infection
12. Sleep deprivation
13. Emotional stress
14. Other concurrent disease (including fibromyalgia)

16. What is the best treatment for the myofascial pain syndromes and fibromyalgia?

1. The patient should be reassured about the benign nature of his or her presentation and favorable prognosis with treatment, whether pain-free or not.
2. The patient should be assessed for evidence of tightness or weakness, both focally and generally, and prescribed a uniquely formulated daily program of gradual stretching (and strengthening).
3. A home program of treatment must stress both flexibility and strength and ideally progress to improved endurance.
4. The clinician and patient must establish mutual goals and objectives, both medical (pain relief, increased ROM, etc.) and social in nature (return to work, sport, or other activity).
5. Return to full function and participation (including return to work) is the major goal of the treatment program, and this goal should be an integral part of the rehabilitation process itself.
6. Sleep restoration is essential, and the use of medication to ensure sleep should be considered.

7. Analgesics, including NSAIDs, should be initiated on a regularly scheduled time-contingency basis. After the patient improves and learns other pain-coping skills, these should be taken as needed or prophylactically prior to engaging in activities that cause discomfort.

8. The use of muscle relaxants probably should be avoided during the daytime, although they may be quite effective at night to promote relaxation and facilitate sleep.

9. The use of narcotics should be kept to a minimum and used for only brief periods in scheduled doses.

10. The use of tricyclics is probably most beneficial in their ability to facilitate sleep but is also effective in patients who are depressed.

11. Physical therapy should initially focus on stretching, strengthening, and restoration of function.

12. Psychosocial factors should be identified and treated in all patients.

13. Adjunctive medications include the use of antianxiety agents, antidepressants, or other psychotropic medications as necessary.

14. Multivitamins, nutritional supplements, and hormone replacement, particularly when endocrine or metabolic dysfunction is present, should be considered additional adjunctive management. Weight reduction and other lifestyle changes (particularly smoking and alcohol) should be made.

15. Injection therapy, using a dilute solution of procaine or lidocaine, are most effective in desensitizing the trigger point, and once a trigger point is injected, the muscle harboring the trigger point should also be gently stretched.

16. The use of TENS, acupuncture, and biofeedback is considered third-line treatment approaches.

17. How long should you continue to treat pain?

The clinician should recognize that the clinical complaint of pain is only the tip of the iceberg and should not be the sole focus of treatment or outcome. Pain really needs to be treated *only* if it interferes with work, play, sleep, or quality of life. More importantly, the clinician should recognize that inadequate treatment of underlying tissue dysfunction may result in recurring symptoms and recurring pain. Pain may be a clue that there is underlying tissue dysfunction, and a careful search for the cause of pain is critical.

18. A patient is alleging disability because of fibromyalgia and/or myofascial pain. How should I go about assessing the degree and significance of disability?

Just as pain and tissue dysfunction are two separate issues and should be treated as such, so too should pain and disability from pain be treated as two separate issues. The clinician should differentiate between disability and impairment and should try to objectify these issues by the use of functional and work capacity evaluations. The clinician should attempt to identify the coping and problem-solving skills of the patient as well as any various psychosocial stressor. Particularly with a patient who has chronic disability, it is critical to involve the family member(s) and make them part of the treatment team.

19. A patient who has a persistent carpal tunnel syndrome is just not getting better. Are there any trigger point syndromes that should be considered as contributing to the persistent symptoms?

There are several. In particular, the infraspinatus, pectoralis minor, subscapularis, and some of the wrist extensors refer into the distribution that is consistent with a median nerve entrapment.

20. A patient has persistent medial joint-line knee pain and a "medial meniscus" problem. Are there any trigger points that can mimic this problem?

Yes. In particular, the vastus medialis. However, the rectus femoris, gracilis, and medial gastrocnemius also can develop trigger points that on occasion create medial knee pain.

21. Are there any trigger points responsible for causing and perpetuating symptoms that suggest thoracic outlet obstruction?

Yes. Any of the muscles normally associated with thoracic outlet obstruction, including, in particular, the scalene muscles and the pectoralis minor. However, it should be kept in mind that the alleged thoracic outlet obstruction can also be due to tightness or weakness of the scapular stabilizers, pectoralis major, infraspinatus, subscapularis as well as the serratus posterior superior and anterior serratus. Thoracic outlet is occasionally associated with rounded shoulders and poor posture, and the muscles that may be contributing to this may be harboring latent or even active trigger points.

22. In a patient with "tendinitis" of his wrist, are there any trigger points that may be causing referred pain to this area?

Yes, several. In particular, the wrist extensors, the supinators, as well as the wrist flexors and pronator muscles. In addition, the shoulder muscles should be evaluated, including the infraspinatus, pectoralis, and subscapularis.

23. Which myofascial trigger points should be considered in a patient with occipital and frontal headaches?

In particular, the suboccipital region, upper trapezius, levator scapulae, sternocleidomastoid, and even some of the jaw muscles (ptergoids and temporalis) and other muscles in and about the head can mimic occipital and temporal headaches.

24. What trigger point should be looked for in a patient having recurring "shin splints"?

"Shin splints" is a term that has been applied to calf tenderness in any of the compartments of the calf, particularly the anterolateral and medial compartments. A presentation with apparent posterior compartment involvement should suggest a myofascial syndrome of the gastrocnemius, soleus, tibialis posterior, or flexor hallucis longus. Anterolateral compartment pain may reflect areas of myofascial pain in the peroneus longus, extensor hallucis longus, or extensor digitorum longus.

BIBLIOGRAPHY

1. Gnatz SM: Referred pain syndromes of the head and neck. Phys Med Rehabil State Art Rev 5:585–596, 1991.
2. Rosen NB: The myofascial pain syndromes. In Andary MT, Tomski MA (eds): Office Management of Pain. Phys Med Rehabil Clin North Am 4:41–63, 1993.
3. Rosen NB: Physical medicine and rehabilitation approaches to the management of myofascial pain and fibromyalgia syndromes. In Masi AM (eds): Bailliere's Clin Rheumatol 10:881–916, 1994.
4. Travell JG, Simons DG: Myofascial Pain and Dysfunction. The Trigger Point Manual. Baltimore, Williams & Wilkins, 1983.
5. Yunus MB: Diagnosis, etiology and management of fibromyalgia syndrome: An update. Compreh Ther 14:8–20, 1988.

67. REFLEX SYMPATHETIC DYSTROPHY

Warren Slaten, M.D., and Kevin O'Connor, M.D.

1. What is reflex sympathetic dystrophy (RSD)?

RSD is a complex disorder with or without antecedent nerve injury, consisting of pain and related sensory abnormalities, abnormal blood flow and sweating, abnormalities in the motor system, and changes in both superficial and deep structures with trophic changes.

2. What conditions can be followed by RSD?

Almost any trauma, minor or major. These include nerve injury, fracture, soft tissue injury such as wrist sprain or rotator cuff strain, or even an injection. Medical conditions such as cerebrovascular accident or myocardial infarction can also lead to RSD.

3. What are some of the terms used to denote RSD?

Sympathetically maintained pain syndrome   Sudeck's atrophy
Causalgia   Post-traumatic osteoporosis
Algodystrophy   Chronic traumatic edema
Shoulder-hand syndrome   Traumatic vasospasm
Sympathalgia

4. What central mechanisms have been postulated to explain the pathogenesis of RSD?

The gate-control theory, the turbulence theory, and the wide dynamic range theory.

5. Describe the gate-control theory.

The gate-control theory postulates that input from large diameter fibers inhibits input from small, unmyelinated pain fibers, preventing central processing of the pain input. In RSD, it is believed that the large diameter fibers are injured, with relative sparing of the small, unmyelinated nociceptive fibers, so the pain input from the smaller fibers is unmodulated.

6. The turbulence theory.

The turbulence theory suggests that nerve injury causes formation of altered nerve input, creating "turbulence" which modifies the brain's perception of normal cutaneous afferent activity.

7. And the wide dynamic range theory.

This theory suggests that large type-A myelinated afferent fibers are sensitized during trauma by type-C unmyelinated fibers. The afferent fibers are excited by sympathetic activity and then induce more pain.

8. Name two peripheral mechanisms postulated to explain RSD.

Artificial synapse theory
Spontaneous discharge theory

9. What is the artificial synapse theory?

At the site of nerve discontinuity, sympathetic efferent fibers propagate impulses to the somatic sensory afferents. This depolarization results in a perception of pain centrally and causes a release of pain-sensitizing substances peripherally.

10. What is the spontaneous discharge theory?

This theory postulates that after nerve injury, regenerating axons result in excessive numbers of sodium and calcium channels and α-adrenergic receptors. These channels discharge spontaneously, and circulating catecholamines augment this activity, resulting in hyperalgesia and abnormal chemosensitivity.

11. Which of these theories explains the development of RSD?

Well, none of them fully explain the mechanism of RSD. The hyperalgesia, vasomotor instability, trophic changes, emotional component of symptoms, onset after peripheral and central events, and spread of pain away from the area of initial injury are a wide constellation of signs and symptoms that do not fit into any one theory.

12. What symptoms and signs are found in each of the stages of RSD?

Acute stage—burning pain, edema, increased nail and hair growth, and hyperthermia or hypothermia (3–6 months)

Dystrophic stage—pain becoming more intense and spreading proximally (sometimes crossing the midline), cold insensitivity, brawny edema which may include fusiform digits, hyperhidrosis, decreased ROM, mottled skin, brittle nails, and early atrophy and osteopenia (late)

Atrophic stage—pain subsides; skin is pale or cyanotic, with a smooth and shiny appearance and feels cool and dry; bone demineralization progresses with muscle atrophy and contractures

13. How is the pain described in RSD?
The pain is described as **dysesthetic**—it is often out of proportion to the inciting injury. Though it may radiate in a dermatomal or nerve distribution, it is more often diffuse and non-dermatomal. The pain usually starts in the distal aspect of the limb and, with progression, spreads proximally. Allodynia (pain to a benign stimulus, such as light touch or a breeze) is characteristic.

14. What clinical criteria are used to diagnose RSD?
The following criteria used are those described by Kozin:
  a. Pain and tenderness in an extremity
  b. Signs and symptoms of vasomotor instability
  c. Swelling of the extremity
  d. Dystrophic skin and nail changes
Definite RSD syndrome: a, b, c, and d
Probable: a, b, and c
Possible: a and b or c
Doubtful: a only

15. How does the clinical presentation and course of RSD differ in children?
Frequently, there is no preceding neurologic or traumatic event, and the lower extremity is more often affected. The bone scan results are more variable and, when positive, show decreased rather than increased uptake. Osteoporosis is rare, and the prognosis is generally favorable.

16. Which diagnostic tests can be used to establish the diagnosis of RSD?
X-rays, triple-phase bone scan, sympathetic blockade, thermography.

17. What are the findings in the triple-phase bone scan in patients with RSD?
The blood flow and blood pool phases may show asymmetric uptake between limbs, while the static phase (most sensitive) shows increased periarticular uptake.

18. What x-ray findings are typical in RSD?
In the initial stages, x-rays may be normal. Periarticular osteoporosis may be found in later stages.

19. Are there abnormal laboratory findings in RSD?
No. All are within normal limits (including calcium, phosphorus, and alkaline phosphatase).

20. Is there one or a combination of diagnostic tests that definitively diagnoses RSD?
No. Laboratory tests, x-rays, and triple-phase bone scan are helpful, but the diagnosis is established on clinical grounds.

21. What other diagnoses should be considered in the differential diagnosis of RSD?

Infectious arthritis	Rotator cuff tear
Systemic lupus erythematosus	Peripheral neuropathy
Rheumatoid arthritis	Local trauma
Scleroderma	Paraneoplastic syndrome
Conversion reaction	

22. What are the principles for treating RSD?
  1. Early recognition and diagnosis.
  2. Early, aggressive treatment to break the cycle of sympathetic activity and pain.
  3. Use of sympathetic blocking agents, including oral agents and sympathetic blocking injections.

4. Symptomatic management, including pain management, avoiding contractures, and edema control.

5. Psychologic support, including patient education, relaxation training, and counseling.

23. Which drugs can be used to treat RSD?

Tricyclic antidepressants	Propranolol
Anti-adrenergic agents	Nifedipine
Prednisone	Calcitonin
NSAIDs	Topical capsaicin
Carbamazepine	Gabapentin

24. Which modalities are used in physical therapy to treat RSD?

TENS to modulate inhibitory control of afferent input may provide some pain relief.

Contrast baths (alternating cold and hot water) for the affected extremity is believed to address the vasomotor component of the patient's symptoms.

Edema control measures, including elevation and gradient compression.

Desensitization techniques may increase the patient's tolerance of normal sensory input and decrease hyperesthesias.

Ultrasound provides pain relief with an inhibiting effect on the paracervical sympathetic ganglia.

25. What injection techniques are used to treat the patient with RSD?

Upper extremities—Bier block and stellate ganglion blocks.

Lower extremities—epidural block and lumbar sympathetic blocks.

26. What is a Bier block?

In this technique, guanethidine or reserpine is infused intravenously into the affected limb, followed by a pressure tourniquet around the affected limb at 100 mmHg above systolic blood pressure. These agents, which decrease sympathetic activity, are then allowed to circulate in a high concentration in the affected limb, until the tourniquet pressure is decreased.

27. How is a stellate ganglion block performed?

The trachea is moved to one side, and the needle is inserted between the trachea and carotid artery. When it reaches the vertebral body, the needle is moved slightly lateral. Then, 3–5 ml of an anesthetic, such as mepivacaine 0.5% or bupivacaine 0.25%, is infused into the stellate ganglion.

28. What signs and symptoms suggest an effective stellate ganglion block?

Pain relief, Horner's syndrome (miosis, ptosis, nasal congestion, and anhidrosis), and an increase in the skin temperature of the extremity. The patient needs to know that benefit from an injection is often short-lived (24–48 hours), and repeat injections every 5–7 days may be required.

29. Which patients with RSD would be good candidates for surgical paravertebral sympathectomy?

If after 4–6 stellate ganglion injections the patient is still getting significant relief from injections but the relief is not lasting, then he or she may benefit from surgical sympathectomy. If injections have stopped having any effect, even temporary, then benefit from surgery is less likely. With surgery, risks to be considered include the possibility of sympathalgia, a painful condition of muscle fatigue and pain which is usually temporary, and Horner's syndrome, which may be permanent.

30. What is the prognosis for patients with RSD?

Guarded. Early diagnosis and treatment improve the prognosis, but there is no definitive treatment at this time.

BIBLIOGRAPHY

1. Babur H: Reflex sympathetic dystrophy. J Neurol Orthop Med Surg 12:46–59, 1991.
2. Bonica J: Causalgia and other reflex sympathetic dystrophies. Postgrad Med 53:143–148, 1983.
3. Kozin F: Reflex sympathetic dystrophy syndrome. Bull Rheum Dis 36:1–8, 1986.
4. Raj P, Kelly J, Cannella S, McConn K: Multidisciplinary management of reflex sympathetic dystrophy. Pain Digest 2:267–273, 1992.
5. Schwartzman R, McLellan T: Reflex sympathetic dystrophy—a review. Arch Neurol 44:555–561, 1987.

68. TENDINITIS

Mark D. Klaiman, M.D., and Joseph Shrader, P.T.

1. What are the important structures making up a tendon?

Tendon is a specialized connective tissue comprised primarily of closely packed collagen **fibrils**, forming **fascicles**, which are surrounded by a connective tissue sheath, or **epitenon**. The **paratenon** is the outermost sheath and is lined in some tendons by a synovial membrane that produces synovial fluid, thereby reducing friction as the tendon glides. The blood supply to the tendon originates at musculotendinous and bone–tendon junctions, but it is primarily derived from vessels in the paratenon that penetrate the epitenon.

2. What factors contribute to a tendon's failing?

The tensile strength of a healthy tendon can be more than double that of its attached muscle, but tendon is most vulnerable to failure when:

1. Tension is applied quickly.
2. Tension is applied obliquely.
3. The tendon is tense before trauma.
4. The attached muscle is maximally innervated.
5. The muscle group is stretched by external stimuli.
6. The tendon is weak in comparison to its muscle.

A variety of factors are known to influence the metabolism of tendon, including age, exercise, temperature, nutrition, hormones, immobilization, and, of course, injury.

Reference: Barfred T: Experimental rupture of the Achilles tendon: Comparison of various types of experimental rupture in rats. Acta Orthop Scand 42:528–543, 1971.

3. What is tendinitis?

Traditionally, tendinitis referred to nonspecific painful conditions involving tendon, its connective tissue sheaths, or the insertion of tendon to bone (enthesis). With improved understanding of these injuries, it has become clear that "tendinitis" is not a single clinical or pathologic condition, but rather a spectrum of injuries with often different clinical presentations, distinct histopathology, and predictably different clinical and functional outcomes.

4. How are tendon injuries classified?

Tendon injuries can be considered from a pathologic or functional standpoint. At least three overlapping pathologic conditions exist; inflammation, degeneration, and rupture. Inflammation of paratenon alone is called **paratenonitis**, whereas involvement of paratenon lined with synovium is **tenosynovitis**. The term **tendinitis** is reserved for injuries and inflammation specifically involving tendon. **Tendinosis** is a condition describing intratendinous degeneration and atrophy in the presence of little inflammation. Chronic inflammation often leads to tendinosis and may ultimately be associated with structural weakening and tendon rupture. A subgroup of patients also present with acute exacerbation of symptoms superimposed on chronic inflammation;

tendon biopsy often reveals inflammation of the paratenon and concomitant tendon atrophy, leading to the term **paratenonitis with tendinosis**.

Classification of Tendon Injuries

INJURY	DEFINITION
Paratenonitis/tenosynovitis	Inflammation of the paratenon; pain, swelling, local tenderness.
Tendinitis	Tendon trauma with associated vascular disruption and inflammation; may be acute, subacute, or chronic.
Tendinosis	Noninflammatory, intratendinous atrophy and degeneration often associated with chronic tendinitis; palpable nodule may be present over tendon.
Paratenonitis with tendinosis	Often an acute injury superimposed on chronic tendinitis.
Partial/complete rupture	Often acute inflammation, swelling, and pain superimposed on chronic inflammation and tendinosis.

5. Describe a functional classification of tendinitis.

A functional classification of traumatic tendinitis is particularly useful, as the degree of disability correlates well with the extent of injury. This grading system also provides objective parameters for following treatment and rehabilitation.

Functional Scale of Tendinitis

GRADE	SYMPTOMS
1	Mild pain after exercise, resolving within 24 hrs
2	Minimal pain with exercise, not interfering with activity
3	Pain that interferes with activity
4	Pain caused by activities of daily living
5	Constant rest pain that interferes with sleep

6. How common are musculoskeletal soft tissue injuries?

In the United States, it is estimated that these injuries constitute 30–50% of athletic injuries seen in the outpatient setting. In general, musculoskeletal disorders occur at the same rate in both men and women and increase in incidence with age.

7. Are some tendons more vulnerable than others in particular sports?

Common Tendon Injuries

INVOLVED TENDON	ACTIVITY/SPORT	INJURY CLASSIFICATION
Achilles	Running	Achilles paratenonitis, rupture
Posterior tibialis	Running	Posterior tibialis tendinitis
Patella	Basketball, volleyball, running	Patella tendinitis (jumper's knee), paratenonitis, rupture
Abductor pollicis longus Extensor pollicis brevis	Cycling	DeQuervain's tenosynovitis
Extensor carpi radialis brevis	Tennis	Lateral epicondylitis-insertion tendinitis (tennis elbow)
Common wrist flexors	Golf, tennis	Medial epicondylitis-insertion tendinitis (golfer's elbow)
Supraspinatus (rotator cuff)	Baseball, swimming, weight-training	Supraspinatus tendinitis (impingement syndrome, paratenonitis, rupture
Biceps brachii	Baseball, swimming	Bicipital tendinitis

8. What factors may contribute to the development of tendinitis?

Intrinsic variables	Extrinsic variables
Age	Training errors/poor technique
Flexibility imbalance	Environmental conditions
Muscle imbalance/weakness	Equipment factors
Anatomic malalignment	
Genetic predisposition	

9. What causes tendinitis?

Direct trauma is a common cause of soft tissue injury, but the majority of sport- and occupational-related soft tissue injuries are related to indirect factors resulting in overuse or cumulative trauma disorders. Musculotendinous structures are vulnerable to failure from sudden overloading, as with forceful muscular contractions, particularly when weakened due to concurrent illness (connective tissue disorders) or medications (steroids). More commonly, repetitive overuse leads to an insidious onset of pain, inflammation, and ultimately, structural failure. Not uncommonly, a cycle occurs in which structural maladaptions in the damaged tissue are continually subjected to abusive forces, leading to further injury and chronic inflammation.

10. A patient who has had shoulder pain off and on for years comes to your office complaining of a flare of tendinitis. What else could it be?

More often than not the clinical picture is suggestive of tendinitis; however, when symptoms are refractory to appropriate therapies, the diagnosis becomes challenging. A variety of bony and soft tissue structures may produce pain that mimics tendinitis, including ligaments, cartilage, synovium, nerve, bursae, muscle, bone and joints.

Differential Diagnosis of Common Tendon Injuries

CONDITION	DIFFERENTIAL DIAGNOSIS
Lateral epicondylitis	Radial collateral ligament sprain
	Wrist extensor muscle strain
	Olecranon bursitis
	Radial-capitellar degeneration
	Radial tunnel syndrome
	Cervical radiculopathy
Supraspinatus tendinitis	Subacromial bursitis
	Bicipital tendinitis
	Glenohumeral instability
	Glenoid labrum tears
	Rotator cuff tear
	Degenerative joint disease
	Myofascial pain
Patella tendinitis	Infra/prepatellar bursitis
	Patellofemoral pain syndrome
	Chondromalacia patellae
	Osgood-Schlater's disease
	Plica syndrome
	Meniscus tear
	Ligament sprain
	Degenerative joint disease
Achilles tendinitis	Pre/retrocalcaneal bursitis
	Achilles tendon tear
	Flexor hallucis longus tendinitis
	Medial tibial stress syndrome
	Lumbosacral radiculopathy

11. What are the important features of the clinical evaluation for tendinitis?

A **good clinical history** often leads to a correct diagnosis. The mechanism of injury should be established. Since pain is the most common presenting symptom for patients with tendinitis, a detailed pain history provides diagnostic clues but also establishes a baseline to which treatment outcome can be compared. Relevant questions pertain to the onset of pain, its intensity, quality, location, and duration. Factors that alleviate or aggravate symptoms should be established, as well as details of all failed and successful treatments, including all diagnostic procedures and pain medications. Training errors or changes in duration or intensity of exercise are commonly discovered in athletes with overuse injuries.

The **directed physical exam** employs the principles of inspection, palpation, provocative, and functional testing. The patient is observed for obvious pain, abnormal posturing, and splinting of painful areas. Involved regions are examined for erythema, swelling, or edema. Joint ROM and muscle length testing provide valuable information about musculotendinous unit inflexibilities, structural malalignments, articular involvement, or, simply, restrictions limited by pain. Provocative testing focuses on the reproduction of pain with predictable movements.

Finally, **functional testing** not only provides diagnostic information but may highlight biomechanical errors that can be addressed in rehabilitation.

12. Is imaging necessary?

For the majority of clinical situations, the diagnosis of acute or chronic tendinitis can be made without the use of expensive and often unnecessary diagnostic aids. Laboratory tests may be required to confirm a clinical suspicion of rheumatic or metabolic disease, infection, or malignancy. Routine x-rays provide little insight into the nature of soft tissue injuries and should be reserved only to rule out bone or joint involvement when symptoms persist despite appropriate treatment. MRI is currently the best way to assess soft tissues but is very expensive. Unless there is suspicion of complete tendon rupture and impending surgical intervention, this test should be used selectively. Ultrasonography is a less expensive method of assessing soft tissues but is less sensitive and technically difficult. CT defines the bony skeleton well but provides little detail of soft tissues.

13. Describe the principles of inflammation and pain control.

Limiting inflammation early after injury is critical. If left unchecked, chronic inflammation, inadequate tendon healing, and prolonged functional disability may ensue. Key principles for controlling inflammation and pain are described in the mnemonic **PRICEMM**.

P = Protection
R = Relative rest
I = Ice
C = Compression
E = Elevation
M = Modalities
M = Medications

14. What role does immobilization play in controlling symptoms?

Immobilization allows for rest and protection but may result in unwanted side effects, including adaptive shortening and disuse atrophy of the musculotendinous unit and surrounding soft tissues, joint contracture, loss of ROM, and a decline in general fitness. Bracing, splinting, or taping may be prescribed during this early period of rehabilitation to facilitate pain-free movement while protecting the tendon.

15. Ice or heat?

In general, ice (cryotherapy) is used more frequently in the acute stages of inflammation, particularly during the first 72 hours. It is probably the most effective anti-inflammatory modality, and its benefits include local vasoconstriction, decreased swelling, and relief of pain and muscle spasm.

Moist heat causes local vasodilatation, increased metabolic rate, and results in a reduction of pain and muscle spasm. It also promotes increased collagen extensibility and, for this reason, is often used prior to stretching and progressive resistive exercises. The use of heat, whether superficial or deep, is generally avoided during the first 72 hours after injury as it may increase tissue swelling.

For the symptoms of chronic inflammation and pain, heat or ice may be used based on patient tolerance and preference.

16. When are NSAIDs used in tendinitis?

NSAIDs are commonly prescribed to reduce pain and inflammation of both acute and chronic injuries. The main mechanism of action is through the inhibition of prostaglandins, which are potent mediators of inflammation. Currently, there is little scientific evidence supporting the use of any one drug over another, and the efficacy of these medications for the treatment of soft tissue injuries has yet to be established through well-designed studies. This is particularly the case for chronic injuries, in which the actual degree of inflammation is suspect. There does, however, seem to be some support for the use of these agents during the first 72 hours after injury.

17. Why bother with therapy if a steroid injection can reduce pain faster?

The use of corticosteroid injections for overuse injuries remains controversial. These drugs do initiate potent anti-inflammatory actions and pain relief, but unfortunately, patients frequently receive injections in place of rehabilitation, resulting in incomplete treatment, recurrent pain patterns, and chronic inflammation. Injection therapy should be used as a therapeutic modality only with the goal of facilitating rehabilitative efforts.

Spontaneous tendon ruptures have been reported following injections, particularly if steroid is mistakenly injected into major weight-bearing tendons such as the Achilles or patella tendons. For this reason, 2–3 weeks of restricted activity is recommended following injections.

Corticosteroid Injection Therapy: Dos and Don'ts

DOS	DON'TS
Preinjection trial of rehabilitation	Intratendinous injections
Inject in peritendinous tissue	Multiple injections (> 3 in 1 year)
Restrict activity for 2–3 weeks postinjection	Injection in infection or acute trauma
Use caution around weight-bearing tendons	Injection prior to activity

18. How important is stretching?

Stretching is critical for successful rehabilitation of tendinitis. Following injury, the resting length of the musculotendinous unit may shorten, causing earlier loading of the tendon as its affected joint is taken through ROM. This increases the risk of re-injury. Stretching may have a positive effect on tendon healing by promoting alignment of newly formed collagen fibers and may also directly increase the tensile strength of tendon.

With careful instruction, stretching can be started during the first treatment session. It should be emphasized that sustained, static stretching is the optimal way to promote tendon length. Bouncing or ballistic movements should be avoided. Home stretching should begin early but only after the patient has demonstrated thorough compliance and understanding of all techniques. It is often helpful to set stretching goals, as patients may become disinterested in this portion of rehab.

19. Which treatments are available to help promote healing of a tendon?

In addition to ice and heat, the physical therapist may use a combination of modalities, including ultrasound, phonophoresis, massage, or electrical stimulation.

Ultrasound is a modality that converts electrical energy into an acoustical waveform, which is then converted into heat as it passes through tissues of varying resistances. As a deep heating modality, it encourages regional blood flow and increases connective tissue extensibility. Nonthermal effects include molecular vibration, which increases cell membrane permeability, thereby enhancing metabolic product transport. For these reasons, ultrasound is commonly used just prior to therapeutic exercise. When ultrasound is used in combination with corticosteroids, salicylates, or local anesthetics, in an attempt to encourage transdermal penetration of these compounds, it is referred to as **phonophoresis.**

Massage has been used commonly to promote healing. Transverse friction massage, applied directly over the healing tendon, may break up inter-layer adhesions and scar tissue, provide analgesia, and increase local blood flow.

High-voltage electrical stimulation has been advocated to reduce swelling, inflammation, and pain. **Transcutaneous electrical nerve stimulation** (TENS) may play a role in reducing pain by influencing nerve conduction along pain pathways.

20. What exercises are commonly prescribed to encourage tendon healing?

Progressive loading is the basic ingredient of all strength training programs and is essential for successful and complete tendon rehab. Therapeutic exercises include stretching, progressive resistive strengthening, and joint and/or soft-tissue mobilization. These are designed to increase the resting length of and progressively load the musculotendinous unit.

Commonly prescribed strengthening exercises include isometrics and isotonics. **Isometrics** are prescribed initially, as they allow for easily controlled "light" loading of the injured tendon and reduce the risk of overloading. **Isotonics** are prescribed after the patient completes a regimen of painfree isometrics. Isotonics are characterized by lengthening (**eccentric**) contractions or shortening (**concentric**) contractions. **Isokinetic** exercise, another form of resistive exercise, allows the speed of muscular contractions, measured by the angular velocity of the respective joint, to remain constant.

To prevent deconditioning during rehabilitation, patients should be instructed on safe, painfree alternative forms of aerobic exercise. Cross-training is an effective and popular method of maintaining or improving fitness while recruiting a broad range of muscle groups.

21. Does "no pain, no gain" hold true during rehab?

Pain should be used as an important guide for exercise intensity and tolerance. During tendon rehabilitation, pain almost always indicates *excessive* tendon overload and *risk* for cumulative trauma. However, as pain intensity is highly subjective and variable among patients, it is recommended that patients progress through specific incremental tendon loading protocols driven primarily by their perception of pain and discomfort.

22. Can a patient return to his or her previous level of activity once the symptoms are gone?

No. This is a common mistake made by many patients with tendinitis. Three criteria must be satisfied in addition to full, painfree ROM:

1. The musculotendinous unit must be progressively strengthened to at least 80–90% of the contralateral limb.

2. Patients must achieve a level of fitness, agility, and skill appropriate for their occupation or sport. To accomplish this, drills must simulate the specific demands of the involved activity.

3. Intrinsic and extrinsic factors must be addressed. The therapist must be aware of intrinsic structural deficits associated with common tendonopathies. If these deficits cannot be adequately treated through therapeutic exercise, alternative techniques that may include bracing, taping, or other protective strategies may be necessary. Extrinsic variables must also be addressed prior to resumption of activity and include training errors, inappropriate equipment (e.g., footwear), improper mechanics, and inadequate warm-up or stretching.

23. When is surgery necessary?

Most tendon injuries can be managed nonsurgically, but surgery should be considered if pain and functional impairments persist despite at least 6 months of intensive therapy. A variety of surgical procedures exist for chronic tendon injury, based on the nature and extent of the lesion. In general, these share the common goals of removing chronic granulation tissue, stimulating neovascularization, decompressing tendon, and inducing healing through direct tendon incisions (tenotomy). Currently, however, there are few well-controlled studies attesting to the efficacy of these procedures. In addition, undesirable surgical outcomes, including persistent pain, hypertrophic scarring, and postoperative immobilization atrophy and weakness, are not uncommon.

BIBLIOGRAPHY

1. Basmajian JV, Wolf SL: Therapeutic Exercise. Baltimore, Williams & Wilkins, 1990.
2. Buschbacher RM: Musculoskeletal Disorders—A Practical Guide for Diagnosis and Rehabilitation. Boston, Andover Medical Publishers, 1994.
3. Curwin S, Stanish W: Tendinitis: Its Etiology and Treatment. Lexington, MA, Collamore Press, 1984.
4. Drez D (ed): Therapeutic Modalities for Sports Injuries. Chicago, Year Book Medical Publishers, 1989.
5. Herring SA: Rehabilitation of muscle injuries. Med Sci Sports Med 22(4):453–456, 1990.
6. Leadbetter WB, Buckwalter JA, Gordon SL (eds): Sports-Induced Inflammation: Clinical and Basic Science Concepts. Park Ridge, IL, American Academy of Orthopedic Surgeons, 1990.
7. O'Connor MFG, Sobel JR, Nirschl RP: Five-step treatment of overuse injuries. Physician Sportsmed 10:128–142, 1992.
8. Renstrom P, Leadbetter WB (eds): Tendinitis, vol I and II. Clin Sports Med 11(3–4): 1992.
9. Saal JA: Rehabilitation of the injured athlete. In Delisa JA (ed): Rehabilitation Medicine: Principles and Practice. Philadelphia, J.B. Lippincott, 1993, p 1131.
10. Woo SL, Buckwalter JA: Injury and Repair of Musculoskeletal Soft Tissues. Park Ridge, IL, American Academy of Orthopaedic Surgeons, 1988.

VIII. Rehabilitation of Other Chronic Conditions

69. CANCER REHABILITATION: GENERAL PRINCIPLES

Fae H. Garden, M.D., and Theresa A. Gillis, M.D.

1. Why is cancer rehabilitation necessary?

Advances in early detection and treatment allow more people with cancer to live longer. An estimated 4 million people have survived 5 years or more with a diagnosis of cancer. These cancer survivors frequently are left with physical deficits and psychosocial problems that diminish their quality of life. Over 80% of persons with lung, colorectal, and prostate cancer report having gait problems. Significant problems in activities of daily living (ADL) and vocation also exist. Up to 50% of persons with cancer may meet the diagnostic criteria for clinical depression. With early rehabilitation intervention, the disability caused by cancer and cancer therapy can be minimized.

2. Who are the members of the typical cancer rehab team?

Team members include the nurse, physical therapist, occupational therapist, social worker, speech and language pathologist, psychologist, primary oncologist, chaplain, and dietician. A physiatrist can evaluate medical rehabilitation issues and assist with diagnosis and management. Rehabilitation issues may include fatigue, nutrition, neurogenic bowel and bladder management, pain control, body image, prosthetic and orthotic fitting, and management of spasticity and weakness.

3. What are the potential adverse effects of cancer surgery on nutrition?

Surgical procedures such as **radical neck dissection** or **glossectomy** can impair mastication, swallowing, taste, and smell. Patients undergoing **gastrectomy** or **bowel resection** can develop gastric stasis, diarrhea, steatorrhea, megaloblastic anemia, malabsorption, and deficiency of vitamins B_{12}, D, and A.

4. What are the adverse effects of radiation therapy on nutrition?

Radiation treatment to the head and neck area can produce alterations in taste and in saliva production. Food texture and sensation alterations can occur from irradiation of the oral mucosa. Radiation to the stomach and intestines can cause acute nausea, cramps, and diarrhea. Patients with radiation damage to the intestines are usually started on lactose-free, low-residue oral diets. If ≥20% of body weight has been lost, parenteral nutrition is recommended.

5. How does chemotherapy affect nutrition?

Antimetabolite drugs, such as methotrexate, inhibit the metabolism of folic acid which is necessary for the synthesis of DNA. The resultant folic acid deficiency can result in macrocytic anemia, leukopenia, and ulcerative stomatitis. The antimetabolites 5-fluorouracil and 6-mercaptopurine prevent nucleic acid synthesis by interfering with thiamine in DNA synthesis. Clinical thiamine deficiency is associated with paresthesias, neuropathy, and heart failure. Vitamin K deficiency results from long-term treatment with adjunctive antibiotics, such as moxalactam disodium, leading to a pronounced bleeding tendency.

6. How does cancer or cancer treatment affect female sexual function?

During or following cancer treatment, sexual dysfunction can occur. The emotional effects of a mastectomy can have a negative impact on sexual response. Fear of partner rejection can lead to the avoidance of sexual intercourse. Women who have undergone pelvic surgery need to be counseled about the possible need for vaginal dilators to prevent stenosis as well as the possibility of bleeding with intercourse. Some women may need to use artificial vaginal lubrication and try changes from their customary sexual positions. Side effects of chemotherapy and radiation therapy, including nausea, fatigue, hair loss, and weight changes, can produce additional psychological and physical roadblocks to resuming sexual activity.

7. What are some sexual dysfunctions that occur in male patients undergoing cancer treatment?

Impotence, retrograde ejaculation, and infertility can result from damage to the vascular or nerve pathways following surgical treatment for prostate cancer. If permanent sterilization is anticipated, preoperative and pretreatment discussion of reproductive concerns, including sperm banking, should be undertaken. Sexual rehabilitation can include the use of erectile assistive devices and surgical reconstruction of the phallus.

8. What is paraneoplastic syndrome?

When tumors produce signs and symptoms at a distance from the tumor or its metastases, they are referred to as paraneoplastic syndrome, or remote effects of malignancy. By definition, these syndromes should not be produced as a direct effect of the tumor of its metastases. Paraneoplastic syndromes develop in a minority of cancer patients. Paraneoplastic syndromes caused by the production of polypeptide hormones are the most frequent and include:

1. ACTH/Cushing's syndrome
2. Syndrome of inappropriate secretion of antidiuretic hormone (SIADH)
3. Hypercalcemia
4. Hypocalcemia
5. Hypophosphatemia osteomalacia
6. Calcitonin production by tumors
7. Hypoglycemia

9. Discuss the manifestations of hypercalcemia in cancer patients.

Hypercalcemia is common in cancer patients, occurring in approximately 10% of patients. Not all cases are associated with bone metastases. Tumor types associated with hypercalcemia include breast cancer, lung cancer, and multiple myeloma. Clinical manifestations of hypercalcemia include polyuria, nocturia, and polydipsia. Symptoms of anorexia, easy fatigability, and weakness also occur. Late symptoms of hypercalcemia include apathy, irritability, depression, mental obtundation, nausea, vomiting, vague abdominal pain, constipation, and pruritus.

10. What causes pain in cancer patients?

The most common cause of pain is tumor invasion of bone from either a primary or metastatic lesion. Compression or infiltration of peripheral nerves by tumor is the second most frequent cause. Acute pain can also occur because of treatment, such as postradiation plexopathy or myelopathy. Chemotherapeutic agents such as vincristine and vinblastine may cause dysesthesias. Cancer pain occurs in 51% of all patients and 74% of those with advanced or terminal disease.

11. Discuss the appropriate use of medications in managing cancer pain?

The World Health Organization recommends the step-wise use of nonopioid analgesics, adjuvant drugs, and opioids. Aspirin and nonsteroidal anti-inflammatory drugs are useful to control the pain of bone metastases because they are potent prostaglandin synthetase inhibitors. Corticosteroids produce analgesia by preventing the release of prostaglandin and are helpful in reducing pain from tumor infiltration of nerves and spinal cord. Adjuvant therapy includes tricyclic antidepressants, which block reuptake of serotonin in the CNS. Carbamazepine and phenytoin may

be effective in the treatment of neuropathic pain. Narcotic analgesics include (from weakest to strongest) codeine, oxycodone, and morphine. Morphine is often improperly underused in the treatment of severe cancer pain. Transdermal preparations and narcotics with longer half-lives than morphine are also available. Demerol (meperidine) is not recommended for the treatment of cancer pain due to its short duration of action and its potential for adverse CNS effects on repeated use.

12. Describe some neurostimulatory and neuroablative procedures that are used in the treatment of cancer pain.

Neurostimulatory procedures include transcutaneous and percutaneous electrical nerve stimulation. This technique is indicated in the treatment of painful disesthesias from tumor infiltration of a nerve. Dorsal column stimulation of the spinal cord has limited use in treatment of deafferentation pain in the chest, midline, and lower extremities. **Neuroablative procedures** include nerve root rhizotomy, which can be used to treat somatic and deafferentation pain from tumor infiltration of the cranial and intercostal nerves. Neuroablative procedures to the spinal cord include tractotomy of the dorsal root entry zone lesions, cordotomy, and myelotomy.

13. What psychological interventions can be used to manage cancer pain?

Psychological techniques may enable patients with cancer to regain a much-needed sense of personal control. Mental imagery, hypnosis, relaxation, biofeedback, and other cognitive or behavioral methods can directly relieve pain as well as anxiety, which enhances analgesia.

14. What is Pancoast's syndrome?

Pancoast's syndrome is caused by carcinomas in the superior pulmonary sulcus. The tumor produces pain in the distribution of C8 and T1–T2 nerves as well as a Horner's syndrome. A shadow can be sometimes be seen on chest films at the apex of the lung. Patients with Pancoast's syndrome usually complain of severe, unrelenting pain that often begins the shoulder and vertebral border of the scapula. Radiation and surgery are recommended treatments.

15. What is the most common form of radiation-induced spinal cord damage?

Transient myelopathy, which may occur in patients being treated for head and neck tumors or lymphoma. The syndrome typically develops after a latent period of 1–30 months, with the peak incidence for onset of symptoms at 4–6 months after completion of treatment. Clinical onset is marked by electric shock sensation, or paresthesia, that radiates from the cervical spine to the extremities. These paresthesias usually occur in a symmetric fashion. Diagnostic studies, such as myelography and CT scans, are typically normal. The syndrome usually resolves in 1–9 months after onset.

16. What is delayed myelopathy?

This irreversible condition typically occurs 9–18 months after completion of radiation treatment. The latent period for delayed myelopathy decreases with increased radiation dose and is also shortened in children. Functional deficits depend, for the most part, on the level of neurologic injury.

17. You are seeing a patient with suspected postradiation brachial plexopathy. How can this be distinguished from plexopathy due to tumor infiltration?

Horner's syndrome (ptosis, enophthalmos) and pain are more common in neoplastic plexopathies. Edema of the affected extremity is more common in radiation plexopathy. Electrodiagnostic findings such as myokymic discharges and abnormal sensory conduction studies are more common in patients with radiation plexopathy.

18. Many patients undergoing cancer treatment have low platelet counts. Does the presence of thrombocytopenia affect the exercise prescription?

Exercise in the presence of thrombocytopenia can increase the risk of intra-articular bleeding. In general, platelet levels < 10,000/mm^3 preclude exercise therapy. The risk of intracerebral bleeding becomes significant below this level. Some centers allow active aerobic, but not resistive, activities in patients with platelet counts between 10,000–20,000/mm^3. Both chemotherapy and radiotherapy can cause thrombocytopenia.

19. How do cancer amputees differ from dysvascular or traumatic amputees?

Patients with cancer often face functional declines associated with chemotherapy. Many sarcoma patients are treated with pre- and postoperative chemotherapy protocols, with the attendant risks of anemia, fatigue, nausea and cardiovascular toxicity while recovering from the amputation. Prosthesis fitting can also be complicated in patients who are receiving chemotherapy due to weight fluctuations caused by anorexia and edema. Irradiated skin is often less tolerant to prosthesis contact. All patients should be considered for prosthetic prescription, but special attention must be given to the cancer treatment protocol when planning fabrication, fitting, and training. Cosmetic prosthesis should be offered to patients unable to use a functional limb.

20. What is meant by "limb salvage"? What procedures does this entail?

Limb salvage describes efforts toward maintaining a functional extremity and avoiding amputation in the treatment of sarcomas and bone metastases from other tumors. The plan may employ the use of reconstruction techniques with custom or modular segmental prostheses and/or allograft or autograft transfer of bony or muscular tissues. Limited resections of muscle groups, compartments, or partial bones may be necessary.

Partial resections of the sacrum, pelvis, scapulae, and femur (e.g .,Girdlestone procedure) are frequently seen. Cemented prosthetic hip and knee components and intramedullary rods of the humerus and femur are very common. Rehabilitation must be tailored to address intact and unstable structures.

21. What is the Van Ness procedure?

Tibial rotationplasty is used in the pediatric population to provide a functional "knee" joint after resection of tumors about the knee. The neurovascular structures about the knee must be free of tumor, and the popliteal vessels, sciatic nerve, and saphenous vein must be intact. The remaining distal tibia is rotated 180° and reattached to the femoral shaft, with the ankle serving as the knee joint. The quadriceps are joined to the gastroc-soleus complex, while the hamstrings are connected to the ankle dorsiflexors.

22. When is the Van Ness used? Are there alternatives?

The advantages to the Van Ness procedure include preservation of femoral shaft length, particularly for very young children, as the rotated tibial growth plate is intact. At skeletal maturity, the patient has a substantial residual limb for prosthetic fitting. The skin of the foot tolerates prosthetic wear very well. The limb appearance is unusual but acceptable by owners. A custom below-knee prosthesis is necessary.

As an alternative to rotationplasty, amputation and segmental endoprosthesis has advantages and disadvantages as well. Expandable endoprostheses must be used in children, with frequent lengthening at regular intervals, and these devices have a high rate of mechanical failure and loosening. Energy expenditure during gait following rotationplasty and above-knee amputation has been studied, two separate studies were unable to show statistically significant differences in energy expenditure/cost between these two patient groups.

23. What is an internal forequarter amputation? Does it really exist?

No. Actually, the correct term is en bloc upper humeral interscapulothoracic resection, much more easily referred to as a Tikhoff-Lindberg resection.

24. How is the Tikhoff-Lindberg procedure done?

The procedure is appropriate for some tumors of the shoulder region which were previously subject to forequarter amputations. Resection of the proximal humerus, partial or total scapulectomy, and claviculotomy are required, with a humeral endoprosthesis implanted and fixed to the remaining clavicle or chest wall.

Early rehabilitation should avoid humeral motion, and after acute healing is complete, passive range beyond 90° abduction and adduction should not be attempted. Patients may choose to wear slings for additional support, particularly if the arm is large. Immediate postoperative compression with elastic bandages may delay lymphedema development and permit early fitting with custom garments. Very limited passive shoulder motion remains, and the limb is essentially non-weight-bearing and nonlifting. Patients can retain active elbow motion and excellent hand and forearm function. A soft shoulder prosthesis allows a more cosmetic clothing fit.

25. What are the most common malignant bone tumors?

Carcinomas metastatic to bone account for > 40 times more cases than all primary bone tumors combined. Breast cancer accounts for most bone metastases, with an incidence of bone metastases in this disease of 50–85%. Prostate carcinoma is the most common primary tumor for metastatic lesions in men, with bone metastases occurring in > 90% of patients with advanced disease. Lung, renal, bladder, thyroid, and bowel primaries each have an incidence of bone metastases of 20–40% at autopsy.

Myeloma is the most common primary malignant tumor of bone in adults, arising within the bone marrow from plasma calls. Osteosarcomas, Ewing's sarcomas, and chondrosarcoma are the most common tumors arising from bone tissue itself. In children, osteosarcoma, Ewing's sarcoma, and primitive neuroectodermal tumors (in descending order) are the most predominant primary malignant bone tumors.

26. When is a bone susceptible to pathologic fracture?

Pathologic fractures occur in 10–30% of patient with metastases and are seen most frequently in the long bones, particularly the femur and humerus. Bone strength is determined by the cortical and trabecular structure. Cortical destruction increases susceptibility of bone to torsional/rotational forces. The guidelines most frequently cited for increased risk of fracture are as follows:

1. Cortical bone destruction affecting ≥ 50% of the circumference as seen on anteroposterior and lateral radiographs or cross-sectional CT
2. Lytic lesions ≥ 2.5 cm in the proximal femur
3. Pathologic avulsion fracture of the lesser trochanter of the femur
4. Persisting or increasing pain with weight-bearing despite completion of radiotherapy

These estimates of fracture risk are used synonymously as indications for prophylactic fixation. An inherent limitation to this list is that tumor extent can be underestimated by radiographs.

27. What rehabilitation methods may be used in managing bone metastases?

Some patients receive prophylactic fixation of metastatic lesions, employing internal fixation, methylmethacrylate and modular prosthesis, or other hardware. After operative management, restoration of mobility and self-care through a rehabilitation approach is essential.

The most painful bone metastases are treated with radiotherapy. During radiation, bone is placed at increased risk of fracture due to hyperemic softening of bone and necrosis of tumor cells, and complete reossification may not occur until 6 months or more after treatment. In theory, therefore, precautions and reduced load-bearing may be indicated for many months. During periods of greatest risk, and for nonsurgical candidates, unloading affected bones with assistive devices, braces, or immobilizers is recommended. Activity restrictions and adaptive equipment for ADLs should be addressed by physiatrists.

28. What are the most common initial symptoms caused by metastases to the spine?

Four symptoms characterize the clinical picture of spinal cord compression: pain, weakness, autonomic dysfunction, and sensory loss including ataxia. Pain is usually the initial symptom and can manifest as central back pain with or without radicular pain.

29. Does the pain of spinal cord tumor differ from the pain caused by a herniated intervertebral disc?

The pain caused by an epidural tumor is described as being worse when the patient is lying down. Patients may complain of being awakened from sleep several times during the night, and some may describe a need to sleep in a sitting position. Radiographs of the spine can reveal bony abnormalities at the painful site of suspected cord compression.

30. When should one consider epidural spinal cord compression in a cancer patient with back pain?

Always! The spine is the most common site for skeletal metastases, regardless of the primary tumor. Early diagnosis is essential, as the outcome is related to patient function at diagnosis—i.e., if a patient is paraplegic at diagnosis, he or she will remain so after treatment. Epidural spinal cord compression (ESCC) from metastasis occurs in 10–33% of cancer patients, and in 10% of these patients, cord compression is the presenting manifestation of malignancy.

31. When evaluating for spinal metastases, what radiologic studies are indicated?

In patients with cancer or high suspicion for malignancy or ESCC, magnetic resonance imaging (MRI) is often the first diagnostic test. Plain films and bone scan are of additional help in planning for surgical intervention and radiation therapy.

In patients with back pain but without cancer or a high suspicion for malignancy, radiographs are often obtained when a patient does not respond to therapy. Although the vertebral body is usually the site first affected by metastases, 30–50% of cancellous bone here must be destroyed before change is seen on plain film. Therefore, destruction of the pedicle is usually discovered first on anteroposterior films. If back pain persists and radiographs are normal, bone scintigraphy or MRI is indicated. The sensitivity of bone scans for metastases is high. MRI clearly delineates epidural disease.

32. What are some primary spinal cord tumors?

Ependymomas and astrocytomas are the usual intramedullary (located in the substance of the cord tumors) tumors. Extramedullary tumors include neurofibromas and meningiomas. Most malignant lesions affecting the spinal cord are metastases from various primary tumors. Extradural spinal cord compression is a common neurologic complication of systemic malignancy.

33. What disability results after radical neck dissection? How is this best managed?

The spinal accessory nerve is usually sacrificed during radical neck dissection, causing loss of trapezius function. The scapula rotates upward and abduction is limited to only 60–70°. Shoulder pain frequently results, and lifting and overhead activities become impossible. Strengthening the levator scapulae, rhomboideus, and serratus anterior muscles may help stabilize the scapula, allow improved shoulder elevation, and reduce pain. Attempts to strengthen the deltoids, supraspinatus, or infraspinatus should be discouraged, as this only increases pain and further overworks the disadvantaged muscles. Pectoralis muscle contracture aggravates the protracted shoulder and results from lack of pull from the opposing trapezius. Therefore, pectoral stretches and maintenance of good scapular positioning is crucial. Some patients reduce their discomfort through use of a figure-of-eight orthosis.

34. How do brain tumor patients differ from brain injury patients?

Most patients with primary brain tumors experience rapid improvement in function following tumor excision. Normal brain tissue has been compressed by tumor, so with pressure relief, recovery can be dramatic and the patient may return to normal function. However, many tumors recur, and with repeated excisions and invasion of normal tissue by tumor, further functions are lost. Radiation and chemotherapy can further limit recovery through lost plasticity and cognitive effects. Despite advances in treatment, most patients with glioblastoma multiforme or high-grade astrocytomas survive 2 years or less; therefore, rehabilitation goals should encompass this pattern of decline.

35. What is the most common primary brain tumor? Metastatic tumor?

Gliomas comprise about 60% of all primary CNS tumor. The most common tumors that metastasize to the brain are **carcinomas** of the lung and breast. Most brain metastases involve the cerebrum, with the frontal lobe being the most common site. Metastases to the cerebellum are less frequent, and those to the brainstem are the least frequent.

36. What rehabilitation needs are greatest among brain tumor patients?

Deficits experienced by brain tumor patients are clearly related to the involved structure. Cognitive deficits are quite prevalent and also related to the site of lesions. Neurobehavioral changes may be the most prominent problems faced by patients with tumors. Memory losses, reasoning and problem-solving skills, decreased energy or initiative, and inability to return to work are cited more frequently by family members as problems than difficulty with ambulation, bowel or bladder dysfunction, ADLs, or aphasia

37. Describe the neuropsychological abnormalities found in patients with brain tumors.

The scope of cognitive effects ranges from subtle attention and motivational problems to frank delirium and clouding of consciousness. These deficits can be due to the primary effects of tumor or secondary effects of treatment. Patients with rapid-growing tumors, such as glioblastoma multiforme, exhibit behavioral and cognitive deficits secondary to rapid destruction of white matter tracts, increased intracranial pressure, and metabolic deficits. Patients with slow-growing tumors often do not demonstrate neuropsychological deficits, possibly due to a reorganization of cognitive functions to other brain regions.

Following radiotherapy to the brain, 14% of patients show subacute cognitive effects occurring 1–4 months after treatment; this effect is due to a reversible demyelination, and gradual improvement in functional status over the next 2–3 months distinguishes this condition from signs of early tumor recurrence. Up to 18% of neurologically normal cancer patients who receive chemotherapy have cognitive deficits after chemotherapy is discontinued. These deficits include impaired visual perception, verbal memory, and judgment.

38. Describe some available treatments of breast cancer.

Over the years, standard treatment of breast cancer has evolved from radical mastectomies to breast-conservation strategies. Modified radical mastectomies spare the pectoralis major muscle but include axillary dissection. Other surgical options include lumpectomy, segmental mastectomy, or total mastectomy with or without axillary dissection. Varying combinations of radiotherapy, hormonal therapy, and adjuvant chemotherapy have further reduced mortality.

39. Describe a postoperative rehabilitation program for women who have undergone mastectomy.

In general, postmastectomy patients without reconstruction are allowed to perform range of motion to 40% of abduction and flexion immediately after surgery. Some physicians prefer the use of abduction slings or pillows immediately postoperatively with the goal of ensuring painfree movement within this range. Immediate therapies can safely consist of hand pumping, wrist and elbow range of motion, positioning techniques, and postural exercises. When surgical drains are removed, active assisted range of motion can be increased. At this point, wall-climbing, wand, and overhead pulley exercises are added. When all sutures have been removed, more aggressive range is pursued to the patient's limits of pain.

40. Define postmastectomy lymphedema.

Postmastectomy lymphedema is a collection of lymph in the interstitial tissues, resulting in a functional overload of the lymphatic system. The edema is usually confined to subcutaneous fat and skin. The problem usually follows radical mastectomy and is likely caused by the excision of lymph channels, radiation, and inflammation of involved tissues with coagulation of lymph and fibrosis. It affects 25.5–38.3% of patients having axillary node and radiation therapy.

41. What conservative management techniques are used for postmastectomy lymphedema?
Elevation, massage, and exercise of the distal musculature have been advocated. Compression of the effective extremity with elastic bandages may be sufficient, but refractory edema will require the use of a pneumatic pump. The initial pump session should be monitored closely for patient complaints of shortness of breath and pain. If improvement in limb circumference results, the patient should be fitted for a custom pressure gradient support sleeve to be worn daily. Both intermittent uniform and differential sequential compression sleeves have been employed.

BIBLIOGRAPHY

1. Bonica JJ: Treatment of cancer pain: Current status and future needs. Adv Pain Res Ther 9:589–616, 1985.
2. Byrd R: Late effects of treatment of cancer in children. Pediatr Clin North Am 32:835-851, 1985.
3. DeLisa JA, Miller RM, Melnick RR, et al: Rehabilitation of the cancer patient. In DeVita VT, Hellman S, Rosenberg SA (eds): Cancer: Principles and Practice of Oncology, 2nd ed. Philadelphia, J.B. Lippincott, pp 2155–2188.
4. Dropcho EJ: Central nervous system injury by therapeutic irradiation. Neurol Clin North Am 9:969–988, 1991.
5. Fallowfield LJ, Baumm M, Maguire GP. Effects of breast conservation on psychological morbidity associated with diagnosis and treatment of early breast cancer. BMJ 293:1331, 1986.
6. Garden FH, Grabois M (eds): Cancer rehabilitation. Phys Med Rehabil State Art Rev 8(2):229–433, 1994.
7. Gerber L, Lampert M, Wood C, et al: Comparison of pain, motion, and edema after modified radical mastectomy vs local excision with axillary dissection and radiation. Breast Cancer Res Treat 21:139, 1992.
8. Harper CM, Thomas JE: Distinction between neoplastic and radiation-induced brachial plexopathy, with emphasis on the role of EMG. Neurology 39:502–506, 1989.
9. Kaplan HS: A neglected issue: The sexual side effects of current treatments for breast cancer. J Sex Mar Ther 18:3–19, 1992.
10. Lehmann JF, DeLisa JA, Warren CG, et al: Cancer rehabilitation: Assessment of need, development and evaluation of a model of care. Arch Phys Med Rehabil 59:410–419, 1978.
11. Levinson SF: Rehabilitation of the patient with cancer or human immunodeficiency virus. In DeLisa JA (ed): Rehabilitation Medicine: Principles and Practice, 2nd ed. Philadelphia, J.B. Lippincott, 1993, pp 916–933.
12. Mandi A, Szepesi K, Morocz I: Surgical treatment of pathologic fractures from metastatic tumors of long bones. Orthopedics 14:43–50, 1991..
13. Meyers CA, Abbruzzese JL: Cognitive functioning in cancer patients: Effect of previous treatment. Neurology 42:434–436, 1992.
14. Ragnarsson KT: Principles of cancer rehabilitation medicine. In Holland JF (ed): Cancer Medicine. Philadelphia, Lea & Febiger, 1993, p 1054.
15. Williams F, Maly B: Pain rehabilitation: 3. Cancer pain, pelvic pain and age-related considerations. Arch Phys Med Rehabil 75: 1994.

70. CANCER REHABILITATION: THERAPEUTIC CONSIDERATIONS

Subhadra Lakshmi Nori, M.D., and Ann Burkhardt, M.A., O.T.R./L.

1. Which two important laboratory tests should be reviewed before prescribing an exercise program for cancer patients?
White blood cell count (absolute neutrophil count) and platelet count. When the WBC count is depressed due to chemotherapy, patients are generally too weak to participate in a therapy program and may be especially susceptible to infection. When platelet counts are reduced in response to chemotherapy and radiation therapy, patients are at risk for bleeding into a muscle compartment or joint if the level of physical activity is excessive or if aggressive range of motion exercises are imposed.

2. What is the role of rehabilitation in the management of a bone marrow transplant recipient?

Rehabilitation intervention emphasizing prophylactic general conditioning exercises and aerobic therapeutics should be initiated before the transplant. A physiatry consultation should be obtained early on for optimal team surveillance of transplant patients during the intensive care/post-bone marrow transplant phase. Special emphasis should be placed on each of the following areas:
- Skin integrity preservation
- Monitoring and maintenance of joint range of motion
- Establishment of an optimal bowel and bladder program
- Incentive spirometry program and deep breathing exercises
- Nutritional surveillance
- Formulation of a "sitting schedule" and mobility program
- Close tracking of platelet count and WBC to determine appropriateness and timing of exercise
- Functional activities and ADLs

3. What major caveats must the rehab practitioner be aware of when treating the bone marrow transplant patient?

Since bone marrow suppression generally occurs within the first 10 days of treatment, patients are at extreme risk for development of infections and pneumonia. During all the early activities related to therapy, rigid adherence to isolation precautions is strictly enforced.

4. What is graft versus host disease (GVHD)?

GVHD occurs in two forms: acute and chronic. Patients who have survived 100 days following bone marrow transplant are at greatest risk for chronic graft versus host disease. Approximately 40% of patients undergoing allogenic bone marrow transplant develop this symptom complex, which may involve multiple organ systems, most notably the musculoskeletal system. Skin induration, dermatologic lesions, fascial induration, and joint contractures are often dreaded features of chronic GVHD.

5. How can rehabilitation help the patient with chronic graft versus host disease?

By offering general flexibility exercises, stretching exercise, functional mobility tasks, and aerobic exercises, the patient's functional outcome and quality of life can be greatly enhanced.

6. What rehabilitation strategies may be used in the cancer patient following spinal stabilization?

Once stabilization is complete, mobilization in and out of bed can be done. In bed activities, log rolling is useful for repositioning and for preparing for transfer activity. For transfers in and out of bed, spinal bracing may be indicated if the patient has multilevel involvement.

7. What spinal stabilization bracing options exist for cancer rehab patients? What are the salient features?
- Halo traction brace: immobilization of the cervical spine
- Body jacket: stabilization of thoracic regions
- Philadelphia collar: limited stabilization of upper cervical segments
- Sternal occipital mandibular (SOMI): cervical spine stabilization
- Jewitt Knight-Taylor orthoses: thoracolumbar region stabilization

8. What is TRAM?

It is an acronym for transverse rectus abdominis muscle reconstruction procedure. This surgical technique is a common and very effective breast reconstruction procedure. It involves resection of the skin, subcutaneous tissue, and a portion of the rectus abdominis muscle along with the rectus sheath, and transfer to the chest for shaping into a breast mound.

9. What is the cardinal complication of TRAM that physiatrists must deal with?
Weakened abdominal musculature.

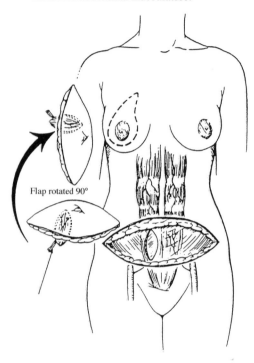

Flap rotated 90°

Transverse rectus abdominis muscle flap breast reconstruction in which the skin, subcutaneous tissue, and a portion of the rectus abdominis muscle and rectus sheath are removed from the lower abdomen and transferred to the chest for shaping into a breast mound. (From Miller MJ, Ross MR: Pregnancy following breast reconstruction with autogenous tissue. Cancer Bull 45:546–548, 1993, with permission.)

BIBLIOGRAPHY

1. Burkhardt A, Weitz J: Oncological applications for silicone gel sheets in soft tissue contractures. Am J Occup Ther 45(5):460–462, 1991.
2. DeLisa JA, Miller RM, Melnick RR: Rehabilitation of the cancer patient. In DeVita VT, Hellman S, Rosenberg CA (eds): Cancer: Principles and Practice of Oncology, 2nd ed. Philadelphia, J.B. Lippincott, 1993.
3. DeVita VT, Hellman S, Rosenberg CA (eds): Cancer: Principles and Practice of Oncology, 2nd ed. Philadelphia, J.B. Lippincott, 1993.
4. Duncan A: Incidence, recovery and management of serratus anterior muscle palsy after axillary node dissection. Phys Ther 63(8):1243–1247, 1983.
5. Gerber L, Lampert M, Wood C: Comparison of pain, motion and function after modified radical mastectomy versus local excision with axillary node dissection and radiation. Breast Cancer Research and Treatment 21:139–145, 1992.
6. Grant J, Young MA, Christianson J, et al: Graft vs. Host Disease Following Bone Marrow Transplant: A Physiatric Challenge (abstract). Arch Phys Med Rehabil 77(9):1996.
7. James MC: Physical therapy for patients after bone marrow transplantation: Phys Ther 67(6):946–952, 1987.

71. REHABILITATION OF THE INDIVIDUAL WITH HIV AND AIDS

Stephen F. Levinson, M.D., Ph.D.

1. Why have a chapter on AIDS in a book on rehabilitation?

For two major reasons—first, HIV and AIDS are major causes of disability, and second, patients traditionally seen for rehabilitation may be infected with HIV. It is crucial that all rehabilitation professionals be familiar with the many faces of disability that may result from HIV and its complications.

2. What is the difference between HIV infection and AIDS?

AIDS is the final stage of a prolonged infectious process caused by the human immunodeficiency virus (HIV). HIV specifically infects T4 lymphocytes, ultimately overpowering the body's ability to replenish the supply. Many people do not develop AIDS until 8–10 years after becoming infected with HIV. A few individuals have never developed AIDS, despite being infected for more than a decade. As defined by the Centers for Disease Control and Prevention (CDC), only individuals who have had an AIDS-indicator condition or a CD4 count < 200/mm³ (normal range, 400–1600) actually have AIDS.

3. Can I catch AIDS from one of my patients?

Transmission can only occur from direct contact with infectious fluids, such as blood, and fluids contaminated with blood, breast milk, and semen. Because open wounds are often contaminated by blood and because the integrity of mucous membranes may be compromised, contact with these tissues is also thought to pose a small risk.

4. What can I do to protect myself when I see HIV-infected patients?

Your risk of contracting HIV will be negligible if you follow **universal precautions** with **every** patient you see.

5. When should a test for HIV be ordered?

First of all, you need to obtain the full consent of the patient, in writing, and to provide follow-up counseling. Testing for HIV should be considered whenever you suspect that a patient's symptoms may be related to infection. Of course, testing should also be offered to anyone who requests it. The **enzyme-linked immunosorbent assay (ELISA)** is used as a screening test, with the **western blot test** being used for confirmation.

6. What should I know about the medications used to treat HIV infection?

AIDS treatments themselves are often a cause of disability. The antiretroviral **zidovudine** (AZT) causes chronic fatigue, bone marrow toxicity, and mitochondrial myopathy. Other dideoxynecleosides include **didanosine** (DDI), which causes less marrow and myotoxicity but is associated with peripheral neuropathy and acute pancreatitis, and **zalcitabine** (DDC), which is associated with a dose-dependent severe painful neuropathy. Protease inhibitors, perhaps the most promising class of antiretroviral drugs, have been shown to dramatically slow and even reverse viral activity when used in combination with other agents. These drugs are toxic, however, and the long-term effects and potential to cause disability are unknown.

7. How often is disability associated with HIV infection?

The best evaluation of this, though not comprehensive, is from the AIDS Time-Oriented Health Survey (ATOHS). In an interim analysis of men with AIDS, 41% reported difficulty with

mobility, 29% with ADLs, and 56% with instrumental ADLs (IADLs). Of those with symptomatic HIV but not AIDS, 15% reported difficulties with mobility, 11% with ADLs, and 28% with
IADLs. For purposes of comparison, only 2% of seronegative controls reported difficulty with
mobility, 3% with ADLs, and 4% with IADLs.

8. What are the causes of disability in HIV infection?

Pneumocystis carinii pneumonia (PCP), the presenting feature in 60% of AIDS cases, is
eventually seen in 85%. Kaposi's sarcoma is a lymphoendothelial malignancy seen in approximately 23%. The dark purple lesions may be found anywhere on the skin, as well as in oral, lymphatic, and visceral sites. Dysphagia and edema are common, with pain being a particular
problem when lesions involve the feet. Other causes of disability include cardiac and gastrointestinal disorders, rheumatologic disorders, and chronic fatigue and general debility related to
chronic illness. Neurologic disorders, however, are the most frequent cause of disability.

9. What sorts of cardiac and gastrointestinal disorders are seen in persons with HIV infection?

HIV cardiomyopathy is exceedingly common and usually asymptomatic. The potential for
limited cardiac function must be kept in mind when planning a rehabilitation program. Diarrhea
and malabsorption disorders are very common in patients with AIDS and in some patients with
HIV. The causes may be multifactorial and management difficult. Good nutrition is very important; supplementation may be required. Swallowing disorders may develop in conjunction with
neurologic deficits, the Sicca syndrome (which involves diminished salivation and lacrimation
and associated drying of mucous membranes), and candidal or herpetic pharyngitis. Evaluation is
with an oral motor examination and videofluoroscopy. Treatment is symptomatic with a modified
swallow and, where necessary, hyperalimentation

10. What are the causes of chronic fatigue and general debility?

Chronic fatigue is a common feature of HIV infection that may be present long before the
development of immune dysfunction. Common causes of fatigue include fibromyalgia, pulmonary dysfunction, anemia, encephalopathy, endocrine dysfunction, myopathies, cardiomyopathy, psychiatric disorders, depression, and side effects of medications. Care must be taken to
prevent contractures, decubiti, venous thromboembolism, compression neuropathy, and other
complications seen in debilitated patients.

11. Is exercise useful in persons with HIV?

As in the management of any disease complicated by chronic fatigue, exercise, energy conservation, and pacing of activities can be helpful in building endurance and maintaining sufficient
capacity to perform daily activities.

12. What are the types of arthritis seen in HIV, and how are they treated?

Psoriasis-associated arthritis, Reiter's syndrome, and reactive arthritis have all been described. An AIDS-associated arthritis has also been found that may be chronic or transient, with a
predominance of lower limb involvement. Treatment is with nonsteroidal antiinflammatory drugs
(NSAIDs), physical modalities, and, if indicated, local steroid injections.

13. Discuss the myopathies seen in HIV.

Autoimmune polymyositis may occur at all stages of infection but is often an early manifestation and is usually steroid-responsive. It is subacute in onset and presents with proximal
muscle weakness and thigh pain on exertion. Zidovudine can cause a **mitochondrial myopathy**
that presents with the insidious onset of myalgias, tenderness, and weakness. **HIV wasting syndrome** presents with the insidious onset of symmetrical proximal muscle weakness that mainly
affects the lower extremities at first. Its cause is not fully known.

The role of exercise in HIV-related myopathies has not been fully determined. However, energy
conservation and avoidance of overuse or high-resistance eccentric contractions should be stressed.

14. What neurologic complications are seen in HIV infection?

Neurologic disorders often result from concomitant opportunistic infections and malignancies. The deficits seen and the disabilities that result are reflective of the sites of involvement.

15. What are some of the causes of cognitive dysfunction in HIV?

HIV dementia	CMV encephalitis
Cryptococcal meningitis	Tuberculin and aseptic meningitis
Cerebral vasculitis	Iatrogenic encephalopathies
Focal CNS disorders of any kind	

16. What is the AIDS dementia complex?

AIDS dementia complex is a term that describes the diffuse cognitive impairment eventually seen in up to 65% of those with AIDS. When seen earlier in the course of disease, cognitive dysfunction may be the result of a subacute encephalopathy, thought to be the result of cytomegalovirus (CMV) encephalitis. Most often, AIDS dementia is insidious and associated with an HIV encephalopathy that can be found in up to 90% of cases at autopsy.

17. List the focal neurologic impairments seen in HIV.

Hemiparesis and other focal motor and sensory deficits

Ataxia	Aphasia	Dysarthria
Swallowing disorders		Cranial nerve defects

Movement disorders

Hemichorea-ballismus	Segmental myoclonus
Parkinsonism	Postural tremor
Dystonia	

Visual loss due to CMV retinitis

18. What causes these focal and other neurologic deficits?

Infection

Cerebral toxoplasmosis
- Most common cause of multifocal mass lesions
- Presents with ring-enhancing hypodense lesions on CT
- May also cause encephalopathy and meningoencephalitis

Cytomegalovirus (CMV)
- Coinfection may play a role in subacute encephalitis
- May cause subacute progressive polyradiculopathy and myelitis
- Retinitis is a relentless cause of blindness found in 20–25%
- Treatment with ganciclovir or foscarnet may slow progression

Progressive multifocal leukoencephalopathy (PML)
- Insidious, rare, usually fatal disorder caused by JC virus
- 2–4 month median survival, though 10% of cases are benign

Herpes simplex virus (HSV)
- HSV-I may cause acute encephalitis
- HSV-II may cause self-limited meningitis
- Both associated with myelitis and autonomic dysfunction

Varicella zoster virus (VZV)
- Causes nerve palsies, encephalitis, transverse myelitis, leukoencephalopathy, ascending myelitis

Epstein-Barr virus (EBV)
- Causes encephalitis, acute cerebellar syndrome, acute psychosis, transverse or ascending myelitis
- May play a role in pathogenesis of primary CNS lymphoma

Bacterial or fungal brain abscesses

Malignant lesions
  Lymphoma
    • Second most common mass lesion; found in 1.5% of cases
  Metastatic Kaposi's sarcoma
  Paraneoplastic syndromes
Cerebrovascular disorders
  Thrombotic   Embolic
  Hemorrhagic   Vasculitic
Possibly multiple sclerosis

19. How can focal neurologic deficits be managed?
The management of focal deficits requires an aggressive, comprehensive team approach specific to the deficits observed. Maintenance of quality of life and adaptive support to meet the patient's short- and long-term personal goals despite new impairments is the guiding principle of rehabilitation interventions.

20. What are some of the causes of spinal cord dysfunction in HIV infection?

Vacuolar myelopathy   Viral myelitis
Meningitis   Varicella-zoster
  Aseptic   Herpes simplex
  Cryptococcal   Cytomegalovirus (CMV)
  Lymphomatous   HTLV-I-associated tropical
Spinal tuberculosis (Pott's disease)   spastic paraparesis
Multiple sclerosis(?)

21. Define vacuolar myelopathy.
Vacuolar myelopathy is a spinal cord disorder seen in 11–22% of persons with AIDS. It is strongly associated with HIV dementia and has an identical pathology. Patients present with progressive paraparesis, ataxia, posterior column loss, spasticity, and neurogenic bladder and bowel.

22. How is spinal cord dysfunction managed?
The rehabilitation approach should take into account the prognosis and concomitant cognitive dysfunction. Gait disturbances may be managed with gait aides, wheelchairs, and orthotics. As vacuolar myelopathy generally occurs in advanced AIDS, over-rehabilitation (planning for expected further decline in function) is often indicated—provided the patient is emotionally ready. Home modifications and adaptive equipment should emphasize comfort and simplicity. Sphincter disturbances should be evaluated early, with initiation of a plan to establish continence with minimal reliance on indwelling devices.

23. Which neuropathies are seen in HIV infection?

Distal symmetrical   Drug-induced neuropathies
  polyneuropathy   Vitamin B12 deficiency
Autonomic neuropathy   Segmental herpes zoster
CMV polyradiculopathy   Compression neuropathy
Inflammatory demyelinating   Mononeuritis simplex/multiplex
  neuropathies   associated with vasculitis

24. What is distal symmetrical polyneuropathy?
Distal symmetrical polyneuropathy is a prominent feature of AIDS, being symptomatic in 18% and detectable by EMG in 35%. It involves symmetrical axonal degeneration with patchy demyelination and is seen in advanced disease, being present in virtually all cases at autopsy.

25. What drugs are commonly associated with neuropathies in AIDS?

Didanosine	Vincristine	Dapsone
Zalcitabine	Rifampin	Ethambutol
Isoniazid		

26. Discuss the inflammatory demyelinating neuropathies?

HIV infection has become a significant cause of inflammatory demyelinating neuropathies and must always be considered in the differential diagnosis of these conditions. **Acute inflammatory demyelinating polyneuropathy** (AIDP) is clinically indistinguishable from other forms of Guillain-Barré syndrome. **Chronic inflammatory demyelinating polyneuropathy** (CIDP) presents similarly but without rapid recovery. **Demyelinating autoimmune conditions** are often seen early in HIV and exhibit a relapsing and remitting course. Both the medical and rehabilitation management are the same as in the idiopathic forms.

These neuropathies must be distinguished from **progressive polyradiculopathy**, which occurs late in AIDS and is highly correlated with CMV. Presenting as a subacute ascending flaccid paraparesis, it is rapidly fatal but may respond to ganciclovir if it is started within the first 24–48 hours.

27. How can HIV-related neuropathies by managed?

Pain may be managed with first-generation tricyclic agents (e.g., amitriptyline), physical modalities, transcutaneous electrical nerve stimulation (TENS), and footwear modifications. Ambulatory aids, orthotics, and adaptive equipment may be helpful in the management of proprioceptive loss and symptomatic motor weakness. Light resistive exercise may be instituted if the lesions are incomplete and stable.

28. Describe the clinical features and management of HIV in children.

The incubation period in children is generally much shorter than in adults, with a median age of onset at 7–9 months. Common features include failure to thrive, diarrhea, and organomegaly. HIV encephalopathy is seen in 40–90% of symptomatic children. It is characterized by delayed developmental milestones, impaired cognition and expressive language, spastic diplegia, ataxia, and other cerebellar abnormalities. There are three subtypes—subacute-progressive, progressive-plateau, and static. It often improves with antiretroviral treatment. The rehabilitation management is similar to that of spastic diplegic cerebral palsy.

29. What about the psychosocial and vocational aspects of HIV?

Central to the rehabilitation of any individual is the relationship of the patient to his or her social support systems. For the person with HIV, the caregiver plays a crucial role as AIDS develops and debility increases. People with HIV infection are often able to work for years before the severity of disability or the medical complications of AIDS interfere. Prior to the development of symptoms, 70–90% of seropositive individuals are employed. Even during the first year after the development of AIDS, less than one-third leave the workforce. Specific problems faced by many individuals with HIV include workplace discrimination, diminished work capacity, and potential loss of health insurance benefits. Fortunately, Americans with HIV are protected from discrimination by the Americans with Disabilities Act (ADA), though enforcement may be difficult when legal proceedings can outlast the patient's health.

30. What is the future of HIV rehabilitation?

The future of AIDS is anyone's guess. Unfortunately, for the near future it seems that, at best, we may learn to control only the symptoms of AIDS, much as we can control only the effects of diabetes without curing the underlying disease process. Rehabilitation professionals may find themselves faced with countless individuals who are otherwise healthy but have residual disabilities. Fortunately, the principles of rehabilitation in HIV disease are similar to those in other disorders; hence, rehabilitation professionals are well prepared to meet this challenge.

BIBLIOGRAPHY

1. Levinson SF, O'Connell PG: Rehabilitation dimensions of AIDS: A review. Arch Phys Med Rehabil 72:690–696, 1991.
2. Levinson SF: Rehabilitation of the patient with cancer or human immunodeficiency virus. In DeLisa JA, Gans BM, et al (eds): Rehabilitation Medicine: Principles and Practice, 2nd ed. Philadelphia, J.B. Lippincott, 1993, pp 916–933.
3. Mukand J (ed): Rehabilitation for patients with HIV disease. New York, McGraw-Hill, 1991.
4. O'Dell MW, Dillon ME: Rehabilitation in adults with human immunodeficiency virus-related diseases. Am J Phys Med Rehabil 71:183–190, 1992.
5. O'Dell MW (ed): HIV-Related Disability: Assessment and Management. Phys Med Rehabil State Art Rev 7(suppl):S1–S232, 1993.
6. Simpson DM, Tagliati M: Neurologic manifestations of HIV infection. Ann Intern Med 121:769–785, 1994.

72. MEDICAL AND REHABILITATIVE MANAGEMENT OF RHEUMATIC DISEASES

Jeanne E. Hicks, M.D., and Jay P. Shah, M.D.

DIAGNOSIS, MEDICAL, AND REHABILITATIVE TREATMENT

1. How do you distinguish between noninflammatory and inflammatory arthritis?

Noninflammatory arthritis is usually *not* associated with acute onset, fever, increased white blood cells (WBC) count, erythrocyte sedimentation rate (ESR), redness, and heat in a joint. The joint fluid has $\leq 2000/mm^3$ (WBCs), there is no extra-articular or systemic involvement, and x-rays are characteristic of a slow, progressive degenerative process. The most common noninflammatory arthritis is osteoarthritis.

Inflammatory arthritis is associated with an acute onset of redness, heat, swelling of joints, elevated ESR, joint fluid WBC count $\geq 50,000/mm^3$, extra-articular and systemic involvement, and x-rays with soft-tissue swelling and sometimes erosions.

2. Name the four distinct groups of inflammatory arthritis.

1. Inflammatory connective tissue disease: polyarteritis nodosa, juvenile rheumatoid arthritis, systemic lupus erythematous (SLE) dermatomyositis-polymyositis, mixed connective tissue disorders
2. Inflammatory crystal-induced disease: gout, pseudogout
3. Inflammation induced by infectious agents: bacterial, viral, tuberculous, fungal arthritis
4. Seronegative spondyloarthropathies: ankylosing spondylitis, psoriasis, Reiter's disease, inflammatory bowel disease

These arthropathies may be symmetrical or asymmetrical in distribution of their joint involvement.

3. What is the mechanism of action of aspirin?

Aspirin has always been the foundation of management of rheumatic disorders with the attendant symptoms of pain, fever, and inflammation. It blocks the synthesis of prostaglandins in the anterior hypothalamus, which is responsible for its **antipyretic effect**. It is a prostaglandin synthesis inhibitor, which is responsible for its **anti-inflammatory effect**.

4. What is the mechanism of action of nonsteroidal anti-inflammatory drugs (NSAIDs)?

NSAIDs suppress inflammation through the inhibition of prostaglandin synthesis and, in addition, inhibit leukocyte migration and the cyclo-oxygenase effect on platelets.

5. List the toxicities associated with chronic NSAID use.

Gastrointestinal bleeding, pancreatitis, hepatotoxicity, decreased renal blood flow, allergic interstitial nephritis.

6. Are any adverse effects associated with long-term methotrexate use?

Gastrointestinal toxicities such as stomatitis and dyspepsia are most common. Pulmonary and hepatic toxicity, though, are the main concerns. Pulmonary hypersensitivity occurs in 2–6% of patients and may be life-threatening, but it is usually reversible. Transaminitis occurs in 67%, but cirrhosis is rare. Teratogenicity is a known side effect. Pretreatment liver biopsy is recommended in patients with a previous history of alcohol abuse.

7. What is the rationale for using slow-acting antirheumatic drugs (SAARDs) and cytotoxic agents in the treatment of rheumatoid arthritis (RA)?

In some cases, there is a need to treat RA aggressively early in the disease process, before cartilage damage occurs. This is particularly true in patients with high-titer seropositive RA. To that end, the early use of SAARDs and especially cytotoxic agents, such as methotrexate, represents a more aggressive approach to the medical management of RA.

8. Do low-dose steroids cause muscle atrophy?

In the past, clinicians seemed to worry about muscle atrophy occurring only with high-dose steroids (prednisone > 15 mg/day), but it has now been shown, in RA patients, that atrophy of muscle also occurs with low doses of prednisone, 5–12.5 mg/day. Patients with RA frequently have low-dose steroids in their treatment regimens, whereas those with stable active polymyositis and SLE often need low- or high-dose steroids, depending on their disease activity. All these diseases cause muscle atrophy from the systemic disease itself plus low patient activity levels. It is important that patients, even on low doses of steroids, be on active isometric and isotonic strengthening programs to help decrease muscle atrophy.

9. Why is it important to measure function in arthritis patients?

Arthritis patients have physical impairments that affect their day-to-day ability to function, and treating the patient with a rheumatic disease means addressing this function as well as controlling the pain and inflammation. Raising or maximizing the patient's functional level by appropriate rehabilitation strategies is an important component in the management of the disease. Measuring their function during medication adjustment and rehabilitation reveals the patient's progress and helps indicate, along with medical parameters of disease activity, when treatment regimens need adjustment.

10. How do you measure function in arthritis patients?

1. **Standard objective physical measures:** These consist of range of motion (ROM) testing, manual muscle testing, dynamometry strength testing (grip and pinch meter, isokinetic machine determination of isometric and isokinetic peak torque, and muscle endurance measures), 50-ft walk time, and ergometry aerobic testing.

2. **Functional assessments:** Global and multidimensional self-report questionnaires of function in the physical, psychosocial, and vocational realms.

3. **Biomechanical assessments:** Analysis of lower-extremity gait characteristics can be done by visual gait analysis, stride analyzers, and sophisticated motion-analysis systems in laboratories with capabilities of analyzing forces across joints and joint moments.

11. What is a global functional assessment? Which one is commonly used in RA?

A global assessment gives a general level of physical function without taking into consideration multidimensional areas of function. The common one used for RA is the Steinbrocker assessment, devised in 1949 and revised by the American College of Rheumatology in 1990. It consists of four levels of global function: independent, functional with assistive devices, needs the help of another person to function, or totally dependent on others.

Steinbroker Global Assessment

1. No limitations (independent)
2. Adequate for normal activities despite joint discomfort or limitation of movement
3. Inadequate for most self-care and occupational activities
4. Largely or wholly unable to manage self-care; restricted to bed or chair

From Schumacher HR Jr (ed): Primer on the Rheumatic Diseases. Atlanta, Arthritis Foundation, 1993.

12. What is a multidimensional functional assessment?

Many functional assessments now exist for the arthritis population that measure function in a number of dimensions: physical, psychosocial, and vocational. These assessments generally are self-report questionnaires. Most have been validated in the RA population. Additional question-naires are available to assess other specific areas, such as fatigue, depression, and altered sleep patterns in rheumatic disease patients. All these assessments are useful in evaluating function over time and can be used as outcome measures in medical trials assessing the effect of new drugs on disease control. In the latter case, they are usually used with other standard measures of disease activity (ESR, joint count) and function (50-ft walk time, manual muscle test, grip strength).

Assessments Measuring Physical Health Parameters

	MOBILITY	SELF-CARE ROLES		COMMUNICATION
ACR	Global	Global	Global	O
Lee	+++	+	O	O
Katz	+	+	O	O
HAQ	++	+++	+	O
AIMS	+++	++	++	+
Jette	++	++	++	+

Abbreviations: ACR = American College of Rheumatology; HAQ =Health Assessment Questionnaire (Stanford); AIMS = Arthritis Impact Measurement Scale.
Symbols: + = few questions in this area; ++ = moderate number of questions in this area; +++ = many questions in this area; O = no questions in this area.

Assessments Measuring Psychosocial Health Parameters

	SOCIAL INTERACTION	LEISURE/GROUP ACTIVITY	MENTAL HEALTH
ACR	O	O	O
Lee	O	O	O
Katz	O	O	O
HAQ	+	O	O
AIMS	++	++	++
Jette	+	+	O
MAC	++	++	++

MAC = McMasters.

13. Intra-articular temperature is normally lower than body temperature. What effect does application of superficial heat have on soft-tissue and joint temperature in arthritis?

Superficial moist heat applied for 3 minutes causes elevation of the soft-tissue temperature by 3°C to a depth of 1 cm and significantly increases the temperature of hand and knee joints. Superficial heat causes decreased soft-tissue pain by acting on pain receptors and by relieving muscle spasm. It also increases collagen extensibility, allowing for more effective stretching programs, but it is associated with increased collagenase enzyme in the rheumatoid joint, an enzyme which causes increased joint destruction. Therefore, it is best if cold is used on acutely inflamed joints and heat reserved for subacute or chronic joints.

14. What are the benefits of deep heat?

Deep heat alone can penetrate and heat even the hip joint and its deep capsular structures. In the presence of decreased motion of the shoulder and hip joints in a subacute or chronic stage, deep heat is useful to increase tendon extensibility prior to a stretching exercise program.

15. What are the benefits of cold treatment on an acutely inflamed joint?

In treating the acutely inflamed or early subacute joint, the goal is pain relief. The use of cold seems most logical because it can increase the pain threshold, relax surrounding spastic muscles, and is associated with decreased indicators of inflammation (collagenase and WBC count) in the joint fluid.

16. List the contraindications to cold treatment.

Raynaud's phenomenon, cold hypersensitivity, cryoglobulinemia, or paroxysmal cold hemoglobinuria.

17. What are the effects of prolonged rest?

Rest is an accepted treatment for inflammatory rheumatic disease, but prolonged rest can have detrimental effects. It stiffens periarticular structures, reduces cartilage integrity, and decreases cardiovascular fitness, muscle mass and strength, bone mass, and coordination.

18. Name the factors to consider in designing an exercise program for patients with inflammatory RA.

1. Assessment of local or systemic involvement
2. Stage of joint involvement
3. Type of pain
4. Preparation for exercise
5. Age of patient
6. Compliance
7. Sequencing of exercise

19. Name the beneficial effects of exercise programs for patients with rheumatic diseases.

1. Increases and maintains joint motion
2. Reeducates and strengthens muscles
3. Increases static muscle endurance
4. Increases aerobic capacity
5. Decreases the number of swollen joints
6. Enables joints to function better biomechanically
7. Increases bone density
8. Increases overall patient function and well-being

20. List the signs of excessive exercise in patients with rheumatic diseases.

Postexercise pain of > 2 hours
Undue fatigue
Increased weakness
Decreased strength
Increased joint swelling

If any or all of these problems occur after exercise, the program should be reassessed and appropriate adjustments made. The type of exercise, its duration, and intensity need to be reevaluated periodically in light of the disease stage and particular condition of various joints.

21. Compare the indications and contraindications of passive exercise in patients with rheumatic disease?

The main purpose of passive exercise is to provide range of motion (ROM) to joints that are incapable of moving and at risk for developing contractures. Passive exercise provides some stretch and compression to muscles and acts as a pump to enhance venous return. This form of exercise is beneficial for patients with severe weakness due to polymyositis or neuropathic disease, stroke, peripheral neuropathy, and vasculitis. Passive exercise is generally contraindicated in an acutely inflamed joint. Patients with acute joints may passively put their joints through an arc of motion once daily to prevent the development of joint contracture, but passive motion with many repetitions increases joint inflammation. This repetitive form of passive motion should be avoided in the presence of an acute joint.

22. When should you avoid forceful stretching of a tendon or joint?

Forceful tendon stretching should be avoided when it is inflamed, very tight, or loose. Forceful stretching of an inflamed tendon can increase inflammation and may initiate tendon sheath fluid accumulation. Forceful stretching of a very tight tendon can be painful, and rupture might occur at the musculotendonous junction. Rupture can occur with quick forceful stretching of lax tendons, as in SLE (particularly of the patellar and Achilles tendons). For a tight, noninflamed tendon, prolonged periods of stretch are more effective in lengthening tendon without causing undue pain.

Forceful joint stretching should be avoided if there is a moderate or large effusion, the joint is inflamed, or there is joint laxity. Forceful stretching in the presence of joint effusion can cause capsular rupture. Even repetitive passive ROM with no stretching of an inflamed joint increases inflammation. Forceful stretching of joints with much ligamentous and capsular laxity can cause joint subluxation (common in RA, juvenile RA, and SLE).

23. Which type of exercise—isotonic, isokinetic, or isometric—is least likely to increase inflammation in an inflamed joint?

Isometric exercise is associated with the least joint inflammation and juxta-articular bone destruction.

24. What are the advantages of an isometric exercise strengthening program in patients with rheumatic disease?

Isometric exercise is ideally suited for restoring and maintaining strength in patients with decreased strength from rheumatic diseases and for the recovery phase of dermatomyositis/polymyositis. An advantage of isometrics is that maximal muscle tension can be generated with minimal work, muscle fatigue, and joint stress.

25. Before prescribing isotonic exercise for a patient with rheumatic disease, what clinical criteria must be met?

Patients with inflammatory arthritis may begin isotonic exercise with low weights (1–2 lbs) when they are over the acute inflammation period.

26. What effect do knee and hip effusions have on surrounding muscle?

Hip effusions in RA patients have an inhibiting effect on contraction of the gluteus medius muscle. Likewise, knee effusions inhibit contraction of the quadriceps. This diminishes the effect of muscle-strengthening programs. It also allows for overpull by the stronger, less-atrophied hamstring muscles and makes the knee prone to flexion contraction. When the effusion is removed and the strengthening program reinitiated, the patient is able to increase the strength of the adjacent joint musculature compared to when the effusion was present.

It is recommended that moderate to large knee effusions, easily detected by clinical exam, be removed in rheumatic disease patients prior to initiating a quadriceps-strengthening program. It is harder to detect hip effusion clinically, but if you are unable to strengthen the gluteus medius muscle and the patient has pain with exercise, you may wish to check the hip by plain film or ultrasound. Removal of a hip effusion is sometimes difficult, and it should be done by a professional skilled in this procedure.

27. What factors contribute to fatigue in patients with rheumatic disease?

Medication, chronic inflammation, anemia of chronic disease, abnormal posture and gait, decreased aerobic capacity, abnormalities of the sleep cycle, atrophy of muscle secondary to disease or chronic pain, and cardiovascular pulmonary problems. Fatigue is difficult to quantify because a decrease in overall stamina, true muscle fatigue, and lack of motivation all result in an inability to complete tasks.

28. Name some appropriate techniques for joint protection.

Elements of a Joint Protection Program

Avoid prolonged periods in the same position	Reduce joint pain
Minimize stress on particular joints by pro-	Unload painful joint
moting good posture	Avoid joint overuse during acute periods of pain
Maintain ROM	Use appropriate adaptive equipment and splints
Maintain strength	when necessary
Maintain good joint alignment	Modify tasks to decrease joint stress

29. Why are orthotics prescribed in the rheumatic disease patient?

To decrease pain, to decrease inflammation, to improve joint alignment, and to improve function.

30. Which are the most common areas for braces in arthritis?

Wrist-hand, Foot-ankle, and Neck/back/knee.

31. Discuss the key reasons for referring patients with rheumatic disease for surgery.

Pain due to joint destruction by inflammatory or degenerative arthritis is probably the commonest cause for surgical intervention. It is important to assess whether the patient with joint pain has had adequate medical and rehabilitative intervention before surgical referral, and pre- and post-operative muscle-strengthening exercises help improve the surgical outcome of the joint replacement.

Decreased function due to pain and biomechanical inefficiency of joints is the second reason for surgery. Suspicion of a **pending extensor tendon rupture**, particularly in the RA hand, or actual **tendon rupture** is another valid reason for surgery. Elective tendon realignment and MCP replacement in RA should be carefully considered with the view toward increasing hand function. Likewise, tendon realignment of the hand in SLE should be considered only if function will clearly be increased.

Deformity alone is not a usual reason for surgery, as much deformity can be present and fairly good function maintained. Synovectomy for pain is still done in RA. Arthrodesis of unstable joints in a functional position, particularly the thumb, is also useful.

32. When is arthrodesis indicated for an arthritic patient? Joint replacement?

Arthrodesis	*Joint Replacement*
Persistent pain	Persistent pain
Instability with mechanical joint destruction	Loss of critical motion in joint
Disease progression	Significantly compromised functional status

RHEUMATOID ARTHRITIS

33. Following total hip arthroplasty (THA), what hip movement restrictions and weight-bearing precautions must be followed by the patient?

Following THA, patients must avoid excessive flexion (> 90°) and internal rotation and abduction of the hip for 6 weeks postoperatively. Ambulation training with a walker or crutches may start on postoperative day 2 or 3. Weight-bearing precautions depend on the type of prosthetic device used:

• Cemented THA: Weight-bearing as tolerated
• Bony-ingrowth THA: Toe-touch weight-bearing for 6 wks, then advance to weight-bearing as tolerated

34. Name the seven criteria used by the American College of Rheumatology (ACR) to establish the diagnosis of RA.

1987 ACR Revised Criteria for the Classification of Rheumatoid Arthritis

CRITERION	DEFINITION
1. Morning stiffness	Morning stiffness in and around the joints, lasting at least 1 hour before maximal improvement
2. Arthritis of ≥ joint areas	At least 3 joint areas simultaneously have had soft-tissue swelling or fluid (not bony overgrowth alone) observed by a physician. The 14 possible areas are right or left PIP, MCP, wrist, elbow, knee, ankle, and MTP joints.
3. Arthritis of hand joints	At least 1 area swollen (as defined above) in a wrist, MCP, or PIP joint
4. Symmetric arthritis	Simultaneous involvement of the same joint areas (as defined in criterion 2) on both sides of body (bilateral involvement of PIPs, MCPs, or MTPs is acceptable without absolute symmetry)
5. Rheumatoid nodules	Subcutaneous nodules over bony prominences, on extensor surfaces, or in juxta-articular regions, observed by a physician
6. Serum rheumatoid factor	Abnormal amounts of serum RF demonstrated by any method for which the result has been positive in < 5% of normal control subjects
7. Radiographic changes	Changes typical of RA on posteroanterior hand and wrist radiographs, which must include erosions or unequivocal bony decalcification localized in or, most marked, adjacent to the involved joints (osteoarthritis changes alone do not quality)

PIP = proximal interphalangeal joint; MCP = metacarpophalangeal joint; MTP = metatarsophalangeal joint.
Adapted from Arnett FC, et al: The American Rheumatism Association 1987 revised criteria for the classification of rheumatoid arthritis. Arthritis Rheum 31:315, 1987.

For classification purposes, the patient is considered to have RA if he or she satisfies at least 4 of these 7 criteria. Criteria 1–4 must have been present for at least 6 weeks. Patients with 2 clinical diagnoses are not excluded. Designation as classic, definite, or probable RA is not to be made.

35. Describe the common articular distribution of RA.

It can symmetrically involve all joints except the distal interphalangeal (DIP) joints of the hands and metatarsophalangeal (MTP) joints of the feet. It can also affect the axial joints of the cervical spine.

36. What are the x-ray hallmarks of RA?

The distribution of early and late x-ray findings are proximal and bilaterally symmetrical. The early x-ray abnormalities are soft-tissue and juxta-articular osteoporosis. Later changes include joint-space narrowing and cartilage and bony erosions.

37. Describe the pathomechanics of a "swan neck" deformity.

The "swan-neck" deformity results from contracture of the interosseous and flexor muscles and tendons of the fingers, resulting in a flexion contracture of the MCP, hyperextension of the PIP, and flexion of the DIP joints. It commonly occurs in RA, although it may be seen due to ligamentous laxity in SLE and polymyositis. This deformity, when reducible, can be corrected with a ring splint.

38. What are boutonnière and mallet deformities?

The boutonnière deformity consists of hyperflexion of the DIP and hyperextension of the PIP joints. The mallet deformity is hyperflexion at PIP. These are commonly seen in RA.

39. Which joint is most likely to develop contractures in a patient with long-standing RA?

Although the shoulder has several joints that make it highly mobile, it is most susceptible to joint contracture in a patient with long-standing RA. The capsule, bursae, and tendons may be inflamed and painful, leading to decreased use of the shoulder, which quickly results in loss of ROM and contracture.

40. Why should you splint an acutely inflamed joint in a patient with RA?

There is no evidence that wearing splints prevents deformities from occurring in patients with RA. However, they should be provided to patients with an acutely inflamed joint to immobilize the joint and thereby reduce pain and inflammation. Other patients with acute joints, particularly those with juvenile RA, also benefit from splinting by decreasing their pain and inflammation.

41. A patient with a long history of RA presents with sudden onset of unsteady gait, paresthesias, and neck pain. You must obtain a lateral x-ray of the cervical spine to rule out what condition?

Atlanto-axial subluxation is common in RA. It may occur with up to 9–10 mm of subluxation with no neurologic findings. However, neurologic findings may occur early. Whenever neurologic findings do occur, it is important to repeat the cervical spine x-ray and compare it to previous ones. In the presence of neurologic findings, surgery to reduce the deformity may be indicated. A neurologic consult is definitely indicated.

42. What common forefoot abnormalities occur in patients with RA?

About 50% of patients with RA have forefoot problems, such as widening of the metatarsal area, prominent MTP joints due to subluxed metatarsal heads, hammertoe deformities, and hallux valgus of the great toe. They also have midfoot problems with a decreased medial longitudinal arch. Hindfoot pronation is a common finding.

43. You are asked to prescribe proper footwear for the patient described in the preceding question. What shoe characteristics should your prescription contain?

In general, proper footwear for RA patients should include a shoe wide and deep enough to accommodate a soft insole or molded orthotic device without applying pressure over the toes. The upper part should be made of leather to allow proper ventilation and molding around the forefoot. The sole of the shoe should be either a crepe wedge or conventional heel-sole combination with a shank support system. If the sole-heel material is too soft, a flotation effect can occur at the ankle which can cause hindfoot pain. Metatarsal relief, a good arch support, and a firm heel counter to help control pronation at the hindfoot should be included.

44. Name some typical gait characteristics observed in patients with RA of the feet?

Gait velocities are usually slower and stride lengths decreased. Gait is characterized by shorter periods of single-limb stance and longer periods of double-limb support. Heel contact is prolonged, which extends into the second double-limb support or weight-release phase of stance.

45. What key muscles should be strengthened and stretched in RA?

Strengthened	*Stretched*
Foot intrinsics	Toe extensors, peroneus, gastrocnemius
Quadriceps	Hamstrings, hip flexors, iliotibial band
Finger, wrist extensors	Hand intrinsics

Certain key muscles around joints affected by RA should be strengthened and stretched to encourage muscle balance. Certain muscles become weaker than others, and an overpull of the stronger muscles around an RA joint may influence the creation of deformity or flexion contractures. For example, a weak atrophied quadriceps with overpull of the stronger hamstrings can create a flexion contracture of the knee.

46. List the indications for synovectomy in RA patients.
- To relieve pain and inflammation associated with chronic swelling uncontrolled by medication
- To retard the progression of joint destruction
- To prevent and retard tendon rupture

SPONDYLITIS

47. What is an enthesitis?
An inflammation at the site of a tendon or ligament attached to bone. It is pathognomonic of the spondyloarthropathies.

48. Name the four disorders that make up the spondyloarthropathies.

Ankylosing spondylitis	Psoriatic arthropathy
Reiter's syndrome	Enteropathic arthropathy

49. List the triad of disorders that make Reiter's syndrome.
Urethritis, conjunctivitis, arthritis. Reiter's syndrome, or reactive arthritis, typically follows a bout of urethritis or diarrhea 2–4 weeks previously (the urethritis may persist) and is presumed to involve the migration of bacterial antigens into these sites, where an inflammatory response ensues.

50. Which joint must be affected before establishing a diagnosis of one of the spondyloarthropathies?
The *sine qua non* of spondyloarthropathies is **sacroiliitis**. Initial abnormalities of the sacroiliac joint include superficial bony erosions and eburnation. Later, the erosions enlarge, and there is progressive sclerosis and focal narrowing of the articular space. At advanced stages, there is extensive sclerosis and focal ankylosis. Eventually, complete ankylosis of the synovial and ligamentous portions of the sacroiliac space results.

51. Describe the clinical test used to measure the progression of spinal involvement in ankylosing spondylitis (AS).
The Wright-Schöber test can measure the progression of motion limitation in AS. This test measures the distraction on anterior spinal flexion above the level of the posterior iliac spine. On anterior flexion, a restriction of 5–10 cm is considered normal. Readings below this indicate significant spinal restriction.

52. What is an appropriate exercise program for a patient with ankylosing spondylitis?
The joint and spinal motion loss, muscle weakness, and decreased endurance seen in AS is less severe in patients who participate in an active and consistent ROM, stretching, strengthening, and aerobic exercise program, as well as maintain good posture. To be effective, the program must be done for the entire course of this chronic disease.

Posture advice includes sleeping on a firm mattress with no pillow or a very thin pillow; lying prone for 15–20 minutes twice a day; sitting upright in a chair that reaches to the thoracic level; having an eye-level computer; and placing reading materials on an eye-level stand.

A twice-daily **ROM stretching program** should be done for the large peripheral joints most affected by AS (shoulder and hips), and **spinal extension exercises** should be done using the corner-pushup exercise. **Strengthening** of the shoulder, hip, and spinal extensor muscles should be done. **Aerobic exercise** in the pool (laps using a snorkel) encourages spinal extension. **Sports** that involve heavy contact should be avoided, and those encouraging spinal extension should be recommended (archery, table tennis, and badminton). Sports or activities that encourage spinal flexion should be discouraged (golf, bicycling, bowling, crochet).

OSTEOARTHRITIS

53. Discuss the pathophysiology of osteoarthritis (OA).

The normal joint provides an extremely smooth bearing surface, permitting virtually frictionless movement of one bone over another within the joint; second, it distributes load, preventing concentration of stresses within the joint. OA, or **degenerative joint disease**, affects the diarthrodial joints, with the primary abnormality residing in the articular cartilage, synovium, subchondral bone, ligaments, or neuromuscular apparatus. The marked changes that occur are cartilage wear and tear, decreased joint space, and osteophyte formation.

54. What joints does osteoarthritis typically involve?

In primary or idiopathic OA, the joints affected are, in order of decreasing frequency, the knees>first MTP joints>DIP>CMC>hips>cervical spine>lumbar spine. It spares the elbows and shoulders, except in cases caused by injury, fracture, or occupation-related tasks.

55. Osteoarthritis in which joints is most likely to lead to disability?

Significant disability in OA is caused by involvement of the large weight-bearing joints, the **hip** and **knee**. **CMC joint** involvement in the hand causes pain and limitation in functional activities, particularly those of a repetitive nature. However, splinting of the CMC joint reduces pain and allows for a very functional thumb.

56. Which foot problems are most commonly encountered in osteoarthritis?

Hallux valgus, with or without bunions; hallux rigidus with cocked toes; metatarsal head calluses; abrasions on the dorsum of the toes.

POLYMYOSITIS

57. Name the four criteria for diagnosis of polymyositis.
1. Symmetrical muscle weakness
2. Electromyography (EMG) with myopathic pattern
3. Elevated creatine kinase (CK)/aldolase
4. Muscle biopsy with inflammation of muscle

58. What is an appropriate exercise program for a patient with polymyositis?

In the past, exercise for patients with polymyositis was not recommended due to fear that it would cause muscle inflammation. Currently, it has been shown that a 1-month isometric exercise program can increase strength in patients with **inactive** or **stable active myositis** without causing sustained CK elevations. Patients with significant muscle atrophy and very weak muscles seem not to respond to a 1-month program. It is reasonable, therefore, to place patients with **chronic** or **stable active disease** on a 3×-a-week or even daily isometric program consisting of 6–10 isometric contractions, each held for 6 seconds, with a 20-second recovery time between contractions. The main muscles to exercise are the deltoids, biceps, hip abductors, extensors, and quadriceps. Those patients who also have distal weakness (20–40%) may wish to exercise wrist and hand muscles and ankle dorsiflexors/plantar flexors. A significant proportion of patients with inclusion body myositis have both proximal and distal weakness. In chronic and stable active disease, isotonic exercise with 1-lb weights 3× a week and low-level aerobic pool programs can also be done. Exercise programs should be reassessed if there is increased muscle weakness and soreness along with significant CK rises.

For patients with **very active** or **active unstable myositis**, only a few isometric contractions 3× a week should be done. If myositis patients have access to a pool, this is the best place for them to exercise.

Stretching exercises to maintain ROM should be done by all patients. Adult patients frequently lose significant shoulder motion. Children lose motion quickly in shoulders, elbows, hips, knees, and sometimes wrists and ankles. Calcium deposits in the soft tissues around the joints in childhood dermatomyositis make these patients particularly prone to loss of joint motion.

59. How can you stabilize the knee in the presence of a very weak quadriceps mechanism?

Patients with polymyositis often develop very weak quadriceps muscles and begin to fall when their strength is in the MRC 3/5 or below level. Although weakness is generally symmetrical in a proximal distribution in these patients, one quadriceps may be weaker than the other. Bracing the limb with the weakest quadriceps dramatically decreases the incidence of falling. The brace used is a short-leg Klenzak locked in 5° plantar flexion to create a stabilizing extension moment at the knee. This brace may also be used if there is concomitant plantar flexor weakness, as the lock position at 5° will prevent tripping on the toes. Do not put a dorsiflexion assist on a brace when the quadriceps is weak; a flexion moment will be created at the knee and make it less stable. If the hip flexors are very weak, this brace may be too heavy for the patient to clear the floor. A lighter plastic brace fixed in plantar flexion may be tried but is not as effective as the metal upright anchored with a metal plate into a firm heel-countered shoe. Braces that create a hyperextension moment at the knee should be used with caution in patients with joint involvement from arthritis, as knee pain can be increased due to the hyperextension force.

SYSTEMIC LUPUS ERYTHEMATOSUS (SLE)

60. What are the criteria for the diagnosis of SLE?

1982 Revised Criteria for Classification of SLE

CRITERION	DEFINITION
Malar rash	Fixed erythema, flat or raised, over the malar eminences, tending to spare the nasolabial folds
Discoid rash	Erythematous raised patches with adherent keratotic scaling and follicular plugging; atrophic scarring may occur in older lesions
Photosensitivity	Skin rash as a result of unusual reaction to sunlight, by patient history or physician observation
Oral ulcers	Oral or nasopharyngeal ulceration, usually painless, observed by a physician
Arthritis	Nonerosive arthritis involving 2 or more peripheral joints, characterized by bilateral tenderness, swelling or effusion
Serositis	Pleuritis—convincing history of pleuritic pain or rub heard by a physician or evidence of pleural effusion; *or* Pericarditis—documented by ECT or rub or evidence of pericardial effusion
Renal disorder	Persistent proteinuria > 0.5 gm/d or > 3+ if quantification not performed; *or* Cellular casts—may be red cell, hemoglobin, granular, tubular, or mixed
Neurologic disorder	Seizures—in the absence of offending drugs or known metabolic derangements; *or* Psychosis—in the absence of offending drugs or known metabolic derangements
Hematologic disorder	Hemolytic anemia—with reticulocytosis; *or* Leukopenia—< 4,000/mm^3 total on two or more occasions; *or* Lymphopenia—< 1,500/mm^3 on two or more occasions; *or* Thrombocytopenia—< 100,000/mm^3 in the absence of offending drugs
Immunologic disorder	Positive LE cell preparation; *or* Anti-DNA: antibody to native DNA in abnormal titer; *or* Anti-Sm: presence of antibody to Sm nuclear antigen; *or* False-positive serologic test for syphilis known to be positive for at least 6 months and confirmed by *Treponema pallidum* immobilization or fluorescent treponemal antibody absorption test
Antinuclear antibody	An abnormal titer of antinuclear antibody by immunofluorescence or equivalent assay at any point in time and in the absence of drugs known to be associated with "drug-induced lupus" syndrome

Adapted from Tan EM, Cohen AS, Fries JF, et al: The 1982 revised criteria for the classification of systemic lupus erythematous (SLE). Arthritis Rheum 25:1271–1277, 1982.

The proposed classification is based on 11 criteria. A person is said to have SLE if any 4 or more of the 11 criteria are present, serially or simultaneously, during any interval of observation.

61. Which sex is overwhelmingly affected by SLE?

SLE is primarily a disease of young women. Its peak incidence occurs between ages 15–40, with a female:male ratio of ~ 5:1.

62. What are the typical musculoskeletal manifestations of SLE?

Arthralgias are the most common presenting manifestations of SLE. These patients may develop arthritis with joint deformities (Jaccoud's arthritis) and muscle pain and weakness. They often have very significant ligamentous laxity, which can lead to dislocation of the shoulder, significant knee instability, and swan-neck deformities of the hands. The laxity makes them prone to tendon rupture during sports activities, particularly of the Achilles and patellar tendons.

63. Describe an appropriate exercise program for a patient with SLE.

Patients with SLE have prominent fatigue, and significantly decreased aerobic capacity has been shown in patients with mild SLE. These patients should be on an aerobic exercise program. Aseptic necrosis of the knee and hips often occurs due to the disease itself or steroids. An isometric and isotonic strengthening program for the quadriceps and hip musculature is important to help maintain biomechanical integrity.

FIBROMYALGIA

64. What are the common manifestations of fibromyalgia?

Fibromyalgia syndrome (FMS) is a myofascial pain syndrome characterized foremost by muscle point areas tender to pressure (**trigger points**). These areas are predominantly located in the neck, shoulder, and lower back, but also in the arms and legs. FMS is accompanied by sleep disturbance (decreased REM sleep time) and fatigue. It is also associated with decreased aerobic capacity by bicycle ergometry testing. In recent years, it has been noted that FMS can be seen in up to 70% of patients with chronic fatigue syndrome.

According to the 1990 criteria of the American College of Rheumatology, a patient is said to have fibromyalgia if both of the following criteria are satisfied. The presence of a second clinical disorder does not exclude the diagnosis of fibromyalgia.

1990 ACR Criteria for the Classification of Fibromyalgia

History of Widespread pain (for at least 3 months)

    Pain is considered widespread when all of the following are present: pain in the left side of the body, pain in the right side of the body, pain above the wrist, pain below the wrist. In addition, axial skeletal pain (cervical spine or anterior chest, or thoracic spine or low back) must be present. In this definition, shoulder and buttock pain is considered as pain for each involved side. "Low back" pain is considered lower segment pain.

Pain in 11 of 18 tender point sites in digital palpation.

    Occiput: bilateral, at the suboccipital muscle insertions
    Low cervical: bilateral, at the anterior aspects of the intertransverse spaces at C5–7
    Trapezius: bilateral, at the midpoint of the upper border
    Supraspinatus: bilateral, at origins, above the scapular spine near the medial border
    Second rib: bilateral, at the second costochondral junctions, just lateral to the junctions on upper surfaces
    Lateral epicondyle: bilateral, 2 cm distal to the epicondyles
    Gluteal: bilateral, in upper outer quadrants of buttocks in anterior fold of muscle
    Greater trochanter: bilateral, posterior to the trochanteric prominence
    Knee: bilateral, at the medial fat pad proximal to the joint line.

Digital palpation should be performed with an approximate force of 4 kg. For a tender point to be considered "positive," the subject must state that the palpation was painful. "Tender" is not to be considered "painful."

Adapted from Wolf F, Smythe HA, Yunus MB, et al: The American College of Rheumatology 1990 criteria for the classification of fibromyalgia: Report of the multicenter criteria committee. Arthritis Rheum 33:160–172, 1990.

JUVENILE RHEUMATOID ARTHRITIS

65. Name the common problems seen in juvenile rheumatoid arthritis.
Decreased joint motion and strength
Limb-length discrepancies
Gait abnormalities

66. You are asked to evaluate and recommend a treatment plan for a 5-year-old boy with pauciarticular juvenile RA. Describe an appropriate exercise program and its rationale.
Children with juvenile RA quickly lose strength around inflamed joints, and motion of the joint is compromised at an early stage. ROM and a few isometric exercises are done even when the joint is acute. Incorporating exercise into play routines is important. Use of the tricycle can increase lower-extremity motion, strength, and conditioning. Pool programs are very helpful. The parent should be instructed in the importance of exercise and incorporate it into the child's daily routines.

ACKNOWLEDGMENT

Thanks is extended to Lula Russell, who was responsible for editorial assistance in organizing this manuscript.

BIBLIOGRAPHY

1. Hicks JE: Approach to diagnosis of rheumatoid disease. Arch Phys Med Rehabil 69:S-79, 1988.
2. Hicks JE: Exercise in patients with inflammatory arthritis and connective tissue disease. Rheum Dis Clin North Am 16:845–870, 1990.
3. Hicks JE: Exercise in rheumatoid arthritis. Phys Med Rehabil Clin North Am 5(4):701–728, 1994.
4. Hicks JE: Rehabilitating patients with idiopathic inflammatory myopathy. J Musculoskel Med (Apr): 41–54, 1995.
5. Hicks JE, Gerber L: Rehabilitation of the patient with arthritis and connective tissue disorders. In DeLisa J (ed): Principles and Practice of Rehabilitation Medicine. Philadelphia, J.B. Lippincott, 1992, pp 1047–1081.
6. Hicks JE, Gerber L: Surgical and rehabilitation options in the treatment of the rheumatoid arthritis patient resistant to pharmacologic agents. Rheum Dis Clin North Am 21(1):19–39, 1995.
7. Hicks JE, Gerber LH: Rehabilitation in the management of patients with osteoarthritis. In Moskowitz RW, Howell DS, Goldberg VM, Mankin HJ (eds): Osteoarthritis: Diagnosis and Medical/Surgical Management, 2nd ed. Philadelphia, W.B. Saunders, 1992, pp 427–464.
8. Hicks J, Nicholas J, Swezey R (eds): Handbook of Rehabilitative Rheumatology. Bayville, NY, Contact Associates, 1988.
9. Klippel JH, Dieppe PA (eds): Rheumatology. London, C.V. Mosby, 1994.
10. Schumacher HR Jr (ed): Primer on the Rheumatic Diseases. Atlanta, Arthritis Foundation, 1993.

73. REHABILITATION IN CHRONIC RENAL FAILURE

Sally S. Fitts, Ph.D., and Diana D. Cardenas, M.D.

1. What is renal failure?
Renal failure is the inability of the kidney to maintain normal fluid and solute homeostasis. It is associated with loss of the kidney's ability to filter and eliminate metabolic waste products and to produce hormones that prevent renal anemia and bone disease and regulate blood pressure. **Chronic renal failure** (CRF) is usually associated with irreversible damage to the kidney and irreversible loss of kidney function. The course of CRF varies depending on any underlying

disease but progresses eventually to **end-stage renal disease** (ESRD), which requires chronic dialysis or transplantation to maintain life. The incidence and causes of ESRD vary from country to country and are changing with our aging population, but in the United States, diabetes mellitus accounts for 36%, hypertension 30%, chronic glomerulonephritis 11%, polycystic kidney disease 3%, and other or unknown causes 16%.

2. How is renal failure treated?

When dialysis is needed (in ESRD), patients choose between hemodialysis and peritoneal dialysis. **Hemodialysis** requires a permanent blood access (usually in the forearm) for external filtering of blood through an artificial kidney (usually 3–4 hours, 3 times per week). **Peritoneal** dialysis requires a permanent intraperitoneal catheter for 4–5 daily exchanges of dialysate fluids to remove waste and fluid. Hemodialysis may result in an intermittent pattern of post-dialysis fatigue and recovery and fluid gain between dialysis sessions; peritoneal dialysis maintains a more steady state. Kidney **transplantation** is the optimal treatment for many CRF patients, yet has side effects resulting from immunosuppressive drugs, such as cyclosporine or prednisone (weight gain, osteodystrophy, and psychological effects).

3. What are the metabolic consequences of renal failure?

CRF and its treatment affect every organ system. The metabolic consequences include anemia, post-dialysis fatigue, hypo- or hypertension, sleep disorders, headache, muscle cramps, renal bone disease (osteodystrophy), peripheral neuropathy, and increased risk of heart disease. These problems continue and may progress despite dialysis to control uremia and electrolyte concentrations, but they are reversed by successful transplantation. Recent efforts to improve dialysis adequacy should reduce mortality and morbidity. The leading causes of death among dialysis patients are cardiac arrest and other cardiovascular complications.

4. Discuss the forms of renal bone disease seen with dialysis.

Renal osteodystrophy is a generic term encompassing all skeletal disorders occurring in CRF patients. High-turnover bone disease (**osteitis fibrosa**) is more common with hemodialysis (50–60%) than peritoneal dialysis, and low-turnover bone disease (**osteomalacia**) is more common with peritoneal dialysis (60–70%). However, both can occur in some patients.

Secondary **hyperparathyroidism** causes increased bone resorption (**osteopenia**) and increased bone formation with increased unmineralized bone matrix (osteitis fibrosa). Three stages are recognized in the progression of secondary hyperparathyroidism in CRF: (1) compensatory, showing an increase in parathyroid hormone (PTH) with normal (or low) serum calcium and only subclinical skeletal changes; (2) hypercalcemia, with an increase in calcium secondary to hyper-secretion of PTH; and (3) osteitis fibrosa cystica, with severe symptomatic bone lesions (brown tumors, not seen in routine radiographic studies) that are preventable or treatable by parathyroidectomy. PTH affects cortical (e.g., distal radius) more than trabecular (e.g., spine) bone, and these effects are cumulative over many years. Excessive calcium supplementation may produce painful extraskeletal (soft-tissue) calcifications.

5. How do metabolic changes and their secondary effects impact quality of life?

ESRD and its treatment affect every aspect of life—diet, work, recreation, sex, and sleep. Symptoms of ESRD include fatigue, decreased exercise tolerance, sleep disorders, headache, muscle cramps, chills, myopathy, renal bone disease, and increased risk of heart disease, all of which can limit function and reduce quality of life. The time required for dialysis treatments and, for many patients, post-dialysis fatigue severely limit the time and energy available for work and recreation.

Surveys have shown that dialysis patients' subjective quality of life is as good as that reported by the normal healthy population. However, objective quality of life measures, such as employment and exercise tolerance, indicate substantial deficits among dialysis patients.

6. How is exercise tolerance influenced by the metabolic effects of CRF?

Exercise tolerance of persons on dialysis (tested by bicycle ergometry) is only about 50% of that among the general population. In dialysis patients over age 60, fatigue was the most frequent reason given for activity limitations, with dialysis patients being more limited in their ability to climb stairs, walk, and perform heavy work around the house than were a control group matched for age, race, sex, and cardiac problems.

The low rate of employment among dialysis patients has long been attributed to reduced exercise capacity, and the reduced exercise capacity, to renal anemia. However, these explanations have been challenged recently as correction of anemia does not restore normal exercise tolerance or physical activity. Because exercise training fails to increase the physical capacity of dialysis patients as much as predicted by their hematocrit increase, some other metabolic limitation is implicated. Extremely low oxygen extraction rates, even in exercise-trained and nonanemic CRF patients, have been attributed to a defect in the muscles' aerobic metabolism. The decreased muscle mass, decreased capillary density in muscles, and a lower proportion of type 2 muscle fibers in dialysis patients are similar to changes in muscle morphology that result from prolonged physical inactivity (disuse) in the absence of ESRD.

7. How is erythropoietin used in treating the anemia of renal failure?

Anemia was almost universal among CRF patients until the development of **recombinant human erythropoietin (EPO)** in the 1980s. EPO treatment replaces the hormone normally produced by the kidneys to induce red blood cell production. Currently, most ESRD patients take EPO to maintain a hematocrit near the target value of 35%, although some nephrologists recommend a higher (near-normal) target hematocrit.

Correction of anemia with EPO clearly improves exercise capacity and subjective quality of life in patients with renal failure. Exercise is another way for dialysis patients to improve anemia, and athletic patients can maintain a normal hematocrit. Many investigators have found improvements in strength and functional status when anemia is treated with EPO.

8. How should patients with renal failure be evaluated for an exercise program?

Early intervention for prevention of disability prior to initiation of dialysis is optimal to maintain employment, relationships, and physical activity, but most patients can benefit from an exercise program at any time. Physical therapy evaluation and treatment are not always needed but can facilitate recovery from transplantation or hospitalization for any other reason.

Most guidelines for aerobic exercise recommend a training heart rate, but this is not useful for people taking beta adrenergic blocking medications to control hypertension, because these medications blunt the normal exercise-induced increase in heart rate. As an alternative, perceived exertion is recommended as a guide for exercise intensity. Each patient should be evaluated by his/her physician before beginning any exercise program. Once specific risks have been ruled out, the risks of not exercising are even greater than the risks of exercising.

Almost every CRF patient can engage safely in mild stretching and strengthening exercises, and many are capable of performing a total of 30 minutes of physical activity daily. Patients should be selected more carefully for strenuous aerobic exercise.

The safest time for diabetic patients to exercise is during dialysis when blood glucose is "clamped" by dialysate. For all patients, the risk of exercise-induced hyperkalemia is lowest when potassium levels are "clamped" during dialysis. Protection of the dialysis during exercise is important for all patients. Specific guidelines for exercise during dialysis are given in reference 9. Peritoneal dialysis patients must avoid abdominal pressure when full with dialysate, but should do abdominal strengthening and back stretching exercises partway through an exchange when only half full.

Frequent monitoring is important for the early identification of medically significant changes in exercise tolerance, minor injuries which can discourage the habit of regular exercise, or the need to advance individual goals. Patients should keep an exercise diary of activity, intensity, and duration.

9. What are the benefits of exercise for CRF patients?

The benefits of exercise include all the benefits for the general population, plus additional benefits related to the special challenges of renal failure. Regular exercise increases muscle strength, flexibility and endurance, increases bone and ligament integrity, increases stroke volume in the heart, decreases resting heart rate, increases pulmonary ventilation, increases high-density lipoproteins, decreases triglycerides, increases muscle mass, and decreases percent body fat. Increasing strength, flexibility, and endurance enables the accomplishment of work and enjoyment of recreation that were previously more challenging or impossible.

Physical exercise can slow, stop, or reverse the progressive deconditioning that often characterizes the course of CRF, thus improving quality of life by preventing progressive frailty, maintaining independence, avoiding nursing home placement, and speeding patients' recovery from illness, surgery (including transplant), and post-dialysis fatigue.

Regular aerobic exercise improves blood pressure control, often reducing medication requirements, and reduces cardiac risks, both of which are serious problems for many CRF patients. Exercise training improves glucose tolerance and insulin sensitivity. Regular exercise reduces depression, hostility, and anxiety and improves sleep, mood, mental alertness, weight control, self-image, and the sense of responsibility for and control over one's own health. Aerobic exercise during dialysis reduces the frequency of symptomatic hypotensive episodes, chills, and muscle cramping and increases the ease of fluid removal.

10. What are the difficulties/challenges of exercise for chronic renal patients?

Post-dialysis fatigue makes a person want to rest, but excessive rest leads to progressive deconditioning which then lengthens the time required to recover from post-dialysis fatigue. Regular exercise is the key to breaking out of this spiral of decline into disability. The time constraints of dialysis mean there is less time available to be physically active, so the habit of regular exercise becomes even more important to balance the forced inactivity required for dialysis treatments. Peritoneal dialysis patients often find exercise difficult because of their feeling of fullness. Dialysis is a life-saving treatment, but many patients need rehabilitation services to resume living fully. Despite their limitations, exercise is an important way for people with CRF to improve the quality of their lives.

BIBLIOGRAPHY

1. Akiba T, Matsui N, Shinohara S, et al: Effects of recombinant human erythropoietin and exercise training on exercise capacity in hemodialysis patients. Artif Organs 19(2):1262–1268, 1995.
2. Delmez JA: Renal osteodystrophy and other musculoskeletal complications of chronic renal failure. Primer on Kidney Diseases. National Kidney Foundation, 1994.
3. Evans RW, Bader B, Manninen DL: The quality of life of hemodialysis recipients treated with recombinant human erythropoietin. JAMA 263:825–830, 1990.
4. Fitts SS, Guthrie MR: Six-minute walk by people with chronic renal failure: Assessment of effort by perceived exertion. Am J Phys Med Rehabil 74:54–58, 1995.
5. Guthrie MR, Cardenas DD, Eschbach JW, et al: Effects of erythropoietin on strength and functional status of patients on hemodialysis. Clin Nephrol 39(2):97–102, 1993.
6. Harter HR: Exercise in the dialysis patient. Semin Dial 7(3):192–198, 1994.
7. Kutner NG, Cardenas DD, Bower JD (eds): Maximizing Rehabilitation in Chronic Renal Disease. New York, PMA Publ. Co., 1989.
8. Life Options Rehabilitation Advisory Council: Exercise for the Dialysis Patient: A Comprehensive Program. Madison, WI, Medical Education Institute, 1995.
9. Painter P: The importance of exercise training in rehabilitation of patients with end-stage renal disease. Am J Kidney Diseases 24(Suppl 1):S2–S9, 1994.
10. Suzuki M, Tsutsui M, Yokoyama A, Hirawawa Y: Normalization of hematocrit with recombinant human erythropoietin in chronic hemodialysis patients does not fully improve their exercise tolerance abilities. Artif Organs 19(2):1258–1261, 1995.

IX. Pediatric Rehabilitation

74. GENERAL AND NEUROMUSCULAR REHABILITATION IN CHILDREN

Frank S. Pidcock, M.D., and James R. Christensen, M.D.

1. Should every child born with myelomeningocele have it surgically repaired?

Advances in surgical care and antibiotics have taken away the need for haste in decisions regarding surgery. Charney et al. reported the relationship between time of surgery and eventual outcome in 110 newborns with myelomeningocele. They found no significant difference in mortality, development of ventriculitis, developmental delay, or worsening of paralysis among groups that were surgically repaired within 48 hours, 3–7 days, and 1 week to 10 months of life.

The fact is that currently most myelomeningoceles are surgically repaired shortly after birth and the children survive. Studies that look at functional outcome suggest that adults with myelomeningocele have difficulty achieving independence from parents, finding suitable living accommodations, and landing a reasonable job. The environmental support systems available to the child appear to be at least as important in determining life satisfaction as the severity of the medical condition.

2. Do Apgar scores predict cerebral palsy or mental retardation?

The Apgar score was developed to quickly identify the newborn infant in need of resuscitation and has little predictive significance for the development of neurologic problems—unless it is depressed at 15–20 minutes after birth. In a large multicenter collaborative project, 4.8% of surviving infants had Apgar scores of < 3 out of 10 at 1 minute. In this group, the risk of cerebral palsy was only 1.7%. However, 15% of infants who had 5-minute Apgar scores of ≤ 3 had cerebral palsy. A score of < 3 at 15 minutes was associated with mortality in about 53% of cases with a risk for cerebral palsy of 36% in survivors.

3. Is cerebral palsy caused by obstetrical misadventure?

Unfortunately, the perception that cerebral palsy is caused by something that went wrong at birth has been a part of popular folklore since its initial description by William John Little in 1868. This issue has since been scrutinized carefully by many epidemiologists. An association between asphyxia at birth and the development of cerebral palsy was detected in only about 3–13% of cases. Furthermore, cerebral palsy rates have not shown a decrease despite major improvements in obstetrical and neonatal care between the 1950s and the 1970s.

4. What are the earliest signs of Duchenne muscular dystrophy?

Early diagnosis of Duchenne muscular dystrophy (DMD) is desirable because its X-linked recessive mode of inheritance places the family at risk for giving birth to additional cases. The early developmental history is normal with age-appropriate achievement of milestones, such as raising head from prone and sitting independently. In retrospect, there is often a history of difficulty in arising from the floor, frequent falls, or an abnormally loud thud when walking. Neck flexor muscles are involved early, and these children have a characteristic difficulty in raising their heads when supine. These subtle deviations are regarded as permissible in the child who is just beginning to ambulate and go unnoticed or are attributed to clumsiness. Around age 3–6 years, the lag in motor development becomes inescapable. The child shows difficulty with climbing stairs, develops a waddling gait to compensate for proximal weakness with lordosis, and develops toe-walking to maintain the center of gravity over the feet and to prevent collapse at the knees.

5. Where is the genetic abnormality in Duchenne muscular dystrophy?

The Xp21 site on the short arm of the X chromosome. The surprise is the enormous size of the gene, which spans 2.3 million base pairs of DNA. It in turn codes for dystrophin, a muscle-specific protein of leviathan size. The specific function of this protein is still being determined, but it is believed to be a component of the muscle cell membrane.

6. What musculoskeletal condition is common to preadolescent female gymnasts and professional football lineman?

Spondylolysis. It is the probable result of nonunion of a stress fracture of the posterior elements of the lumbar vertebrae brought on by repetitive high-stress hyperextension activities. The L5 vertebra is most commonly involved, but any spinal segment may be affected. Spondylo-listhesis refers to slippage of one vertebra on the one below it and, if severe, may compress spinal nerve roots, causing an impingement syndrome. Just remember that *spondylo* means spine, *lysis* means a breakdown, and *listhesis* slips off your tongue.

7. When do you worry about idiopathic adolescent scoliosis?

Although idiopathic scoliosis is the most common form of childhood scoliosis, other causes must be considered before the diagnosis is made. These include relatively minor problems, such as a leg-length discrepancy or poor posture, as well as serious conditions such as vertebral and spinal cord tumors, osteoid osteomas, and spondylolisthesis. Muscle spasms and hysteria are other conditions that may present as a scoliosis.

Since idiopathic scoliosis is generally a painless condition, a report of **pain**, especially at the convexity of the scoliotic curve, must be taken seriously, and further evaluations to determine an etiology are mandatory. Other red flags which signal the need to evaluate a child in greater detail are onset before puberty and presentation in a male.

8. What degree of spinal curvature is of concern in cerebral palsy, muscular dystrophy, and idiopathic scoliosis?

The degree of curvature determines the recommended treatment. In muscular dystrophy, surgical stabilization should be done before the decline in vital capacity makes surgery risky. This occurs when the patient's vital capacity falls below 35% of expected, which equates to a curvature of 35° or more. Surgery when vital capacity is < 25% of expected may lead to postoperative ventilator dependence. In cerebral palsy, correction of scoliosis depends on the stiffness of the back and ability to straighten it.

Degrees of Curvature	Idiopathic	Muscular Dystrophy	Cerebral Palsy
1–20°	Observation	Observation	Observation
20–40°	Brace	Surgery (sooner if rapidly progressive)	
> 40°	Surgery		Surgery (may wait until 60° or more in some cases)

9. Are there signs that help distinguish fractures resulting from child abuse versus accidental trauma?

Nonaccidental trauma to children unfortunately continues to be a serious health problem. A high index of suspicion backed up by appropriate medical findings is very important. Fractures suggestive of abuse include:

Multiple fractures in various stages of healing

Growth plate fracture

Transverse metaphyseal fracture ("bucket-handle" fracture) near the growth plate of femur, tibia, and humerus

Spiral fractures of long bones

Unusual locations of fracture (posterior rib, sternum, scapula)

An important nonskeletal associated finding in child abuse is retinal hemorrhages. The optic fundi must be examined in suspicious cases because of the malignant nature of the syndrome and the significant risk of fatality following repeated episodes.

10. What is the Wee-FIM?

It's not just a small functional independence measure (FIM). Developed in 1987, the WeeFIM is a measure of functional abilities and the need for assistance associated with disability in children age 6 months to 7 years. It can be used above the age of 7 as long as the child has delays in functional abilities. There are six subdomains which include items that are rated on a 7-point ordinal scale (from dependence to independence).

11. What is the COAT?

COAT stands for **Children's Orientation and Amnesia Test**. It is a 16-item test of orientation and memory designed for children recovering from traumatic head injury. It assesses three areas: general orientation, temporal orientation, and memory. A score within 2 SD of the mean for age is defined as the end of the period of post-traumatic amnesia (PTA) or the interval when the brain is unable to store and recall ongoing events. The duration of PTA has been correlated with prognosis. In a controlled study by Rutter, children with PTA of < 1 week were doing well 2 years 3 months following injury. Persistent psychiatric problems were noted in approximately 50% of children with PTA for > 1 week. Greater than 3 weeks of PTA was associated with significant educational problems related to attention deficits and disinhibition.

12. Why are the neonatal reflexes an important part of the examination of infants suspected of having neurologic disorders?

The neonatal or primitive reflexes are part of the bundled software with which we are born. These provide a temporary set of automatic instructions for protecting the defenseless newborn in the hostile extrauterine world. These include the Moro reflex, asymmetric tonic neck reflex, tonic labyrinthine reflex, positive supporting, rooting, palmar grasp, plantar grasp, automatic neonatal walking, and placing. As the brain completes its myelination and the ability to control movements increases during the first year, the child needs to be able to control voluntary movements. If the neonatal reflexes persist beyond 4–6 months of age or manifest themselves in a mandatory fashion which "locks" the child in specific positions, they become chains that bind rather than rails to guide the child on the path to independent movement. Therefore, their presence in a persistent or obligatory fashion is one of the earliest clues of impairment to the motor control centers of the nervous system.

13. How do the asymmetric (ATNR) and symmetric (STNR) tonic neck reflexes differ?

The ATNR is one of the classic neonatal reflexes that gradually fades away by age 6 months to allow independent reaching and head-turning. It is a fencer's pose: head turned toward the opponent with rapier extended, and opposite arm flexed at the elbow with finger pointed toward the shoulder.

In contrast, the STNR is the only reflex that is not present at birth and again absent at the first birthday. It provides postural stability as the child makes the precarious transition from crawling to standing. Think of it as the "Aesop's fables" reflex: when the child's neck is flexed, the arms flex and the hips extend, recalling the "dog and the bone." If the neck extends, the arms extend and the hips flex, a perfect position for steadying oneself before attempting to pull up to stand, reminiscent of the "fox and the grapes."

14. Is a 3-year-old nonambulatory girl with spastic cerebral palsy going to walk?

A valuable rule of thumb to remember is the association between independent sitting and eventual ambulation. A child with spastic diplegia or quadriplegia who sits by age 2 will eventually walk. If independent sitting is not achieved by age 4, then walking is not achieved. Between ages 2 and 4, eventual ambulatory status cannot be predicted if the child is not sitting.

15. What is the earliest age at which a child can learn to operate an electric wheelchair safely?

Children attain the cognitive and perceptual skills required to safely drive a motorized wheelchair around 3 years of age. Since exploration of surroundings through movement is one of the chief means of learning in early life, introduction of an alternative to ambulation for children for whom mobility is severely limited is desirable as early as possible. Don't forget that a child in a wheelchair requires the same vigilant supervision as any other rambunctious toddler.

16. What is SCIWORA?

SCIWORA is a medical acronym that stands for "spinal cord injury without radiographic abnormality." About 20% of children under age 12 years having serious spinal cord injury do not have evidence of fracture or dislocation. The inherent elasticity of the fibrocartilaginous spine and its surrounding soft tissue in the growing child is believed to account for the phenomenon. Fifty percent of children with SCIWORA have delayed onset of paralysis up to 4 days following injury. Therefore, every effort should be made at the time of presentation to rule out potential spinal instability with tomograms and controlled flexion extension radiographs.

17. Does outcome after traumatic brain injury (TBI) follow the general pediatric brain injury rule that "outcome is better with earlier insults" (due to plasticity of the developing CNS)?

Unfortunately, for younger children, this does not seem to be the case. While some studies using narrower age ranges have shown no significant differences with age, others have shown that older children and adolescents do better than younger children.

Why does this not follow the general rule in pediatric brain injury? There are many possible explanations. Plasticity, which is so important in recovery from focal brain injuries (i.e., infantile strokes), may be at a disadvantage due to the diffuse nature of the injuries. The younger brain may be more susceptible to the effects of trauma due to its different physical (i.e., less myelinated) and neurochemical (i.e., increased excitatory amino acids) properties. Also, mechanism of injury is different depending on age, which may result in differences in the primary injury.

18. Which groups are most at risk for injuries and therefore the focus of any injury prevention strategies in the rehab setting?

While the care and treatment of the patient with traumatic injuries are improving, prevention is the most effective intervention. Prevention should be given highest priority by any professional working with children.

Trauma is the major cause of childhood morbidity and mortality, and head trauma is the single most important determinant of the severity of injury and outcome. The incidence of TBI is highest in males aged 10–29 years, with the peak incidence between 15–19 years. A shocking statistic is that the estimated cumulative risk of brain injury for children through age 15 years is 4% in boys and 2.5% in girls.

Injury does not occur randomly across the population. Race and socioeconomic status are major determinants of risk. Death rates for unintentional injury among children < 15 years old vary with race, ranging from highest to lowest frequent, Native Americans, African-Americans, whites, and Asian-Americans. For all races, injury death rates are inversely related to income level.

One of the most significant risk factors for a head injury is a history of previous head injury. This means that patients in a rehab setting are at higher risk for injury, which further highlights the importance of and need for injury prevention.

19. What injury prevention strategies are most effective?

The main principles of brain injury prevention include:

1. Anything that can decrease the amount and rate of energy transfer will decrease the severity of injury to the brain, if not prevent it entirely.

2. Strategies that rely as much as possible on "passive" or automatic strategies are likely to be more effective than those based solely on behavioral change, especially since behavior changes are most difficult to achieve in the population at most risk (e.g., adolescents, the poor, and the intoxicated).

3. Strategies and recommendations should be focused and specific (e.g., don't say "be careful"—instead say "use a car seat, buy and use a bike helmet, and throw out the baby walker!").

Because of the limitations of education and other strategies in isolation, prevention will need to be approached from multiple simultaneous angles—passive strategies, education, financial incentives (e.g., bicycle helmet coupons/subsidies), and "mandatory use" legislation. However, the first step is for all professionals working with children to remember the need and importance of prevention.

20. What is the most frequent cause of diffuse hypotonia in infants and children?

The differential diagnosis of hypotonia in the pediatric age range is long and includes abnormalities of every part of the neuromuscular system, from the brain to the neuromuscular junction and muscle: e.g., infantile botulism, spinal muscular atrophy, congenital myasthenia gravis, congenital myopathies/muscular dystrophies, and a host of other uncommon disorders. However, 80% of children evaluated for hypotonia will have a developmental or acquired disorder of the CNS.

21. In patients with cerebral palsy, which joint is most susceptible to structural change?

Subluxation and dislocation of the **hip joint** is the most common and serious structural change in patients with cerebral palsy. This is an acquired deformity and not a congenital dislocation. Due to the combination of the abnormal pull of spastic muscles (especially the adductors), femoral torsion, and weight-bearing, subluxation generally becomes apparent by about age 3 years, with secondary acetabular dysplasia occurring after age 5 years. Progression to dislocation of the hip occurs almost exclusively in the total body-involved, nonambulatory patient. It is important to perform serial examinations and x-rays on patients at risk for hip deformities to allow for early diagnosis and treatment. If left untreated, the subluxed or dislocated hip will become painful and lead to functional impairments (gait and hygiene problems).

22. Should you be concerned if a newborn presents with an isolated Klumpke's palsy?

Yes! Dr. Eng teaches that she has never observed an isolated Klumpke's palsy secondary to birth trauma. While the lower plexus may be involved, it is essentially always seen in conjunction with upper plexus injury. If a true isolated lower plexus injury is observed in a neonate, one must rule out other causes, such as spinal cord injury, outlet tumors (rare), and anomalous brachial plexus (very rare).

23. What is the most common peripheral neuromuscular disorder affecting infants? Is it really associated with all of the "fibs and positive sharp waves" you heard about in medical school?

Spinal muscular atrophy (SMA) type 1, which affects the anterior horn cell and is present in infancy (Werdnig-Hoffman disease), is the answer. Although electrodiagnostic evaluation of SMA demonstrates significant membrane instability with numerous fibrillations and positive waves, clinical studies do not report an overabundance of these findings. In fact, if fibrillation potentials are profuse, think of other disorders, such as type I hypotrophy with central nuclei, mitochondrial myopathy, or storage diseases.

24. In children, when do motor nerve conduction velocities (MNCV) approach adult values?

MNCV parallel the development of myelination. Myelination begins at about the 15th week of conceptional age. After birth, there is a direct relationship between conceptional age (defined as gestational age plus age from birth) and MNCV, which is independent of birth weight. By 3–5 years, MNCV has reached adult values.

25. Is there such a thing as executive function in children?

The executive system is described as those mental processes necessary for formulating goals, planning how to achieve them, and carrying out the plans effectively. Executive function can also be thought of as those processes that allow mental flexibility—the ability to mentally initiate and sustain thoughts and plans appropriately, inhibit unwanted thoughts and actions, and yet mentally "shift gears" when appropriate. Remember the mnemonic **ISIS**—initiate, sustain, inhibit, shift.

Executive dysfunction is commonly seen in children after closed head injury (as it is in adults). As with many other functions, it is developmental in nature and may become more obvious (and testable) with increasing age.

BIBLIOGRAPHY

1. Charney EB, Weller SC, Sutton LN, et al: Management of the newborn with myelomeningocele: Time for a decision-making process. Pediatrics 75:58–64, 1985.
2. Eng GD: Rehabilitation of children with neuromuscular diseases. In Molnar GE (ed): Pediatric Rehabilitation. Baltimore, Williams & Wilkins, 1992, pp 374–375.
3. Ewing-Cobbs, et al: The Children's Orientation and Amnesia Test: Relationship to severity of acute head injury and to recovery of memory. Neurosurgery 27:683–691, 1990.
4. Hresko MT: Thoracic and lumbosacral spine. In Steinberg GG, et al (eds): Ramamurti's Orthopaedics in Primary Care. Baltimore, Williams & Wilkins, 1992.
5. Rivara FP: Epidemiology and prevention of pediatric traumatic brain injury. Pediatr Ann 23:12–17, 1994.

75. CEREBRAL PALSY

Edward A. Hurvitz, M.D.

1. What is cerebral palsy?

Cerebral palsy is a static encephalopathy caused by an insult to the immature brain, leading to a global dysfunction which always includes problems with motor function. Although definitions vary, the onset of injury is usually limited to the prenatal, perinatal, or immediate postnatal period. It is important to note that the lesion resulting in cerebral palsy is static, i.e., it does not become worse. However, as children grow, their muscles may become tighter, and as they age, they may have increasing functional deficits, but neither of these problems is related to increasing loss of cerebral function. They are generally secondary effects of spasticity and other primary problems.

2. What causes cerebral palsy?

Causes include an intraventricular hemorrhage in the premature infant or episodes of anoxia, but usually, the cause is unknown. Congenital brain malformations, intrauterine infections, and trauma can be considered. Risk factors include prematurity, low birth weight, history of fetal deprivation, history of fetal wastage, abnormal presentation, and associated malformations, among others.

3. How do you diagnose cerebral palsy?

Clinical diagnosis based on the criteria mentioned in Question 1 is the most common way. In less severe cases, developmental delays and the manifestations of spasticity may not be present for up to a year. Infants may, in fact, be initially floppy. The common complaints are developmental delay, trouble feeding, and the legs crossing over each other and feeling stiff (scissoring).

Sometimes, cerebral palsy can "go away," especially if the diagnosis is made in the first year of life.

The most important thing to determine is that there is *no loss of milestones*, which would indicate a degenerative disorder, hydrocephalus, or even a tumor. Metabolic testing to rule out other diagnoses is often indicated. An MRI or brain CT scan in a child who is developmentally delayed but is making gains and who is known to have been premature is of questionable value in most cases.

Part of the diagnosis is a description of the clinical manifestations: **Spastic diplegics** have legs involved more than arms, **spastic quadriplegics** have total body involvement, and **spastic hemiplegics** have only one side involved. Some children are athetoid or ataxic rather than spastic, or they may have a combination of these symptoms. Pure ataxia is rare and is usually associated with a problem in the posterior fossa.

4. What are the most common questions parents ask?
Will my child walk?
Doesn't having CP mean that you are retarded?
What should I be doing now?

5. Well, will their child walk?
The best indicator of how the child is going to do is how the child *is* doing. Molnar used sitting balance at age 2 as an indicator of future walking; Badell described similar criteria for spastic diplegics. Bleck listed seven primitive reflexes and found that a child whose response was abnormal for two of these reflexes by age 12 months had a poor prognosis for walking. These were:

Should be Absent	Should be Present
Asymmetric tonic neck reflex	Parachute reaction
Symmetric tonic neck reflex	Foot placement
Moro response	
Neck righting reflex	
Extensor thrust	

Trahan and Marcoux identified topography of the impairment, presence of the Moro or asymmetric tonic neck reflex, presence of seizures, and ability to sit at 12 months as indicators of ambulation by age 6. Walking in these studies includes use of a walker and crutches.

6. What does the gait look like?
Children with hemiplegia will **toe walk** with plantar flexion and excess knee flexion on the involved side and their involved arm held in flexion synergy. Diplegic children often have bilateral equinovarus deformity, knees that are flexed and in valgus, and "scissoring" (feet crossing in front of each other with each step). Rotational problems, including femoral anteversion and tibial torsion, will cause internal rotation of the feet.

7. Is cerebral palsy associated with mental impairment?
Not necessarily. Cerebral palsy covers a wide spectrum of clinical presentations. Many children have normal to above-normal cognition, while others are severely impaired. Mental deficiency is noted in approximately 50–75% of these children. About one-third of diplegic children have some degree of mental impairment, but many have perceptual-motor deficits.

8. What should the parents be doing?
The parents should listen carefully to their medical professionals, remain calm, and obtain early intervention services for the child. The law requires that every state provide education for every child and appropriate services for children with special needs. The parents should contact their local school district, inform them that they have a child with special needs, and have the child evaluated. The family will have an IFSP (individual family service plan), or if the child is older than 3, an IEPC (individualized education planning committee) with the staff from the

school, and determine the child's service eligibility. Children under 3 generally receive physical and/or occupational therapy once to twice a week.

9. Should you worry about seizures?

Many children with cerebral palsy have seizures. Children with spastic quadriplegia are most prone, followed by those with spastic hemiplegia. There is no need for a baseline EEG; evaluation and management can wait until there are symptoms.

10. What kind of visual problems occur?

Strabismus is a common problem in cerebral palsy, due to an imbalance in the eye musculature. It is often treated with ophthalmologic surgery. **Hemianopsia** may be present with dense hemiplegia with a middle cerebral artery lesion.

11. What kind of problems does spasticity cause?

Spasticity is a common manifestation of the upper motor neuron syndrome. The most prominent finding is **hypertonicity** of the musculature, which is defined as increased resistance to passive stretch. Spasticity interferes with the ability to perform ADLs by impairing motor control. (Removing spasticity improves motor control but does not normalize it—other aspects of the upper motor neuron syndrome are also involved.) Spasticity can cause **contractures** secondary to muscle tightness, especially in the gastroc-soleus group, hamstrings, adductors, hip flexors, biceps, and wrist flexors. **Hip dislocation** can occur due to tight adductors. Spasticity can also cause difficulty with seating and interfere with caretakers' ability to do transfers and other aspects of care.

12. What should be done about the hips?

In children with tight hip musculature, especially the adductors, the hips should be followed with plain x-rays on a regular basis (every 1–1.5 years). Hip dislocation is a common problem, occurring in 25–30% of the children. Orthopedic procedures, such as adductor tenotomies or derotational osteotomies, help prevent dislocation. Surgical reduction of a dislocated hip is indicated for ambulatory children or for nonambulatory children with pain or seating difficulties. In younger children, hip dislocation can lead to improper development of the hip joint and painful arthritis in young adulthood. In spastic quadriplegic children with very high tone, hip dislocation is very common. Unfortunately, results of surgical repair have been variable in this group and may not be indicated.

13. What can be done about the other limbs and joints affected by spasticity?

Spasticity tends to lead to loss of ROM in a joint due to tight musculature, especially in muscles that cross two joints. In cerebral palsy, it is complicated by growth; bones grow faster than muscles, leading to greater loss of range. The main joints at risk are the ankles (plantarflexion) and the knees, hips, elbows, and wrists (flexion contractures).

The first line of treatment is **stretching exercises**. **Serial casting** and **orthoses** are used, especially for the ankles, knees, and elbows. Casting can be combined with **nerve blocks**. If these methods fail, **orthopedic surgery** is indicated for muscle and tendon lengthening. Muscles that are lengthened will lose about a grade of strength. As children grow, the muscle continues to fail to keep up with bone growth, and all of the interventions (including surgery) will need to be repeated.

14. When are spasticity medications used?

Spasticity medications (diazepam, baclofen, dantrolene) are indicated for the treatment of **generalized spasticity**. They are useful in severely involved children to aid with hygiene and prevent mass extensor spasm. Their use to improve general mobility on a long-term basis is more controversial. They are occasionally used to see if the child might be a candidate for a rhizotomy or other more extensive interventions.

Each drug has its own complications. Diazepam (Valium) and baclofen are sedating, baclofen and dantrolene (Dantrium) cause hepatic problems, and baclofen lowers the seizure threshold. Dantrolene is a current favorite because it avoids the seizure and sedation issue with the other drugs, but liver function tests must be monitored.

15. What are nerve/motor point blocks?

Motor point/nerve blocks are indicated for spasticity affecting specific muscle groups. They are commonly done to decrease scissoring due to adductor spasticity, equinovarus foot deformity during gait, and hamstring tightness. Phenol and, less commonly, alcohol are neurolytic. They basically cause a chemical neurectomy that is effective for 3–6 months. An electrical stimulator is usually used to identify the proper location for injection. An aggressive stretching and gait training program is indicated after the procedure.

Botulinum toxin affects the neuromuscular junction with essentially the same results. It has been used extensively for ocular muscles and to treat torticollis. It is a much simpler, better tolerated procedure than phenol injections, and the effects and time course are essentially the same. Many ongoing studies are further clarifying its use in children with cerebral palsy and other spastic conditions.

16. When is a rhizotomy indicated, and what can it do?

The selective dorsal rootlet rhizotomy is a neurosurgical procedure designed to decrease the excitatory input to the motor neuron, thereby decreasing spasticity. It was popularized in the United States by Warwick Peacock in the early 1980s for children with cerebral palsy. The procedure consists of a laminectomy and exposure of the cauda equina. The dorsal roots are electrically stimulated, and various criteria are used for determining which parts of the root contain more fibers involved with abnormal reflexes. These rootlets are then severed. This technique allows for decreased tone without sacrificing significant sensation.

The ideal patient is a young child (ages 3–8) with spastic diplegia who is quite ambulatory with a spastic gait. Generally, any child who could make significant functional gains if the spasticity was reduced could benefit, as well as children with significant seating problems. Children with poor head and trunk control and children who use spasticity for functional purposes (e.g., extensor spasms to stand) are poor candidates for the procedure. After surgery, the children require an extensive physical and occupational therapy program to recover from postoperative weakness and to maximize functional gains.

17. When should orthopedics be consulted? Neurosurgery?

The rhizotomy decreases spasticity, but it has no effect on shortened, contracted muscles. Orthopedic surgery can lengthen muscles and change the biomechanics of gait through tendon transfers, but it does not change the basic neurology. Using both rhizotomy and orthopedic surgery in combination is often required to gain greatest improvement in gait. Gait lab analysis is useful in many cases for determining the appropriate interventions.

18. What else is out there for spasticity?

The **baclofen pump** delivers baclofen directly to the spinal cord, performing a chemical, adjustable rhizotomy and minimizing side effects. Of course, implanted devices have their own problems, and they need to be filled on a regular basis. The pump is used in some centers for children who are rhizotomy candidates. **Therapeutic electrical stimulation** uses different protocols of muscle stimulation through the night, which is the time of greatest muscle growth. Results on both of these methods are still pending.

19. Who were Karel and Berta Bobath?

The Bobaths began treating children with cerebral palsy in the 1940s. He was a neurologist, and she a physical therapist. The Bobath treatment program is based on normalizing movement patterns and inhibiting abnormal reflexes. Most therapists incorporate some of their techniques in treatment, along with a neurodevelopmental approach that encourages the child to sit correctly before they crawl, crawl correctly before they stand, etc.

20. What are tone reducing AFOs?

Ankle-foot orthoses (AFOs) aid in gait by controlling the equinus or equinovarus deformity. The older type consisted of two metal sidebars going into the shoe. Most AFOs today are custom-molded plastic, and they may be capable of dorsiflexion if constructed with an articulated ankle joint. Tone-reducing AFOs (TRAFOs) have certain features designed to decrease abnormal reflexes, including a foot plate that extends past the toe to discourage toe flexion and a metatarsal support to discourage stimulation to a particularly reflexogenic area of the foot. They are most effective during gait, but use during rest helps prevent contracture.

21. Discuss some of the seating issues in cerebral palsy.

The goals of seating are proper postural alignment, comfort, and mobility. Positioning should protect the joints and skin, support the trunk and pelvis to prevent deformity, and discourage abnormal reflexes. Extensor reflexes can be inhibited by keeping the hips, knees, and ankles in at least 90° angles. Head support can discourage the asymmetric tonic neck reflex. Power chairs are important mobility devices for many children.

22. What kind of swallowing and nutritional problems are present?

Children with cerebral palsy may have difficulty with swallowing, speech, and drooling due to oral motor control problems. Dysphagia can lead to difficulty with adequate nutrition or aspiration. A dysphagia team, usually involving speech/language pathologists, occupational therapist, and/or dietitian, evaluate the child clinically as well as with a fluoroscopic swallow study using different consistency of food. Fiberoptic endoscopic evaluation of swallowing gives a better view of the sequence and timing of swallowing, as well as the amount of residual food left with each swallow. Interventions include positioning and dietary changes, usually involving soft foods over liquids and full solids. Swallowing evaluations are helpful to resolve conflicts between families and the school about safety and appropriateness of oral feeding. With severe aspiration or caloric need problems, a gastrostomy tube is indicated. If the aspiration is asymptomatic, placement of a G-tube is somewhat controversial and less of an absolute indication.

23. How can kids who have communication problems be helped?

Speech problems are often accompanied by spasticity, decreased coordination, and choreoathetosis. Augmentative communication devices must compensate for lack of speed and accuracy. Special switches have been developed to improve access to technology, as well as software that allows for greater options with fewer demands for accurate keyboard use.

24. What other equipment should be considered?

Various ADLs may require specialized seating. There are feeder seats, car seats, corner seats, and bath seats. Prone or supine standers are used to encourage weight-bearing and standing activities. If children have difficulty sleeping at night, supine liers can position them more comfortably. Computers are important for school and recreation. An assisted technology assessment can aid with access problems. Specialty equipment may be commercially available or custom modified.

25. Describe some of the adapted recreational options for an individual with cerebral palsy.

Most recreational activities can be adapted, depending on the resources and willingness of the community. Special Olympics offers the child a chance to participate in peer-level athletic competition. There are many adapted horseback-riding programs. Horseback-riding has several therapeutic advantages, including stretching the adductors and strengthening head and trunk control, as well as being fun. Computers can open up many recreational opportunities. In today's world, a child who is severely impaired can interact on an even plane with others through the Internet.

26. What are some of the critical psychosocial issues to address?

Children with cerebral palsy are at high risk for development of psychological and behavioral problems. Like other children with disabilities, they often have difficulties with peer interaction and other issues of social competence. Higher functioning kids will have more awareness of disability with resultant adjustment issues. Vocational issues, long-term care concerns, advocacy training, and access to proper resources are all factors to be considered when managing a family with a child who has cerebral palsy.

27. What interventions are scientifically proven and universally accepted in the treatment of children with cerebral palsy?

The obvious answer is, nothing. The real answer is, a loving, caring family environment. It works for everyone else, so why not kids with cerebral palsy?

28. What is the best thing I can say to this family?

A family needs to hear that there will be support for them down the road, from their doctor, and from their community. The physician should demonstrate this by listening to the family's concerns, providing medical information, and providing access to resources. They also need to know that cerebral palsy has a wide spectrum of clinical presentations and functional prognoses, and that the effort they put in can make a positive difference in the final outcome.

BIBLIOGRAPHY

1. Bleck EE: Orthopedic Management of Cerebral Palsy. London, Mac Keith Press, 1987.
2. Cornell MS: The hip in cerebral palsy. Dev Med Child Neurol 37:3–18, 1995.
3. Kuban KCK, Leviton A: Cerebral palsy. N Engl J Med 330:188–193, 1994.
4. McLaughlin JF, Bjornson KF, Astley SJ, et al: The role of selective dorsal rhizotomy in cerebral palsy: Critical evaluation of a prospective series. Dev Med Child Neurol 36:755–769, 1994.
5. Molnar GE: Cerebral palsy. In Molnar GE (ed): Pediatric Rehabilitation. Baltimore, Williams & Wilkins, 1992, pp 481–533.
6. Sussman MD (ed): The Diplegic Child: Evaluation and Management. Rosemont, IL, American Academy of Orthopedic Surgeons, 1992.
7. Trahan J, Marcoux S: Factors associated with the inability of children with cerebral palsy to walk at six years: A retrospective study. Dev Med Child Neurol 36:787–795, 1994.

76. NEURAL TUBE DEFECTS

Subhadra Lakshmi Nori, M.D., Ann Burkhardt, M.A., O.T.R./L., and Steven A. Stiens, M.D.

1. List the four types of neural tube defects (dysraphism).

Neural tube defects (NTDs) are failure of neuralization of the primitive neural tube between the 3rd and 4th week in utero.

1. **Spina bifida:** failure of vertebrae to fuse posteriorly, with defective neural tube causing injury to rootlets

2. **Meningocele:** open wound in the back with direct exposure of meninges

3. **Myelomeningocele:** spinal cord, nerves, and meninges exposed

4. **Spina bifida occulta:** least severe type, as the defect is occult, and there is no neurologic damage. Radiographs demonstrate defects closure of posterior vertebral arches (typically L5 and S1).

2. What methods are available for the diagnosis of NTDs?

Ultrasound screening prenatally for dysraphism (sensitivity 96–100%, specificity 30–80%). Determination of alpha-fetoprotein levels (AFP) and acetylcholinesterase levels in amniotic fluid (15–16 week gestation). Estimation of AFP in maternal serum may also help.

3. **What other CNS defects are associated with spina bifida?**

   Congenital hydrocephalus: 80% of children with spina bifida have associated congenital hydrocephalus. Causes include:

   Arnold-Chiari syndrome—herniation of cerebellar tonsils through the foramen magnum, obstructing CSF flow

   Aqueductal stenosis

   Dandy-walker complex (cystic dilatation of fourth ventricle)

   Failure of development of subarachnoid space

   Acquired hydrocephalus: due to infection with toxoplasmosis, cytomegalovirus, mumps, rubella, varicella, etc.

   Tethered cord syndrome: spinal cord becomes attached to the defective site. Thickened cord and filum terminate cause traction injury, resulting in weakness and spasticity, as well as paraplegia or quadriplegia.

   Syringomyelia: 40% of patients with NTD have cavitation of spinal cord. Progressive motor/sensory loss results.

4. **What causes spina bifida? What is its incidence?**

   The actual cause is unknown. Some implicated factors include economic status, alcohol use, vitamin A deficiency, and folic acid deficiency. Spina bifida occurs in 1 in 1,000 live births in the U.S., and its incidence increases with family history. Some geographic areas are known to have higher incidences, and the maternal use of valproic acid increases its incidence.

5. **Why and how is hydrocephalus treated?**

   Hydrocephalus causes blockage of cerebrospinal fluid pathways, leading to increased intracranial pressure and ventricular dilatation. CNS tissues become thin and overstretched. In the compensated hydrocephalus, the ventricular system dilates, increasing head circumference and resulting in intellectual impairment and defective language function. Surgical placement of a shunt becomes necessary to relieve pressure and to prevent brainstem herniation.

6. **How is the level of motor paralysis assessed in a child with spina bifida?**

   Objective muscle testing is difficult in a child, so attention should be paid to major muscle groups, e.g., in thoracic paralysis, the legs are flaccid, assuming a frog-leg position. No spontaneous movements are seen in the lower extremities. With midlumbar paralysis, the hips are in flexion abduction; with low lumbar paralysis, ankles are in dorsiflexion. Note that sensory levels may not always correspond to motor levels.

7. **What is the prognosis for walking in spina bifida?**

   It depends on the degree of paralysis, medical complications, and intellectual factors. Congenital hip dislocations or subluxation require surgery. For proper hip alignment, a hip abduction orthosis with a ratchet joint set at 15° of abduction is necessary. Patients with high-thoracic-level paralysis can benefit from a thoracic-hip-knee-ankle-foot orthosis (THKAFO), primarily for home-based ambulation. Lumbar-level children may attain limited community ambulation with crutches. Low-lumbar level paralysis requires AFOs. Patients with sacral level defects who have foot and claw-toe deformities achieve good ambulation with high-top shoes. Grade 0–3 iliopsoas motor strength is associated with partial or complete reliance on wheelchair.

8. **Are there any special ambulation devices to assist a child with myelomeningocele?**

   Two different types of mobility devices are available:

   1. **Swivel walker** or **parapodium** is used at age 1 for standing and crutchless walking. It has a low energy requirement. This device has a standing frame with foot plate.

   2. **The reciprocating gait orthosis (RGO)** is a hip-knee, ankle-foot orthosis with a cable attached between the hips. The child must also use crutches.

   Both these devices cost five times as much in energy consumption as wheelchair ambulation.

9. What orthopedic problems are encountered in a child with myelomeningocele?

Kyphosis is seen in 10–20%, most commonly in the lumbar spine. Kyphectomy is most commonly used for correction.

Scoliosis is seen in 42–90% of children with NTD. Rapidly progressive scoliosis heralds syringomyelia in the cervical spine. A Milwaukee brace or thoracolumbosacral orthosis (TLSO) is used to correct curves under 45°. Surgical correction is necessary for curves beyond 45°. The optimal age for surgery is 12 years.

Hip dislocations are common in high lumbar paraplegics, but hip-positioning devices and physical therapy may prevent this. Acetabular correction may become necessary.

Congenital club foot may be treated by various options, including ROM exercises, bracing, and triple arthrodesis.

10. How is bowel incontinence managed? (See also Neurogenic Bowel.)
1. Increase fiber and bulk in diet
2. Small dosages of laxatives for regularity
3. Maintain a consistent daily time for bowel movement
4. Reflex emptying techniques such as digital stimulation for reflexic, manual evacuation for areflexic.
5. Strengthening of accessory muscles for relaxation or expulsion

11. Is intelligence affected in a child with myelomeningocele?

On formal IQ testing, they generally score low: 10–15% have speech deficits, and 13–16% have sensory-neural impairments. Verbal performance may be better than quantitative. Vision, motor, and perceptual deficits are common. Overall, the mild deficits do not preclude normal educational settings, independent living, and work.

12. At what age should physical and occupational therapy be initiated for a child with NTD?

Therapy should be started *as early as possible* and should include sensory motor stimulation, training of caregivers, specialized positioning devices, and ROM exercises to prevent contractures.

13. In a child with hydrocephalus and Arnold-Chiari malformation with right-sided neglect, what aspect of rehabilitation needs to be emphasized?

Once shunt malfunction is ruled out, occupational therapy should be initiated to promote the use of the limb during gross motor activities such as crawling, weight-bearing on the extremity, and proprioceptive kinesthetic stereognostic stimulation. Anticipatory guidance promotes a normal developmental sequence.

BIBLIOGRAPHY

1. Charney EB, Melchionni RN, Smith DR: Community ambulation by children with myelomeningocele and high level paralysis. J Pediatr Orthop 11:579–582, 1991.
2. Crandall RC, Birkeback CR, Wintor BR: The role of hip location and dislocation in the functional status of the myelodysplastic patient: A review of 100 patients. Orthopaedics 12:675, 1989.
3. Hoppenfeld S: Congenital kyphosis in myelomeningocele. J Bone Joint Surg 49B:276–280, 1967.
4. Kurtz LA, Scull SA: Rehabilitation for developmental disabilities. Pediatr Clin North Am 40:629–643, 1993.
5. Lie HR, Borjeson MC, Lagerkvist B, et al; Children with myelomeningocele: The impact of disability on family dynamics and social conditions, a Nordic study. Dev Med Child Neurol 36:1000–1009, 1994.
6. McDonald CM, Jaffe KM, Mosca VS, Shurtloff DB: Ambulatory outcome of children with myelomeningocele: Effect of lower-extremity muscle strength. Dev Med Child Neurol 33:482–490, 1991.
7. McDonald CM: Rehabilitation of children with spinal dysraphism. Neurosurg Clin North Am 6(2): 393–412, 1995.
8. Molnar GE, Taft PT: Pediatric rehabilitation: Part II. Spina bifida and limb deficiencies. Curr Probl Pediatr 7:3–33, 1977.
9. Muller EB, Nordwall A, Oden A: Progression of scoliosis in children with myelomeningocele. Spine 19:147–150, 1994.
10. Phillips DL, Field RE, Broughton NS, Monolaus MB: Reciprocating orthoses for children with myelomeningocele: A comparison of two types. J Bone Joint Surg 77:110–113, 1995.

77. PEDIATRIC AMPUTATION AND LIMB-DEFICIENT CHILDREN

Subhadra Lakshmi Nori, M.D., and Lisa Daley, M.D.

1. What are the frequent causes of acquired amputation in children?
Motor vehicle accidents
Home accidents (e.g., burns, fireworks)
Malignancy of long bones (e.g., osteogenic sarcoma, fibrosarcoma)
Vascular insufficiency, gangrene
Neurologic disorders (e.g., neurofibromatosis) with associated nonunion of fracture

2. Name the most common congenital deformity of the leg.
Absence of the fibula. Children with fibular absence have shortening of the extremity and anterior bowing of the tibia. The involved foot is held in valgus. However, the patient can walk with or without a prosthesis. If leg-length inequality is severe, a Syme's amputation may be performed with fitting of a Syme's prosthesis.

3. What are the advantages of intraoperative prosthetic fitting for a lower-extremity amputee?
Intraoperative prosthetic fitting of a lower-extremity amputee was devised to enable an amputee to begin walking soon after surgery. Other advantages include decreased edema and calf pain. In general, a teenager or young adult undergoing amputation for a tumor may benefit from this approach. A younger child is not a good candidate because they may not be mindful of weight-bearing restrictions on a prosthesis or increased physical activity, which may put the stump at risk. Other poor risks for using an intraoperative prosthesis include immunocompromised children, insensate limbs, and infection.

4. What would you initially prescribe for an upper-extremity amputee?
The child with an upper-limb deficiency is fitted with a prosthesis when the child begins to achieve sitting balance and attempts grasping activities at 6 months of age. The initial prosthesis has a passive mitt in which the infant can practice placing objects.

Most children with congenital upper limb amputations have below-elbow limb deformity. A prescription for a below-elbow amputee would include an exoskeletal double-walled socket with a figure-of-eight harness and a voluntary opening terminal device.

5. Describe the special considerations in the prescription of a prosthesis for an infant with a lower-extremity amputation.
The first prosthesis in the lower-extremity amputee has some variation from the standard above-knee system. At the time when the child attempts symmetric sitting balance, at about 6 months of age, it is beneficial to have a light-weight stubby prosthesis in place, with weight-bearing capacity when the infant begins to pull to stand several months later. The above-knee amputee receives a prosthesis without a knee joint initially. An articulated knee joint is prescribed at about 3–3.5 years of age or when the child demonstrates satisfactory gait pattern with the prosthesis.

Suspension systems are also important in the lower-extremity amputee. A suction socket is not prescribed until a child can assist in donning a prosthesis, at about 5 years of age. The pelvic belt is an acceptable way to suspend an above-knee prosthesis. SACH feet are available in a wide range of sizes. The below-knee amputee may use a patellar tendon-bearing prosthesis with a supracondylar cuff. Caution should be taken in using this type of suspension, since one-third of limb-deficient children develop dislocatable patellae. Other suspension systems can also be used with success.

6. What are the indications for surgical conversion of a limb?

Conversion of a deformed extremity into an acceptable residual limb may be necessary in the traumatic amputee when there is persistent infection or scarring prohibits use of a prosthesis. In the congenital limb-deficient patient, indications for conversion include severe leg-length discrepancy, congenital webs or flexion contracture, feet in positions unsuitable for weight-bearing, or malrotation of the limb. Small appendages attached to the deformed extremity should be removed cautiously, since they may prove useful in the control of a prosthesis. In the lower extremity, conversion is performed when the child attempts to stand. Upper extremity conversion is rarely required.

7. What is a myoelectric prosthesis? What are its advantages and disadvantages?

Electrodes are placed on the muscle of the stump, and with contraction, an electromyographic signal is generated. This is sent to a processor for amplification. This signal controls the functions of the hand, such as opening and closing, elbow flexion and extension, and pronation and supination of the electric wrist.

Advantages	Disadvantages
Appearance/cosmesis	Weight
Freedom from harnessing	Cost
Increased grip strength	Tight fit
	High maintenance

8. Is parental support important for the limb-deficient child?

Parents should be counseled to cope with the feelings of anger, frustration, and guilt at having a child with a disability. Optimum treatment of a child amputee can be obtained if the parents fully understand and participate in the treatment program. With cooperation of the entire family, carry-over of training at home and attendance at follow up appointments is more consistent.

9. Does the juvenile amputee experience phantom pain?

Patients with acquired amputation retain some awareness of the amputated part. Some amputees report this sensation as uncomfortable or painful. The older the child is at amputation, the greater the chance that he or she may experience phantom pain, especially if the procedure is performed after age 10. Congenital limb-deficient children do not develop phantom sensation or pain, even after the surgical conversion of the limb.

10. How do you determine if the fit of a prosthesis in an infant is comfortable?

Comfort is a major concern in prosthetic fitting. An infant cannot tell you that wearing the socket is painful or that there is excessive pressure in an area, and the signs of skin irritation may not be present. However, to avoid pain, infants may assume gait deviations to relieve pressure from the area. Parents and therapists should be aware of these signs of poor fit.

11. How often should a juvenile amputee be followed in the prosthetic clinic?

The frequency of clinic visits depends on the child's growth pattern and amount of wear on the prosthesis. Parents should be trained to identify prosthetic malfunction. They should also be aware that the prosthesis needs adjustment as the child grows. In the upper limb, harness size and lengthening of the forearm require frequent follow-up. In the lower limb, congenital deformities may result in impairment of residual limb growth, so the prosthesis may not need to be changed as frequently as with an acquired residual limb with an intact epiphysis. In general, follow-up should be every 3 months at first. A new prosthesis may be required annually until age 5 years, then every 2 years between the ages of 5–12, then every 3–4 years until adulthood.

12. Is the alignment of a child's lower-extremity prosthesis the same as that for an adult?

No. The prosthesis for a toddler has to be aligned differently. A person with a lower-extremity prosthesis needs to feel comfortable in standing and full weight-bearing on the entire sole of the prosthetic foot during midstance. When toddlers first learn to walk, they ambulate with their hips flexed, abducted, and externally rotated, knees flexed, and feet flat on the floor. Therefore, the alignment of the child's first prosthesis must be flexed, abducted, and externally rotated enough in relation to the prosthetic foot to accommodate the toddler's natural stance and gait pattern. If the prosthetic alignment does not accommodate this pattern, the child will feel unsteady on his or her feet and ambulation will be difficult.

13. What is Amelia? Meromelia?

Amelia is the complete absence of one or more limbs. **Meromelia** is the partial absence of a limb. These can be further subdivided into terminal (transverse) and intercalary, each of which may have horizontal or longitudinal deficits (preaxial [radial or tibial] or postaxial [fibular or ulnar]). These groupings are part of the revised Frantz and O'Rahilly classification, which is the most common classification for describing congenital limb deficiencies.

14. In child amputees, the disarticulation level of amputation is preferred. Why?

The goal is preservation of the epiphyses to allow maximum limb growth and to avoid bony overgrowth that can occur in amputations performed through the shaft of a long bone.

15. What is bony overgrowth?

Bony overgrowth is a phenomenon virtually unique to the child amputee. It occurs in approximately 12% of children with acquired amputations but seldom in congenital limb deficiencies. Bony overgrowth is appositional bone formation at the end of an amputation of a long bone. The overgrowth may grow faster than the overlying skin and soft tissue, leading to ulceration, cellulitis, and osteomyelitis. It has a predilection for the humerus, fibula, tibia, and femur (in descending order of frequency). The best option for treatment is surgical revision.

BIBLIOGRAPHY

1. Banerjee S: Rehab Management of Amputees. Baltimore, Williams & Wilkins, 1982.
2. Challenor Y: Limb deficiencies in children. In Molnar G (ed): Pediatric Rehabilitation, 2nd ed. Baltimore, Williams & Wilkins, 1992.
3. Hubbard S: Myoelectric prosthesis for the limb deficient child. Phys Med Rehabil Clin North Am 2:4, 1991.
4. Patton J, et al: Prosthetic components for children. Phys Med Rehabil State Art Rev 5(2):245–265, 1991.
5. Setoguchi Y: The Limb Deficient Child. Springfield, IL, Charles C Thomas, 1982.

X. Rehabilitation of Special Populations

78. BURN REHABILITATION

Elizabeth A. Rivers, O.T.R., R.N., and Steven V. Fisher, M.D.

1. What is a burn and what different agents can cause it?

A burn is a permanent destruction of tissue proteins by an external agent. Thermal, electrical, chemical, and radiation energy cause burns. Heat injury accounts for 85–90% of civilian burns; frostbite, chemical, and electrical burns comprise most of the remainder. In the deepest burns, protein coagulation causes cell death. Lesser burned tissue has a surrounding area of stasis with potentially reversible changes, and very superficial burns have an area of hyperemia with little cellular compromise.

2. How common are burns?

Each year, about 1% of the populations sustains a burn. Annually, of every 70 burned adults, 1 is hospitalized. Home-related accidents account for one-third of all burn injuries. Over 2.5 million burn and fire-related injuries occur each year in the United States and Canada, affecting mostly young children and older adults. Burns are the number one cause of accidental deaths in children under 2, the second cause for those under 4, and the third leading cause for all those under 19. Every day, emergency rooms treat over 100 children for kitchen and scald burns.

3. How are burns classified?

First degree	Only the outer layers of epidermis are injured, sparing deeper layers. Erythematous, but no blistering.
Second degree	
Superficial partial thickness	Involves epidermis, but most of basal layer remains. Blistering.
Deep partial thickness	Involves the dermis; only the basal layer lining skin appendages remains. Blistering.
Third degree (full thickness)	Total destruction of epidermis and dermis.

The degree of burn describes the depth of the injury. Most injuries are of varying depths.

4. What factors can affect the severity or recovery from burns?

Patient age, total body surface area, associated injuries, and, to a lesser extent, burn depth and associated illnesses determine the severity of burn injury. The very young and the very old do not tolerate illness and trauma, particularly burn trauma, as well as those in the "prime" of life (10–50 years of age). Persons at the extremes of age are more fragile physiologically. They poorly tolerate massive fluid shifts and infectious complications associated with the burn and its treatment.

5. Which is the worst kind of burn?

Electrical burns are often deceptively deep, causing serious multiorgan damage relative to resistance, conductivity, and subsequent heat production.

6. Outline the clinical findings and treatments for the various degrees of burn injury.

Assessment and Treatment of Burn Injuries

DEPTH OF INJURY	HEALING TIME	PAIN	WOUND OUTCOME	TREATMENT MODALITIES
Superficial epidermis (1st degree)	1–5 days	Painful for 1-3 days Ibuprofen* or acetaminophen gives adequate analgesia	No sequela	Elevation decreases pain of limb Keep wound clean Aloe or other moisturizer reduces dry skin and itching If needed (usually in electrical injuries), therapy to prevent PTSD
Superficial dermis (2nd degree/ superficial partial-thickness)	14 days	Painful for 5–14 days Acetaminophen with codeine or oxycodone gives adequate analgesia for wound care, exercise, and sleep	Possible pigment changes	Wound care Active exercise Protective garments Sunscreen Therapy to prevent PTSD
Deep reticular dermis (2nd degree/ deep partial-thickness	21 days for spontaneous healing If grafted after 10–14 days, less scar formation will be noted, with improved functional outcome, less pain, and shortened hospital stay	Very painful until closure Methadone or oral morphine continuously for baseline pain control Parenteral or instant-release oral morphine and/or oxazepam and midazolam for dressing changes and stretching exercises	Probable pigment changes Reduced skin durability Severe scarring Sensory changes Apocrine changes Edema in dependent limbs	Wound care Antiinflammatories, analgesics, antipruritics Active exercise Elevated positioning/ orthotics External vascular support garments Moisturization and lubrication Daily living skills Psychological therapy Therapy to prevent PTSD
Subcutaneous tissue (3rd degree/ full-thickness)	Graft needed, or if small, undermine to approximate with primary closure Variable healing time	Nonpainful initially due to destruction of nerve endings Pain medication as above Carbamazepine, phenytoin, or amitriptyline	Same as above Additional sweating loss Possible loss of finger- or toenails Possible additional sensory loss Alopecia over grafts Areas of cultured epithelial autograft show permanent fragility, loss of temperature control, dry blisterable skin with changed sensation	Same as above Postop positioning/ immobilization Possible need for NSAIDs or etidronate disodium to prevent heterotopic ossification (controversial early treatment) Therapy to prevent PTSD Very slow weaning from analgesics and anxiolytics Vibration for pruritus

(Continued on following page.)

Assessment and Treatment of Burn Injuries (Continued)

DEPTH OF INJURY	HEALING TIME	PAIN	WOUND OUTCOME	TREATMENT MODALITIES
Muscle, tendon, bone (4th degree) [Old term in disfavor and rarely used]	Amputation or reconstructive surgery, such as flaps, needed Healing time variable	Nonpainful initially due to destruction of nerve endings Chronic pain treatment for neuromas and phantom limb pain and later bone spicules	Variable Early amputations with closure using noninjured tissue shortens hospital stay, decreases pain, and and improves prosthesis fit	Same as above Deep tendon massage Adapted equipment Prosthetic fitting if indicated

* Ibuprofen has the dual action of inflammation reduction at injury site and pain reception reduced at the CNS level.
PTSD = post-traumatic stress disorder; NSAIDs = nonsteroidal anti-inflammatory drugs.

7. How do electrical and chemical burns differ from thermal burns?

Conduction **electrical injury** is very different from thermal injury. The heat produced from electrical conduction is directly related to the current, resistance, and duration of current flow. Unlike thermal burns, electrical injuries often cause severe damage around underlying bone and in surrounding tissues. As the cross-sectional area decreases, the current density increases, thereby increasing the resistance and heat. For these reasons, the location of the thermal injury will be very different in electrical injuries; the wound may initially look minor but be very deep and devastating, resulting in limb loss. The incidence of neuropathies is higher, as is the incidence of post-traumatic stress disorder.

Although the etiology of **chemical burns** is different from that of thermal burns and the extent and depth of burn may be initially underestimated, the rehabilitation needs are similar. The healing burn may contract more than expected because of the depth of injury.

8. What is the "rule of nines"?

The rule of 9's is a convenient and fairly accurate way of estimating adult total body surface area (TBSA). The head, each arm, front of upper chest, back of chest to waist, abdomen, buttocks, front of leg, and back of leg each comprise 9% of the body and the perineum is 1%. A child's head represents a larger percentage and the legs a smaller percentage than in the adult.

Burn centers document the extent of a burn by a detailed chart, such as the Lund-Bowder. As a rough estimate, the patient's palm print, excluding the fingers, is approximately 0.5% of TBSA.

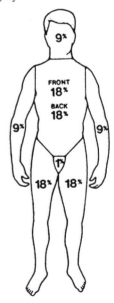

9. When is it time to graft?

Skin grafting is a method of achieving wound coverage by transferring tissue from an uninjured source. A burn wound that will not heal in 18–21 days typically requires skin grafting, since the final functional and cosmetic result of a skin graft is superior to the poor-quality skin covering obtained by spontaneous wound healing. Early wound closure reduces pain, length of hospital stay, wound infection, risk of scarring, and medical complications. Therefore, grafting, begins as soon as the patient is medically able to undergo the procedure.

10. What accommodations can the rehab program make to enhance the take of skin grafts?

The major goal of burn care is wound closure. All efforts to optimize the "take" or adherence of the graft are valuable. Some rehabilitation efforts are suspended during this period while the graft is immobilized for a minimum of 3–5 days postsurgery. Antigravity positioning of the affected limb optimizes graft take and maximizes functional outcome. For extremity grafts, immobilize the joint just proximal and just distal to the graft. Grafted areas placed in a dependent position in the first few days can develop subgraft edema with loss of the graft. For lower-extremity burns, many factors contribute to timing of ambulation, including surgeon preference, previous cellulitis, complicating medical problems, age, and quality of skin graft. From a rehabilitation perspective, "the earlier the better" without sacrificing the skin graft is the rule for movement. The overall rehabilitation process should continue on the nongrafted areas of the patient.

11. Do I need to look at the burn to determine the rehabilitation program?

Yes, you do. Not only should you see the wounds with the dressings off, but at least once a week you should see them with the surgeon while the wounds are exposed for care. The surgical and rehabilitation teams execute a comprehensive review of the healing process, pertinent range of motion, plans for therapy, and surgical procedures. This is an opportunity for the patient to participate with the team in overall planning. This minimizes the patient's focus on isolated problem areas.

Air-flow beds, positioning, and splining for the postoperative period should be discussed preoperatively. A decision concerning resuming exercises, ambulation, and other activities should be made as a team at the time of wound inspection. During visualization of the wounds, the rehabilitation plan is updated and the new goals are communicated to all concerned, including the patient.

12. What structures and functions are permanently altered in burned skin?

Consequences of Burn Injury by Depth of Burn

	ABSENT OR IMPAIRED MORPHOLOGY	WOUND CONSEQUENCES
Epidermis	Stratum basale	Source for proliferating cells
	Stratum spinosum	Decreased protection
	Stratum granulosum	Increased water loss
	Stratum corneum	Water loss, microorganism growth, entry of noxious agents
	Melanocytes	Repeated sunburn
Dermis (does not regenerate)	Altered collagen	Decreased tensile strength
	Increased collagen	Scarring
	Aging collagen	Altered surgical response
Nerves	Affected	Pruritus/paresthesias
	Absent	Decreased sensation, trauma, and burn risk
Vascular system	Impaired	Impaired (especially venous return)
	Absent	No healing (depends on area)
	Fragility	Reinjury risk
Basement membrane zone	Basal decidua and densa	Blisters
	Rete pegs and dermal papillae	Blisters, fragility
Epidermal appendages	Sweat ducts	Impaired thermoregulation
	Sebaceous glands	Loss of duct, sweat, and oil glands
	Hair follicle	Loss of hair root, resultant alopecia
Fingernail bed	Basal cells for proliferation absent	Malformed or absent nail

Adapted from Johnson CL: Wound healing and scar formation. In Campbell MK, Covey MH (eds): Topics in Acute Care and Trauma Rehabilitation. Frederick, MD, Aspen, 1987, 1(4):1–14.

13. Why do I have to worry about heterotopic ossification?

Heterotopic ossification (HO) is the ectopic formation of bone usually observed around joints and tendons. It is probably multifactorial, and its incidence in the burn population is variably reported to up to 23%. The location does not necessarily correlate with area of burn, but it is more common in larger burns and in patients whose wounds remain ungrafted for long periods of time. The early recognition and therapy using only active range of motion within the painfree arc is considered optimal for HO following a burn (see also the chapter on heterotopic ossification).

14. Can neuropathies be prevented?

The incidence of peripheral neuropathy is estimated at 15–30% in healed burn patients. Neuropathy occurs more commonly in patients with > 20% TBSA burns. Electrical burns exhibit a higher incidence of neuropathy. The etiology may be infectious, metabolic, nutritional, toxic, or drug-induced. Neuropathies caused by stretch and pressure from improper positioning or tight bulky dressings are preventable. The most commonly injured sites are the peroneal nerve at the fibular head and ulnar nerve at the elbow. Proper positioning to eliminate stretch and pressure to the brachial plexus will also reduce brachial plexopathies.

15. When an amputation is planned, is longer or bigger better?

Most surgeons are initially conservative in amputations and attempt to salvage all possible length. This is wise since demarcation of the possible level of limb salvage may not be immediately determined. However, definitive amputation should be planned with a physiatrist who is familiar with prosthetic fitting and function. **Longer is not necessarily better.** Excess fragile tissue may in fact be detrimental to proper fitting of a prosthesis. A stiff phalangeal remnant that is tender, lacks subcutaneous padding, or is covered with thin epithelium can interfere with hand function much more than an amputated digit.

16. Burn patients may take large amounts of narcotics for pain control. When should you suspect addiction?

Burn pain severity cannot be predicted but is influenced by the burn depth, location, patient age, gender, ethnicity, education, occupation, history of drug or alcohol abuse, and psychiatric illness. A burn medication protocol includes long-acting narcotics for background pain, short-acting opiates for procedural pain, as well as anxiolytics. Drug metabolism is markedly accelerated after a large burn. All medications including narcotics are quickly metabolized. It is surprising to inexperienced physicians when a severely burned child needs 40 mg of morphine an hour for pain during the second month of hospital care, but large doses are appropriate.

Studies have shown that the patient's perception of pain is often greater than the burn staff believe it to be, suggesting that the patient has been undermedicated. New narcotic addiction is rarely observed secondary to pain protocols for hospitalized burn patients. Wound healing is not the appropriate time for treatment of drug or alcohol abuse. Outpatient treatment when the patient is free to focus on life changes is more likely to be beneficial.

17. Is patient-controlled analgesia a reasonable choice for burn patients?

When the patient controls the pain medications received, frequency, vigor, and duration of supervised exercise improve. Patient-controlled analgesia (PCA) with IV morphine assists the patient to recover a sense of control. In many instances, the total dose of analgesic is actually reduced when a PCA pump is used. Patients with inadequate pain control learn to make submaximal efforts during exercise, focus (waste energy) in exhibiting pain behavior to get more drugs, and are less invested in self-care. Since narcotics are constipating, initiate a bowel program as part of patient management.

18. Is pruritus in a burned patient a bad sign?

Full-thickness burns do not hurt initially. As they debride, nerve endings deep in the wound are exposed. Once the open wound has reepithelialized or the area is grafted, itching, a form of pain, becomes problematic. Antihistamines aid in decreasing the histamine response. The antidepressant doxepin hydrochloride (Sinequan), has strong antihistamine properties and is prescribed for depression, commonly seen in burn patients, as well as pruritus.

19. A burned child on the unit has become obstreperous. What does this mean?

Children have pain and often few words to communicate it. Studies have indicated that children were given inadequate pain medication because it was believed they did not have pain.

When children do not receive sufficient pain medications, they become depressed, withdrawn, obstreperous (which is noisily defiant and stubborn), and difficult to focus toward independence.

20. Can scar tissue that develops over burned areas be prevented?

A hypertrophic scar is a hard, red, collagenous bundle of connective tissue raised above the surface of the burn wound. Myofibroblasts remain active in this hyperemic, dynamically remodeling wound 24 hours a day until some unknown factor causes their regression some 6–36 months after healing. The patient, family, and burn team must accept the challenge of continuing and prolonged round-the-clock diligence to achieve flat, soft, mobile, supple, light-colored, durable scars. Good outcomes can be expected if the people involved can maintain intensity, tenacity, and persistence greater than the scar tissue. A sense of humor is helpful to diffuse anger during this rigorous period.

21. Why are burns disfiguring?

Disfigurement is a change from normal tissue contour, color, and texture that can contribute to disability and handicap. Scarring is only a part of disfigurement, but a part that the rehabilitation team can help minimize. However, even after the wound is mature, hypopigmentation, hyperpigmentation, wrinkling of thinned skin, tethering of healed skin to underlying muscle, fascia, or tendon, and puckering of skin are noticeable sequelae. Pigmentation can be altered somewhat by reconstructive surgery, as can puckered skin or wrinkles. However, plastic surgery is more the art of camouflage than restoring original skin qualities to burned tissue. Patients often accept a friend's "myth" information about scar control rather than participate in rigorous rehabilitation programs. There are no magic treatments, ointments, vitamins, or minerals that will eliminate disfigurement. Friction massage on well-healed tissue helps remodel scars and prevents adhesions.

Cosmetic products enhance appearance and self-confidence for both male and female patients. These should never be considered unnecessary or frivolous. Especially if the patient has public contact at work, improved appearance will increase self-esteem and future successes. Accessories for camouflage, such as wigs, scarves, fashion gloves, adaptive clothing, and prosthetic foam covers, may be needed. Protection from sunburn is an additional benefit from camouflage make-up applied over the face, ears, nose, and neck.

22. Can the whirlpool help burn healing?

No. Whirlpools circulate water that can float dressings off. Although a time-honored tradition, generally accepted by patients and doctors alike, the whirlpool may actually be deleterious. Problems include bacteria multiplying in filters, skin maceration, potential damage to exposed joints or tendons, edema, and rebound stiffness.

23. Whirlpools are still useful for burn wound debridement. Right?

There is significant disagreement concerning submersion for mechanical burn debridement. Most burn centers use a spray technique that is easier on the medical team and, from a rehabilitation point of view, causes less edema, less rebound stiffness, and less pruritus. It moistens bandages to facilitate removal and provides gentle mechanical removal of exudate. Whatever means is used, adequate analgesia and a skilled, flexible technician are appreciated. Water should be 100° F and the duration of the bath limited. Avoid chilling, which further increases the already hypermetabolic load.

24. How far will the patient's own skin grow to cover a burn wound?

Epithelial cells proliferate from the remaining dermal rete pegs and dermal appendages (hair follicles and sebaceous glands). In full-thickness burns, the epithelium must migrate from the periphery. The cells migrate under a variety of stimuli, but no matter what the stimulus, the total distance they can migrate is about **1 cm**, growing at a rate of about 1 mm a day. Dead cells need to be removed to prevent vertical build up of skin cells.

25. Does eschar provide a protective covering for healing skin?

Dead dermis that remains attached to the wound bed is called **eschar** (pronounced *es-kar*, not *es-shar*). Eschar is not coagulated serum, bits of desiccated silver sulfadiazine, or other debris left on the wound after cleansing. It may be called scabs or any other descriptive name you choose. Since the wound cannot heal without white blood cells, platelets, and adequate levels of oxygen, ascorbic acid, zinc, copper, and growth factors, it must be kept free of eschar and significant infection, and blood flow must be optimized. All eschar should be removed as feasible. Cover clean open wounds with biological dressings to prevent desiccation.

26. Are pressure garments useful in preventing disfiguring scars over burned areas?

Pressure garments are elastic vascular support apparel. Patients sometimes believe wearing pressure garments will magically prevent disfigurement. Healed superficial burns or sheet grafts return to an appearance near the original, but most burns remain evident to an observer unless the person wears a covering make-up.

Vascular support garments protect the fragile maturing burn wound from trauma and promote smooth remodeling if worn around the clock. They help decrease itching, reduce edema, lessen hypertrophic scars, and speed wound healing. If external supports are to be effective, they must not be worn out, or out of fit, as is too often the case. They should be worn 24 hours a day. Initially after grafting or healing, a soft, slightly compressive garment, such as an Isotoner glove or bicycler's pants, toughens the healing area and prepares the patient for tighter supports, such as Tubigrip cotton and rubber or custom-measured Spandex garments.

All elastic support garments tend to tent over concave body contours, allowing these to fill in with scar tissue. Without diverse, interesting contours, the human body would look like a snowman and romance would be dead. Therefore, felt or silicone materials are used as inserts in support garments or as an overlay to push the garment into the appropriate contours, thereby reducing scarring and contracture bands. This helps restore original flexibility and appearance. Therefore, keeping the "kinks" is kinky.

27. What about therapeutic positioning?

Since edema is "glue," elevated, antigravity, antideformity positioning is essential. Alert patients accomplish their positioning program in planned activities, sitting, and walking. When patients are adequately sedated, they do not move enough to prevent decubiti and contractures or to enhance venous and lymphatic return. Proper positioning counteracts contracture by maintaining correct length of connective tissue. A series of individualized positions is designed to decrease pain and improve function. Positioning and splinting, however, never replace active exercise.

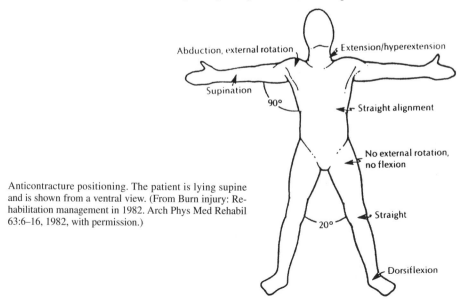

Anticontracture positioning. The patient is lying supine and is shown from a ventral view. (From Burn injury: Rehabilitation management in 1982. Arch Phys Med Rehabil 63:6–16, 1982, with permission.)

28. What is the best way to splint a typical clawed burned hand?

Since the usual clawed burned hand presents with hyperextension of the metacarpopha-langeal (MCP) joints, flexion of the proximal and distal interphalangeal joints (PIPs and DIPs), thumb adduction, and external rotation, an effective means of splinting is with a resting wrist-hand-finger orthosis with the wrist in slight extension, the MCPs in 40–90° of flexion, the PIPs and DIPs in full extension, and the thumb in palmar abduction.

29. How about CPM?

Continuous passive motion machines (CPM) decrease pain and increase recovery in ortho-pedic injury and are gaining popularity within the burn community. Technology is rapidly making improved machines with multiple functions available. Most of the machines can be set to pause at the end range to resemble slow prolonged stretch. Individuals who have burns involving multi-ple joints, comatose patients, and patients who refused active motion because of pain, swelling, or anxiety benefit from use of CPM in addition to customary physical and occupational therapy.

If on the first morning repetition, the burned patient is unable to flex the shoulder beyond 135°, use of a night **shoulder CPM** may be indicated. **Elbow CPMs** can statically maintain shoulder motion at 90° or above in a chair or bed while moving the elbow slowly through a pain-less range of motion. Since the machine provides low-load stretching and auto-reverse, there is little risk of trauma. **Hand CPMs** speed rehabilitation, prevent contractures, and do not interfere with healing. This passive finger motion with elevation is adequate to decrease hand edema. Adaptations can be made to block MCP or PIP motion or achieve composite MCP and PIP or DIP flexion. **Lower-extremity CPMs** are rarely needed for burn rehabilitation, since walking is a comfortable and nearly universally encouraged exercise.

30. A face mask is used to cover the disfigurement. Right?

No! Clear face or neck orthoses do not prevent infection either. These orthoses attempt to preserve normal face or neck contours, decrease itching, protect from sunburn, and, with adapta-tion, preserve corneal humidity with eye domes. A transparent facial orthosis worn 20 hours a day, to allow time for hygiene and eating, during the maturation phase of wound healing is one method to prevent distortion of facial contours. Fitting a transparent total-contact orthosis is a therapist-intensive four-step process, the most import of which is fitting the mask in a way that modifies scars, restores facial contours, and prevents eversion of the eyelids and lips.

31. Are there special considerations in a face burn microstomia?

A facially burned person can eat Big Macs again without adaptations. As with all other con-tractures, prevention is better than cure. Microstomia splints can prevent horizontal lip contrac-ture. Cheek pouches must be stretched with soft or solid cylinders several times a day. These also stretch the vertical oral opening. The inability to have dental work and the extreme difficulty of intubation for anesthesia are not motivating reasons for burn survivors to do their facial exercises. However, the inability to be understood by friends and family as well as the obvious cosmetic changes and difficulty kissing are hopefully motivating to the patient.

32. Are there any adverse effects of waterbeds?

A waterbed with wave action is not the most effective way to overcome problems of bedrest for burned patients.Waterbeds increase kyphotic chest positioning in bed, decrease full-chest ex-pansion during respiration, increase itching from warmth and sweating, obstruct antigravity posi-tioning devices, and require so much effort to exit that the patient may stay in bed.

33. How can bed positioning be used to minimize contractures?

Severely burned patients may be on bedrest for 5 or more days. Proper and varied bed posi-tioning decreases edema, minimizes contracture development, prevents dislocations, neu-ropathies, and decubiti, and prevents complications of bedrest such as pneumonia or phlebitis. The typical anticontracture bed positioning method consists of:

Neck extension (no pillow)
Shoulders abducted to 90° and forward flexed 15°
Elbows lacking 15° of extension and supinated
Wrists and hands in functional position
Hips extended and abducted 10° without external rotation
Knees in extension
Ankles at neutral
Consider all burned areas when planning positioning; no single position totally prevents contractures. Burn team members and the patient must communicate openly to provide time for medical treatments, occupational therapy and physical therapy, and appropriate rest periods.

34. No pain, no gain? Does this hold true for burn rehab, too?

"Walk? I've been burned. It hurts when I put my legs down," is commonly heard by burn therapists. Most importantly, this is not a time to skimp or reduce pain medications. The rehabilitation professional's job is teaching the patient that pain decreases with repetition; motion gets better as edema fluid is actively pumped out of extremities. Sleep improves with increased activity; complications such as pneumonia, phlebitis, and debilitation of bedrest are avoided; and people feel better doing activities independently. Once the patient experiences success and is provided with choices such as grippers, reciprocal pulleys, bike exercise, or work stimulation activity that gives the person control of the duration and frequency of activity, the battle is over.

If needed, tilt-table positioning begins before grafting is completed. Despite intravenous lines, a bladder catheter, chest tubes, and feeding tubes, tilt-table exercise combined with functional activities distracts the person from wanting to return to bed. People also learn that although pain was important to get them to the treatment center, it now can be tuned down through a variety of behavioral interventions, such as hypnosis, imagery, relaxation, and music. Family members and the patient supply important information about the individual's past and present thoughts, feelings, wants, needs, and learning style which contribute to more effective rehabilitation. Patient and family education decreases apprehension and improves motivation for those with readiness and ability to learn.

35. List the rehabilitation goals for outpatient burn care.

1. Assist in non-narcotic analgesia
2. Maintain wound closure
3. Prevent infection
4. Control edema
5. Regain joint and skin mobility
6. Regain strength and endurance
7. Facilitate resumption of family roles
8. Resume independent self-care
9. Fit total-contact, stretching orthoses to minimize hypertrophic scars
10. Learn compensation techniques for exposure to friction, trauma, ultraviolet light, chemical irritants, extremes of weather or temperature
11. Develop awareness of sensory changes
12. Fit prostheses
13. Develop a plan for return to part-time modified or full-time work, school, or play
14. Continue counseling to deal with the psychological stresses of living with permanently changed appearance, altered ability levels, and difficulties with stress symptoms

36. Discuss the psychological effects seen in burn patients.

There can be serious long-term psychological effects of a burn. Normal responses to a major burn injury include crying, degrees of fear, depression, grief, and loss of hope. Discharged patients report that it takes months of being at home before they can cope, as they did before the injury, with emotions and activities that require concentration. Distractibility gradually subsides.

Impatience, irritability, and frustration are common. Psychological adjustment for returning to work in an area where the injury occurred must be considered. Few people will return easily to the injury site. In addition, patients note that sexuality and sexual counseling is a crucial problematic issue that is their least attended need. Outpatient counseling provides interventions for depression, anger, grieving, and changed sexual function. Premorbid drug or alcohol abuse is best aggressively managed in an outpatient setting.

37. What are the criteria for post-traumatic stress disorder?

There is a high incidence of post-traumatic stress disorder (PTSD) among recently burned patients. This syndrome is defined in the DSM-IV with the following criteria:

1. Person exposed to trauma
2. Trauma is re-experienced
3. Avoidance of stimuli associated with the trauma and numbing of general responsiveness
4. Persistent symptoms of increased arousal
5. Duration of disturbance > 1 month
6. Disturbance causes clinical distress or impairment

The burn patient responds to a recognizable stressor that evokes the distress symptoms. In addition, he or she experiences vivid, intrusive dreams or recollections of the incident. Other frequently noted characteristics are an exaggerated startle response, impaired memory, concentration problems, avoiding cues of the accident, withdrawal from normal social interaction, and withdrawal from chores at home, tasks at work, or participation in work.

Treatment is aimed at giving the patient as many choices as reasonably possible during recovery, thereby relieving a sense of helplessness. Stress reduction strategies and goal-directed individual counseling are also beneficial. Short-term pharmacologic intervention is appropriate.

38. When should a burn patient return to work?

Return to work at the earliest possible time maximizes the benefits of peer support, routine, and work, although few people will return easily to the site of injury. Considerations for return to work include

1. Open wounds (these are not permitted in food handlers)
2. Skin fragility
3. Heat and cold intolerance
4. Chemical sensitivity
5. Decreased standing tolerance
6. Reduced coordination, dexterity, strength
7. Sensory impairment
8. Post-traumatic stress disorder
9. Reduced endurance
10. Visual impairment
11. Prosthetic training complete

Rating permanent impairment is a physician's function. Disability or handicap is related to performance loss, preinjury age, education, economic and social situation, sex, and the burned person's attitude toward recovery. The physician has the final responsibility in determining when it is medically safe for the person to return to work. Appraising the extent of the burn injury and objectively estimating residuals that affect performance are most accurate when based on objective evaluation and experienced prediction.

39. What equipment or techniques are required to protect the person with healing burns in the outdoor environment?

Prevent cold injuries:
• Keep vehicle well-maintained
• Blankets, extra mittens, warm clothing, candles, snacks
• Insulated, waterproof boots

- Hats or insulated hood
- Multiple-layer, nonrestrictive clothing
- Wind-resistant fabric
- Avoid vasodilating drugs such as alcohol and vasoconstricting drugs such as cigarettes

Prevent sun exposure injuries:
- Work in shaded area
- Apply sunscreen
- Wear light-colored lightweight nonrestrictive clothing
- Sandal shoes
- Cool flap hat or wide-brimmed hat
- Battery fan, spray bottle
- Sunglasses
- Drink more fluids
- Avoid vasoconstricting drugs such as cigarettes

40. Do children really return to school after being burned?

School and play are the work of children. After an injury a child needs to go back to school as soon as possible despite injuries, splints, scars, and ongoing therapies. Early reintegration promotes a positive body image and prevents maladaptive, inappropriate behavior. There are professionals in every school system whose job it is to include the child in regular school activity.

A summer camp is an important exercise for burn survivors to assist them in healing their emotional scars and to improve their quality of life. After their injury, contact with other burned kids dilutes the pain of being the only kid who looks different.

BIBLIOGRAPHY

1. Achauer BM: Reconstructing the burned face. Clin Plastic Surg 19(30):623–636, 1992.
2. Campbell MK, Covey MH (eds): Topics in Acute Care and Trauma Rehabilitation: Burn Trauma. Frederick, MD, Aspen, 1987.
3. Fisher SV, Helm PA (eds): Comprehensive Rehabilitation of Burns. Baltimore, Wilkins & Williams, 1984.
4. Heimbach DM, Engrav LH: Surgical Management of the Burn Wound. New York, Raven Press, 1984.
5. Helm PA, Kevorkian CG, Lushbaugh M, et al: Burn injury: Rehabilitation management in 1982. Arch Phys Med Rehabil 63:000, 1982.
6. Jordan CL, Allely R, Gallagher J: Self-care strategies following severe burns. In Christiansen C (ed): Ways of Living. Bethesda, MD, AOTA, 1994.
7. Kloth LC, McCulloch JM, Feedar JA: Wound healing: Alternatives in management. In Wolf SL (ed): Contemporary Perspectives in Rehabilitation. Philadelphia, F.A. Davis, 1990.
8. Richard RL, Staley MJ: Burn Care and Rehabilitation: Principles and Practice. Philadelphia, F.A. Davis, 1994.
9. Ward RS: Pressure therapy for the control of hypertrophic scar formation after burn injury: A history and review. J Burn Care Rehabil 12:257–262, 1991.
10. Watkins PN, Cook E, May SR, Ehleben CM: Psychological stages in adaptation following burn injury: A method for facilitating psychological recovery of burn victims. J Burn Care Rehabil 9:376, 1988.

79. GERIATRIC REHABILITATION

Barry D. Stein, M.D., and Gerald Felsenthal, M.D.

1. What does the aging population mean to rehab medicine?

Adults who need rehabilitation are often older than 65 years. In 1990, nearly 13% of the U.S. population (> 30 million) were ≥ 65 years of age, and their number is increasing all the time. By the year 2020, 17% (52 million) of the U.S. population may be > 65.

The subgroup of those aged ≥ 85 years will increase the most by 2020; from the current 3.3 million to 7 million. These oldest people have the greatest prevalence of functional impairments, with greater use of health care resources. The percentage of people with mobility or activities of daily living (ADL) impairments greatly increases between ages 65–85. In the United States, 70–80% of the elderly population live in the community and not in nursing homes.

2. What are the effects of normal aging on the various systems?

Heart and lungs: Decreased cardiac reserve, contractile function, and pulmonary vital capacity, along with increased blood pressure, are mainly due to **disease**, not aging. Some age-associated changes include left-ventricular hypertrophy, decreased beta-adrenoceptor-mediated cardiovascular responses, cardiac dysrhythmias with exercise, and possible limited left-ventricular filling due to increased pericardial and myocardial stress.

Skin: We wrinkle more. With the decreased blood flow, epidermal renewal, skin sensations (pain, touch, temperature), elasticity, and moisture, pressure sores and infection are more likely.

Hydration and urinary system: We get less thirsty and have decreased thirst perception, resulting in potential dehydration and constipation. Elderly bladders often have a smaller capacity and larger post-voiding residual (PVR) volume. Prostatic hypertrophy, in men, can worsen PVRs. So, the result is more frequent trips to the bathroom at night, frequency, hesitancy, and retention. Renally excreted drugs are more toxic in people with reduced renal function.

Fat: As we age, our bodies lose muscle and gain fat—an increase from 15% fat at age 30 to 30% fat at age 80. The aged have more retention of fat-soluble drugs with greater side effects.

Temperature regulation: The elderly are more susceptible to hyperthermia and hypothermia and may have a blunted temperature response to infection.

3. How does aging affect the components of the neuromusculoskeletal system?

Bones: Peak bone mineral density drops after the mid-30s. The hips develop a valgus deformity, with widening of the base of stance.

Muscles: Total body muscle mass, muscle cross-sectional area, and muscle fiber numbers decrease. There is a longer twitch contraction, slower rate of relaxation, and increased fatigability. Muscle strength decreases throughout the body. Diminished muscle strength in limb girdle muscles, especially hip extensors, results in more difficulty in arising. Decreased grip and triceps strength means more difficulty in using a cane or walker.

Neurologic system: Nerve conduction velocity decreases. There is increased postural sway, decreased righting reflexes, and increased reaction time with age. There is loss of upward gaze and occasional loss of ankle jerks and vibratory sense in the feet. Older people's center of gravity on standing shifts to behind the hips, due to changes in posture. To reduce the chance of loss of balance, assistive devices (such as a cane) may be needed.

4. What factors should be considered in writing an exercise prescription for an elderly patient?

A physiatrist should review the goals of exercising, the patient's diagnosis, any contraindications to exercise (i.e., untreated or unstable cardiovascular disease), and any precautions (such as monitoring the heart rate and blood pressure due to cardiac precautions).

The exercise prescription should include warm-up and cool-down exercises as well as lower training intensities than in younger patients. Exercise testing for those individuals with known cardiac disease or with two or more risk factors has been recommended by the American College of Sports Medicine. In a rehabilitation setting, those recovering from stroke, fracture, or other major diagnoses may be monitored by pulse, blood pressure, and exertion responses to exercises.

5. What factors should you consider in prescribing medicines for older persons?

An older person has changes in liver and kidney function, absorption, and body distribution of medications, often making the effects and side effects of drugs more prominent. One important reason for unwanted medication effects is **polypharmacy**. This may be from multiple illnesses, multiple physicians, substance abuse, patient confusion, nonprescription drugs, or herbal compounds used in addition to prescription medicines. Asking the patient or family member to bring in all medications, vitamins, and other nonprescription products from the home for medical review can be a critical factor in streamlining medication use. Elderly patients in a rehabilitation program often demonstrate significant improvement in function only after changing their medication regimen.

6. Should any special measurements of function be used in the elderly?
In addition to other assessment tools used in PM&R, consider:
- **Mini-Mental State Exam**, a 30-point scale measuring attention, orientation, recall, calculation, and visual perception.
- **Geriatric Depression Scale**, a 30-point scale for common symptoms of depression.
- Other scales for **cognition** and **mood**.
- Specific **gait** and **balance** tests, which show a person's mobility function better than neuromuscular testing in a typical physical examination.

7. Describe some abnormal changes of gait that occur with aging.
In addition to the normal aspects of aging, changes can develop that reflect weakened musculature and altered posture. Men often develop a wider base of support and small steps. Women may develop a "waddling" gait with a small base of support. There is a shorter "swing" phase of walking, with more time that both feet are contacting the ground. With postural changes, the energy cost for walking is greater. Illness superimposed on a person's functional loss can result in additional gait deviations.

8. List some gait deviations that are attributable to disease.

Gait Deviations with Illness

Circumduction	Stroke
Scissoring	Upper motor nerve disease
Festinating	Parkinson's disease
Ataxia	Cerebellar disease Cervical spondylosis Vitamin deficiency
Apraxia	Stroke Normal-pressure hydrocephalus
Waddling	Muscle weakness

9. How serious are falls?
Falls are the most feared problem of elderly people, after the fear of loss of independence. One-third of the elderly have falls or near-falls. Injuries occur in 10–20% of falls, and fractures occur in 3–5%. Like congestive heart failure, falls are a **symptom** and may be a **sign** of one or more serious problems.

The physiatrist needs to be aware of the causes of falls as well as their rehabilitation. One should try to implement educational, preventive, and corrective measures (such as added assistants and adjustments to the home environment). If a fracture results in sufficient loss of functional ability, that person cannot return home safely.

Falls can also cause new problems, even if there is no fracture or painful bruising. A fall often causes fear of falling, with a resulting "shut-in" attitude: social isolation, immobility, and increased weakness. These, in turn, increase the chance of yet another fall.

10. What are some causes of falls in the elderly?

The mnemonic **IDEAS** is a useful guide to investigating the reasons for falls.

I ILLNESS	D DRUGS	E ENVIRONMENTAL	A AGING	S SOCIAL/LIFESTYLE
Strokes	Benzodiazepines	Poor lighting	Decreased:	Isolation
Syncope	Anticholinergic	Uneven surfaces	Vision	Bedrest
Parkinson's	drugs	Slippery surfaces	Strength	Exercise
disease	Many tricyclics	Obstacles (trip/fall)	Balance	Nutrition
Dementia	Many antipsychotics	Poor weather	Reaction time	Alcoholism
Delirium	Bladder detrusor	Crime (assault and	Motor control	Other drug abuse
Depression	anticholinergic	battery)	Hearing	Shoe style
Arthritis	drugs			
Paraparesis	Antivertigo drugs			
Previous leg	Barbiturates			
fractures	Other potentially			
Normal pressure	CNS-depressing			
hydrocephalus	drugs			

11. What are the risk factors for fractures in the older person?

Osteoporosis and falls.

12. How do fractures in the elderly differ from those seen in younger populations? Why?

Generally, hip and pelvic fractures tend to occur in older persons and humeral and Colles' fractures in younger people. This difference in fracture site may be due to younger people's walking faster and having faster protective responses than older people. Having a faster walking speed and then tripping with arms outstretched may result in upper-extremity fractures. A slower walking speed with a fall straight down may result in a fracture at the pelvic or hip region. Major fractures is one of the most common reasons for a temporary stay in a comprehensive inpatient rehab setting or a subacute rehab service.

13. How prevalent is pain in the elderly? How does it differ in this population?

Serious pain is a common problem, affecting 75% of nursing home residents. Musculoskeletal pain is the most common type of pain you will encounter. In your evaluation, remember secondary gain or hidden agendas in the elderly (loneliness, family vacations) and specific problems found frequently in the older population (hearing loss, dementia, delirium, depression, and underreporting of symptoms). Radiographic and laboratory tests can be complicated by agitation, contractures, and inaccessible veins. Physical medicine techniques should be the cornerstone of treatment of musculoskeletal pain in the elderly, due to the greater risk of medication in this age group.

14. Name four common reasons for neuromusculoskeletal spinal pain in the elderly.

- Spondylosis—present in up to 82% of persons by their 50s
- Cervical disc degeneration—most commonly C5–6 > C6–7 > C4–5
- Cervical spondylitic myelopathy—most common reason for spinal cord dysfunction over age 55
- Lumbosacral spinal stenosis—common; look for:
  1. Bilateral symptoms worse when standing or walking
  2. Sitting or flexing the spine while standing relieves symptoms

15. List the common reasons for neuromusculoskeletal limb pain in the elderly.

A. Shoulder—present in at least 25% of the elderly
  1. Cervical spondylosis
  2. Arthritis of the acromioclavicular joint
  3. Rotator cuff tendinitis or tears, with or without radiculopathy

    4. Cervical radiculopathy of C5 and/or C6
    5. Chronic tendinitis or bursitis
    6. Medical problems such as after myocardial infarction or with reflex sympathetic dystrophy
  B. Elbow, wrist, hand
    1. C7 radiculopathy
    2. Medial or lateral epicondylitis
    3. Median or ulnar nerve entrapment
    4. deQuervain's tenosynovitis
    5. Arthritis, especially of the first carpometacarpal joint
    6. Carpal tunnel syndrome, sometimes with arthritis
  C. Hip and pelvis
    1. Arthritis
    2. Trochanteric bursitis
    3. Radiculopathy at L5 or S1
    4. Falls with fractures
  D. Knee
    1. Arthritis
    2. Trauma (sometimes even trivial) leading to meniscal tears and/or ligamentous strain
    3. Bursitis (there are > 30 bursae about the knee)
  E. Ankle and foot
    1. Painful calluses
    2. Tarsal tunnel syndrome
    3. Tibialis posterior tenosynovitis
    4. Metatarsalgia
    5. Plantar heel spur

16. What considerations are appropriate for an elderly person with arthritis?

Joints in the elderly, even without arthritis, may have decreased ROM due to loss of elasticity in the tendons, ligaments, and capsules surrounding the joint. ROM exercises for joints should be done initially at a few degrees of stretch and be gentle. The patient may resist needed assistive devices such as canes because of the stigma of disability. If he or she can be shown that pain is reduced with the use of the device, the patient may at least use it privately, although perhaps not publicly.

Minimum ROMs for Major Joints

UPPER EXTREMITY		LOWER EXTREMITY	
Shoulder:	90° abduction	Hip:	90° flexion
	Touch lower back (internal rotation)		Extension to neutral
	Touch back of head (external rotation)	Knee:	110° flexion
Forearm:	45° pronation		Extension to neutral
	45° supination	Ankle:	Dorsiflexion to neutral
Wrist:	45° flexion		
	30° extension		
Hand:	Finger flexion to within 1 inch of palm		

17. What exercises or modalities are appropriate for an elderly person with spinal osteoporosis?

Acute symptomatic osteoporosis from vertebral fractures can be treated with brief bedrest and physical modalities. Flexion exercises for this population are not recommended due to the possibility of vertebral wedge fractures.

18. What factors can complicate the elderly person's recovery from stroke?

Older persons are at greater risk of institutionalization after stroke than younger persons. Multi-infarct dementia, cardiovascular disease, impaired auditory and visual abilities, polypharmacy, osteoarthritis, skin ulceration, and social stress can greatly affect the older stroke patient's recovery.

19. How does traumatic brain injury in the elderly differ from that in younger persons?

The most common cause of traumatic brain injury (TBI) in those > 65 years of age is **falling**. Alcohol is often a precipitating factor. As with stroke, concurrent illnesses, including fractures and seizures, can increase the severity of the illness. Avoiding the possibility of another fall is a major goal to prevent further TBI and fractures. Family involvement is critical in optimizing recovery. Reemployment is usually not a goal in the elderly.

20. Peripheral neuropathy becomes prevalent with aging. Tell me more.

Approximately three-quarters of the elderly have decreased vibratory sense and/or ankle muscle stretch reflexes. Muscle atrophy is often seen. Electrodiagnostic changes in the aged are found. Appropriate exercise in the elderly is successful in strengthening neuropathic muscles. Energy conservation and carefully graded exercises are also important.

21. What is post-polio syndrome?

More than 50% of persons who had paralytic poliomyelitis develop progressive fatigue, pain, loss of function, and, occasionally, muscle atrophy 30–40 years after the initial episode. This is called post-polio syndrome and requires interdisciplinary care, including strengthening, conservative pain treatment including physical medicine techniques, orthoses, psychological care, and sometimes a pulmonologist's evaluation.

22. What are the issues to consider in the older patient with spinal cord injury?

Survivors of spinal cord injury (SCI) over 55 years old are more likely to have medical problems. Greater age is statistically associated with lesser skills in SCI with bathing, dressing, complex transfers, and stair climbing. Psychological and social issues in aging are compounded by a SCI.

23. And with multiple sclerosis?

Age-related losses in lower motor nerve innervation, muscle atrophy, and decreased cardiopulmonary reserves compound the weakness and fatigue of multiple sclerosis (MS). Exercise for general fitness is important. Elderly persons with MS have to cope with such problems as additionally diminished special senses, impairments of genitourinary and gastrointestinal systems, decreased skin sensation, cognitive impairment, and affective disorders. Psychological issues of aging compound the psychological, vocational, financial, and recreational issues with MS.

24. How are hearing and vision affected in aging?

There is a 25–50% incidence of significant hearing loss in persons > 65 years of age. Often people refuse hearing aids because of sound distortion, uncomfortable fit, impaired finger dexterity to use or adjust, or vanity. Decreased hearing is also associated with paranoia.

Vision is a major factor in balance, with impaired vision increasing the risk of falling. Impaired vision concurrent with a mobility problem, such as stroke or amputation, is especially challenging. Social isolation and reduced self-image can result from impairments in hearing and vision. Visual rehabilitative services can alleviate some of the disability from cataracts, age-related macular degeneration, glaucoma, and diabetic retinopathy.

25. Describe the geriatric foot and lower extremity circulation.

The geriatric foot is more than simply an issue for the shoe salesman, and lower-extremity problems with painful, functional loss will be seen in your patients. Bony disfigurement, arthritis, neural entrapment syndromes, diabetic neuropathy, muscle problems, and skin problems can cause pain and injury. Proper foot care by the patient, including appropriate shoes with appropriate orthoses as needed and, for diabetic patients, regular skin inspection, is part of the spectrum of care. Skin ulceration needs careful, aggressive care. Those patients with insufficient vision to inspect their feet or with lack of dexterity, cognitive skills, or emotional desire to care for their feet will need another person's assistance.

26. What are some common causes of urinary incontinence in the elderly?

Common Causes of Transient Urinary Incontinence

POTENTIAL CAUSES	COMMENT
Delirium (confusional state)	In the delirious patient, incontinence is usually an associated symptom that will abate with proper diagnosis and treatment of the underlying cause of confusion.
Infection (symptomatic urinary tract infection	Dysuria and urgency from symptomatic infection may defeat the older person's ability to reach the toilet in time. Asymptomatic infection, although more common than symptomatic infection, is rarely a cause of incontinence.
Atrophic urethritis or vaginitis	Both may present as dysuria, dyspareunia, burning on urination, urgency, agitation (in demented patients), and, occasionally, incontinence. Both disorders are readily treated by conjugated estrogen administered either orally or locally.
Pharmaceuticals Sedative hypnotics	Benzodiazepines, especially long-acting agents such as flurazepam and diazepam, may accumulate in elderly patients and cause confusion and secondary incontinence. Alcohol, frequently used as a sedative, can cloud the sensorium, impair mobility, and induce a diuresis, resulting in incontinence.
Diuretics	A brisk diuresis incuded by loop diuretics (furosemide, ethacrynic acid, and bumetanide) can overwhelm bladder capacity and lead to polyuria, frequency, and urgency, thereby precipitating incontinence in a frail older person.

Adapted from Agency for Health Care Policy and Research: Urinary Incontinence in Adults: Clinical Practice Guidelines, no. 2. Rockville, MD, U.S. Public Health Service, 1992, p 7.

27. Who benefits from rehabilitative services?

Matching patients to the most appropriate intensity and location of care for their needs is not an exact science. Patient goals should be functionally significant and achievable in a reasonable amount of time. Motivation in the elderly is often more successful when concrete goals (getting out of bed or to the toilet) are emphasized instead of abstract goals (improving balance or dexterity). Knowing what the patient values is the key to integrating patient and team goals successfully. Management, rather than cure, of the multiple impairments of the older person is emphasized.

Problems with bladder or bowel incontinence and/or dementia *may* preclude successful rehabilitation to the community and result in institutionalization.

28. Name three factors that are important determinants in ultimate discharge to a noninstitutional setting.

ADL status

Cognitive, judgment, and safety status

Social support system

Often, these factors have not reached their potential until a rehabilitative program has been tried with the patient. The amount of frailty of the patient, family expectations, and resources are considered. Each patient should therefore have a plan tailored to their needs.

BIBLIOGRAPHY

1. Clark GS, Siebens HC: Rehabilitation of the Geriatric Patient. In DeLisa JA (ed): Rehabilitation Medicine: Principles and Practice, 2nd ed. Philadelphia, J.B. Lippincott, 1993.
2. Cummings SR, Nevitt MC: A hypothesis: The causes of hip fractures. J Gerontol 44:M107–111, 1989.
3. Felsenthal G, Garrison S, Steinberg F (eds): Rehabilitation of the Aging and Elderly Patient. Baltimore, Williams & Wilkins, 1994.
4. Felsenthal G, Stein BD: Rehabilitation of dysmobility in the elderly: A case study of the patient with a hip fracture. In Brody SJ, Paulson LG (eds): Aging and Rehabilitation II: The State of the Practice. New York, Springer, 1990.
5. Felsenthal G, Stein BD: Principles of Geriatric Rehabilitation. In Braddom R (ed): Textbook of Physical Medicine and Rehabilitation. Philadelphia, W.B. Saunders, 1996.

80. WOMEN'S ISSUES IN REHABILITATION

Martin Z. Kanner, M.D., and Melinda-Ann B. Roth, M.D.

1. Who was Pomona, and why is she important to physiatrists?

Pomona was the Greek goddess of fruit trees. Quite appropriately, this symbol of fertility lends her name to a mnemonic that covers the majority of women's conditions treated by physiatrists:

P = **P**regnancy and postpartum

O = **O**steoporosis

M = **M**astectomy rehabilitation

O = **O**steoarthritis

N = **N**erve pain (carpal tunnel syndrome)

A = **A**thletic injuries

In addition, females have fibromyalgia in much greater numbers than males.

2. Why do women have back pain during pregnancy?

As the body adapts to the growing fetus, stresses are placed on the back, hips, and pelvic joints. Back pain is produced by a combination of factors including the dramatic weight gain, a shift in the center of gravity as the fetus fills the abdominal cavity, and laxity of the pelvic, abdominal, and paraspinal muscles. Instability of the sacroiliac joint or the development of osteitis condensans ilii may also cause back pain during pregnancy. Sciatica frequently develops due to the shift of the fetus toward the sciatic notch as pregnancy progresses.

3. Are any of the conventional physical therapy modalities contraindicated during pregnancy?

Ultrasound, electrical stimulation, and intermittent pelvic traction may carry certain risks for the fetus. On areas other than the back or pelvis, however, all of the conventional modalities may be used safely.

4. Should a previously active woman continue to exercise during pregnancy?

Yes. Continuing physical activities as much as possible during pregnancy is to be encouraged, provided that appropriate modifications are made to avoid jeopardizing the fetus' health or the viability of the pregnancy. Certain activities that may be engaged in safely during the first and second trimester, however, should probably be avoided during the third trimester.

5. What are the limitations, restrictions, and contraindications of exercise during pregnancy?

During pregnancy, large concentrations of circulating estrogens and relaxin prepare the uterus and pelvis for delivery by enhancing ligamentous laxity. This same laxity is found in other collagen-containing structures. (Witness, for example, the frequent development of venous varicosities during pregnancy.) Thus, specific stretching exercises, particularly to the knees, should be avoided during pregnancy. The ligaments may become "overstretched" due to their abnormally lax state.

During aerobic exercise, increased oxygen demands by the peripheral musculature may lead to blood flow shifting away from the gravid uterus, creating transient fetal hypoxia. Therefore, the pregnant athlete should keep her target heart rate at about 60–70% that of her previously attained aerobic peak. High impact aerobics, exercises in the supine position, and scuba diving should be avoided.

6. How can the physiatrist help the postpartum woman?

After pregnancy, the stretched and weakened muscles of the abdomen and pelvis may require reconditioning. Some women actually develop diastasis recti. Physiatrists can prescribe specific exercise programs, including strengthening exercises for the abdomen, Kegel exercises for the weakened vaginal walls, and strengthening of the pubococcygeal muscles in a progressive program. Special weighted cones have been devised to aid in the strengthening of these muscles and to take advantage of the well-established principle of progressive resistive exercise. Strengthening of these muscles also helps in eliminating or reducing postpartum stress incontinence.

7. List seven areas of special consideration in the pregnant spinal-cord-injured woman.

1. **Autonomic dysreflexia** (if the lesion is above T6) may occur in response to noxious stimuli below the level of the injury, such as labor and delivery. This can be treated either by blood pressure-lowering medication (remember to keep the head up) or, if severe, by giving epidural anesthesia and performing a cesarean section.

2. **Bladder** management is affected as the uterus enlarges and presses against the bladder, affecting its ability to fill. Urinary tract infections become more frequent, and their treatment may cause vaginal yeast infections that require treatment. Women who perform intermittent catheterization will likely find this more difficult, as their enlarging abdomen obstructs their view and reach.

3. **Bowel** management may require a change as pregnancy tends to slow the bowel and may cause changes in food and fluid intake and general activity level.

4. **Mobility**—specifically transfers, pressure relief, and manual wheelchair propulsion—are variably affected depending on the injury level and weight gain. Most patients require additional assistance in the last months of pregnancy. Manual wheelchair users will be more apt to develop carpal tunnel syndrome during pregnancy.

5. **Spasticity** may become problematic during labor and delivery if it interferes with positioning for vaginal delivery. Medications used to treat spasticity should be reviewed during pregnancy to assess fetal risk.

6. **Skin breakdown** can occur as increased size and weight impair mobility and pressure relief. There also has been reported dehiscence of episiotomies.

7. Significant **lower-extremity edema** and **thrombophlebitis** are greater concerns because of bilateral lower-extremity paralysis.

8. What are the special considerations in the pregnant traumatic-brain-injured woman?

Bowel, bladder, spasticity, and mobility considerations are much the same as in the spinal-cord-injured woman. Special considerations regarding mobility in these women also extend to those who are ambulatory, as their balance will be affected by their forward-shifting center of gravity, putting some at a greater risk of falls.

9. What osteoporosis-related complications does the physiatrist treat?

The physiatrist frequently treats nonpainful and painful conditions related to osteoporosis, including postural abnormalities, loss of flexibility, and pain syndromes following compression fractures of the vertebrae and ribs. The physiatrist frequently aids in the rehabilitation of patients who have sustained osteoporotic fractures of the humerus and radius. These patients may develop, respectively, frozen shoulders or peripheral nerve injuries. Often it is the physiatrist who directs the care of the post-hip fracture patient in a progressive ambulation program.

10. Can exercise increase bone density? Reduce fractures?

Without question, a decrease in weight-bearing activity leads to a decrease in bone density. Other studies have shown that appropriate weight-bearing exercises can successfully increase bone mineral density or, at least, slow the loss of bone mineral density.

Although intuitively logical, it is uncertain whether an exercise regimen leading to increased bone density actually leads to a decreased number of fractures. Inappropriate exercise, such as programs emphasizing flexion of the spine, may actually lead to an increase in vertebral fractures, as this increases the load on the vertebral body.

11. Name the most common sites of osteoporotic fractures.

Thoracic and lumbar spine (500,000/yr)
Hip fractures (300,000/yr)
Wrist fractures (200,000/yr)
Miscellaneous fractures (including ribs, humerus, and ankles) (300,000/yr)

12. Which fracture site is the most serious?

In terms of morbidity and mortality, **hip** fractures are the most feared. Some 15–25% of women who sustain hip fractures lose independence within the first year. Fifty percent require nursing home placement, and of these, half remain in a nursing home after 1 year. There is a 12–20% mortality rate, either directly or due to complications after hip fracture.

13. Describe simple preventive measures to reduce the risk of falls in osteoporotic women.

To prevent falls, measures such as handrails for stairs, both indoors and out; good, safe, stable lace-up Oxford shoes; avoidance of high heels; well-lit stairwells, removal of household hazards such as throw rugs and loose electrical cords, and use of tub benches and toilet-seat grab-bars are simple and inexpensive. Interestingly, instruction in tai chi in certain nursing homes and other group settings appears to enhance a patient's balance and decrease falls.Of course, the use of assistive devices for ambulation, including standard walking canes, walkers, tripod and quadriped canes, are all helpful preventive measures, although these are usually resisted on an emotional basis by patients.

14. Why do more women develop osteoarthritis than men?

Osteoarthritis is a degenerative condition of the bones, joints, and disks, and by definition degenerative conditions worsen over time. Women in the United States have a life expectancy of 79.7 years compared with 72.8 years for men. In 1992, of all people in the United States over age 65, 67.8% were female. By the year 2000, this percentage is projected to reach 70.5%. Therefore, not only are there **more women** in the geriatric age category than men, but they have a **longer lifespan** over which to manifest degenerative changes.

15. Are there special considerations in treating osteoarthritis in women?

Yes. Frequently, osteoarthritis coexists with osteoporosis in the geriatric-age woman. Spinal extension exercises that may **help** women with osteoporosis may **aggravate** exiting spinal nerve roots by decreasing the size of neural foramina. By the same mechanism, the extension braces used in treating women with osteoporotic fractures may aggravate osteoarthritic spurs.

16. After mastectomy, what complications might a woman expect?

The most common reasons that mastectomy patients present to physiatrists postsurgically include painful scar formation, lymphedema, frozen shoulder, and weakness in the upper extremity on the side of the mastectomy. Fortunately, over the years, less radical and more limited surgical procedures have evolved, and there has been a greatly decreased frequency of lymphedema. In the past, the lymphedema, in conjunction with a frozen shoulder, often led to reflex sympathetic dystrophy.

17. How can a physiatrist help in the rehabilitation of the postmastectomy patient?

For painful **scars**, the physiatrist can frequently prescribe a physical therapy program for use at home, which includes the use of topical anesthetics such as fluoromethane spray, counter-irritants such as capsaicin, and friction massage with and without cocoa butter directly to the scar line. The use of compressive gradient pumping devices, followed by manual massage distally to proximally and the use of elastic wraps in the same direction, frequently is helpful in reducing **lymphedema**. Range of motion exercises, wand exercises, upper body ergometers, and shoulder wheels are helpful in overcoming **restricted shoulder movement**. Although superficial heating modalities may safely supplement all of the aforementioned activities, the use of ultrasound is contraindicated.

18. Does carpal tunnel syndrome occur more frequently in women?

Yes. Women constitute 75% of all cases. Additionally, the peak occurrence of carpal tunnel syndrome corresponds to the age of menopause.

19. Why?

Several theories have been postulated:
- Women have smaller wrists and therefore a smaller space through which the median nerve must travel.
- Hormonal influences may cause swelling of soft tissues in the wrist and lead to fluid retention, particularly in women using birth control pills, during pregnancy, and during menopause.
- More women than men are engaged in light assembly-line work and in clerical positions that require repetitive wrist movement.
- Recreational activities of many women may include needlecrafts, gardening, and ceramic work, which involve frequent wrist movement.

20. How do the goals in training and rehabilitation of the female athlete differ from those of the male athlete?

As a general rule, female athletes should not seek to develop the large bulky musculature of their male counterparts. Without the use of anabolic steroids, this is simply not an attainable goal in the female athlete due to genetic and hormonal differences. Rather, females should focus more on the development of muscle tone, flexibility, agility, and speed.

21. What condition in the female athlete should alert the physiatrist to other concurrent medical conditions?

Amenorrhea. Physicians treating highly competitive female athletes, especially gymnasts, long-distance runners, triathletes, as well as ballet dancers, should be sensitive to the possible presence of **eating disorders**. These young women sometimes seek to achieve dramatic weight reduction by combining restrictive dietary control (bulimia and/or anorexia) with excessive exercise. When too great a loss of adipose tissue occurs, these athletes lose the estrogen-producing potential of their fat cells, leading to derangement of the pituitary/ovarian axis and premature (often permanent) cessation of menses. Ironically, amenorrhea may predispose women to osteoporosis, despite hours of weight-bearing exercise performed by the female athlete.

22. What is fibromyalgia syndrome?

Fibromyalgia syndrome is a common form of generalized muscular pain and fatigue involving the muscles and fibers of connective tissues. For reasons not fully understood, this syndrome has a strong female predominance of > 85% in most series. The typical patient is a middle-aged woman who complains of chronic fatigue, generalized diffuse muscular pain, sleep disturbance, and other accompanying psychophysiologic abnormalities, including headaches, abdominal pain, urinary frequency, and alternating constipation and diarrhea.

23. How does fibromyaliga differ from fibromyositis?

Although the terms were frequently used interchangeably in the past, it is now recognized that fibromyositis is discrete and well-localized, frequently follows trauma or overuse to certain specific muscles, and is not accompanied by the variety of systemic complaints described for fibromyalgia.

24. Can specific laboratory tests be used to diagnose fibromyalgia?

No. Frequently, these patients have already undergone a wide variety of studies and have seen a number of specialists before coming to the physiatrist. Fibromyalgia is basically a diagnosis by exclusion. The telltale sign is the widespread number of stereotypical "tender points" in combination with systemic complaints.

25. How do you treat fibromyalgia?

Exercise: Many fibromyalgia patients resist exercise on the grounds that they are constantly "tired" and need rest. This mentality should be discouraged by prescribing a specified exercise program, particularly emphasizing stretching and aerobic activities.

Physical therapy: The adjunctive use of physical therapy modalities for brief periods of time often helps the patient overcome her fear of increased pain with activity. Physical therapy programs should be active rather than passive.

Medication: The long-term use of narcotic agents should be avoided. Nonsteroidal anti-inflammatory drugs should be used on an episodic or as-needed basis. The regular use of antidepressant medications, particularly those providing nighttime sedation, may be useful.

ACKNOWLEDGMENT

Special thanks to Research Assistant, Dmitry Tuder, Second Lieutenant, USAF.

BIBLIOGRAPHY

1. Agostini R: Medical and Orthopedic Issues of Active and Athletic Women. Philadelphia, Hanley & Belfus, 1994.
2. Artal R, Buckenmyer PJ: Exercise during pregnancy and postpartum. Contemp Ob-Gyn (May):62–90, 1995.
3. Berger K, Bostwick J III: A Woman's Decision: Breast Care, Treatment, & Reconstruction, 2nd ed. St. Louis, Quality Medical Publishing, 1994.
4. Birge J, Morrow-Nowell N, Proctor EK: Hip fractures. Clin Geriatr Med 10:589, 1994.
5. Bouxsein AL, Marcus R: Overviews of exercise and bone mass. Rheum Dis Clin North Am 20:787, 1994.
6. Breske S: Bone-fide PM&R for osteoporosis. Adv Rehabil (Feb):15–49, 1995.
7. Clark SL, Cotton DB, Lee W, et al: Central hemodynamic assessment of normal term pregnancy. Am J Obstet Gynecol 161:1439, 1994.
8. Edwards BJ, Perry HM III, et al: Age-related osteoporosis. Clin Geriatr Med 10:575, 1994.
9. Miller RS, Iverson DC, Fried RA, et al: Carpal tunnel syndrome in primary care: A report from ASPN. J Family Pract 38:337, 1994.
10. Schumacher HR Jr (ed): Primer on the Rheumatic Diseases, 10th ed. Atlanta, Arthritis Foundation, 1993.
11. Tanaka S, Wild DK, Seligman PJ, et al: The US prevalence of self-reported carpal tunnel syndrome. Am J Public Health 84:1846, 1994.
12. Travell JG, Simons DG: Myofascial Pain and Dysfunction: The Trigger Point Manual. Baltimore, Williams & Wilkins, 1992.
13. Verduyn WH: Spinal cord injured women: Pregnancy and delivery. Paraplegia 24:231–240, 1986.
14. Wolfe LA, Oktoke PJ, Mottola MF, et al: Physiologic interactions between pregnancy and aerobic exercises. Exerc Sport Sci Rev 17:295, 1989.

81. INDUSTRIAL REHABILITATION

Frank J. E. Falco, M.D., and Francis P. Lagattuta, M.D.

1. What role does the physiatrist play in industrial medicine?

The physiatrist acts as the primary care doctor for workers with musculoskeletal injuries. In industry, the physiatrist ideally becomes involved before any actual injuries occur by educating the workforce on prevention and proper ergonomics. The physiatrist treats the injured worker from the initial injury through the recovery process. Early intervention by the physiatrist or industrial medicine specialist can reduce morbidity and disability from work-related injuries and effect early return to work. The physiatrist possesses the expertise in injury pathophysiology and rehabilitation which results in the most comprehensive management of work-related injuries.

2. Who makes up the rehab team in industrial medicine?

The physiatrist is the leader and facilitator of the interdisciplinary rehabilitation team. The team can consist of a physiatrist, occupational nurse, rehab nurse, physical/occupational therapist, attorney, insurance adjustor, and employer. Although some of the members on the industrial medicine team are different from those on the traditional rehab team, the goal of promoting physical, psychological, mental, vocational, avocational, educational, and social development in the injured person is the same.

3. What are the most common work-related injuries?

The two most common work-related injuries are low back pain and repetitive strain or cumulative trauma disorders of the extremities. **Low back pain** affects 2–4% of the working population yearly; 80% of the working population will probably have an episode of low back pain at least once during their working years.

Cumulative trauma disorders involve primarily carpal tunnel obstruction and ulnar nerve entrapment at the elbow, but also include lateral epicondylitis, low back, neck and shoulder pain as the most frequent problems. Obviously, any area of the body can be involved in a cumulative trauma or repetitive strain injury, and the clinician should always assess the job, the patient, and the way the patient performs the job.

4. Who are NIOSH and OSHA?

These two organizations work hand in hand in providing safety standards in the workplace. **NIOSH**, the National Institute of Occupational Safety and Health, establishes all guidelines and requirements for the work environment, individual jobs, and material handling. **OSHA**, the Occupational Safety and Health Administration, enforces these guidelines and standards in the workplace at the state and federal levels.

5. How does the Americans with Disabilities Act affect preplacement examinations in the workplace?

The Americans with Disabilities Act (ADA) was passed into law in 1990. Title I of the ADA addresses workplace discrimination and disabled individuals. The ADA prohibits any inquiries or preplacement examination to determine any degree of disability until after a job has been offered to the individual. Any medical evaluation given after employment must apply to *all* initial employees and the information is kept confidential, except for making necessary accommodations, safety purposes, or ADA investigations. An employer cannot withdraw a job offer based on a disability uncovered by a subsequent evaluation.

6. Why is medical imaging overused in industrial medicine?

The compensation of a work-related injury is greatly influenced by the presence or absence of objective pathoanatomy. Medical imaging is one of the most common means used by clinicians to "objectively" evaluate work-related injuries. However, the clinical significance or insignificance of an anatomical "abnormality" (functional deficits) also needs to be considered in determining the degree of compensation.

7. How useful are plain x-rays in identifying workers at risk for spine injury?

X-rays had been used in the past as a routine screening tool to identify workers at risk for spine injury. However, because of the high frequency of abnormal x-ray findings in the general population, the general consensus is that lumbar spine x-rays have a low predictive value for injury in the workplace.

8. What is the role of MRI in industrial rehabilitation?

MRI is currently the best choice for detecting soft-tissue musculoskeletal injuries. The MRI allows for evaluation in great detail of the cruciate ligaments of the knee, rotator cuff of the shoulder, intervertebral disc, and other related soft-tissue structures. The high cost prevents the use of MRI as a screening tool.

9. When is CT used in industrial rehabilitation?

The CT scan allows for assessment of osseous lesions in greater detail than MRI but is inferior to MRI in the evaluation of musculoskeletal soft-tissue injuries. CT with contrast can provide additional information not furnished by MRI under certain circumstances. When a CT scan is performed after intrathecal injection of contrast (myelogram), a very accurate measurement of the thecal sac cross-sectional area can be made. This is considered the most precise means of measuring spinal canal dimensions and establishing spinal stenosis. CT-myelography is very helpful in the evaluation of thoracolumbar vertebral fractures for spinal instability and compromise of neural elements within the spinal canal. Rotator cuff tears involving tendons other than the supraspinatus can be successfully evaluated by post-shoulder arthrography CT scan (computed arthrotomography). This technique is considered by many as the choice test for imaging glenoid labrum tears. CT can also aid in the evaluation of stress fractures.

10. How are nerve conduction studies and needle electromyography (EMG) helpful in the assessment of low back pain?

Although x-rays and imaging studies allow for the evaluation of anatomy, electrodiagnosis provides information regarding the physiologic function of nerves and muscles. In contrast to imaging studies, there are no false-positive findings with needle EMG testing. The detection of denervation potentials during an evaluation represents actual abnormal neurophysiology.

EMG is very helpful in determining whether there is motor involvement of a particular nerve root (motor radiculopathy) in the presence of a herniated intervertebral disc and nonspecific leg pain. Nerve conduction studies and EMG can also assist in ruling out other conditions, such as a myopathy, plexopathy, multiple radiculopathy, and peripheral neuropathy.

11. What factors have the strongest association with low back pain (LBP) in the industrial workplace?

Heavy lifting—The rate and severity of work-related back and other musculoskeletal injuries increase significantly when heavy, bulky objects are frequently lifted from the floor.

Lifting technique—Proper lifting technique can decrease the incidence of LBP by one-third.

Strength—LBP is three times greater in workers whose strength is less than the demands of the job.

Vibration—Vibration has been implicated to increase the risk of LBP and herniated disc, especially with whole-body vibration and with long-distance driving.

Smoking—Repetitive strain from chronic coughing and disc degeneration from decreased disc oxygen tension are believed to increase the risk of LBP in smokers.

12. What accommodations in the sedentary sitting position at work can decrease intradiscal pressure?

Sitting has been shown to increase intradiscal pressure more than other sedentary positions, such as standing or lying down. Several simple modifications have been shown experimentally to decrease discal pressure while sitting and include using a chair with a backrest, increasing the posterior inclination of the backrest, using armrests, and using a lumbar support.

13. What is dynamic stabilization? How is it used to treat a worker with a spinal injury that limits job performance?

Spinal stabilization is a rehabilitation program designed to limit pain, maximize function, and prevent further injury by stabilizing spinal segments through muscular control. Stabilization is accomplished through restoration of spinal flexibility, postural reeducation, and strengthening of the torso and extremity muscles. This training program is typically applied to individuals with painful spinal segments such as a herniated disc with associated radiculopathy.

14. When are epidural injections indicated?

Epidural injections can be used both diagnostically and therapeutically in persons suffering from neck and back pain. The best indication for this procedure is an inflammatory radiculopathy, in which the extremity pain can respond dramatically to the powerful anti-inflammatory effects of the steroid. Good results can also be accomplished in elderly individuals with spinal stenosis and spondylosis who have pain presumably from inflammation within the spinal canal.

15. How about selective nerve root (SNR) blocks? What is their role in treating back and neck pain?

The SNR procedure is more selective than the epidural and can determine which root level is the pain generator in complicated cases of radiculopathy. Steroid and anesthetic are injected along the nerve root after correct placement has been identified with radiopaque contrast under fluoroscopy.

Selective nerve root blocks can predict surgical outcome for lumbar radiculopathy lasting > 1 year. In this population, individuals who did not obtain pain relief at 1 week from a SNR block were unlikely to benefit from surgery.

16. When are zygapophyseal (facet joint) injection procedures indicated?

Typically, patients with facet joint syndrome have axial pain greater than extremity pain, which increases with extension of the spine. Flexion-extension acceleration injuries (whiplash) can result in injuries of the facet joints, particularly in the cervical spine. Facet joint injection procedures can be used in the diagnosis and treatment of posterior element injuries or inflammatory arthropathy at the facet joint. These injections are best performed under fluoroscopic guidance to guarantee correct needle placement and avoid inadvertent intravascular or spinal injection.

The sacroiliac joint can produce pain in a similar pattern as symptomatic lumbar facet joints and should be considered in the evaluation and treatment of nonradiating, axial back pain. Sacroiliac joint injections performed under fluoroscopy can help determine if the pain generator is the sacroiliac joint and potentially provide long-term relief.

17. Name the common cumulative trauma disorders.

Carpal tunnel syndrome (median nerve entrapment), lateral epicondylitis (tennis elbow), de Quervain's tenosynovitis, and rotator cuff tendinitis.

18. What role does fibromyalgia play in workers' compensation?

Fibromyalgia is a chronic soft-tissue rheumatologic condition that is not typically caused by a work-related injury but can be exacerbated at work. This controversial diagnosis is more common in women and is characterized by diffuse muscle pain, fatigue, difficulty sleeping, and trigger points in a distinctive distribution. There is a considerable amount of time lost from work with fibromyalgia patients and they have a high degree of perceived disability.

Fibromyalgia symptoms have been reported to increase with certain work activities and are tolerable with other tasks. Typing, prolonged sitting, prolonged standing and walking, stress, heavy lifting, repetitive bending, and lifting exacerbate symptoms. Activities not associated with intensifying symptoms including walking, variable light sedentary work, teaching, light desk work, and phone work. Light sedentary work with varied tasks and allowance for changes in position are best tolerated by persons with fibromyalgia.

19. How important is it to understand the psychological status of the worker in industrial rehabilitation?

The psychological make-up of the injured worker is very important! Workers with conditions such as depression, hypochondriasis, and somatization are less likely to return to work and tend to be unemployed for longer periods of time. The depressed patient is more likely to experience minor injury as incapacitating pain, making treatment more challenging and difficult. Somatization is often the expression of physical complaints in the absence of any significant organic pathology as a way of dealing with emotional or psychological problems.

Preventing chronic pain behavior is just as important as treating the injury. Psychological testing can be helpful in identifying workers with mental conditions that can hamper successful treatment. The **visual analog scale, Mooney pain drawing,** and **Wadell testing** are more objective means of documenting pain behavior or pain experience in addition to formal psychological testing.

20. What are the nonorganic signs of LBP described by Wadell?

Gordon Waddell, a British orthopaedic surgeon, in 1980 described nonorganic signs of LBP that are not associated with lumbar pathology. There are five categories or types of nonorganic physical signs commonly referred to as Waddell signs

1. Tenderness—superficial, nonanatomic
2. Simulation—axial loading, rotation
3. Distraction—straight leg raising
4. Regional—weakness, sensory
5. Overreaction

The presence of any of these individual signs represents a positive finding for that category or type. Three or more types of nonorganic findings present during an evaluation is clinically significant and suggests that disturbances other than physical pathology are contributing to the patient's condition. "Waddell" testing has been used clinically as a simple screen to help identify those individuals that may require a detailed psychological evaluation.

21. What is a functional capacity evaluation?

This is a set of objective task-based measurements of functional performance and endurance. This information is used to estimate a worker's capability to perform a job. Standardized measures are used to direct workers toward new jobs compatible with their abilities. Functional capacity evaluations can also be specifically designed to simulate the performance expectations of an employment goal. Shortfalls in performance can be identified and emphasized in training efforts or job modification.

22. What is a work or job analysis?

Work analysis examines the details of a particular job and helps identify the major physical requirements to perform the job. Many factors are considered during a job analysis, including loads, load dimensions, load distribution, coupling of worker and load, load stability, workplace geometry, temporal factors, complexity of movements, environment, worksite organization, and psychological factors. Potential job-related biomechanical problems can be identified by these evaluations. This information can then be utilized to eliminate or reduce identifiable risk factors for injury by ergonomically redesigning the job.

444 Industrial Rehabilitation

23. Define the term maximum medical improvement (MMI).

An individual reaches MMI when there is no significant change in his or her condition during a course of treatment. A date is recorded in the medical records when an injured worker has reached MMI to establish an endpoint or stability in the course of recovery from an injury or illness with a reasonable degree of medical certainty. An MMI date does not preclude further treatment, and patients can continue to receive necessary medical care. The declaration of MMI allows further assessments to be made regarding likelihood of returning to work, work status, restrictions in the workplace, permanent impairment, and legal settlement of claims. Some states have laws that impose a limit to the time that can elapse from injury to the MMI date for all work-related injuries.

24. What factors affect treatment outcome and return to work for persons with LBP independent of the diagnosis?

Duration of symptoms, length of time out of work, job satisfaction, and psychological factors. Approximately 90–95% of people with LBP recover within 3 months of the injury, and those who don't are at risk of developing chronic pain with a greater probability of disability. The longer an individual with chronic low back pain is out of work, the less likely they will return to work. Poor job satisfaction, depression, hypochondriasis, and somatization have all been reported to adversely affect treatment and return to work.

25. What is an independent medical examination (IME)?

An independent medical examination is an evaluation of the injured worker by a nontreating physician. After evaluating the worker, the physician provides an "unbiased" assessment of the individual through a written report. The report typically comments on the diagnosis, appropriate treatment, prognosis, MMI date, impairment rating, and recommendations such as functional capacity evaluation or vocational rehabilitation. Any and all of these topics are covered in the IME depending on who requests the examination and whether or not the injury is acute or chronic. The IME is sometimes known as the CME, company medical examination.

1. Andersson GBJ, Svensson H-O: The intensity of work recovery in low back pain. Spine 8:880, 1983.
2. Barnsely L, Lord S, Wallis BJ, Bogduk N: The prevalence of chronic cervical zygapophysial joint pain after whiplash. Spine 20:20–26, 1995.
3. Bigos SJ, Battié MC, Fisher LD, et al: A longitudinal, prospective study of industrial back injury reporting. Clin Orthop 279:21–34, 1992.
4. Damkot DK, Pope MH, Lord J, et al: The relationship between work history, work environment and low-back pain in men. Spine 9:395–399, 1984.
5. Gibson ES, Martin RH, Terry CW: Incidence of low back pain and pre-employment X-ray screening. J Occup Med 22:515–519, 1980.
6. Gordon SL, Blair SJ, Fine LJ (eds): Repetitive Motion Disorders of the Upper Extremity. Rosemont, IL, American Academy of Orthopedic Surgeons, 1995.
7. Holbrook TL, Grazier K, Kelsey JL, et al: The Frequency of Occurrence, Impact and Cost of Selected Musculoskeletal Conditions in the United States. Park Ridge, IL, American Academy of Orthopaedic Surgeon, 1984, pp 154–156.
8. McKenzie F, Storment J, VanHook P, et al: A program for control of repetitive trauma disorders associated with tool operations in a telecommunications manufacturing facility. Am Ind Hyg Assoc J 46:674–678, 1985.
9. Silverstein BA, Fine LJ, Armstrong TJ: Occupational factors of carpal tunnel syndrome. Am J Ind Med 11:343, 1987.
10. Stock SR: Workplace ergonomic factors and the development of musculoskeletal disorders of the neck and upper limbs: A meta-analysis. Am J Ind Med 19:87, 1991.
11. Waddell G, McCulloch JA, Kummel E, et al: Nonorganic physical signs in low-back pain. Spine 5:117–125, 1980.

82. WORKERS' COMPENSATION AND REHABILITATION

Norman B. Rosen, M.D.

1. Why are workers' compensation patients so difficult?

"Workers' comp" patients can be among the most challenging to work with. Most are motivated and anxious to return to work, and some even attempt to hide or minimize their disabilities because of their need to work and earn a salary. Unfortunately, individuals sometimes use their symptoms for secondary gain, either consciously or subconsciously. These individuals present with symptom-magnification and symptom-substitution disorders once the initial complaint has been addressed. Persistent symptoms may reflect passivity, dependency needs, passive aggressiveness, depression, anger, anxiety, or even frank malingering.

2. What concurrent emotional factors can lead to symptom magnification?

The key emotional factors to address are the patient's **anger** (and how he or she expresses this), level of anxiety, sense of feeling in control, depression, passivity (or passive dependency), and perceived level of job satisfaction. Frank malingering behavior needs to be identified early and not rewarded inadvertently by the unsuspecting practitioner with time off or some other "reward."

3. How do you deal with a malingerer?

The patient should be started on a gradual and structured **program stressing wellness** recommendations (cessation of smoking, weight reduction, exercise, other lifestyle changes). It is imperative that the clinician **monitor compliance** closely. By validating the patient's complaints with the prescription of a structured "wellness" treatment program, the injured worker starts on the path to recovery. With a less intensive treatment program, the less-motivated individual will be rewarded in terms of more time off from work and responsibility, and this will merely reinforce the manipulative behavior of the malingerer (or the helplessness behavior of the subconscious symptom-magnifier).

In stubborn cases, the clinician should attempt to involve a critical family member or significant other and assess his or her motivation for wellness as well. The clinician should be sure to listen to this person's assessments of the dysfunction presented by the injured worker and inquire as to what this family member thinks is going on and how he or she would correct it. The clinician should also recognize that the immediate family or significant other could be codependents in the process.

4. Is there a difference between symptom magnification disorders, somatization, and malingering?

Yes. **Symptom magnification** may be either a conscious or subconscious need to survive in a stressful environment and may merely reflect a somewhat unsophisticated problem-solving, communication, and negotiation style in a person who feels trapped or overwhelmed by the system.

Somatization reflects a true concern with the body integrity and body function and usually is subconscious (but perceived to be real by the patient).

Malingering is a conscious attempt to deceive for social rewards (money, time off, attention or pity).

5. What are the major disincentives to wellness and early return to work among the workers' comp patients?

1. Injured workers receive partial or complete **immediate wage replacement**; therefore, there is less of a need to return to work rapidly.

2. If recovery is less than complete, there will be a higher financial award (or reward) for any **residual disability** sustained by the patient.

3. Any **attorney compensation** is often dependent on how much permanent disability the patient is ultimately awarded.

Other major disincentives include job dissatisfaction, a poor sense of self-worth and self-esteem, a sense of not being in control of the work situation, and poor problem-solving, communication, and negotiation skills on the part of the worker. Finally, keep in mind that poor problem-solving by the clinician may result in a poorer outcome as well as a prolonged illness and persistent disability in refractory patients.

6. Name seven job-related factors that the clinician should keep in mind when dealing with an injured worker?

1. Age of the patient and the age when most people in that same job generally "burn out."

2. Length of time on the job. Most injuries occur during the first year of injury or at the time when the individual gets "too old" for the particular job or has let himself get out of shape.

3. History of the injury. How did it happen, and have other workers been injured in the same job?

4. Who does the injured worker feel is at fault for this injury?

5. Premorbid level of conditioning.

6. Previous history of injury and recovery times.

7. What is the nature of the job? Are frequent unusual postures required? Repetitive stresses, sustained loads? Frequent breaks allowed? Job satisfaction? Sense of "being in control"?

7. What are the most common facilitators to hasten a rapid return to work?

Reinforcement of job satisfaction

The patient's sense of importance in performing the job

Pay

Seniority

Benefits

Job security

Communication skills (access to supervisors and harmony with coworkers)

Overall motivation for wellness

Willingness to make "lifestyle changes"

Role of family stresses (?)

8. What major errors do clinicians make in dealing with refractory patients?

1. Not recognizing that pain and disability from pain are two separate issues and should be treated as such.

2. Not recognizing the existence of underlying tissue dysfunction (particularly myofascial pain syndromes, entrapment neuropathies, reflex sympathetic dystrophy).

3. Not understanding the job stresses that the patient has to return to and his or her ability to relate with supervisors and coworkers.

4. Not taking the time to explore problem-solving options and to set mutually-agreed-upon goals relative to return-to-work options.

5. Not believing the patient and his or her perceived level of disability.

6. Inability to tactfully (nonconfrontationally) explain to the patient his or her inconsistencies in performance and noncompliance.

7. Failure to place the patient on a structured program and monitoring the patient's compliance as well as determining long-term and short-term goals.

8. Not recognizing the underlying psychosocial, intellectual, and problem-solving skills of the patient.

9. Not recognizing the personality and coping style of the patient as well as communication skills.

9. When the clinician is faced with a repetitive strain or repetitive trauma syndrome, what factors should be explored?

1. Load (weight) and distance of the object from the body's center of gravity
2. Intensity of the activity
3. Frequency of the task, repetitions
4. Speed required to perform the activity
5. Equipment associated with the activity
6. Awkward positions, previous learning of the task
7. Rest periods or changes of work position
8. What adaptations have more senior coworkers made to increase work tolerance and efficiency?

10. In cases of resistant carpal tunnel obstruction, what factors should the clinician always look for?

Hand position in performing the task	Trunk stability while performing the activity
Undetected areas of myofascial pain in the forearm, extensors, and flexors and in the shoulder girdle muscle	Obesity Vibration

11. To determine the maximum weight which is safe to lift, NIOSH has defined the action limit. What is this?

This is the weight that is safe for 99% of males to lift and 75% of females. Another term that is used is **the maximal permissible limit**, and this is the weight that 25% of males and 1% of females are able to lift.

12. Is isokinetic equipment necessary to assess the patient's ability to return to work?

At this point, there is no literature indicating that any particular piece of equipment is more effective in assessing injured workers than taking the time, energy, and interest in trying to work with the injured worker. Cheap equipment and expensive personnel are better than expensive equipment and less-qualified personnel. Isokinetic equipment should always be considered as adjuncts to the clinician's clinical judgment.

13. What are the common characteristics of poor responders or nonresponders to treatment?

Poor compliance with structure, anxiety, depression, overt or covert anger, impulsivity, inability to delay immediate gratification, inability to intellectualize emotional feelings, poor communication, poor negotiation and problem-solving skills, no long-term goals, a sense of being trapped in a job ("going nowhere"), unwillingness to take risks, lack of self-esteem, too much reliance on other's feelings, unwillingness or inability to work through a crisis independently, passivity and helplessness, and frequently, poor problem-solving skills in the caretakers to whom they turn for help.

14. When the clinician makes a determination that the patient or injured worker cannot or should not return to his or her regular job, what should be done? When should this be done?

The sooner the clinician determines that the patient will not be able to function adequately at the former job, the sooner alternative vocational objectives should be identified and pursued. This means returning the worker to a modified job environment, seeking a job change, or retraining. Before recommending an expensive vocational rehabilitation program, it is critical that the patient's psychosocial deterrents to wellness be explored.

15. An injured worker reports difficulty in the workplace. What should be the physician's request to this patient?

To allow the physician to contact the worker's employer or supervisor and to include them as part of the treatment team in order to effect more appropriate problem-solving and negotiation. By talking directly to the supervisor or employer, the physician can get a better first hand feeling for the level of cooperation that these individuals are willing to extend and will be better able to place themselves in the position of the worker.

16. What are the most common causes of recidivism among injured workers?
Incomplete healing or resolution of a previous episode
Failure to comply with the home exercise program
Failure to take medications (if needed)
Failure to resolve the psychosocial aspects of work related stresses

17. What age groups are at higher risk for injuries among laborers?
The oldest group and the youngest group. The latter group lacks the necessary skills, and the former group usually has become deconditioned for the work, frustrated with their job, and are anxious for retirement (any way they can).

18. Patients with low back pain who are fitted with lumbosacral corsets sometimes become dependent on their corsets. How can this be avoided?
The usual muscles that get weak with the wearing of a lumbosacral corset are the abdominal muscles. If all patients are taught abdominal strengthening and how to do an appropriate dynamic pelvic tilt, the abdominal muscles can remain strong and conditioned. In addition, the back extensors should be stretched and strengthened, and low back mobility should be maintained. It is important that, once the acute episode has passed, patients try to go without their corset for less-demanding activities. The patient who has not done well on a conservative management and who is symptomatic deserves a trial of an appropriately fitted lumbosacral corset.

19. When starting a work-hardening program, what single warning should the therapist or doctor give the patient?
That increased pain is to be expected and that this increased pain does not mean that damage has occurred. Rather, it should be considered a "spring-training" effect and will be short-lived. It is often advisable to have the injured worker change routine for a day or so and work on a different part of the body at a lesser degree of performance and then resume the work hardening program the following day. The use of NSAIDs and mild analgesics may improve both work tolerance and exercise tolerance.

20. Is pain in and of itself a contraindication to returning to work?
No. Pain is a necessary concomitant of exercise and vigorous activity and does not reflect a contraindication to work. However, underlying tissue dysfunction should always be carefully looked for (weakness of muscles, tightness of muscles, and imbalance between agonist and antagonist), and an appropriate treatment should be directed toward correcting the underlying dysfunctions. On the other hand, if the patient has persistent pain while at work, appropriate intervention should include (if possible) frequent breaks for stretching and rest, change of routine or task, work analysis for ways to conserve energy, or work simplification and pacing. Taking medications such as acetaminophen or NSAIDs and wearing appropriate supports (back brace, elastic wraps, etc.) should be stressed.

21. How should cumulative trauma or repetitive strain disorders be treated?
Treatment begins with an analysis of the job, the worker, and the technique employed by the injured worker. Ergonomic modifications should be made and treatment directed to all three areas. Other recommendations include the application of ice combined with stretching both prior to and following the task, as well as the use of NSAIDs, analgesics, and external supports. Frequent rests or changes in position should be advised. The clinician taking care of an injured worker often needs to use ingenuity in solving repetitive strain problems. Ergonomists, occupational therapists, and industrial designers may be required if a site needs refabrication with more emphasis on the worker's tolerances.

22. What other dysfunctions should be sought in the patient with a cumulative trauma or repetitive strain disorder?

Myofascial pain and dysfunction is the greater imitator and potentiator of other musculoskeletal dysfunctions. It not only can perpetuate the disorder by causing tightness and weakness of involved muscles but also mimic the suspected disorder through the mechanism of referred pain and tenderness from trigger areas in muscles and tissues. As a result, the focus of attention is usually on the patient's presenting complaint rather than on a remote "trigger point."

23. What are the best ways to control costs involving injured workers?

1. Return the injured worker back to some work or structured situation as quickly as possible—whether pain free or not—while at the same time protecting the injured part with external supports or alternative work situations.

2. Continue to treat the injured worker (from an interdisciplinary standpoint) while assessing whether the modified job will be short-term or long-term and assessing the specific job stressors (physical and emotional) that may result in increased complaints of pain.

3. Encourage the injured worker to get onto vigorous programs of exercise in order to achieve the necessary fitness that is required for this specific job but also to remain healthy in general. This may require changes in adverse lifestyle habits (e.g., smoking, diet, sleep, drugs, etc.).

BIBLIOGRAPHY

1. Bonfiglio RF: LaBan MM, Taylor RS, et al: Industrial rehabilitation medicine management. In DeLisa JA, Gans BM (eds): Rehabilitation Medicine: Principles and Practice, 2nd ed. Philadelphia, J.B. Lippincott, 1993, pp 169–177.
2. Johnson EW (ed): Rehabilitation of the injured worker. Phys Med Rehabil Clin North Am 3(3), 1992.
3. Moore JS, Garg A (eds): Ergonomics: Low-back pain, carpal tunnel syndrome, and upper extremity disorders in the workplace. Occup Med State Art Rev 7(4):593–790, 1992.
4. Rosen NB: The myofascial pain syndromes. Phys Med Rehabil Clin North Am 4:41–63, 1993.
5. Rosen NB: Physical medicine and rehabilitation approaches to the management of myofascial pain and fibromyalgia syndromes. Bailliere's Clin Rheumat 8:881–916, 1994.
6. Rosen NB, Sharoff KA, Khanna VK: The dysfunctional pain patient—Returning to work: A preliminary report. Md Med J 34:605–608, 1985.

83. SPORTS MEDICINE

Joel M. Press, M.D., and Jeffrey L. Young, M.D., M.A.

1. I am a general practicing physiatrist. Why do I need to know about sports medicine?

No matter how narrow a physiatrist's focus of practice, a working knowledge of musculoskeletal anatomy and biomechanical principles is always important for some aspect of patient management. Most patients in the traditional rehabilitation setting with other disabilities will have numerous musculoskeletal problems that need to be addressed. Back, knee, and shoulder pain are common complaints in patients hospitalized for stroke, traumatic brain injury, amputation, spinal cord injury, and arthritis rehabilitation. Sports medicine and sports technology have also been responsible for many of the advances in care for the disabled. For example, adaptation of ski technology led to development of the "flex foot," and racing wheelchairs were the precursors to the lightweight chairs that are used today.

2. What are the most common sports injuries?

Most sports-related injuries are specific to a given sport. High-impact sports that require a lot of jumping and landing on hard surfaces (e.g., basketball, volleyball) predispose athletes to lower-extremity injuries at the knee and ankle (e.g., anterior cruciate ligament tears, meniscal tears, inversion sprains). Upper-extremity activities (e.g., tennis, baseball, racquetball) are more commonly associated with rotator cuff injuries and elbow disorders. Sports that require back hyperextension or repetitive extension (e.g., cheerleading, volleyball, gymnastics, weight-lifting) may predispose participants to back injuries.

Common Sports Injuries Due to Musculotendinous Overload

INJURIES	SPORT(S)
Acromioclavicular ligament sprain	Weight-lifting, gymnastics
Rotator cuff tendinitis	Baseball, tennis, swimming
Medial epicondylitis	Golf, baseball (pitching), tennis (forehand)
Lateral epicondylitis	Tennis (backhand)
deQuervain's tenosynovitis	Rowing, golf
Spondylolyis, lumbar spine	Gymnastics
Trochanteric bursitis	Running
Adductor tendinitis	Hockey
Iliotibial band friction syndrome	Running
Patellofemoral pain	Basketball, cycling, running, soccer, weight-lifting
Achilles tendinitis	Running, basketball
Ankle sprains	Baseball, basketball, soccer
Plantar fasciitis	Running, soccer, tennis
Flexor hallucis tendinitis	Dance

3. When you have not observed the injury, what are important questions to ask the injured athlete?

1. How did you get hurt? (What was the **mechanism** of injury?)
2. Have you been injured there before? (Is this a **reinjury**, implying either inadequate rehabilitation or the progression of chronic microtraumatic injury, or was this an acute macrotraumatic event?)
3. Where else have you been injured? (A **kinetic chain analysis** of injuries often reveals events proximal or distal to the site of acute injury which have rendered the new site more vulnerable to overload.)
4. What treatment did you receive? (An alarming number of musculoskeletal injuries do not receive adequate attention and proper rehabilitation.)
5. What other medical conditions do you have? (Just because the patient is an athlete do not assume that he or she is healthy in all other regards. Many individuals with asthma, cardiac conditions, and metabolic and hormonal disorders are active participants in sports. Treatment regimens need to take this information into account.)

4. What should a sports physiatrist look for in a preparticipation history and examination?

Some of the major goals of the preparticipation examination include:

1. Detection of conditions that will restrict athletic participation, predispose to injury, or limit the level of performance
2. Evaluation of fitness and maturity
3. Determination of general health
4. Establishment of an open physician-athlete relationship for maximal health education
5. Adequately fulfilling medical-legal requirements

The preparticipation history needs to include review of previous neurologic and musculoskeletal injuries and their rehabilitation, a thorough family and personal cardiovascular and respiratory disease inquiry, review of thermoregulatory and endocrine dysfunction, and the presence or absence of unpaired organs.

5. What is PASSOR?
The Physiatric Association for Spine, Sports, and Occupational Rehabilitation is a section of the AAPM&R formed "to foster the growth of the specialty of physiatry in research, education, and the physiatric practice of musculoskeletal medicine with a special emphasis upon spine, sports, and occupational rehabilitation."

6. Describe the important aspects of rotator cuff pathology rehabilitation.
Rotator cuff rehabilitation must address:
    1. Flexibility deficits, particularly in the external rotators and posterior capsule
    2. Joint motion restriction within the sternoclavicular, acromioclavicular, scapulothoracic, and glenohumeral joints
    3. Strength deficits, particularly in the scapular stabilizers (rhomboids, lower and middle trapezii, and seratus anterior) as well as the cuff muscles
Assessment of the entire kinetic chain (e.g., cervical, thoracic, and lumbar spine and upper and lower extremities) is especially important in the overhead athlete. Muscles should be strengthened both concentrically and eccentrically, individually and in groups. Progression should lead to activity/sports-specific conditions to maximize the chances for return to activity painfree.

7. How is tennis elbow treated?
Lateral epicondylitis is the result of repetitive eccentric overload of the extensors and supinators of the wrist. The great majority of cases do not occur in tennis players. Rehabilitation focuses on the stretching tight wrist extensors eccentrically, strengthening the wrist extensors and avoiding aggravating factors. Limitations of motion at the shoulder, poor cervicothoracic posture, and poor "ergonomics" at the workplace must be corrected. Counterforce braces and, occasionally, corticosteroid injections can be helpful.

8. What is biker's palsy?
Entrapment of the ulnar nerve at the wrist at Guyon's canal. It occurs commonly in cyclists because of direct pressure on the ulnar side of the hand with standard handle bars. Sensory and motor symptoms are confined to the ulnar-innervated structures distal to this area, with sparing of the flexor carpi ulnaris muscle and the dorsal ulnar cutaneous sensory patch. Methods of prevention include wearing padded bicycle gloves and the use of "aero-bars" which allow weight-bearing through the forearm.

9. Is surgery always necessary for a meniscal tear of the knee?
No. Meniscal injuries associated with mechanical locking, loss of full range of motion, and persistent pain that limits daily activity will probably require surgical treatment. However, due to the vascular supply to the peripheral 30% of the menisci, there is potential for healing with some meniscal tears. Many meniscal injuries that minimally affect daily activities during the first few weeks after injury can be cautiously watched for symptomatic improvement and possible resolution of symptoms. If symptoms persist after 6–8 weeks, definitive studies (magnetic resonance or arthrogram) and surgical consultation are typically indicated.

10. How is the anterior cruciate ligament (ACL) torn?
The ACL prevents anterior displacement of the tibia with respect to the femur and imparts control over knee rotation. There are a number of ways in which the ligament can be disrupted:
    1. Deceleration of the leg via quadriceps contraction combined with valgus and external rotation forces upon a slightly flexed knee
    2. Sudden internal rotation of a hyperflexed knee
    3. Sudden hyperextension of the knee (landing from a jump)
    4. Backward fall on a flexed knee accompanied by a forceful quadriceps contraction in an attempt to maintain an upright position
    5. Direct blows to the knee (both laterally and medially directed blows will cause ACL disruption if of sufficient force)

11. Can an athlete participate in sports without surgical repair of the torn ACL?

Sometimes. The ACL provides the majority of rotatory stability at the knee. If it is torn, most of that stability to lateral and twisting movements is lost. Most high-level athletes and young recreational athletes who wish to return to the same level of sports competition need surgical repair of the ACL. Reconstructive surgery, typically done with a bone-tendon-bone graft harvested from the distal patella, middle one-third of the patella tendon, and the proximal tibia reestablishes some of the restraint to rotatory instability. Following ACL reconstruction, an aggressive rehabilitation program is required—if the patient is incapable of adhering to or not motivated to follow a comprehensive program (typically 6–9 months), then surgery should be reconsidered. Some patients will do well without surgery and can return to sports activities. Keys to both nonoperative and postoperative treatment include aggressive hamstring strengthening and proprioceptive training.

12. Why are inversion sprains so common in sports?

The ankle mortise is least stable, from an osteologic standpoint, when the foot is plantarflexed. In this position, stability is conferred by the ligaments, particularly on the lateral side. Plantar flexion is accompanied by inversion, which further stresses the lateral structures, rendering them susceptible to injury. In sports like basketball, soccer, football, tennis, and wrestling, which require explosive jumping, running, or lateral movement, the athlete is often on the ball of the foot with the foot in a plantar-flexed position. Eversion sprains are less common due to the greater strength of the medial ligaments and the obligatory coupling of eversion with dorsiflexion, which confers greatest osteologic stability.

13. What is a hip pointer?

A contusion to the iliac crest with subperiosteal hematoma, usually the result of direct trauma. The injured athlete has difficulty walking and standing upright due to the pain and muscular tightening in that area. The true hip joint is unaffected.

14. Why do gymnasts have low back pain?

Gymnastics, like other sports that require a lot of hyperextension of the spine, can place excessive loads on the posterior structures of the spine. In particular, loads are placed on the pars interarticularis (the site of spondylolysis) and on the facet joints. Other sports with a high incidence of low back pain are cheerleading, weight-lifting, and football.

15. What is "little league elbow"?

Little league elbow is the consequence of repeated valgus overload in the skeletally immature elbow. During late cocking and acceleration, medial structures are stretched while lateral structures are compressed. The distraction forces on the medial side may cause enlargement or avulsion of the medial epicondyle and osteochondritis dissecans, while the compressive lateral forces may induce radial head and capitellar growth disturbance, fractures, and articular cartilage breakdown.

16. What are common running injuries?

Most running-related injuries occur in the lower extremities. During running, forces up to three times body weight are placed on the lower-extremity joints 2000 times/mile. In particular, injuries include plantar fasciitis, medial tibial stress syndrome, achilles tendinitis, patellofemoral pain syndrome, and iliotibial band friction syndrome. Stress fractures, another type of overload injury, commonly occur in the tibia, metatarsals, and fibula and less commonly in the femur and pelvis.

17. Which entrapment neuropathies commonly occur in sports?

Entrapment (or compressive) neuropathies are an important cause of pain and limit the ability to participate in sports for many athletes. In the upper body, **thoracic outlet syndrome** can cause unilateral or bilateral dysesthesias in an ulnar and/or median nerve distribution. **Suprascapular nerve entrapment** induces weakness in the supraspinatus and infraspinatus or the infraspinatus alone. **Long thoracic nerve compression** results in shoulder dysfunction via reduced scapular control. **Musculocutaneous nerve entrapment** may result in biceps weakness or, more commonly, reduced sensation in the lateral forearm. Classic entrapment sites for the ulnar nerve are at the level of the cubital tunnel and Guyon's canal, while the level of the bicipital aponeurosis, pronator teres, and carpal tunnel are common sites for compression of the median nerve. In the lower body, important entrapment sites include the piriformis muscle which can compress the sciatic nerve, the fibular head where the common peroneal nerve is vulnerable, and the tarsal tunnel where the distal tibial nerve can be compressed.

18. Why are passive modalities used so much in sports medicine?

Good question. There is no doubt that passive modalities are overused in general in musculoskeletal rehabilitation. Although they may have some benefit in the acute situation, long-term use has not been shown effective for any specific disorders.

19. What does "rehabilitation beyond the resolution of symptoms" mean?

Many musculoskeletal injuries appear to resolve despite whatever treatment patients are given. After treatment of the acute inflammation, symptoms from many ailments disappear, and athletes mistakenly assume it is safe to return to sport. However, stopping rehabilitation at this point is inadequate. Most musculoskeletal injuries in sports are the result of chronic overload where biomechanical alterations have occurred and microtraumatic tissue injury has occurred. These biomechanical changes, consisting of muscle imbalances, inflexibilities, and weaknesses need to be addressed to prevent recurrence of injury.

20. What is a "stinger" or "burner"?

A traction or compression injury to the brachial plexus, probably at the rootlet level. These typically occur in the upper roots and are more common in contact sports, such as football, where head and neck contact result in extraforaminal root compression (college and professional) or increased acromiomastoid distance (high school) with upper plexus tension. Sharp, burning pain is experienced down the arm and generally lasts from seconds to minutes.

21. What is "mallet finger," and how is it treated?

"Baseball finger" or mallet finger is a stretch injury to the terminal extensor mechanism of the distal interphalangeal joint. It often occurs when a ball strikes the tip of an extended finger, suddenly forcing it into flexion and tearing the extensor mechanism or detaching a piece of bone. Treatment usually consists of splinting the distal joint in extension for up to 6–8 weeks.

22. When should you use the philosophy "no pain, no gain"?

In most cases of rehabilitation of musculoskeletal and sports injuries, the patient needs to be careful not to push beyond the limits of pain when significant muscle, tendon, bone, or ligament injury has occurred. Pain often will be a guideline that is approached but not forced past. On the other hand, the healthy patient who wants to "get stronger" is expected to experience some soreness of muscles after lifting the necessary weights to obtain strength gains. The assumption is that in the latter case, muscle has been subjected to systematically applied overload and that adequate recovery time has been given so that full recovery between exercise sessions has been achieved.

23. What sports have an increased risk of a herniated disk?

The usual mechanism of injury to the intervertebral disk is one of flexion combined with rotation. Sports that require these activities repetitively will cause damage to the peripheral annular fibers and ultimately disk herniation. In particular, baseball, golf, and bowling (the number one sport in the United States from a participation standpoint) have an increased risk of disk herniation.

24. What is a musculoskeletal examination?

In a complete musculoskeletal examination, the examiner notes inflexibilities and restrictions at the level of the joints, connective tissue, muscle, and fascia. Strength and dynamic and proprioceptive ability are also assessed. These findings, along with the neurologic exam, give a more complete diagnosis from an anatomic and functional standpoint. Biomechanical deficits and imbalances can be determined which may be important in prescribing a comprehensive rehabilitation program.

25. Give some of the important considerations in rehabilitation of the patellofemoral pain syndrome.

Patellofemoral pain syndrome is often due to poor tracking of the patella into the trochlear groove throughout the full range of flexion and extension. Emphasis needs to be placed upon stretching posterior and lateral structures which may be tight (i.e., the iliotibial band, hamstrings, gastrocsoleus), strengthening structures that directly or indirectly move the patella medially (e.g, medial quads, hip external rotators), proprioceptive retraining of patellofemoral motion (e.g., taping), and strengthening exercises that do not increase patellofemoral joint reaction forces excessively.

26. How does the iliotibial band friction syndrome (ITB) occur?

ITB syndrome is a lateral knee pain syndrome due to overload of the ITB. Pain is produced as the ITB rubs over the lateral femoral condyle, typically between 20–30° of flexion. Pain may also occur over the lateral tibia at Gerdy's tubercle. Causes include running on uneven surfaces, sudden increases in running mileage, and incorrect footwear in either pronators or supinators.

27. What is "turf toe"?

A sprain injury of the plantar capsule of the metatarsophalangeal (MTP) joint of the great toe. It is generally due to excessive forces placed on the MTP joint during push-off or running on hard surfaces (i.e., artificial turf in football and soccer). The athlete complains of pain and swelling of the first MTP joint which worsens with attempted push-off. Splinting for 7–10 days and/or taping to limit dorsiflexion are necessary to prevent further injury.

28. What causes shin splints?

Shin splints or medial stress syndrome, is due to overload of structures in the posteromedial or anterolateral leg. Enthesitis at the attachment of the soleus to the tibia may be the most common cause, but tibial stress fractures, posterior tibialis tendinitis/periostitis, flexor hallucis tendinitis, and tibialis anterior overload injuries may all contribute to the medial tibial stress syndrome.

BIBLIOGRAPHY

1. Bruckner P, Khan K: Clinical Sports Medicine. Sydney, Australia, McGraw-Hill, 1993.
2. Cantu RC, Micheli LJ: ACSM's Guidelines for the Team Physician. Philadelphia, Lea & Febiger, 1991.
3. DeLee JC, Drez D: Orthopedic Sports Medicine: Principles and Practice. Philadelphia, W.B. Saunders, 1994.
4. Fu FH, Stone DA: Sports Injuries: Mechanisms, Prevention, Treatment. Baltimore, Williams & Wilkins, 1994.
5. Harvey JS (ed): Sports medicine. Phys Med Rehabil Clin North Am 4(3), 1994.
6. Nicholas JA, Hershman EB: The Lower Extremity and Spine in Sports Medicine. St. Louis, C.V. Mosby, 1986.
7. Nicholas JA, Hershman EB: The Upper Extremity in Sports Medicine. St. Louis, C.V. Mosby, 1986.
8. Press JM (ed): Sports medicine. Phys Med Rehabil Clin North Am 5(1), 1994.
9. Saal JA (ed): Rehabilitation of sports injuries. Phys Med Rehabil State Art Rev 1:4, 1987.
10. Simon SR: Orthopaedic Basic Science. Elk Park, IL, American Academy of Orthopedic Surgeons, 1994.
11. Weinstein SM, Herring SA: Nerve problems and compartment syndrome in the hand, wrist, and forearm. Clin Sports Med 11(1), 1992.
12. Young JL, Press JM: Rehabilitation of running injuries. In Buschbacher R, Braddom R (eds): Sports Medicine and Rehabilitation: A Sport-Specific Approach. Philadelphia, Hanley & Belfus, 1995.

84. PERFORMING ARTS MEDICINE

Scott E. Brown, M.D.

1. What is performing arts medicine?

Performing arts medicine is practiced by physicians from various medical disciplines who apply expertise in a specialized body of knowledge to the treatment of musicians, dancers, vocalists, and others involved in the lively arts. The focus is on problems that develop from performance, although underlying medical problems often require an individualized treatment approach to reduce their disabling effects. While the field borrows from sports, occupational, and rehabilitation medicine, there are many unique issues to be considered when evaluating and treating performing artists. A seemingly minor medical impairment can cause a career ending disability. The more general field of **arts medicine** includes other aspects, such as music and dance therapy, the biology of music, and therapeutic effects of the visual arts.

2. How many artists actually get injured by performing their art?

In a survey of the members of the International Conference of Symphony and Opera Musicians, 76% reported having had at least one medical problem severe enough to interfere with performance, and 36% reported four severe problems. The annual incidence of injury in students musicians is 5.7/100 male conservatory students and 11.5/100 female conservatory students. In dancers, injury has affected as many as 90% in some studies.

3. Is there such a thing as cellist's scrotum?

No. In the early days of performing arts medicine, many case reports described various syndromes in terms of the specific instrument involved, affected body part, exacerbating activity, or famous musician afflicted—e.g., **flutist's chin** and **Satchmo's syndrome**. The situation became unwieldy with so many eponyms, that a fictitious report of cellist's scrotum was published. Disorders are now described according to the underlying pathology.

4. So what is Satchmo's syndrome?

In light of the preceding question, we now talk about **orbicularis oris rupture** rather than Satchmo's syndrome. This disorder, of course, was named for the great Louis Armstrong who, in later years, "lost his lip" and his high E flat.

5. What are the four categories of risk factors for injury in musicians?

Risk factors unique to musicians can be divided into four general categories:

1. **Physiologic/psychological**—musician response to demands. Gender, genetic predisposition, psychological and anthropometric factors (such as hand size) are generally unmodifiable. Personality traits, coping mechanisms, and stress responses, if inadequate, may predispose to physical injury.

2. **Musical**—technical difficulty, technique. The approach and commitment to music performance can have detrimental effects, including practice habits (warm up, breaks, cool down), sudden changes in practice time, and changes in repertoire, technique, or teacher.

3. **Instrumental/costume**—For adults, instruments are generally one-size-fits-all, but musicians come in all shapes and sizes. Ergonomic compromises may be needed to support and play the instrument or for theatrical effect.

4. **Environmental**—temporal, social, financial. These are situational factors related to audience and venue and include stress related to performance anxiety and playing for critics or judges during auditions. Other factors are cramped orchestra pits, bad lighting and temperature control, dark and smoky clubs, and travel demands. Additional risk factors for injury include general conditioning, diet, sleep, drug use and smoking.

6. Which is the most dangerous instrument?

Keyboard players seem to have the highest reported prevalence of problems, followed by the small strings (violin, viola).

7. Are there special considerations in the physical examination of a musician?

If at all possible, a musician should be examined playing the instrument. Most can bring it with them to the examination, but sometimes, the physician must make a "house call" and observe the environment as a whole. It may also be helpful to perform the exam with the teacher present.

A thorough but directed musculoskeletal and neurologic exam should be undertaken. Underlying medical problems may present earlier in musicians who may be more sensitive to the functional effects of minor impairment early in the course of disease. A careful search for tendon anomalies should be done, especially in string and wind players. Common patterns that can cause difficulties for certain instrumentalists are the **conjoined flexor sublimis tendons** of digits four and five in the left hand of violin players and the same finding in the right hand of clarinet players.

8. What are the most common medical problems diagnosed in musicians?

Overuse syndromes, especially injuries involving the muscle-tendon unit and nerve entrapment syndromes. Specific tendonopathies and ligament strains can be seen more often in certain instruments. The postural and biomechanical demands of most instruments combined with long playing times can create subtle imbalances in strength and range of motion. **Focal dystonia** has accounted for up to 10% of diagnoses of musicians seen in performing arts medicine centers. **Stress** and **performance anxiety** are also common problems that can coexist with or precede physical injury.

9. What is focal dystonia?

Better known as **occupational cramp**, focal dystonia is a movement disorder characterized by sustained, involuntary muscle contractions. Musicians often complain of loss of control, weakness, involuntary flexion and extension of digits or the wrist, difficulty relaxing, difficulty moving fingers off keys, or difficulty with rapidly alternating ascending or descending passages. The problem is usually task-specific and only becomes apparent while playing. Pain is uncommon but may develop as the musician compensates by straining to overcome the abnormal movements. The condition is often refractory to treatment and has completely disabled many artists. It is important to be certain there is no underlying medical condition that can manifest with dystonia (i.e., Wilson's disease or stroke).

10. How can focal dystonia be treated?

Aggressive treatment of other conditions (e.g., tendinitis, nerve entrapment)
Anticholinergic medications such as trihexyphenidyl
Technique retraining to correct the defect of motor coordination
Biofeedback
Movement therapies, such as the Alexander technique (corrective exercises for posture, breathing and muscle relaxation) and Feldenkrais method (lessons of subtle movements for enhancing kinesthetic sense)
Botulinum toxin injection
Splinting during performance

11. What are the common nerve entrapments seen in musicians?

Lederman found 143 peripheral nerve entrapments in a large series of 640 musicians. The most common were consistent with a diagnosis of **thoracic outlet syndrome**, although few if any had characteristic electrodiagnostic findings. Also very common is **carpal tunnel syndrome**. **Ulnar neuropathy** at the elbow is seen in the left upper extremity of fiddle players who hold their arm in constant elbow flexion to play the instrument. If focal dystonia is diagnosed, a thorough search for entrapment neuropathies should be undertaken.

12. What is meant by relative rest?

Relative rest is the cumulative reduction in task performance time that allows some continuation of the activity within the context of a controlled, therapeutic regimen. This can be accomplished by a total reduction of playing time in a day and by playing for short intervals separated by longer breaks. This population tends to ignore admonitions about activity restrictions. Writing out a strict schedule is often the only way to ensure compliance. A simple kitchen timer in the practice room will serve to remind the musician when it's time to take a break. Another method of accomplishing relative rest is to construct a device to relieve the burden of the supporting body part. Straps can be devised for instruments that don't routinely utilize them (i.e., the clarinet). Splints can be fabricated to unload specific regions, such as the thumb in the oboe.

13. How can instruments be modified?

The current design of many instruments is the result of centuries of refinement and adjustment for a desired musical effect. Instrument modification attempts to adapt the instrument to the individual musician. Changes to these designs are not often embraced by the music community, but there are circumstances when making a modification can mean the difference between continuing to play or not. Simple modifications include the use of chin rests or shoulder rests in the violin (viola), switching to a flute with closed key pads, using the angle-head flute (which allows one to maintain the cervical spine in neutral position and keep the arms down at the side), or recessing part of the body of the guitar or viola to reduce the amount of wrist flexion required to reach higher notes. While not strictly an instrument modification, seating should be assessed and optimized given the needs of the musician and the instrument.

14. What are the four categories of risk factors for injury in dancers?

The same general categories for injury can be applied to dancers as for musicians.

1. **Physiologic/psychologic**—Hip structure may preclude a professional career in classical ballet if there is femoral anteversion or an acetabular deformity that limits external rotation at the hip. Some degree of hypermobility may be a plus. Eating disorders can be a serious psychological disorder.

2. **Dance-specific**—performance task demands. The skill of one's partner, who may be responsible for throwing or catching the dancer, and choreography that includes potentially dangerous stunts are examples.

3. **Equipment**—Examples include ballet slippers and pointe shoes with good fit, changed at appropriate intervals (every several weeks in serious dancers) and properly padded if necessary; costumes; or lack of shoes (much modern dance is performed bare-footed).

4. **Environmental**—These include floor surface (wood floor preferable to concrete), cold temperature, aesthetic standards that can produce anxiety, and body image problems and are similar to performance pressures for musicians.

15. What is turnout?

Turnout refers to the total amount of external rotation of the lower extremity. It includes contributions from the hip, knee, and foot. Ideally, for classical ballet, each lower extremity should have 90° of total external rotation so that a total of 180° turnout will be produced. This rarely occurs.

16. How does a dancer cheat to increase the turnout?

Lumbar hyperlordosis. This produces hip flexion, relaxing the Y ligaments and loosening the hip capsule. More hip external rotation can be attained.

Screwing the knee. Hip flexion with capsular laxity can be achieved by flexing the knees while moving into the turned-out position and then straightening the knees after having utilized those few precious degrees of extra hip rotation. As the knees are straightened, the femurs tend to rotate back internally. With the feet already planted on the floor, excess torsional stress is applied to the knee, especially the medial collateral ligament and medial joint capsule.

Toe grab. To stabilize a forced turnout, the toes can be used to grab the floor.

Midfoot hyperpronation. A dancer forcing turnout below the knee may allow subtalar joint eversion and midtarsal abduction, giving the appearance of excessive pronation. The foot rolls over the medial arch and the navicular bone collapses.

17. What is point?

Point (or en pointe) refers to the position of the foot when balancing the body on the tips of the first two toes. **Demi-point** refers to the position when balancing on the ball of the foot. A special shoe is required (called a point shoe) to attain point. A minimum of 90° of plantar flexion of the foot with respect to the leg is required. Demi-point requires a minimum of 90° of dorsiflexion of the first metatarsophalangeal joint.

18. At what age can a dancer begin to work en pointe?

There is some controversy about this. Developing certain skills, including mastering most routine ballet steps and positions, developing strong hip rotators to control and maintain the turnout without cheating, refining balance away from the ballet barre, and strong foot intrinsic muscles, are prerequisites to beginning point work. Some say this should not be done before age 11 or 12, regardless of skill level. Beginning point work before the onset of puberty has not yet been clearly associated with long-term difficulties.

19. Are there unique problems seen in dancers?

Most of the medical literature has focused on the classical ballet dancer. A few common problems are encountered.

Spondylolysis   Snapping hip
Jumper's knee   Anterior compartment knee pain
Shin splints/stress fractures   Posterior ankle impingement
Anterior ankle impingement   Flexor hallucis longus tendinitis
Bunions

20. What causes a snapping hip?

There are two tendons that can create a snapping sensation around the hip joint. Groin pain with a snap during hip flexion and circumduction (ronde de jambe) may be due to a tight **iliopsoas tendon** rubbing across the anterior hip joint. The underlying bursa may also become irritated. Hip flexor stretching, soft-tissue release techniques, and attention to turnout mechanisms, along with NSAIDs, can be effective. Occasionally, bursal injection is necessary. The **iliotibial band** (ITB) can snap across the greater trochanter, causing lateral hip pain and also potentially irritating the underlying bursa. ITB stretching, release techniques and correcting turnout mechanics, along with NSAIDs, are effective. Bursal injection may be necessary for refractory cases. In rare cases, surgery for debridement and tendon lengthening can be considered in the professional dancer.

21. How can you differentiate shin splints from stress fractures?

Shin splints may involve either the anterior or posterior tibialis muscles. More severe dysfunction along this continuum may be a true periostitis. Point tenderness along the tibial shaft should always raise suspicion for stress fracture. Tomograms or a bone scan may be required for diagnosis and to distinguish these entities. A horizontal line seen along the anterior tibia on a lateral or oblique x-ray or tomogram is an especially ominous finding, the so-called dreaded black line, and represents a stress fracture with a high nonunion rate. Dancing must be stopped for at least 6 weeks, with only a gradual return to activity. Follow-up radiographs should be taken to monitor healing. Shin splints without fracture require relative rest with gradual return to activity.

22. Discuss the ankle impingement seen in dancers.

Posterior ankle impingement. The posterior talar tubercle or an os trigonum can be impinged between the distal posterior tibia and the calcaneous when the dancer is en pointe or demi-point (i.e., when the foot is maximally plantarflexed). With repeated compression, the talar tubercle or os trigonum can even fracture. This condition can be confused with Achilles tendinitis or retrocalcaneal bursitis. The latter two problems may be distinguished from posterior impingement when the dancer is on full point, as impingement pain will persist and increase, but bursal or tendon pain may decrease some in a skilled dancer whose balance uses less muscular force. Sometimes, symptoms are due more to compression of soft tissues and a trial of physical therapy (including massage, deep heat, and gastroc-soleus stretching), relative rest, and NSAIDs can be effective. For refractory cases, surgery to remove the os trigonum or chronically inflamed tissue is necessary.

Anterior ankle impingement. With plie, the ankle dorsiflexes and the tibia moves over the foot as the heel is kept on the floor. The tibia can impinge at the talus anteriorly. Over time, bony exostoses form, causing increasing pain. Injection at the front of the ankle joint can reduce symptoms in the early stages. Technique may need to be modified to reduce the depth of plie. Surgery may be required to remove the exostoses.

23. Should bunions be removed surgically?

Bunions are exostoses that can occur in conjunction with hallix valgus deformities of the first metatarsophalangeal (MTP) joint. They are very common in dancers as a result of the forces applied to the first MTP joint and can be exacerbated by poor technique, including faulty point/demi-point and cheating turnout. They should *never* be surgically corrected in a dancer who wishes to continue to perform classical ballet. The hallix rigidus that develops postoperatively will not allow sufficient dorsiflexion of the first MTP joint for demi-point. Although they may be unsightly, symptomatic bunions should be treated conservatively with physical therapy modalities for pain relief, NSAIDs, injection, padding the ballet slipper, and a toe spacer between first and second toe. Poor technique must be corrected.

BIBLIOGRAPHY

 1. Amadio PC (ed): Hand injuries in sports and performing arts. Hand Clin 6:355–549, 1990.
 2. Barringer J, Schlesinger S: The Pointe Book. Princeton, NJ, Princeton Book Co., 1991.
 3. Brown S: Shoulder pain and the instrumental musician. J Back Musculoskel Rehabil 2:16–27, 1992.
 4. Garrick JG, Requa RK: Turnout and training in ballet. Med Probl Perform Art 9:43–49, 1994.
 5. Lederman RJ: Entrapment neuropathies in instrumental musicians. Med Probl Perform Art 8:35–40, 1993.
 6. Norris RN: Applied Ergonomics: Adaptive Equipment and Instrument Modification for Musicians. Maryland Med J 42:271–275, 1993.
 7. Ryan AJ, Stephens RE: Dance Medicine—A Comprehensive Guide. Chicago, Pluribus Press, 1987.
 8. Sammarco GJ: Injuries to dancers. Clin Sports Med 2:457–656, 1983.
 9. Sataloff RT, Brandfonbrener AG, Lederman RJ: Textbook of Performing Arts Medicine. New York, Raven Press, 1991.
10. Solomon R, Minton SC, Solomon J: Preventing Dance Injuries. Reston, VA, American Alliance for Health, Physical Education, Recreation and Dance, 1990.

XI. Medical Complications in Rehabilitation

85. NEUROGENIC BOWEL DYSFUNCTION

Steven A. Stiens, M.D., and Lance L. Goetz, M.D.

"This is a fundamental principle of medicine, that whenever the stool is withheld or is extruded with difficulty, grave illnesses result."

—Maimonides (1135–1204)

1. How are the large intestine and pelvic floor innervated?

Colonic peristalsis is orchestrated by a series of nerve cells linking the brain to the colonic mucosa. The **vagus** (vagabond) nerve courses from the brainstem and innervates the gut all the way to the splenic flexure of the colon. The **nervi erigentes** (inferior splanchnic nerve) carries pelvic parasympathetic fibers from the S2–4 conal spinal cord levels to the descending colon and rectum. The descending colon receives sympathetic innervation from the hypogastric nerve (L 1,2,3). The intrinsic nervous system of the intestine includes the **Auerbach's plexus** (intramuscular myenteric), unmyelinated fibers and postganglionic parasympathetic cell bodies that coordinate peristalsis. Under the mucosa, **Meissner's plexus** relays sensory and local motor responses. The external anal sphincter is supplied by the somatic **pudendal nerve** (S2–4), which innervates the pelvic floor.

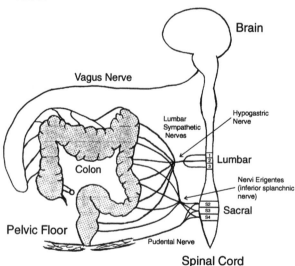

Nerve connections to the colon.

2. What is the "law of the intestine"?

In 1899, two English physiologists, W.M. Bayliss and E.H. Starling, reported that the intestines, even when removed from the body, have an inherent tendency to produce peristalsis toward the anus. This has become known as the "the law of the intestine." Whenever the intestinal wall is stretched or dilated, the nerves in the myenteric plexus cause the muscles above the dilation to constrict and those below the dilation to relax, propelling the contents toward the anus.

3. What is the sequence of normal physiologic processes that lead to defecation?

Reflex activity

1. Giant migratory contractions (GMC) advance stool through the colon to the rectum.
2. Stool distends the rectum as the internal sphincter relaxes (rectal inhibitory or sampling reflex), triggering a conscious "urge."
3. External anal and puborectalis muscle contraction retains stool (holding reflex).

Voluntary activity

1. Relaxation of the external anal sphincter and puborectalis.
2. Contraction of the levator ani, external abdominals, and diaphragm combined with glottic closure elevates intra-abdominal pressure and propels stool out.

4. How are the types of neurogenic bowel dysfunction defined and classified?

Neurogenic bowel is a term that relates colon dysfunction (constipation, incontinence, and discoordination of defecation) to lack of nervous control. The **upper motor neuron (UMN) bowel** results from a lesion of the spinal cord above the conus medullaris and typically manifests as fecal distention of the colon, overactive segmental peristalsis, underactive propulsive peristalsis, and a hyperactive holding reflex with anal constriction and the requirement for mechanical or chemical stimulus to trigger reflex defecation. The **lower motor neuron (LMN) bowel** results from a lesion that affects the parasympathetic cell bodies at the conus, cauda equina, or inferior splanchnic nerve.

5. What patterns of bowel dysfunction are observed with UMN and LMN lesions?

The UMN colon has been described as "spastic" due to the excessive colonic wall activity observed. Surface EMG studies have demonstrated increased muscular activity in the colon after spinal cord injury (SCI). Colonic transit is normal until the descending colon is reached. There, movement is characterized by excessive segmentation waves and less frequent propulsive mass action. The striated muscle of the external anal sphincter, normally under voluntary control, remains tight due to spasticity of the pelvic floor.

The LMN colon tends to be relaxed; no spinal-cord-mediated reflex peristalsis occurs. Slow stool propulsion is coordinated by the myenteric plexus alone, and the anal sphincter has low tone. This produces a drier, rounder (scybalous) stool because the prolonged transit time results in increased absorption of moisture from the stool.

6. What is the internal sphincter?

The internal sphincter is the thick layer of colonic smooth muscle that surrounds the anal canal at the distal rectum. It is the major contributor to the resting pressure of the closed anal canal. Closure is maintained by tonic excitatory sympathetic (L1,2) discharges. Internal sphincter tone is inhibited by anal dilatation by stool (**rectoanal inhibitory reflex**) or digital stimulation. Those experienced in bowel care are frequently able to palpate an increase in internal sphincter tone after defecation, which is a clinical sign that the bowel program is over.

7. What is digital stimulation?

Digital stimulation is a technique for inducing a reflex peristaltic waves from the colon to evacuate stool. Gentle insertion of the entire lubricated gloved finger into the rectum opens the external anal sphincter and provides a stretch stimulus that reduces spastic tone and outflow resistance. Stimulation is produced by rotation of the gloved finger in a firm circular manner, dilating the proximal rectum. It is important to continually maintain contact with the mucosae. Rotation is continued until relaxation of the bowel wall is felt, flatus passes, stool comes down, or the internal sphincter constricts. This maneuver activates peristalsis locally (coordinated by the myenteric plexus) and stimulates conal-mediated reflex peristalsis. Digital stimulation ideally should require no more than 1 minute to generate peristalsis.

8. Describe the bowel program used to facilitate reflex defecation for a person with an UMN bowel.

Persons with UMN injuries need a scheduled trigger of defecation every 1–3 days. Without the ability to feel the stool in the rectum or to easily initiate reflex defecation, a person with SCI must regularly assume the need for bowel movements to predictably eliminate stool and avoid colonic overdistention. The bowel program, or **bowel care**, is a process of facilitated reflex defecation. The reflex is stimulated manually with a finger (or assistive device) inserted in the rectum (digital stimulation) and/or with appropriate chemical stimulus.

The initial trigger is typically a suppository, enema, or mini-enema, which produces a mucosal contact stimulus that initiates conus-mediated reflex peristalsis. The chemical trigger is placed against the mucosa in the upper rectum. After the active ingredients have had time to dissolve and disperse, stool flow begins and is augmented as necessary with digital stimulations. Digital stimulations are repeated every 10 minutes if no stool passes. The end of the bowel program is signaled by cessation of gas and stool flow, palpable internal sphincter closure, or the absence of stool from the last two digital stimulations. Patients frequently "sense" the end of the bowel program. This sensation is possibly mediated by visceral afferents or partial sacral sparing of anal afferents.

9. What events and intervals mark the progress of the bowel program?

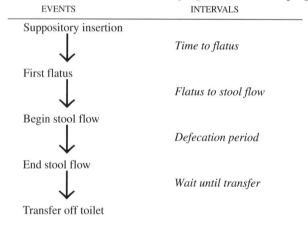

EVENTS	INTERVALS
Suppository insertion	
↓	*Time to flatus*
First flatus	
↓	*Flatus to stool flow*
Begin stool flow	
↓	*Defecation period*
End stool flow	
↓	*Wait until transfer*
Transfer off toilet	

10. What is the gastrocolic reflex?

Feeding induces increased propulsive colonic motility mediated by cholinergic motor neurons. The mechanism of this cholinergic stimulation is yet to be conclusively defined. Proposals include central vagal mediation, intrinsic colon pathways, and humoral mediation via cholecystokinin or gastrin. The reflex may be facilitated by a fatty or proteinaceous meal or blunted by atropine. Some investigators have reported that the gastrocolic reflex is less robust after SCI.

11. Describe techniques to produce defecation and maintain continence in persons with LMN bowels.

Persons with LMN injuries often have more difficulty with their bowel programs due to the absence of spinal reflex peristalsis and low anal sphincter tone. The rectum must be cleared of stool more frequently, usually one or more more times per day, to prevent leakage of stool that cannot be retained by the patulous external sphincter. Some patients wear tight underwear or bicycle pants to support the pelvic floor and help retain stool.

The LMN bowel program usually consists of removing stool with the finger and using digital stimulation to increase peristalsis. Continence is improved by modulation of stool consistency with a high-fiber diet. Plant fibers such as psyllium hydromucilloid "regularize" stool by absorbing excess water and retaining it to prevent dry hard stool.

12. What if the bowel program becomes excessively long, dependent, or complicated by autonomic dysreflexia or intractable bleeding hemorrhoids?

Some persons with long histories of SCI may have limited ability to independently manage their own bowel care, develop difficulty maintaining continence, or evolve excessively long bowel programs with insufficient results. A **colostomy** will offer independent bowel management, less incontinence, and reduced bowel care time, with a resultant improvement in quality of life. A colostomy is generally an elective procedure and is usually reversible, although people with SCI who elect for colostomy seldom have it reversed. Colostomies are often considered if severe bilateral grade 3 decubiti are present. Fecal diversion reduces wound contamination and simplifies care.

13. How can complications related to the neurogenic bowel be prevented?

Complications include hemorrhoids, impaction, colonic diverticuli, rectal prolapse, perirectal abscess, megacolon, and colonic cancer. Current prevention strategies include a high fiber diet to maintain a soft stool. Supporting the pelvic floor with a gel or air cushion to distribute pressure over the entire perineal surface prevents the enlargement of hemorrhoids and maintains closure of the anal sphincter.

Following a regular schedule of bowel programs is important even if stool elimination does not occur each time. Missed bowel programs can contribute to excessive stool buildup, making the stool drier and more difficult to eliminate. Retained stool can overstretch the colon wall, reducing the effectiveness of peristalsis and resulting in longer bowel programs with poor results. Hemorrhoids can be prevented through frequent digital stimulations (to minimize the time necessary for the bowel program) and by avoiding constipation.

14. What laxative preparations should be avoided as chronic medication?

Stimulant laxatives that are **anthraquinone derivatives**, such as senna, aloe, and cascara preparations, should be avoided because they can cause neuropathic damage to the myenteric plexus. Pigments from such laxatives also can stain the colonic mucosa (melanosis coli). Stool softeners, such as docusate sodium and mineral oil, are preferred for ongoing use because neither organ damage nor tolerance develops. Daily fiber supplements containing cellulose, polysaccharide, or psyllium can improve stool consistency if adequate fluid intake is maintained. Chronic suppository use is not known to cause colonic complications. Attempts to wean from suppositories and rely solely on reflex emptying from digital stimulation can be made over time.

15. What medications are used to augment the bowel program?
Oral:
Psyllium hydromucilloid—maintains stool moisture and consistency.
Docusate sodium—a surface-acting emulsifying agent that lubricates and maintains stool moisture.
Cisapride—a prokinetic agent that works locally by facilitating the release of acetylcholine at the myenteric plexus. Used in refractory constipation.
Suppositories to trigger defecation:
Glycerine—mild stimulus, lubricating.
Bisacodyl (phenolphthalein derivative)—a polyphenolic molecule that produces colonic mass action on contact. Provides a stronger chemical stimulus. Bisacodyl may be compounded with a vegetable oil or a potentially faster-acting polyethylene base.
CO_2-generating suppositories—produce reflex defecation in response to colon dilatation. Not uniformly reliable in persons with SCI.
Enemas to trigger defecation:
Theravac mini-enemas (rapid acting)—contain docusate sodium, polyethylene glycol, and glycerine with or without benzocaine (which can reduce the incidence of autonomic dysreflexia by locally anesthetizing the rectal wall).
Bisacodyl enema with a water base.

16. How can diarrhea in patients with neurogenic bowel be managed?

Diarrhea can be related to gastrointestinal infection, food intolerance, or use of antibiotics (most common treatment for a urinary tract infection). Treatment in these cases is similar to that for patients without a neurogenic bowel: antidiarrheal agents, laboratory evaluation for infectious causes (including *Clostridium difficile*, when indicated), and discontinuation of offending agents. Commonly, diarrhea alternating with constipation is related to partial bowel obstruction with flow of diarrhea around an impaction. A rectal exam is essential in evaluating these patients and may relieve the obstruction. Higher impactions are revealed by stool-filled loops of bowel on plain radiographs and require complete evacuation of the bowel, usually with oral magnesium citrate preparations.

BIBLIOGRAPHY

1. Aaronson MJ, Freed M, Burakoff R: Colonic myoelectric activity in persons with spinal cord injury. Dig Dis Sci 30:295–300, 1985.
2. Connell AM, Frankel H, Guttmann L: The motility of the pelvic colon following complete lesions of the spinal cord. Paraplegia 1:98–115, 1963.
3. Glick ME, Meshinpour H, Haldeman S, et al: Colonic dysfunction in patients with thoracic spinal cord injury. Gastroenterology 86:287–294, 1984.
4. Gore RM, Mintzer RA, Calenoff: Gastrointestinal complications of spinal cord injury. Spine 6:536–544, 1981.
5. Menardo G, Baujano G, Corazziari E, et al: Large bowel transit in paraplegic patients. Dis Colon Rectum 30:924–928, 1987.
6. Stiens SA: Reduction in bowel program duration with polyethylene glycol based bisacodyl suppositories. Arch Phys Med Rehabil 76:674–677, 1995.
7. Stiens SA: Neurogenic bowel dysfunction after spinal cord injury. Parapl News 50(1):65–67, 1996.
8. Sun EA, Snape WJ, Cohen S, et al: The role of opiate receptors and cholinergic neurons in the gastrocolonic response. Gastroenterology 82:689–693, 1982.
9. Weingarden SW: The gastrointestinal system and spinal cord injury. Phys Med Rehabil Clin North Am 3:765–779, 1992.

86. UROLOGIC DISORDERS IN REHABILITATION

Inder Perkash, M.D., F.A.C.S.

1. What is meant by a neurogenic urologic disorder? What are some common conditions leading to this disorder?

A neuro-urologic disorder is defined as a loss of voluntary control on initiation of micturition and/or an inhibition of micturition. This loss of control leads to either **retention** and/or **incontinence** of urine. Neuro-urologic disorders usually result from CNS lesions (e.g., cerebrovascular accident, head injury, intracranial tumors, spinal cord injuries [SCI], multiple sclerosis, and myelodysplasia) but may result from peripheral nerve injury as well (e.g., diabetic neuropathy). After a complete SCI lesion, there is usually a total lack of voluntary control on voiding, and as a result, there is usually retention or inadequate voiding.

2. What are the neural pathways linking the bladder to the CNS?

The human bladder is supplied by both the parasympathetic (motor and sensory) and sympathetic nervous systems. The bladder outlet at the pelvic floor is innervated by the somatic nervous system through the **pudendal nerves**.

The micturition center in the spinal cord is localized primarily in the interomediolateral region of **spinal cord segments S2–4**, with S3 being the most important root for bladder innervation. The pelvic parasympathetic nerves (S2–4) innervate the detrusor muscle and carry both motor and sensory fibers. However, the cell bodies of the parasympathetic fibers are located in the bladder wall. In other words, preganglionic fibers originate in the spinal cord, and postganglionic fibers originate in the bladder wall and innervate the bladder through short loops.

The innervation to most striated muscles of the pelvic floor, including those of the periurethral and anal sphincter, is through the pudendal nerve arising from S1–4.

There is ample evidence that the actual organizational center for micturition is localized in the **pontine-mesencephalic reticular formation**. Lesions above this level (suprapontine) are usually associated with detrusor hyper-reflexia, whereas infrapontine lesions are always associated with detrusor sphincter dyssynergia.

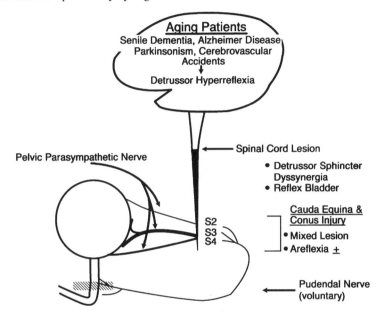

CNS lesions leading to different neurologic bladder disorders. (From Perkash I: Incontinence in patients with spinal cord injuries. In O'Donnell P (ed): Geriatric Urology. Boston, Little, Brown, & Co., 1994, pp 321–325; with permission.)

3. Describe the physiology of micturition.

When the bladder fills to about 100 ml, there is a minimum sensation of filling, but when it fills to about 300–400 ml, there is usually a feeling of fullness sensed by the brain (frontoparietal cortex). This sensation can be depressed and therefore micturition is inhibited. However, one can instantly initiate voiding when desired. Therefore, both initiation and inhibition are under voluntary control of the cerebral cortex, and thus continence is maintained. During vigorous sudden activities, such as jumping, coughing, or dancing, continence is maintained reflexively through the spinal cord, the **holding reflex**.

The bladder's response during filling is to accommodate and not lead to an increase in intravesical pressure. This very high compliance is due to passive viscoelastic properties of the bladder wall and possibly to intact β-adrenergic sympathetic innervation. Any fibrotic changes due to chronic infection and/or a neurologic lesion can reduce compliance and lead to much higher pressures during bladder filling.

4. What happens after spinal cord injury (SCI)?

Below the level of injury, there is complete loss of voluntary control; therefore, initially, there is retention of urine. However, later there is a tendency to develop a hyper-reflexic bladder with spontaneous voiding.

The basic function of local spinal cord reflexes is to hold urine. Normally, any sudden impact in the lower abdomen or strenuous activity, such as dancing or coughing, will lead to an instant reflex contraction of the external urinary sphincter and thus prevent leakage of urine. In spinal cord lesions, however, this **holding reflex** manifests with increased EMG activity of the external urethral sphincter during filling of the bladder or at attempted voiding and thus prevents leakage of urine. In people with SCI, this pathologic reflex is demonstrated by simultaneous cystometrographic and EMG studies of the external urethral sphincter during gradual bladder filling. When detrusor contraction attempts to empty the bladder, there is a reflex external sphincter contraction. This is referred to as **detrusor-sphincter dyssynergia** and is responsible for inadequate reflex voiding in SCI patients.

5. What is the role of sympathetic innervation of the bladder and bladder neck?

Efferent sympathetic nerves to the bladder and urethra originate in the intermediolateral nuclei of spinal cord segments T11–L2 and promote urine storage and continence. These nerves traverse the paravertebral ganglia to the hypogastric plexus to the bladder wall, bladder neck, and posterior urethra. They carry both motor and sensory fibers.

The bladder wall (fundus or body) primarily exhibits β-adrenergic receptors and responds to norepinephrine by relaxing. There is also an abundance of β-adrenergic receptors at the bladder base, which includes the upper trigone vesicoureteral junction. This helps bladder storage by relaxing the bladder muscle.

The bladder neck (vesicoureteral junction) is predominantly supplied with α-adrenergic fibers. There is a high density of α-adrenergic receptors along the bladder neck, particularly in males. This helps to prevent retrograde ejaculation and also helps close the bladder neck during bladder filling. Since α-adrenergic activity leads to closure of the bladder neck, α-adrenergic blockers (α-antagonists) have therefore usually been used to improve voiding by relaxing the bladder neck.

6. What basic bedside neurologic assessments provide initial clinical data for urologic management?

A basic neurourologic clinical exam should include a clear history for difficulty or inability to void. It should also include a quick, general neurologic exam to document any neurologic deficit. The exam should include perianal sensation (touch, pinprick), anal tone and voluntary contraction of the anal sphincter with digital examination, and bulbocavernous reflex (anal contraction with squeeze of the head of the penis). Rectal examination is also important to evaluate possible obstruction due to benign or malignant enlargement of the prostate. Because toe plantar flexors and hip external rotators are innervated by the S1 and S2 segments, their examination provides information on the integrity of sacral motor branches supplying the external urethral sphincter (S2) muscle.

An abdominal examination is important to feel for a distended bladder, as well as palpation before and after attempted voiding. In SCI patients, attempted voiding can be evaluated by suprapubic tapping over the bladder, valsalva maneuver, and credé (suprapubic pressure). However, objective evaluation of micturition problems can only be accomplished by urodynamic testing.

Postvoid residual (PVR) measurements are made by allowing the patient's bladder to fill naturally to capacity and then having the patient attempt voiding voluntarily in a natural position (standing or sitting). Measurement of the voided volume is compared with the residual volume obtained by catheterization or ultrasound. A PVR > 100 ml or more than about 20% of the total voided urine is considered abnormal.

7. How is a routine urodynamic evaluation done?

Because flow rates are difficult to determine in completely paralyzed patients, other objective urodynamic parameters must be used, including **cystometry** and **urethral pressure profiles**. The term **video urodynamics** refers to the simultaneous pressure flow studies with fluoroscopic visualization of the lower urinary tract. Similar studies can also be done using transrectal ultrasonography to simultaneously visualize the lower urinary tract.

Cystometry is the recording of intravesical pressures during bladder filling. It requires introduction of a catheter through the urethra and slow filling of 24–40 ml/min of fluid at body temperature. During bladder filling, intravesical pressure usually does not rise above 20 cm H_2O prior to bladder contraction. In patients with bladder wall fibrosis due to repeated infections, the bladder filling pressure rises more suddenly, and it rises above 20 cm H_2O and at lower volume. Such a situation is noticed because of reduced compliance. Normal persons have a feeling of fullness at around 400 ml, when they feel a desire to void.

It is difficult to study flow rates in patients with SCI, and therefore pressure/flow studies cannot be accomplished. Some information can be obtained by gently tapping the suprapubic area over the bladder, which can lead to voiding. Post-void residuals can then be determined either with ultrasound or by catheterizing the bladder.

8. What is a urethral pressure profile? How is it useful?

A urethral pressure profile (UPP) is the pressure curve provided by the measurement of intraurethral pressure during withdrawal of a pressure sensor along the bladder neck, prostatic urethra, and the rest of the urethra. Profilometry can be performed on an empty or full bladder. Maximal urethral pressure is usually noticed close to the bulbous urethra. The UPP has limited value in patients with neurogenic bladders. In the presence of obstruction, the fall in UPP is more marked just beyond the site of obstruction.

9. What is detrusor compliance?

Compliance is defined as the increase in bladder pressure per unit of volume and is calculated by the change in volume divided by the change in pressure ($\Delta V/\Delta P$). The detrusor wall is composed of roughly equal amounts of muscle and collagen. When the collagen is more abundant, the elasticity decreases, the detrusor becomes stiffer, and the pressure rises faster during filling. Hypertrophic, spastic (neurogenic) detrusor muscle can also have a varying degree of reduced compliance.

10. What is detrusor sphincter dyssynergia?

The normal process of voiding includes a balanced synergy of simultaneous bladder wall contraction and sphincter relaxation. Detrusor sphincter dyssynergia is a pathologic hyperactive holding reflex characterized by the presence of involuntary pelvic floor (urinary sphincter) EMG activity during detrusor (bladder wall) contraction. This is observed in patients with spinal cord lesions below the pons and is absent in those with intracranial lesions. In normal persons, it is sometimes difficult to differentiate involuntary sphincteric activity such as dyssynergia from voluntary contractions to inhibit micturition. A careful evaluation is therefore required to diagnose detrusor sphincter dyssynergia in a patient with a normal neurologic examination.

11. How are the bulbocavernous reflex (BCR) and genitocerebral-evoked potential tested? Why?

Bulbocavernous reflex is a polysynaptic (S2–4) crossed sacral withdrawal reflex and a nociceptive reflex of very constant latency. Clinically, it can be tested by squeezing the glans or clitoris and feeling the contraction of anal sphincter muscle. This reflex is present in all normal persons and in those SCI patients with lesions above the conus. BCR can also be recorded objectively by stimulating the dorsal nerve of the penis and picking up the EMG response (50–200 µV) in the anal sphincter muscle or from the perineal striated muscle.

The **sacral-evoked response** can be obtained either by stimulating the dorsal nerve of the penis with a ring electrode or by placing a stimulating needle on the left or right side of the bulbocavernosus muscle in the perineum to define a unilateral lesion. The first latency (about 12 msec) can be recorded over T4–L1 on the back, which represents the sensory peripheral conduction time. The central conduction time can be recorded at the scalp, which is usually 50 ms. Patients with previously diagnosed neurologic disease or those found to have subtle abnormalities on neurologic screening are candidates for this type of evaluation. The sacral-evoked potential testing and somatosensory-evoked potential testing should not be used as screening tests but rather as objective measurements of the location, presence, and nature of afferent penile sensory dysfunction. The findings of this testing can aid in anatomic localization of the lesion as peripheral, sacral, or suprasacral.

12. Which type of neurourologic dysfunction is typically seen with UMN lesions in SCI patients?

Vesicoureteral dysfunction depends on the site of lesion, preexisting or associated disease such as diabetes mellitus, radiculopathy, enlarged prostate, urethral stricture, and even ethanol abuse. Initially after an acute spinal injury, there is widespread autonomic paralysis (spinal shock phase); this often recovers by 3–6 weeks but can take longer. The reappearance of reflexes below the level of injury heralds the end of the spinal shock. The bladder can easily become overdistended due to neglect during this period. As a result, reflex voiding may not immediately ensue. Later, the appearance of detrusor sphincter dyssynergia leads to intermittent voiding (squirting of urine alternating with retention of urine). Bladder emptying can then be accomplished with intermittent catheterization. Baseline urodynamic testing is usually performed 6–8 weeks after acute injury.

13. What is the best way to provide bladder drainage in patients with acute SCI?

During the first 7–14 days, an indwelling catheter may be left in the urethra for continuous bladder drainage to prevent inadvertent bladder overdistension. A small catheter (F14 or 16) is recommended, which prevents urethral irritation and allows periurethral secretions to drain easily around it. Most patients who have severe injuries require fluid intake/output charting since they are on intravenous fluids.

Intermittent catheterization can be started as early as 7–15 days after injury. Fluid intake may need to be restricted to < 1500 ml/day. The bladder is drained with a straight catheter (F14) every 4 hours with a goal bladder volume of no more than 500 ml. After the establishment of reflex bladder, the patient is evaluated objectively with urodynamic monitoring of intravesical voiding pressures (leak pressure). A cystometrogram (CMG) may need to be repeated to evaluate voiding pressures following the use of anticholinergics to reduce detrusor contractions. Persistently high voiding pressures > 40–50 cm H_2O with sustained rise during CMG may necessitate a further increase in the dosage of anticholinergics. To start, patients are given oxybutynin (Ditropan, anticholinergic), 2.5–5 mg two or three times a day to lower intravesicle pressure to < 40–50 cm H_2O. This also helps to achieve continence between catheterizations, and therefore patients do not have to wear external drainage and leg bags.

14. Which method provides optimal long-term drainage of the neurogenic bladder?

Patients who have a reflex bladder, particularly tetraplegics, cannot catheterize themselves but can wear an external drainage condom, and they should be considered for surgical reduction of outflow obstruction. To reduce outflow resistance and to have them void at low pressure, transurethral sphincterotomy or stenting of the urethral sphincter is considered. This also helps to reduce the autonomic dysreflexia triggered by detrusor sphincter dyssynergia.

A patient with a small retractile phallus with reflex bladder may be considered for a penile implant. Other patients who cannot self-catheterize and have a small retractile phallus may need an indwelling catheter or suprapubic cystostomy.

In female patients who cannot self-catheterize and are incontinent, supravesical diversion, such as a suprapubic cystostomy or bowel pouch, may be considered. Continent reservoirs that can be catheterized through sites on the abdomen area also available. Recently, such patients are also being considered for sacral nerve root implants to accomplish an electrically controlled bladder.

15. What is autonomic dysreflexia? How is this condition treated?

A sudden paroxysmal rise both in systolic and diastolic blood pressures with compensatory slowing of the pulse rate is observed clinically in dysreflexia. It usually happens in patients with spinal cord lesions above T5–6. Symptoms may include a pounding headache and sweating.

Autonomic dysreflexia is commonly precipitated by a full bladder and/or rectum or by other painful stimuli. To relieve the condition, the bladder is emptied by suprapubic tapping and/or immediate catheterization. Immediate blood pressure reduction can also be achieved with nifedipine, 10 mg sublingually, or by chewing the caplets and swallowing them for rapid absorption. Long-term management includes prevention of the triggering mechanism and may require the chronic use of α-adrenergic blockers such as prazosin, terazosin, or a ganglionic blocker. Permanent resolution of dysreflexia (caused by voiding dysfunction) can sometimes be accomplished by transurethral sphincterotomy or following placement of a metallic stent in the posterior urethra.

16. Describe the usual protocol for urologic follow-up of these patients.

Patients with SCI are monitored with radionuclide renal perfusion imaging to evaluate glomerular filtration (GFR), renal plasma flow (RPF), and annual ultrasound of kidney to detect renal parenchymal loss, hydronephrosis, and stones. If hydronephrosis of the kidneys or ureters is noticed or deterioration of the renal function is found, a full work-up including intravenous urogram and voiding cystourethrogram is done. Cystoscopic examination is also done to evaluate outflow obstruction or to rule out other bladder problems such as bladder tumors. A yearly cystoscopic examination is recommended for patients who are heavy smokers or use chronic indwelling catheters.

17. What bladder problems are seen in patients with brain injury?

Following head injury or other intracranial lesions, the bladder is hyper-reflexic, but there is no dyssynergia. Initially, there may be retention of urine, and patients can be managed with an indwelling catheter followed by intermittent catheterization every 4–6 hours. Some patients may have an enlarged prostate which may require treatment later. Involuntary leakage of urine can be controlled with a small dosage of oxybutynin. Inadequate voiding due to internal sphincter resistance can be improved with the use of terazosin, an α-receptor antagonist, starting with a dose of 1 mg at night. Effectiveness of this therapy on voiding needs to be assessed with post-void residual measurements, then gradually increasing the dose as needed over several days. All autonomic drugs are gastrointestinal irritants; therefore, they should be given with meals. Initially patients may not tolerate hypotensive effect; therefore, they are given a low dose until they get used to the drug.

In patients with intracranial lesions such as parkinsonism, the bladder also is hyper-reflexic. The use of drugs (anticholinergics) to manage tremors may lead to retention of urine. In all such patients with detrusor hyper-reflexia, a transurethral resection of the prostate can sometimes result in permanent incontinence.

18. What are the common urinary tract complications of neurogenic bladder? How can they be prevented?

- The earliest changes are noticed as trabeculations seen inside an irregular, thickened bladder wall and even small diverticuli seen on voiding cystographic studies.
- Vesicoureteral reflux has been recorded in 10–30% of poorly managed patients. The presence of reflux is a serious complication since it leads to pyelonephritis and renal stone disease.
- Severe bladder outflow obstruction can result in bilateral hydronephrosis and hydroureters and even an overdistended areflexic bladder.
- Repeated bladder infections can lead to bladder wall changes and marked reduction in the compliance of the bladder.

All of these bladder wall changes can be prevented to some extent by adequately draining the bladder at a pressure below 40 cm H_2O either by intermittent catheterization along with the use of anticholingergic drugs or by timely surgical relief of the outflow obstruction.

19. List the drugs used in the management of bladder problems and their desired effects.

Pharmacologic Manipulation of Bladder Function

DESIRED FUNCTIONAL CHANGE	DRUGS	MODE OF ACTION
Improve bladder emptying		
Facilitate bladder contraction (muscarinic action)	Acetylcholine (clinically not used)	Normal neurotransmitter of the cholinergic receptors. It cannot be used for therapeutic purposes.
	Bethanechol (clinically used)	Limited indications. It should not be used with outlet obstruction or in suspected coronary disease. It could be used in selected patients along with α-sympathetic blockers and in patients with atonic or hypotonic bladder.
Decrease outlet resistance	Prazosin, terazosin, doxazosin (clinically used) Phenoxybenzamine (mutogenic in laboratory animals) Tamsulosin (newer selective blocker	α-Adrenoceptor blockers improve voiding by opening bladder neck.
Improve bladder storage		
Reduce bladder contraction	Atropine, propantheline, oxybutinin	Anticholinergic action (antimuscarinic action).
Increase outlet resistance	Phenylnephrine, ephedrine	Sympathetic agonist response on α-adrenergic receptors.
Improve bladder storage and increase outlet resistance	Tricyclic antidepressants	Central and peripheral anticholinergic effects and also enhances α-adrenergic effect on bladder base and proximal urethra.

BIBLIOGRAPHY

1. Cardenas DD, Hooton TM: Urinary tract infection in persons with spinal cord injury. Arch Phys Med Rehabil 76:272, 1995.
2. Perkash I: Intermittent catheterization failure and an approach to bladder rehabilitation in spinal cord injury patients. Arch Phys Med Rehabil 59:9, 1978.
3. Perkash I: Management of neurogenic dysfunction of the bladder and bowel. In Kottke FJ, Stillwell GK, Lehmann JF (eds): Krusen's Handbook of Physical Medicine and Rehabilitation, 3rd ed. Philadelphia, W.B. Saunders, 1982, p 724.
4. Perkash I: Long-term urologic management of the patient with spinal cord injury. Urol Clin North Am 20:423, 1993.
5. Perkash I: Urologic diagnostic testing. In Lennard TA: Physiatric Procedures in Clinical Practice. Philadelphia, Hanley & Belfus, 1995.
6. Perkash I: Contact laser sphincterotomy: Further experience and longer follow-up. Spinal Cord 34:227, 1996.
7. Reid G, Kang YS, Lacerte M, et al: Bacterial biofilm formation on the bladder epithelium of spinal cord injured patients. II. Toxic outcome on cell viability. Paraplegia 31:494, 1993.
8. Rutkowski SB, Middleton JW, Truman G, et al: The influence of bladder management on fertility in spinal cord injured males. Paraplegia 33:263, 1995.
9. Silver JR, Doggart JR, Burr RG: The reduced urinary output after spinal cord injury: A review. Paraplegia 33:721, 1995.
10. Thyberg M, Ertzgaard P, Gylling M, Granerus G: Effect of nifedipine on cystometry-induced elevation of blood pressure in patients with a reflex urinary bladder after a high level spinal cord injury. Paraplegia 32:308, 1994.

87. COMMON MEDICAL PROBLEMS ON THE INPATIENT REHABILITATION UNIT

James K. Richardson, M.D.

FEVER

1. Does everyone with a fever have an infection?

No, especially on the inpatient rehab unit. An elevated temperature in a patient with C6 spinal cord injury who is situated on the south or west side of the unit in the late afternoon may simply be reflecting impaired autoregulation. Processes that are not infectious, such as connective tissue diseases and deep vein thrombosis/pulmonary embolism, may cause fever. Finally, an elderly diabetic stroke patient may have overwhelming sepsis and not manifest an increased temperature.

2. A patient has a fever but doesn't have pneumonia or a urinary tract infection. What conditions should you consider?

On the inpatient rehabilitation unit, the patient population has traits that predispose them to a number of difficult-to-diagnose fever etiologies.
- Deep venous thrombosis/pulmonary embolism
- Sinus infection in patients with nasogastric tubes
- Osteomyeolitis underlying pressure sores
- Intra-abdominal, retroperitoneal, or paraspinal abscesses in trauma patients
- Blood-borne infection (after transfusions)
- Heterotopic ossification
- Infections related to not-original equipment, such as catheters, feeding tubes, orthopedic hardware, and ventricular shunts
- "Central fever" in patients with brain injury (cooling response to environment good, to acetaminophen poor)
- Drugs

3. List some drugs that commonly cause fever.

Penicillin derivatives	Hydralazine	Propranolol
Sulfonamides	Methyldopa	Procainamide
Thiazide diuretics	Phenytoin	Amphotericin B
Nitrofurantoin	Allopurinol	Quinidine
Isoniazid		

4. Some of my patients have fever now and then. When do I really need to worry?

Three common conditions that are associated with fever on a rehab unit and that can kill rapidly are deep venous thrombosis/pulmonary embolus, bacterial meningitis, and "sepsis syndrome."

5. How is sepsis syndrome diagnosed?

Patients with bacteria in their blood may be just febrile, or febrile and manifesting the septic syndrome, or septic syndrome without fever. The septic syndrome occurs when a blood-borne bacterial infection causes a diffuse vascular endothelial injury with resultant loss of arteriolar tone. As a consequence, there is an elevated heart rate (> 90 bpm), an initially normal and then decreasing blood pressure (< 90 mmHg systolic or a drop of 40 below baseline systolic), loss of organ perfusion, acidosis, and organ-system failure. Clinically, this condition is recognized as hyperventilation (> 20 breaths/min), mental status change, anorexia/nausea/vomiting/diarrhea, and decreasing urine output. The last is the best monitor of the septic syndrome, as the kidneys are exquisitely sensitive to perfusion and pressure changes. It should be recognized that patients with normal urine outputs may still be systematically and seriously infected, but it is unlikely that such patients are developing the septic syndrome.

6. My brain-injured patient has fever, tachycardia, and normal blood pressure, but he is disoriented and can't tell me if he's hungry or not. Now what?

1. Utilize the kidneys. Start an IV of NS or 0.5 NS at 100–150 ml/hr. If the patient does not average > 30 ml of urine/hr, he clearly needs empiric antibiotics and closer monitoring.

2. Check a complete blood count. In the setting of bacteremia/sepsis, most young, non-immunosuppressed patients have a markedly increased white blood cell count with polymorphonuclear (PMN) forms predominating. Keep in mind that some patients, particularly older or immunosuppressed patients, may have normal or abnormally low white cell counts, but the differential usually shows a large percentage of immature forms of PMNs.

3. Check a blood gas, as most septic patients demonstrate respiratory alkalosis superimposed on metabolic acidosis. In other words, the PCO_2 is significantly below 40 mmHg, while the pH is normal or mildly acidotic.

GASTROINTESTINAL DISORDERS

7. About 85% of my patients are intensely constipated, while the other 15% have diarrhea. Anything to worry about here?

Yes, in reality, they may be constipated and leaking liquid stool around a fecal mass. Examine the belly and check a flat plate if you are uncertain before treating the presumed "diarrhea" symptomatically, or you may contribute to the problem.

8. What about colitis due to *Clostridium difficile*?

Many patients on the rehab unit have had complications during their acute course that required antibiotics, and as a result, they are at risk for pseudomembranous colitis caused by *Clostridium difficile*. In diagnosing this condition, the presence of fecal leukocytes is a helpful, fast, and relatively specific finding but not very sensitive, as some patients with clearcut clinical *C. difficile*-associated diarrhea have minimal observable changes. The presence of *C. difficile* toxin in stool is the most reliable diagnostic test. Stool culture for *C. difficile* is nonspecific and positive in 3% of the general population.

9. How do you treat pseudomembranous colitis?

For patients who are not seriously ill, **cholestyramine** to bind the toxin (a 4-gm packet three times daily for 5–10 days) and **metronidazole** (500 mg orally three or four times daily for 10–14 days) to decrease *C. difficile* counts are effective treatments. For the seriously ill patient, oral **vancomycin** (125–250 mg four times daily orally) is recommended instead of metronidazole. Relapses are common on discontinuation of antibiotics, and retreatment may be necessary.

10. Everybody who has had blood loss comes to the rehabilitation unit on t.i.d. iron. Does oral iron allow anemia to resolve more quickly?

If the patient is iron-deficient, yes; if the patient is not iron-deficient, no. However, it very effectively enhances anorexia in most patients when started immediately on a three-times-daily dose.

11. What should I do?

Check the iron indices. If the serum iron to iron-binding capacity ratio is < 0.15, give iron. If it is > 0.20, stop it. If it is in the "gray zone," then consider the situation. Previously well-nourished adult males usually have abundant iron stores. Regularly menstruating women and the poorly nourished usually have depleted iron stores. Remember, mild iron deficiency can occur with a normal mean cell volume, so err on the side of treating such patients. Serum ferritin reflects iron stores nicely if the patient does not have cancer, infection, inflammation, or liver disease, in which case the serum ferritin is falsely elevated.

If you decide to treat, give the patient one dose of iron 0.5 hour before a meal with orange juice or vitamin C in those with reflux esophagitis. Increase by one dose every 5 days until the patient is on a three-times-daily schedule; this should avoid problems with gastric irritation, nausea, and anorexia.

12. Everybody seems to come out of the intensive care unit taking an H2 antagonist such as rantidine. Do all patients have to stay on these medications?

Probably not. Three groups of rehabilitation patients would likely benefit from continued prophylaxis against GI bleeding:

1. Patients with complete T4 and higher spinal cord injuries seem especially prone to upper GI bleeds (possibly owing to unopposed parasympathetic stimulation to the stomach causing excessive release of acid) and benefit from 4–6 weeks of such prophylaxis.

2. Patients with a previous history of peptic ulcer disease or GI bleeding, especially if on anticoagulation, likely benefit.

3. Patients with an acute course complicated by multiple factors associated with GI bleeding, such as ventilator dependence, hemorrhage, shock from any cause, sepsis, multiple trauma, and steroid usage, should likely continue such medications.

There is, however, a potential trade-off in terms of pneumonia risk. As a result, you must use clinical judgment to decide if the patient's risk for GI bleeding is offset by the possible increased risk of pneumonia with the use of H2 antagonists.

13. Abdominal problems are difficult to diagnose in patients with spinal cord injury (SCI). Aside from GI bleeding, what else should I worry about?

• **Pancreatitis** also occurs with increasing frequency in the first 4–6 weeks after SCI; unlike GI bleeding, there is no change in risk depending on the level of injury.

• **Nephrolithiasis** may occur in young men with SCI in association with the hypercalciuria from bone demineralization. Such stones are radio-opaque.

• These patients have slowed bile transit and are at increased risk for **cholelithiasis** and **cholecystitis**.

ELECTROLYTE DISORDERS

14. What is the most common electrolyte abnormality on the rehab unit?

Hyponatremia.

15. How do I tell if the hyponatremia is significant?

Serum sodium is a ratio of total body sodium to total body water—a low serum sodium by itself says nothing about whether total body sodium is too high, too low, or just right. Go see the patient and assess his or her clinical volume status. Distended neck veins, presacral/pretibial edema, orthopnea, and rales all suggest hypervolemia or increased total body sodium. (It should be noted that patients with SIADH or syndrome of inappropriate secretion of antidiuretic hormone, and no other problem affecting their electrolytes have none of these signs and are clinically euvolemic, as they are able to excrete sodium normally.) Postural hypotension, decreased skin turgor, dry membranes, resting tachycardia, and increased blood urea nitrogen (BUN) to creatinine (Cr) ratio (> 20) all suggest hypovolemia and decreased total body sodium.

16. Which other labs should I look at?

Lab Values that Distinguish SIADH from Volume Depletion in Hyponatremia

	SIADH	VOLUME DEPLETION
BUN/Cr	< 20	> 20
Urine osmolality	> 200 mOsm/kg H_2O	> 400 mOsm/kg H_2O
Urine Na	> 40 mEq/hr	< 20 mEq/hr
Fractional excretion of Na	> 2%	< 1%

* Fractional excretion of Na = [(urine Na/serum Na)/(urine Cr/serum Cr)] × 100.

17. Now that I have determined volume, and therefore total body sodium, status with laboratory and physical examination, what's next?

Decreased total body sodium: Consider giving volume with normal saline intravenously. Serum sodium will correct as the kidney senses adequate volume and it stops reabsorbing water in the distal tubule.

Normal total body serum: The patient likely has SIADH, which is usually treated effectively with water restriction to approximately 1 liter/day. A more humane alternative in patients with good left ventricular pump function is ad-lib water and high-salt diet combined with daily furosemide. Obviously, when drugs are contributing or causing SIADH, they should be discontinued or another drug substituted. Finally if the SIADH is severe, then intravenous hypertonic saline and furosemide are likely required; at that point, call for medical consultation.

Elevated total body sodium: The patient likely has a concurrent pathologic process that is making the kidneys believe that the body is hypovolemic, and the lab values will usually reflect avid sodium and water conservation. Examples include congestive heart failure and cirrhosis. Such situations suggest incomplete filling of the arterial tree, either due to deranged Starling forces (e.g., loss of intravascular colloidal osmotic pressure in cirrhosis) or pump dysfunction in heart failure. Fluid restriction is a mainstay of treatment. These situations can have an ominous prognosis—a patient trying very hard to remain a patient—and medical consultation is called for.

18. List some common causes of SIADH.

The major causes of SIADH are so ubiquitous on the inpatient rehabilitation unit that it is almost surprising if some patients do not have it.

- CNS thrombotic or hemorrhagic event
- CNS infection or neoplasm
- Postoperative state
- Psychosis
- Prolonged nausea
- Lung disease
  Pneumonia
  Positive pressure ventilation
  Malignancy
- Drugs
  Carbamazepine
  Chlorpropamide
  Phenothiazines
  Cyclophosphamide
  Amitriptyline
  Other tricyclic antidepressants
  Morphine

19. How quickly should the sodium be corrected?

Correcting the sodium too fast places the patient at risk for acute cerebral shrinkage with mental status changes, and possibly central pontine myelinolysis. It is prudent to correct the sodium by not faster than 10 mEq/L over 24 hours until the sodium reaches 125 mEq/L and then more gradually, being careful to avoid overcorrection.

20. Do any other electrolyte problems occur on the inpatient rehab unit?

Yes, hypercalcemia can occur in young men with recent spinal cord injury. Such patients often have fatigue, apathy, and depression as the most prominent manifestations of hypercalcemia. Therefore, diagnosis in subjects with any kind of brain dysfunction requires a high index of suspicion. Other symptoms/signs include polydipsia, polyuria, nausea and vomiting. Treatment includes mobilization of the patient to the degree possible, disodium etidronate, and a furosemide-induced saline diuresis.

21. Are there any special concerns for patients with diabetes mellitus on the inpatient rehabilitation unit?

Diabetes mellitus is always of concern, but it is particularly tricky to manage in rehabilitation inpatients. In that setting, the patient may go from completely inactive and relatively insulin-resistant to actively involved in an aerobic conditioning program, which renders the patient more insulin-sensitive. The tapering of steroids may have the same effect. In general, it is probably better to be conservative during this time of change and tolerate a few episodes of hyperglycemia than to have recurrent hypoglycemia, especially in patients recovering from any kind of brain damage. Finally, fatal hyperkalemia has developed in patients with diabetes mellitus on nonsteroidal antiinflammatory drugs; therefore, monitor serum K^+ in diabetic patients placed on these agents.

MENTAL STATUS CHANGES

22. The rehab team tells me that my profoundly brain injured patient has mental status changes, but he sure looks the same to me. What should I do?

Work it up. One of the real advantages of a rehabilitation team working with your patient several hours per day is that they become very sensitive to the patient's cognitive and physical abilities. They can detect a drop off in these abilities that is not evident with bedside examination. For example, loss of sitting balance in a low-level, incontinent patient might be hydrocephalus—which normally causes gait ataxia, incontinence, and cognitive dysfunction.

23. How do I work up acute/subacute mental status changes?

1. Think about structural/anatomic causes, metabolic causes, and drugs. A brain imaging study may be ordered to rule out hydrocephalus, edema, and thrombotic or hemorrhagic events.

2. Check the blood for white cell count, as sepsis can cause mental status change; also check the serum glucose, sodium, and calcium, and check the arterial blood gases for alterations in PO_2 and PCO_2. Cerebral hypoperfusion from myocardial infarction or arrhythmia can lead to mental status change. Emboli to the brain may occur, especially in those with atrial fibrillation, valvular abnormalities, myocardial infarction, or recent aortic or coronary catheterization.

3. Meningitis is common in patients who have had neurosurgical procedures, so check the CSF after ruling out hydrocephalus. If your clinical suspicion is high for meningitis, then antibiotics should be started immediately—even if that means that CSF has not already been obtained.

4. If the patient is initially lethargic but recovers nicely within 24 hours, consider the possibility of an unwitnessed seizure.

5. Finally, and most importantly, look for drugs that might be diminishing cognitive function. Check anticonvulsant levels. Also consider the effect of drugs which might have recently been withdrawn, such as alcohol and benzodiazepines.

24. Which drugs might limit the recovery of a brain-injured patient or induce mental status change?

Benzodiazepines (short- and long-acting)
Phenothiazines (major tranquilizers)
Central sympathetic inhibitors (methyl-dopa, clonidine)
Anticonvulsants (phenobarbital/phenytoin)

DYSPNEA

25. What do I worry about when my patient gets short of breath?

You worry a lot about pulmonary embolus (PE). In autopsy series of patients whose cause of death was unknown, PE still tops the list of causes. It is almost impossible to be too aggressive in working up and treating DVT/PE.

Risk Factors for DVT/PE

Age > 50 yrs	Trauma
Bedrest	Obesity
Congestive heart failure	Estrogen administration
Lower extremity weakness	Malignancy
Surgery	History of DVT/PE

26. My patient with dyspnea has a low or intermediate probability ventilation-perfusion scan. What do I do?

Check lower-extremity Doppler/ultrasound studies before subjecting your patient to a pulmonary angiogram or venogram, both of which have risks.

27. What if it is a weekend or night and I cannot get the studies done that I need?

If the patient has risk factors for DVT/PE and the most common symptoms (dyspnea, anxiety) and signs of PE (tachycardia), or a respiratory alkalosis on arterial blood gas in a patient who cannot communicate symptoms, then the patient should be treated empirically with heparin until more definitive workup can be done. Heparin not only prevents further clot formation but has a relaxing effect on pulmonary endothelium after PE, which lessens the resultant perfusion defect and in turn lessens the patient's symptoms. If there is a contraindication to heparin, then transfer the patient to a monitored bed and place an inferior vena caval filter when and if the diagnosis is confirmed.

28. What other causes of acute dyspnea should be considered?

Dyspnea can be an anginal equivalent in any population, but given the percentage of patients with impaired sensation or ability to express themselves, **angina** as a cause of dyspnea is likely even more frequent on the rehabilitation unit. Patients with cervical spinal cord injury, diabetes, and cognitive dysfunctions or aphasia may all have difficulty reporting or sensing typical anginal symptoms. In addition, many patients on the inpatient rehabilitation unit have abundant risk factors for coronary artery disease. Stroke patients have a greater mortality from coronary artery disease than stroke.

One bedside clue that suggests angina is the absence of a **tibial pulse**. If a patient is missing a tibial pulse, then that patient's risk of significant coronary artery disease is > 90%. Missing a leg (and therefore a tibial pulse) due to vascular occlusive disease is another way not to have a tibial pulse, but the rule still applies—vascular amputees are at high risk for coronary artery disease and myocardial infarction.

29. Isn't there at least one relatively benign cause of sudden dyspnea in the inpatient rehabilitation population?

Yes, a **mucous plug** can be a significant problem in rehabilitation populations, who often have weakened expiratory force and cough. Aggressive pulmonary toilet with percussion/postural drainage, assisted cough, and suctioning are usually enough, but at times bronchoscopy and lavage are necessary.

30. Why do so many patients on the rehab service acquire pneumonia during their stay?

The risk factors for hospital-acquired pneumonia include impaired mentation, abnormal swallow, chronic debilitating illness, weak or absent cough, mechanical ventilation or tracheostomy, and possibly the use of H2 antagonists such as cimetidine. The endotracheal tubes and tracheostomy tubes are particularly risky, as they allow microorganisms direct access to the bronchial tree, which quickly becomes colonized.

31. What is a good empiric therapy for hospital-acquired pneumonia while I await culture results?

Patients rapidly become colonized with gram-negative bacilli and *Staphylococcus aureus*, and thus those are the leading causes of hospital-acquired pneumonia. Reasonable empiric coverage includes a third-generation cephalosporin with good activity against *Pseudomonas* and an aminoglycoside.

Also, percussion, postural drainage, saline lavage, and suctioning are at least as important as antibiotics, and probably more important than antibiotics in typical rehabilitation patients who have impaired cough. The antibiotics slow the rate of bacterial proliferation, but the pneumonia must be cleared by the rehabilitation team.

BLOOD PRESSURE ABNORMALITIES

32. Half of my patients have high blood pressure, and the other half have hypotension. What are common causes of hypotension on the inpatient rehabilitation service?

Simple **bedrest** is a common cause of postural hypotension. Loss of postural reflexes is common after 3 weeks in healthy people and after as little as several days to weeks in the elderly and those with major trauma or illness. **Disturbed autonomic function** is another cause and occurs in patients with autonomic neuropathy from Guillain-Barré, diabetes mellitus, certain antihypertensives, and other causes.

33. So my patient is a little light-headed. Is that really anything to worry about?

Yes. Obviously, postural light-headedness can precipitate a fall, but it also can cause stroke and myocardial infarction in those with **systemic vascular disease**. Remember that the coronary arteries fill during diastole, so postural hypotension may be particularly concerning for patients with coronary artery disease. Also, malignant arrhythmias due to autonomic dysfunction can occur in patients with **Guillain-Barré**. Any clinical evidence of tachy- or bradyarrhythmia or fluctuating blood pressure suggests that the Guillain-Barré patient deserves a monitored bed and close observation in an intensive care unit setting. Finally, patients with **diabetes** who have significant autonomic dysfunction are felt to have an ominous prognosis, possibly due to erratic gastric motility, food absorption, and insulin timing.

34. How do I treat postural hypotension?

Mechanical efforts to enhance venous return, such as thigh-high compressive stockings and abdominal binders, are recommended. Moving gradually and pumping the calves are recommended for those who are ambulatory. Graduated use of a tilt table may be necessary for those who are not.

Before starting new medications to improve the situation, look for medications that the patient is taking which may be worsening it. Diuretics, vasodilators, and anticholinergics such as tricyclic antidepressants should be stopped, and an adequate fluid and salt intake allowed.

If further help is needed, sympathomimetic medication such as ephedrine is helpful, particularly acutely, while fluorocortisone (Florinef) is helpful in more chronic situations. The latter medication may take several days to a few weeks to reach its maximal effect, which probably occurs through mechanism other than increasing volume (possibly improving "vascular tone" through an extrarenal mechanism).

35. A lot of my patients are on tricyclic antidepressants (TCAs). Except for anticholinergic side effects, they are safe, right?

The anticholinergic effects, such as dry mouth, constipation, urine retention, postural hypotension, and difficulty with visual accommodation, are usually tolerable, especially with time. More worrisome, however, is the use of TCAs in patients with cardiac conduction abnormalities. In older patients and those with cardiac risk factors, it is prudent to check an electrocardiogram prior to initiating the medication. Evidence of conduction problems, such as prolonged P-R interval or QRS complex widening, is a contraindication for the use of TCAs, which may then result in complete heart block in such patients. There is little evidence to suggest that TCAs are negative inotropes, so they should be relatively safe in patients with impaired left ventricular function. TCAs are actually antiarrhythmic for tachyarrhythmias, but antiarrhythmic medication for tachyarrhythmias has met with mixed success so that the safety of TCAs in this setting is uncertain.

36. What about the other half of my patients who seem to be hypertensive?

There are reasons why a high percentage of patients on the rehabilitation service may have hypertension. **Stroke patients** often have essential hypertension which underlies their disease. In general, blood pressure control goals of patients with recent stroke are modest. Most feel that maintenance of perfusion pressure in the post-stroke period is important, as the arteries in the injured region have lost their ability to autoregulate, and as a result, flow to the area that is markedly pressure-dependent. Therefore, in the hypertensive stroke patient, blood pressures should be lowered gradually during the weeks following the stroke.

Often, patients with closed **head injury** are hypertensive. These are often young patients, and since hypertension exerts its damaging effects over months and years, such patients can usually just be monitored. Should treatment be necessary, therapy that does not interfere with cognitive recovery and/or which helps the patient in some other way should be chosen. For example, clonidine should be avoided in general, and beta-blockers may be a good choice in brain-injured patients with rage reactions or headaches with vascular qualities.

37. Are there any hypertensive emergencies to worry about?

Yes. If your brain-injured patients have blood pressure increases, with any suggestion of change in neurologic status, they should be imaged with CT or MRI to rule out causes of increased intracranial pressure. Of course, malignant elevations of blood pressure can occur in patients with spinal cord injury.

38. Which patients are at risk for autonomic dysreflexia? What causes it?

Patients with spinal cord lesions above T6 are at risk for autonomic dysreflexia. It is caused by some noxious afferent input (usually a distended viscus, such as a full bladder or bowel) into the spinal cord below the level of the lesion, which in turn causes a large autonomic outflow. This outflow, which occurs below the level of the lesion, is unmonitored and therefore not modulated by higher centers in the brainstem and hypothalamus. Therefore, pronounced vasoconstriction occurs below the level of the lesion as the vascular tree has sympathetic, but not parasympathetic, innervation. The vasculature above the level of the lesion has reduced sympathetic tone and dilates appropriately in an effort to decrease blood pressure. As a result, the patient often appears flushed above the level of the lesion, often complains of a pounding headache characteristically behind the eyes, nasal congestion, and sweats.

39. How is autonomic dysreflexia treated?

Prompt treatment is important; blood pressure elevations can be malignant and cause intracranial hemorrhage. Sit the patient upright to reduce blood pressure. Check the bowel and bladder and evacuate these. (It is a good idea to use lidocaine gel during these procedures to minimize further noxious afferent input.) Usually, this is enough and the patient's pressure returns to baseline. If not, treat to control blood pressure while the search for the cause proceeds. Nitropaste is rapid in onset and easily removed should pressure go too low. If this is not effective, sublingual nifedipine or intramuscular or intravenous morphine should be added to the regimen; the latter may be particularly helpful if the patient is in pain or anxious.

40. What are the potential causes of autonomic dysreflexia?

Gastrointestinal—appendicitis, cholecystitis, diverticulitis, ischemic or perforated bowel
Genitourinary—nephrolithiasis, endometriosis, epididymitis
Dermatologic—cellulitis, ingrown toenail, tight-fitting clothes
Vascular—aneurysm, deep vein thrombosis
Musculoskeletal—heterotopic ossification, gout/pseudogout, joint infection

41. Is there any way to identify who is at greatest risk for developing a medical problem, requiring transfer off the inpatient unit and back onto an acute care floor?

Not without a crystal ball. However, some patient characteristics have been associated with an increased risk for transfer to an acute medical service: abnormal vital signs upon admission to the rehab unit, presence of a feeding or tracheostomy tube, impaired renal function, anemia, hypoalbuminemia, and history of DVT/PE.

BIBLIOGRAPHY

1. Bartlett JG: Clostridium difficile: Clinical considerations. Rev Infect Dis 12(suppl 1):S243, 1990.
2. Bone RC: The pathogenesis of sepsis. Ann Intern Med 115:457, 1991.
3. Criqui MHY, Langer RD, Frank A, Feigelson HS: Coronary artery disease and stroke in patients with large vessel peripheral arterial disease. Drugs 42(suppl 5):16–21, 1991.
4. Dombovy ML, Vasford JR, Whisnant JP, Bergstralh EJ: Disability and use of rehabilitation services following stroke in Rochester, Minnesota, 1975–1979. Stroke 18:830–836, 1987.
5. Felsenthal G, Cohen S, Hilton B, et al: The physiatrist as primary physician for patients on an inpatient rehabilitation unit. Arch Phys Med Rehabil 65:375–378, 1984.
6. Goldstein LB, et al: Common drugs may influence motor recovery after stroke. Neurology 45:865–871, 1995.
7. Harkness GA: Risk factors for nosocomial pneumonia in the elderly. Am J Med 89:457, 1990.
8. Linstedt G: Serum ferritin and iron deficiency anemia in hospital patients. Lancet 1:205, 1980.
9. Robinson KM, Sigler EL, Streim JE: Medical emergencies in rehabilitation medicine. In DeLisa JA (ed): Rehabilitation Medicine: Principles and Practice, 2nd ed. Philadelphia, J.B. Lippincott, 1993, pp 792–795.
10. Rose BD: Renal function and disorders of water and sodium balance. In Rubenstein E, Federman DD (eds): Scientific American Medicine. New York, Scientific American, 1994.
11. Roth EJ, Wiesner S, Green D, Wu Y: Dysvascular amputee rehabilitation: The role of continuous noninvasive cardiovascular monitoring during physical therapy. Am J Phys Med Rehabil 69:16–22, 1987.
12. Warkentin TI, et al: Heparin-induced thrombocytopenia in patients treated with low-molecular-weight heparin or unfractionated heparin. N Engl J Med 332:1330–1335, 1995.

88. IMMOBILIZATION AND ADVERSE EFFECTS OF BEDREST

Paul Corcoran, M.D.

1. List the adverse effects of bedrest on the various organ systems.

Muscles	Disuse atrophy
Joints	Contracture, loss of ROM
Bone	Osteoporosis, pathologic fracture
Urinary tract	Infection, calculi
Heart	Deconditioning, diminished cardiac reserve, reduced stroke volume, resting and postexercise tachycardia
Circulation	Orthostatic hypotension, thrombophlebitis
Lung	Pulmonary embolism, atelectasis, pneumonia
Gastrointestinal	Anorexia, malnutrition, constipation, impaction
Skin	Decubitus ulcer
Psychological	Depression, disorientation, anxiety

2. What is a contracture?
Contracture is a limitation of passive joint ROM commonly resulting from a restriction in connective tissue, tendons, ligaments, muscles, and joint elements.

3. What four factors accelerate contracture formation in an immobilized limb?
The mnemonic **BITE** lists these nicely:
B = **B**leeding
I = **I**nfection
T = **T**issue Trauma
E = **E**dema

4. How long is a collagen fiber?

As long as it needs to be. This is why people instinctively stretch after awakening from sleep. We all know how good this morning "ROM exercise" feels, yet hospital routines may deny it to patients for days at a time. Coiled collagen fibers, not required to elongate regularly, become fixed in the shortened position, causing clinical contractures.

5. Which organs and systems are helped by bedrest?

None, but some impaired body parts may receive short-term benefits from temporary rest: e.g., elevating the legs to treat shock or edema, maintaining basal metabolic levels during severe acute myocardial infarction, or briefly resting or splinting inflamed joints after trauma or surgery.

6. How strong is a muscle?

It depends on the workload regularly imposed on it. Muscles must regularly exert 50% of their maximum strength in order to preserve that strength. If a muscle never exerts as much as 50% of its maximum strength, that maximum will diminish.

7. How fast does an inactivated muscle develop disuse atrophy?

Muscles lose about 15% of their baseline strength per week of total inactivity. Thus, 5 weeks of total inactivity costs 50% of the previous strength of the muscle. A plateau is reached at 25–40% of the original strength.

8. What two factors prevent osteoporosis by stimulating osteoblastic activity?

Muscle pull and weight-bearing, both of which are prevented by bedrest.

9. How quickly does osteoporosis begin?

Urinary calcium clearance increases 4–6-fold within 3 weeks after total immobilization. High levels of calcium clearance persist until a new equilibrium is reached at a lower total calcium mass, a process that may take 6 months after complete quadriplegia.

10. Why do patients often complain of backache after bed confinement?

Their intervertebral joints are stiffer, their paraspinal muscles are weaker, and their vertebrae are more osteoporotic; hence the futility of bedrest as therapy for back pain.

11. How does the gravity of bedrest affect urination and defecation?

A basic rule in the plumbing trade is, "S – – t" doesn't run uphill." This rule also applies to the gastrointestinal and urinary tracts. It is no accident that the cloaca of all species is in their nether regions, while the mouth is on top. Every day in modern hospitals, attempts to swallow, urinate, or defecate in the horizontal position continually revalidate the law of gravity. The resulting dehydration, aspiration, constipation, and urinary stasis lead to the familiar UTIs and fecal impactions of bed-confined patients.

12. What is the orthostatic reflex? Why is it lost during bedrest?

Falling blood pressure acts via the carotid baroceptors to signal the medullary sympathetic center to trigger vasoconstriction in the muscular layers of the small arterioles. Like all muscles, these muscles atrophy from disuse when the body remains horizontal and/or weightless. The resulting orthostatic hypotension can cause syncope, with resulting falls and injuries in patients after prolonged bedrest, as well as in astronauts returning from space. The space program prevents this by carefully planned exercises during space missions; the terrestrial health care system has not yet adopted similar preventive exercises for bed-confined patients.

13. What is the most common cause of sudden unexpected death in hospitalized patients?

Acute pulmonary embolism.

14. How does the internal pressure of skin capillaries compare with the external pressure on the skin?

Capillary filling pressures range from about 18 mmHg at the venous end to 35 mmHg at the arteriolar end, or about 0.5 psi. To maintain perfusion and avoid collapse of skin capillaries, the external pressure therefore must be kept below 0.5 psi. This means that a 150-lb patient in bed requires a minimum of 300 sq in of skin area for support. The good news is that this much area is in fact available on the dorsum of the head, trunk, and extremities of a recumbent person. The bad news is that firm V mattresses (e.g., hospital mattresses) prevent equal pressure distribution.

15. Can exercise prevent aging?

The depressing graphs of declining function with advancing age look suspiciously like the graphs of declining function with inactivity. Recent research in geriatrics and exercise physiology has demonstrated that, like the young, the elderly can improve strength and function through activity. Persons who choose a more active lifestyle can significantly retard much of what is erroneously called "the aging process." Maintenance of strength and flexibility can prevent falls. Continued regular sexual activity can diminish male impotence and female vaginal atrophy. Mental stimulation and involvement can retard the changes of Alzheimer's disease as well as those of "normal" aging. The maxim, "use it or lose it," applies to all functions at all ages.

16. Name 10 strategies for minimizing the harmful effects of bedrest.

1. Minimize duration of bedrest.
2. Avoid strict bedrest unless absolutely necessary.
3. Allow bathroom privileges or bedside commode.
4. Stand the patient for 30–60 sec whenever transferring from bed to chair.
5. Encourage the wearing of street clothes.
6. Encourage taking meals at a table (not in bed).
7. Encourage walking to hospital appointments.
8. Encourage passes out of the hospital on evenings and weekends.
9. Order physical therapy and occupational therapy as needed.
10. Encourage daily ROM exercises as a basic part of good nursing care.

BIBLIOGRAPHY

1. Asher RAJ: The dangers of going to bed. BMJ 2:967–968, 1947.
2. Bailey DA, McCulloch RG: Bone tissue and physical activity. Can J Spt Sci 15:229–239, 1990.
3. Berg HE, Dudley GA, Haggmark T, et al: Effects of lower limb unloading on skeletal muscle mass and function in humans. J Appl Physiol 70:1882–1885, 1991.
4. Bortz WM: Disuse and aging. JAMA 248:1203–1208, 1982.
5. Browse NL: The Physiology and Pathology of Bedrest. Springfield, IL, Charles C Thomas, 1965.
6. Coyle EF, Hemmert MK, Coggan AR: Effects of detraining on cardiovascular responses to exercise: Role of blood volume. J Appl Physiol 60:95–99, 1986.
7. Deitrick JR, Whedon GD, Shorr E: Effects of immobilization on various metabolic and physiologic functions of normal men. Am J Med 4:3–6, 1948.
8. Fitts RH, McDonald KS, Schluter JM: The determinants of skeletal muscle force and power: Their adaptability with changes in activity pattern. J Biomech 24:111–122, 1991.
9. Greenleaf JE: Physiological responses to prolonged bed rest and fluid immersion in humans. J Appl Physiol 57:619–633, 1984.
10. Saltin B, Blomquist G, Mitchell JH, et al: Response to exercise after bed rest and after training. A longitudinal study of adaptive changes in oxygen transport and body composition. Circulation 38(suppl 7): VII-1–VII-78.

89. HETEROTOPIC OSSIFICATION

Jay V. Subbarao, M.D., M.S.

1. What is heterotopic ossification?

Heterotopic ossification (HO) refers to the formation of bone in abnormal locations, such as soft tissues. The bone formation is commonly periarticular in location and is classified as either progressive or nonprogressive, the latter being the kind typically seen in rehabilitation. Pathologically, HO is a metaplasia of the mesenchymal cells into osteoblasts. Even on biopsy material, it is very difficult to differentiate the bone formed in HO from callus in a healing fracture. HO should be differentiated from periosteal reaction, which may occur due to any irritation or inflammation close to the long bones.

2. What are some other names used for this condition?

1. Myositis ossificans
2. Para-osteoarthropathy
3. Neurogenic ossifying fibromyopathy
4. Osteosis neuratica
5. Para-articular bone formation
6. Ectopic ossification

3. How often does HO occur?

The reported incidence of HO in patients with spinal cord injury (SCI) varies from 16–53%. However, the incidence reported depends on diagnostic measures used, type of institution (acute or rehabilitation hospital), prospective or retrospective design, full versus limited roentgenographic evaluation, and 6-month versus 1-year follow-up of patients. The literature suggests that clinically significant HO occurs in 20% of patients following head injury and in 20–30% following SCI. The peak incidence is in the first 2 months following the onset of neurologic deficit, and rarely HO occurs long after SCI. In approximately 10% of cases, the HO is massive and causes severe restriction in joint motion or leads to ankylosis.

4. What causes HO?

No one knows the exact etiology of HO. A genetic predisposition has been suspected, but none is confirmed except in the progressive variety. Initial studies have suggested an association with human leukocyte antigens (HLA). There is no laboratory test that can predict which patients are susceptible to HO, although a number of factors are associated with HO formation, including:

- Spasticity
- Pressure sores near joints
- Proliferative osteoarthritis in multiple joints (males)

Complicating matters, HO commonly recurs after resection in these high-risk populations.

5. How do exercise and physical therapy affect HO formation?

After experimental studies noted that bleeding and hematoma preceded the formation of HO, exercise and physical therapy were implicated in causation of HO. Thus some have postulated that an injudiciously aggressive physical therapy program may cause trauma and bleeding into the soft tissues, leading to HO. However, this is not supported by the clinical experience. For example, an SCI patient who undergoes stretching of the hamstrings with similar force on both sides rarely shows clinical evidence of hematoma or other soft-tissue hemorrhage, and even if HO were to form, it usually involves only one joint. Also, HO occurs in only 20% of SCI patients, while all SCI patients undergo similar rehabilitative exercise programs. It seems safe to reason also that if HO is going to occur, it is less likely to occur in a joint that is mobilized than one that is immobilized.

6. There is soft tissue all over the body, so can bone form anywhere?

In neurologically compromised patients, HO commonly is noted around proximal joints, but when HO occurs, it is always in an area impaired by the neurologic deficit, i.e., below the level of lesion. Upper extremities are more commonly involved in patients with brain injury than with SCI. The hip joint is a very common site, followed by the knee. The shoulder is more commonly involved than the elbow. Bilateral involvement is sometimes seen. Interestingly, just because HO occurs at the hip or knee does not necessarily mean that HO formation will occur all along that extremity. And do not forget that always HO is periarticular.

7. How can I tell if HO exists when I make daily rounds?

This is not easy. While the joint involved may initially present with erythema, swelling, and intense pain, the most pathognomonic finding is the gradual loss of range of movement (ROM) in the involved joint. To determine if stiffness, e.g., in the knees, is due to bedrest, check the ankle and hip on the same side. Generally, they are not as limited as the knee, or for that matter, the opposite knee is also not as stiff as the one that is red and swollen. Patients with HO rarely have accompanying systemic findings such as fever or leukocytosis.

8. Should any redness around the joint make me think of HO then?

Watch out! Other condition may resemble HO, including cellulitis, deep vein thrombosis, hematoma, abscess, septic arthritis, and all other acute inflammatory processes. To complicate things, there are reports that deep vein thrombosis may coexist with HO. Also, check for edema distal and proximal to the joint and for spasticity in that extremity, as these may influence the diagnosis and future management. Often the existence of HO is suggested by the therapist who notes decreasing ROM of the involved joint.

9. Can I rely on any laboratory tests to detect HO?

In most patients with HO, elevation of **serum alkaline phosphatase** (SAP) is commonly noted. However, the elevated SAP is also seen in healing fractures and surgical procedures involving the bone. Surprisingly, elevation of SAP does not correlate directly with the rate of bone formation or the number of HO lesions. It is useful, yet imperfect, if the level increases from baseline in a patient with suspected HO.

10. What about x-rays?

Roentgenograms do reveal the presence of bone formation, but they are always negative in the first 2 weeks. Orthopedic surgeons have graded HO based on x-rays, but it is not of great relevance to the physiatrist because it does not assess loss of function.

11. Are any imaging procedures helpful?

Radionuclide bone imaging involves injecting ^{99m}Tc-methylene diphosphonate followed by imaging in **three phases**. First, pictures are taken after injection, then within 2 minutes, and finally 2 hours later to document evidence of hyperemia as shown by pooling of contrast around the suspected joint. Phases 1 and 2 are very sensitive and often positive in early stages of HO, and therefore the test is effective for early detection. In fact, even phase 3 may be positive for up to 4 weeks prior to your seeing any noticeable changes in the plain x-ray. I depend on the triple-phase bone scan in deciding my management strategies, especially surgery.

12. Once HO is suspected, what is the treatment?

1. Passive and active range of movement (ROM)
2. Positioning joint in optimal functional position
3. Anti-inflammatory drugs
4. Ultrasound
5. Cryotherapy
6. Radiation to the involved joint
7. Manipulation of involved joint
8. Medications to arrest HO progression (etidronate disodium, EHDP)
9. Surgical resection

13. Is joint rest helpful or not? What about physical therapy?

Although restricted motion is the pathognomonic sign for HO and although rest is associated with loss of motion, in the acute phase **short-term rest** is nonetheless essential to minimize the inflammatory changes as well as the possibility of further microscopic hemorrhages which may lead to hematoma and HO formation. As controversial as it sounds, immobilization of the involved joint for up to 2 weeks is very acceptable.

Physical therapy for gentle-active or active-assistive movement through painless ROM should be prescribed. If the patient does not have voluntary movement, gentle passive ROM within the painless arc should be performed. It is essential to monitor the response of the joint to treatment. If there is any increase in redness and swelling, joint motion should be discontinued. If ROM is continuously decreasing, immobilizing the extremity in a functional position is recommended; in the worst scenario, if the HO formation continues and the joint becomes ankylosed, it at least will be in a functional position. More aggressive movement of the joint is initiated as soon as the inflammatory responses subside in approximately 2 weeks. The patient must participate in general conditioning and ROM exercises to the uninvolved joints to prevent loss of their function. At present, there are no studies regarding the role of the continuous passive movement machine in the management of HO, but such an intervention is intriguing.

14. How does EHDP work?

Studies have shown that HO occurs within 15 weeks after total hip replacement and that the occurrence has plateaued by 4–6 months after surgery. In a double-blind study, patients were treated with etidronate disodium (EHDP, Didronel), 20 mg/kg body wt for 2 weeks, and then 10 mg/kg body wt/day for an average of 14 months. In that study, 10% of patients treated with EHDP and 30% of patients treated with placebo had developed clinically significant HO lesions at 9-month follow-up after stopping the treatments.

EHDP is commonly used to control new bone formation. Studies suggest that it inhibits growth of hydroxyapatite crystals by preventing the precipitation of soluble amorphous calcium phosphate. EHDP also slows the rate of osteoblastic and osteoclastic activity. These studies were done in laboratory animals, and unfortunately, clinical studies in humans have not proved conclusively that EHDP controls HO formation.

HO is a self-arresting process with an unclear natural history. We do not know how long this process continues, so if we treat it, we cannot tell if HO stopped because of the treatment or died off on its own.

15. Does EHDP dissolve any of the bone already formed by HO?

No.

16. Are any other medications used to manage HO?

Anti-inflammatory medications, such as indomethacin, have been used in the management of HO, but most of the studies were in total hip arthroplasty patients and varying degrees of success were reported. The ability of indomethacin to inhibit prostaglandin synthesis is considered a primary mechanism of action. Indomethacin, 25 mg three times a day for 6 weeks, is a commonly prescribed dosage. Medications such as ibuprofen and aspirin have also been tried.

17. Since we cannot do anything once HO forms, can we prevent it?

A number of treatments (EHDP, ibupofen, and indomethacin) have been used for prevention also, mostly in the total hip arthroplasty population, but their effectiveness in patients with SCI or brain injury is unproven. The use of EHDP preoperatively before the resection is recommended. Prophylactic radiation has been used in patients with neurologic disorders but has not been vigorously tested and has the theoretical risk of skin breakdown.

18. Can we crack it?

It is not uncommon to find studies recommending manipulation of ankylosed joints under anesthesia. Manipulation is commonly done in patients with nonneurologic conditions, such as burns and post-traumatic myositis ossificans. The use of manipulation following a neurologic injury may be justified when a patient has a residual functional extremity, but manipulation is not without risk. Experimental studies in rabbits have shown that forcible manipulation has produced HO in the quadriceps. Other reports, however, indicate that manipulation promotes function without increasing the HO. Be careful, however, as HO is often stronger than osteoporotic bone; manipulation of HO is not recommended in SCI patients, as these patients often have extensive osteoporosis and any forcible manipulation may result in pathologic fracture of the long bones.

19. When is surgical resection indicated?

Surgical intervention is required in only a very small percentage of patients and is aimed at enhancing a specific function. In either SCI or brain-injured patients, the main indication for surgical intervention should be a very clearly defined **functional limitation** which can be corrected by surgery. If there is opportunity for further neurologic return, surgical intervention can be delayed for up to 1.5–2 years. In the SCI patient, surgery is generally not recommended for at least 1 year after onset of HO. Surgical intervention is not for excising the HO entirely, preventing recurrence, achieving complete ROM in that joint, or arresting progression.

Prior to surgery, the HO progression should be arrested, as evidenced by normal or decreasing serum alkaline phosphatase, lack of increased uptake and hyperemia in the triple-phase bone scan, and an x-ray showing evidence of "mature bone." Entrapment of the neurovascular bundle in the HO mass should be excluded. Clinically, the patient should not have any evidence of inflammatory signs or joint pain. If there is any source of infection in the skin or urine, it should be treated prior to surgery. The patient's spasticity should be controlled. A general conditioning and stretching program to promote speedy recovery should be started prior to surgery.

The literature supports the use of prophylactic EHDP or anti-inflammatories for at least 2 weeks prior to surgery and continuing the medication postoperatively until the bone scan activity has subsided.

20. What types of surgical procedures are used?

Wedge resection or excision. Excision is not meant to remove all the new bone formed. Excision of HO in patients following total hip arthroplasty is generally done within the first 6 months. Wedge resection is commonly utilized in hip, knee, and elbow joints.

21. Describe the postoperative course.

The postoperative mobilization should be well-monitored and maintained while promoting good wound healing and hemostasis. The positioning of the joint postoperatively depends upon the type of function desired, e.g., increase in flexion or extension. The joint should be mobilized within 48 hours after surgery to facilitate effective drainage of the hematoma. Superficial infection often occurs in these patients. It is essential that the patient be involved in functional activities as soon as possible to prevent complications, such as urinary tract infection, pressure ulcers, and deconditioning from immobilization.

Postoperative x-rays invariably show some amount of new bone formation, and recurrence after surgery is very common. Considering that the aim of surgical intervention is improvement of function, outcome measures should be based, not on the x-rays, but instead should assess the functional gains.

ACKNOWLEDGMENT

The authors thanks Ms. Vaunda Bray of the Hines Comprehensive Rehabilitative Services, Hines, Illinois, for her assistance in preparing this chapter.

BIBLIOGRAPHY

1. Chantraine A, Minaire P: Para-osteo-arthropathies: A new theory and mode of treatment. Scand J Rehabil Med 13:31–37, 1981.
2. Citta-Pietrolungo T, Alexander M, Steg N: Early detection of heterotopic ossification in young patients with traumatic brain injury. Arch Phys Med Rehabil 73:258–262, 1992.

3. Ebraheim N, Kim K, Jackson WT, Kane JT: Heterotopic ossification and pseudoarthrosis in the shoulder following encephalitis: A case report and review of the literature. Clin Orthop 219(Jun):219–298, 1987.
4. Freed JH, Hahn H, Menter R, Dillion T: The use of the three phase bone scan in the early diagnosis of heterotopic ossification. Paraplegia 20:208–216, 1982.
5. Garland DE, Razza BE, Water SRL: Forceful joint manipulation in head injured adults with heterotopic ossification. Clin Orthop 169:133–138, 1982.
6. Garrison SJ: Update on heterotopic ossification in spinal cord injury. Curr Concepts Rehabil Med 5(1): 1–35, 1989.
7. Lal S, Hamilton B, Heinemann A, Betts HB: Risk factors for heterotopic ossification in spinal cord injury. Arch Phys Med Rehabil 70:387, 1989.
8. Michelsson JE, Ravschning W: Pathogenesis of experimental heterotopic bone formation following temporary forcible exercising of immobilized limbs. Clin Orthop 178(Jun):265–272, 1983.
9. Orzel JA, Rudd TG: Heterotopic bone formation: Clinical, laboratory, and imaging correlation. Clin Sci 26(2):125–132, 1985.
10. Stover SL: Heterotopic ossification after spinal cord injury. In Bloch RF, Basbaum M (eds): Management of Spinal Cord Injuries. Baltimore, Williams & Wilkins, 1986, pp 284–301.
11. Stover SL, Garland DE, Nilsson OS: Symposium: Heterotopic ossification. Clin Orthop 263(Feb): 1–120, 1991.
12. Stover SL, Niemann KMW, Miller JM: Disodium etidronate in the prevention of postoperative recurrence of heterotopic ossification in the spinal cord injured patient. J Bone Joint Surg 58:683–687, 1976.
13. Subbarao JV: Pseudoarthrosis in heterotopic ossification in spain cord-injured patients. Am J Phys Med Rehabil 13:88–90, 1990.
14. Subbarao JV, Nemchausky BA, Gratzer M: Resection of heterotopic ossification and didronel therapy— Regaining wheelchair independence in the spinal cord injury. J Am Paraplegia Soc 10:3–7, 1987.
15. Varghese G, Williams K, Desmet A, Redford J: Nonarticular complication of heterotopic ossification: A clinical review. Arch Phys Med Rehabil 72:1009–1013, 1991.

90. SPASTICITY

Richard T. Katz, M.D.

1. What is spasticity?

Spasticity is one of the most important impairments of individuals with CNS disease. A widely accepted definition of spasticity is: "a motor disorder characterized by a velocity-dependent resistance to movement associated with exaggerated phasic stretch reflexes (tendon jerks), representing one component of the upper motor neuron syndrome." **Tone** is the sensation of resistance you feel as you test the patient's passive range of motion at the bedside (while they are relaxed).

2. What causes spasticity?

Spasticity is probably due to neural mechanisms, although other etiologies have been suggested. The alpha motor neuron (the nerve cell that controls muscle contraction) is hyperexcitable. That is, less synaptic excitatory input is needed to cause the alpha motor neuron to fire or reach threshold. This is akin to a pot being "almost ready to boil." Very minimal input into the system can cause it to go awry. Spasticity can be caused by a wide variety of diagnoses that damage descending motor tracts (but not just the corticospinal tracts) at the cortical, subcortical, brainstem, or spinal cord level. Examples include stroke, degenerative diseases, multiple sclerosis, head injury, cerebral palsy, spinal cord injury, space-occupying lesions, and transverse myelitis.

3. Is spasticity a single disease with increased tendon jerks as its manifestation? If I had a magic pill to cure spasticity, would the patient be cured?

Sorry but no. Spasticity is just one component of the **upper motor syndrome**, which has a host of features. Reflexes run amok (like the Babinski response seen upon stroking the bottom of the foot). There is a velocity-dependent increased resistance to stretch observed with passive range. There is a loss of cutaneous reflexes (remember, one of the clinical presentations of multiple sclerosis is hyperactivity in the lower extremity stretch reflexes and loss of the superficial abdominal reflex). There is loss of precise autonomic control (quadriplegics often suffer from autonomic hyperreflexia in which an overdistended bladder or bowel can cause life-threatening changes in blood pressure and heart rate). There are also changes in the way motor units fire. Normally, as a person tries to increase the strength of contraction, preferentially more motor units are recruited early on, and then later, the motor units fire faster and faster. All this is disturbed in the patient with upper motor neuron syndrome.

Upper Motor Neuron Syndrome

Abnormal behaviors (positive symptoms)	Performance deficits (negative symptoms)
Reflex release phenomena	Decreased dexterity
Hyperactive proprioceptive reflexes	Paresis/weakness
Increased resistance to stretch	Fatigability
Reduced cutaneous reflexes	
Loss of precise autonomic control	

Spasticity in the cerebral palsy patient has a clinical presentation distinct from that in the spinal cord injury patient. This reflects different types of damage to components of the motor system, including the corticospinal, vestibulospinal, and reticulospinal tracts.

4. I think I recognize spasticity when I see it, but how do I quantify it?

Now here you have a problem. There is no uniform and useful way of quantifying the severity of spasticity. Most people use a crude scale named the Ashworth Scale. Spasticity can also be measured with torque devices that stretch a limb and test how much angular "resistance" occurs. These are very complex issues that at this point have only research applications. Finally, people have tried to quantify spasticity using a host of electrical tests related to the H reflex and F wave. Again, these are useful only in a research protocol. Basically, the clinician has to base an evaluation of spasticity on the clinical examination (heightened tone and decreased range of motion [ROM] which can be increased with prolonged stretch), the Ashworth Scale, and the presence and/or severity of intermittent "spasms."

Clinical Scale for Spastic Hypertonia (Modified Ashworth Scale)

0	No increase in tone
1	Slight increase in muscle tone, manifested by a catch and release or by minimal resistance at the end of the ROM when the affected part(s) is moved in flexion or extension
1+	Slight increase in muscle tone, manifested by a catch, followed by minimal resistance throughout the remainder (less than half) of the ROM
2	More marked increase in muscle tone through most of the ROM, but affected part(s) easily moved
3	Considerable increase in muscle tone, passive movement difficult
4	Affected part(s) rigid in flexion or extension

5. Do I treat everyone who has spasticity?

A definite no. Patients should be treated only when their spasticity interferes with present function or the potential for future function or when the condition is painful. Ask yourself some simple questions: *Does the spasticity cause a gait disturbance?* Some people "walk on their tone," and if you decrease their extensor "synergy," they might be unable to ambulate successfully. Some people stand with their hypertonicity. In both cases the tone is serving a purpose for the patient. *Do spasms interfere with lifestyle?* Some spinal-cord-injured patients are literally thrown out of their chairs by flexor spasms; others may have adductor spasticity that causes a scissoring gait or precludes successful catheterization. Finally, *will treatment be beneficial?* Spasticity is often very difficult to treat (such as in the severe stroke patient), and the clinician should be convinced that the potential benefits of treatment clearly outweigh the possibility of side effects or drug toxicity.

6. Where do I start in treating the patient with spasticity?

Start with two basic foundations.

1. A **daily stretching program** is important and can have a significant effect that lasts for several hours after stretch due to synaptic changes that occur within the spinal cord circuitry.

2. **Avoid noxious stimuli.** Unwanted stimuli from an overdistended bowel or bladder, pressure sores, or ingrown toenails play an important role in the local spinal circuitry of spasticity. Even an overly tightened leg bag may be a problem.

Therapists also can use certain "facilitation" techniques (e.g., Bobath, Brunnstrom) to "overcome" tone while they teach patients to relearn certain movements. Topical cold and anesthesia sometimes may have useful short-term effects.

7. What is the role of drugs in treating spasticity?

Drugs are most useful in the patient who has mild to moderate tone, but even then, the drugs are only mildly to moderately effective. In a severely brain-injured patient with drastic spasticity and marked dystonic posturing, the drugs simply do not work, and the cognitive side effects are very displeasing . The ideal patient for drugs is often the patient with less severe spasticity, whether due to spinal cord dysfunction (e.g., spinal cord injury or transverse myelitis) or brain dysfunction (cerebral palsy, stroke, or brain injury).

8. Is baclofen the most effective drug?

It is surprising that baclofen (Lioresal) is used for as many indications as it is, because it is not a "wonder" drug. Baclofen is an analog of the inhibitory neurotransmitter, γ-aminobutyric acid (GABA), and binds to a recently discovered and less-well-characterized "B" receptor. Agonism at this site inhibits calcium influx into presynaptic terminals and suppresses release of excitatory neurotransmitters. Baclofen is probably the drug of choice in **spinal forms of spasticity** and may help to improve bladder control. Whereas diazepam is generally contraindicated in patients with cerebral injury because of its marked cognitive side effects, baclofen is significantly less sedating. Unfortunately, its efficacy in cerebral spasticity is unimpressive, although it continues to be used for this purpose. GABA is a potent inhibitory neurotransmitter, so sudden discontinuation of baclofen can lead to seizures and hallucinations.

9. Diazepam is an antianxiety agent. Why use it for spasticity?

Diazepam (Valium) facilitates postsynaptic effects of GABA but has no direct GABA-mimetic effect. It exerts indirect mimetic effect only when GABA transmission is functional. Available before baclofen was introduced, diazepam has proved to be a successful treatment for spastic hypertonia in **spinal cord injury** as well as other spinal forms of spasticity. It is generally unsuitable for patients with brain injury (traumatic or vascular) due to its ability to cause significant cognitive impairment. Nonetheless, it has a good track record and an extremely large index of safety.

10. Doesn't dantrolene sodium have the ideal mode of action?

In a word, yes. Dantrolene sodium (Dantrium) reduces muscle action potential–induced release of calcium into the sarcoplasmic reticulum, decreasing the force produced by excitation-contraction coupling. Thus, it is the only drug that acts right where we want it—at the spastic muscle. Dantrolene sodium seems to have more effect on fast than slow muscle fibers and next to no effect on smooth or cardiac muscle. It is the preferred agent for **cerebral forms of spasticity,** such as hemiplegia or cerebral palsy, but may be a useful adjunct to the treatment of spinal forms of spasticity. Generally, the spastic muscles are affected far more than nonspastic muscles, and so there is no weakness in spared muscles. Dantrolene sodium may be mildly to moderately sedative.

11. What is the drawback to dantrolene?

Dantrolene sodium was initially embraced with a tremendous amount of excitement which was dampened when a small number of patients developed severe hepatic insult and died. However, there do not seem to be many new cases of this irreversible liver damage, which is puzzling. Hepatotoxicity may occur in ~1% of patients but generally occurs as a reversible and transient elevation in liver function tests. The severe and fulminant hepatotoxicity that has been described may have been overstated.

12. What about tizanidine?

Tizanidine is not currently available in the United States, but trials are underway and it is available in Europe. Tizanidine is a imidazoline derivative (like clonidine) and has an agonistic action at central α-2 adrenergic receptor sites. It facilitates the action of glycine, an inhibitory neurotransmitter, and prevents the release of excitatory amino acids. It is equivalent to baclofen as an antispastic agent in both **cerebral** as well as **spinal forms of spasticity**. Tizanidine is better tolerated than diazepam in patients with chronic hemiplegia, and multiple sclerosis patients have shown significant benefit in several large double-blinded studies.

13. Is clonidine an effective spasticity drug in spinal-cord-injured patients?

Yes, but it is not highly dramatic. Clonidine, a more traditional antihypertensive agent, has recently been shown to be fairly effective in controlling spasticity for patients with **spinal cord injury**. Clonidine is an α-2 adrenergic agonist that can cause improved locomotor function in a spastic paraparetic. However, spinal-cord-injured patients have unstable autonomic nervous systems, and the side effects of clonidine include syncope, hypotension, nausea, and vomiting. An adhesive patch (Catapres-TTS) is available for week-long transdermal delivery.

14. What is the most significant advance in the treatment of spasticity in recent years?

Intrathecal baclofen delivered via a subdermal pump. A pump can be implanted subcutaneously in the abdominal wall, with a catheter surgically placed into the subarachnoid space. In this manner, higher dosages of baclofen can be placed near the spinal cord—the desired site for action of the drug—while largely avoiding the CNS side effects associated with increased oral intake. The pump may be refilled on a monthly basis by transcutaneous injection. Eligible patients are those who are significantly disabled by their spasticity and have failed more conservative measures.

15. Who should be considered for intrathecal baclofen? What are its drawbacks?

The ideal patient generally has **spinal spasticity** with some preserved function below the level of the lesion. This is an expensive treatment—approximately $6,500 for the pump alone, plus another $3,000/year for the drug itself, plus surgical costs. Therefore, patients are generally given a trial run with an external pump and a catheter inserted percutaneously into the subarachnoid space. Dosage is initiated at 25 μg/day and may be titrated to an average of 400–500 μg/day or more.

The most common side effects are drowsiness, dizziness, nausea, hypotension, headache, and weakness. Problems with the delivery apparatus are not common but include tube dislodgment, disconnection, kinkage, and blockage. More serious complications include infection, skin breakdown, or spinal headaches due to cerebrospinal fluid leakage around the catheter. The pump may be refilled on a monthly basis and lasts about 5 years. Patients may also note a beneficial effect on bladder function.

16. Drugs act in a general manner. What if the effect of spasticity is more focal?

If the problem is focal, short- and long-term solutions may be considered, including chemical neurolysis and casting.

17. Discuss the use of phenol blocks.

Chemical neurolysis, or **phenol block**, uses 2–6% aqueous phenol solutions to chemically disrupt nerves within a trunk or at the motor point where it attaches to muscle. The phenol causes protein coagulation and axonal necrosis, leading to denervation which may last 3–6 months. Phenol blocks may cause dysesthesias and causalgia due to destruction of sensory fibers. This problem may be circumvented by performing open phenol nerve blocks in a surgical suite. Phenol blocks are relatively easy and quick to perform and last several months, so they can be performed widely and repeatedly.

18. Which sites have traditionally responded to phenol blocks?

Musculocutaneous blocks may be useful in the hemiplegic with upper-extremity elbow flexion synergy or the C5 quadriplegic who has elbow flexion unopposed by a paretic triceps. Median nerve blocks may help the hemiparetic patient with a flexed wrist or fingers curled in the palm. Obturator blocks have been used in the patient with scissor gait, a frequent concomitant of cerebral palsy. Hip flexor spasms or flexor contractures may be prevented by performing paravertebral lumbar spinal nerve block (although these require a high level of skill). Tibial nerve block can help the patient with an equinovarus posture (pointed foot turned inward) during gait.

19. Describe how a phenol nerve block is administered.

Nerve blocks can be performed with a 22-gauge Teflon-coated needle with a bared bevel. The hub of the needle is connected to an electrical stimulator, which delivers a square pulse of approximately 0.1 msec once or twice per second. With surface stimulation, you can approximate the site of the nerve by watching for a visible twitch in the desired muscle. After the needle is inserted, the needle is gradually moved until only the minimal current (~ 1 mA) is necessary to obtain a maximal twitch in the desired muscle(s). At this point, the phenol is injected. Motor point blocks may require multiple injections into a single muscle. As commonly practiced, aspiration should be done before injection to avoid intravascular administration of the drug.

20. How is botulinum toxin used?

Recently, botulinum toxin has been used in the spastic patient to weaken dystonic muscles in an analogous manner to its use in blepharospasm, strabismus, cervical dystonia, and focal dystonia. However, studies are only preliminary toward its use in the spastic patient. Advantages include direct treatment of muscles, although it is not precisely localizing. Because spastic muscles may require large dosages, the high cost of this agent remains a significant impediment.

21. What role does casting play in treating the spastic patient?

Casting is another focal technique that can be done frequently in a patient with focal contracture due to spasticity. Limbs can be stretched and then casted in a lengthened position. Casts are changed every few days or weeks to stretch contracted structures gradually. Casting is limited, however, in that it can only achieve mild increases in joint range. To achieve more dramatic increases, one must incorporate a surgical release procedure.

22. Name several other forms of hypertonicity that may be confused with spasticity.

1. Decorticate rigidity
2. Decerebrate rigidity
3. Parkinsonian rigidity (cogwheel rigidity)
4. McArdle's disease (type 5 glycogenosis)
5. Contracture

23. How do you distinguish between decorticate and decerebrate rigidity?

- Decorticate rigidity
  Hypertonic upper-extremity flexion
  Hypertonic lower-extremity extension
- Decerebrate rigidity
  Hypertonic extension of both upper and lower extremities

24. When is orthopedic surgery an option for the spastic patient?

A long list of orthopedic surgical procedures has been proposed for spastic patients, predominantly for those with **cerebral** insult. The orthopedic surgeon should consider several questions before considering surgical intervention:

(a) *When was the insult to the CNS?* Traumatic brain injury patients continue to change for up to 2 or more years. Surgery prior to this may be premature.

(b) *Are the "spastic changes" dynamic or static?* Dynamic refers to loss of range due to spasticity, while static refers to "contracture" due to intrinsic changes within the muscle.

(c) *What are the goals of surgery: functional or static improvement?* A highly functional stroke patient may require a complicated series of lengthenings and transfers to improve hand function, whereas a severely impaired patient with cerebral palsy may need a simple adductor release to facilitate perineal hygiene.

(d) *What is the residual sensorimotor function of the limb in question?* A functionally opening hand without adequate sensory feedback is a useless hand.

The surgeon often incorporates multichannel electromyography (EMG) or poly-EMG during gait or upper extremity motion to help determine which muscles are most spastic. The surgeon must then determine what type of procedure will best restore abnormal forces: tenotomy or neurectomy eliminates deforming forces, tendon transfers redirect deforming forces, tendon lengthening diminishes deforming forces, and fusions stabilize deforming forces.

25. List the available orthopedic options for upper extremity spasticity.

Orthopedic Interventions for the Spastic Upper Extremity

Shoulder
    Adducted or internally rotated shoulder: pectoralis major/subscapularis tendon release
    Painful shoulder subluxation: biceps tendon sling
Elbow
    Flexor spasticity: step-cut lengthening of brachioradialis, biceps, and brachialis
    Extensor spasticity: V-Y lengthening of triceps
Wrist and hand
    Flexor spasticity:
        Fractional lengthening of flexor digitorum superficialis/flexor digitorum profundus
        Step-cut lengthening of flexor pollicis longus
        Over-lengthening of flexor carpi radialis, flexor carpi ulnaris
        Flexor-pronator origin release
        Sublimis to profundus transfer
    Thumb-in-palm deformity: release of thenar, adductors, and flexors

26. What orthopedic surgeries are useful for lower extremity spasticity?

Orthopedic Interventions for the Spastic Lower Extremity

Functional deformities
    Limb scissoring: obturator neurectomy
    Crouched gait: iliopsoas recession, hamstring lengthening
    Stiff knee gait: selective quadriceps release in select patients
    Equinovarus foot: tendo-Achilles lengthening, SPLATT, release of extrinsic/intrinsic toe flexors
    Spastic valgus foot: release and transfer of peroneus longus
Static deformities
    Hip adduction contracture: release adductor longus, gracilis
    Hip flexion contracture: release of sartorius, rectus femoris, tensor fascia lata, iliopsoas, pectineus
    Hip extension: release proximal hamstrings
    Knee flexion contracture: release distal hamstrings
    Knee extension: VY-plasty to lengthen quadriceps
    Foot: as for functional deformities, other options include release of planta fascia and triple arthrodesis

27. What is SPLATT?

The SPLATT procedure—split anterior tibial tendon transfer—is an especially effective treatment for the equinovarus foot. The SPLATT procedure involves splitting the tibialis anterior tendon distally. Half is left attached to its site of origin, while the distal end of the lateral half of the tendon is tunneled into the third cuneiform and cuboid bones. This provides an eversion force that balances the spastic inturning at the ankle, giving the patient a solid platform on which to place weight during gait. Achilles tendon lengthening is often performed in conjunction with the SPLATT procedure to decrease the toe-pointing equinus posture. These procedures can dramatically improve the gait pattern of a hemiplegic patient.

28. How does dorsal rhizotomy work?

Rhizotomy refers to the surgical section of nerve roots. Cutting the anterior (motor) nerve root is undesirable, as it causes denervation atrophy which predisposes to pressure sores. Cutting the posterior (sensory) nerve root seems preferable, as it decreases the sensory input to the spinal cord circuitry. By selectively sectioning nerve rootlets rather than entire dorsal roots, the neurosurgeon can decrease the amount of spastic tone while minimizing sensory loss necessary for skin protection and motor control.

Selective dorsal rhizotomies are open procedures that require laminectomy. Twenty-five to 80% of the posterior rootlets are cut, often under the guidance of electrophysiologic studies. The precision with which electrophysiologic studies guide the surgeon in which roots to cut is at best unclear.

29. Dorsal rhizotomies are effective for children with cerebral palsy. Right?

Although there was a wave of initial enthusiasm over dorsal rhizotomy, careful scrutiny of the literature begs caution. It is unclear whether the child with cerebral palsy between 3–8 years of age (the most frequent age for the procedure) has a better long-term result than the child who does not have the surgery but has the same intensity of physical therapy. In the short term, children with cerebral palsy who have dorsal rhizotomy do show significant improvements in ambulation.

BIBLIOGRAPHY

1. Brown P: Pathophysiology of spasticity [editorial]. J Neurol Neurosurg Psychiatry 57:773–777, 1994.
2. Katz RT: Management of spastic hypertonia. Am J Phys Med Rehabil 67:108–116, 1988.
3. Katz RT, Rymer WZ: Spastic hypertonia: Mechanisms and measurement. Arch Phys Med Rehabil 70:144–155, 1989.
4. Katz RT (ed): Spasticity. Phys Med Rehabil State Art Rev 8:441–611, 1994.
5. Katz RT: Spastic hypertonia. Phys Med Rehabil Clin North Am,1995 (in press).
6. Katz RT, Rovai G, Brait C, Rymer WZ: Objective quantification of spastic hypertonia: Correlation with clinical findings. Arch Phys Med Rehabil 73:339–347, 1992.
7. Lance JW: Symposium synopsis. In Feldman RG, Young RR, Koella WP (eds): Spasticity: Disordered Motor Control. Chicago, Year Book Medical Publishers, 1980.
8. Lance JW, McLeod JG: Disordered muscle tone. In Physiological Approach to Clinical Neurology. Boston, Butterworth, 1981.

91. PRESSURE ULCERS

Michael M. Priebe, M.D.

1. The axiom goes, "Where there is no pressure, there is no ulcer." What is it about pressure that causes ulceration?

Tissue ischemia. When tissues are compressed between a bony prominence and an external surface, capillaries are compressed and blood flow is obstructed, leading to ischemia. However, pressure is not the only contributor to ischemia.

2. Name some other factors leading to pressure ulcers.

Shear forces, elevated tissue temperature, maceration, malnutrition, anemia, altered mental status, altered sensation, decreased mobility, and smoking.

3. How much pressure is too much?

Kosiak, in his classic 1961 study of the etiology of pressure ulcers, found a clear relationship between pressure and time in producing tissue changes in rat muscle. Constant pressure of 35 mmHg applied for up to 4 hours did not cause microscopic changes in the muscle fiber of neurologically intact and paraplegic rats, but 70 mmHg applied for 2 hours did produce moderate microscopic changes. In general, the more pressure applied, the shorter the duration needed to produce tissue changes. He also found that alternating pressure, in which the tissue was relieved of pressure for 5-minute intervals every 5 minutes, showed consistently less ulcer potential or no change compared to tissue subjected to an equivalent amount of constant pressure.

While Kosiak's experiment is very important in understanding the pathophysiology of pressure ulcers, it still does not answer the question of how much pressure is too much. Theoretically, mean arteriolar perfusion pressure is 32 mmHg, and when exceeded, blood flow will cease (although this is very hard to measure clinically).

4. What are the primary objectives of pressure management?
• Even distribution of pressure
• Minimize shear forces
• Frequent pressure relief

5. Which tissues are most sensitive to pressure?

This is a great exam question. Tissues vary in their sensitivity to pressure. Interestingly enough, muscle is the most sensitive and skin is most resistant to pressure-induced ischemia. This explains, in part, the natural history of many deep pressure ulcers: a single insult—usually sustained high pressure over a bony prominence—leads to tissue ischemia and necrosis, which is worse at the muscle–bone interface. The affected area appears clinically as an area of induration, erythema, and warmth, but with intact skin. Within a few days to a week, even with complete pressure relief, the wound opens, revealing a deep crater filled with necrotic tissue.

6. If muscle is the most sensitive tissue to pressure, why do surgeons use muscle flaps (myocutaneous flaps) to close large pressure ulcers?

Myocutaneous flap procedures are based on the basic surgical principle of minimizing deadspace. Myocutaneous flaps do not provide a "cushion" as mistakenly assumed. They provide well-vascularized tissue to fill the large deadspace left after resection of a pressure ulcer. In fact, within a year or less, the bulk of the muscle in a myocutaneous flap has often atrophied due to chronic pressure. However, the blood supply is still intact, and the wound remains healed.

Another benefit is that the surgeon is often able to move the suture line—a very vulnerable region due to the formation of scar tissue which has very poor tensile strength initially—away from the site of maximum pressure.

7. Where are pressure ulcers most likely to develop?
They develop most commonly over areas of bony prominence:

Sacrum (most common)	Scapulae	Coccyx	Malleoli
Ischii	Heels	Trochanters	

8. What other factors determine ulcer location?
The location is often predictable and depends on the individual's activity level. Persons who spend much or all of the day lying in bed most often develop pressure ulcers over the sacrum, trochanters, and heels. Persons who are sitting develop pressure ulcers over the ischii, coccyx, and trochanters. The location of a pressure ulcer often suggests its origin, thereby allowing for focused interventions for treatment and prevention.

9. How does sitting put pressure on the trochanters?
Trochanteric pressure ulcers commonly occur when a person uses a wheelchair with a sling seat. Sling seats "squeeze" the hips when you sit down, causing increased pressure over the trochanters. Use of a solid seat insert will minimize this effect.

The sling seat may also lead to the development of a pelvic obliquity, which causes excessive pressures on the ischium and trochanter on the low side. A pelvic obliquity in turn often contributes to the development of scoliosis.

10. How are pressure ulcers classified?
Location
Size
Depth

11. Are all pressure ulcers created equal?
No. Like everything else in medicine, there is a grading system. The National Pressure Ulcer Advisory Panel defines pressure ulcer stages as follows:
- **Stage I:** Nonblanchable erythema of intact skin, the heralding lesions of skin ulceration. Note that reactive hyperemia can normally be expected to be present for one-half to three-fourths as long as the pressure occluded blood flow to the area. Hyperemia should not be confused with a Stage I pressure ulcer.
- **Stage II:** Partial-thickness skin loss involving the epidermis and/or dermis. The ulcer is superficial and presents clinically as an abrasion, blister, or shallow crater.
- **Stage III:** Full-thickness skin loss involving damage or necrosis of subcutaneous tissue that may extend down to, but not through, underlying fascia. The ulcer presents clinically as a deep crater with or without undermining of adjacent tissue.
- **Stage IV:** Full-thickness skin loss with extensive destruction, tissue necrosis or damage to muscle, bone, or supporting structures (e.g., tendon or joint capsule). Note that undermining and sinus tracts may also be associated with Stage IV pressure ulcers.

12. What is the best treatment for a pressure ulcer?
Once again, there is no right answer. Every patient is different, and every wound unique. There are, however, a few principles to guide the treatment approach.
1. **Prevention is paramount.** As with most things in life, an ounce of prevention is worth a pound of cure. In the case of pressure ulcers, an ounce of prevention may be worth a pound of flesh. Careful attention to risk factors allows early detection of persons at risk for developing a pressure ulcer so that preventive efforts can be made.
2. **Wounds must be adequately cleansed and debrided before healing can occur.** Eschar, the tough, leathery, or dry matter covering a wound, is not a beneficial natural dressing

that can be left in place. Not only does the eschar prevent proper staging of the wound, but it also harbors bacteria and prevents the formation of granulation tissue and epithelialization of the wound. Chronic, nonhealing pressure ulcers without eschars should also be debrided to stimulate the acute wound-healing cascade.

3. **A moist wound environment provides the optimal conditions for cell migration and mitosis.** Adequate oxygen in the wound bed increases local resistance to infection and enhances collagen formation. A dry wound impedes the healing process. A good blood supply is necessary to provide nutrients and oxygen to the wound and remove toxins and waste products.

4. **The underlying systemic and systematic problems that initially led to the development of the ulcer must be corrected.** This principle is the one most often ignored. Biologic, psychosocial, and environmental problems must be addressed to maximize the rate of healing and minimize the risk of recurrence.

13. Which is the best way to debride a pressure ulcer?

The fastest, and often most effective, is surgical, or "sharp," debridement. Small wounds may be debrided at the bedside, but extensive wounds should be debrided in the operating room. This is often necessary early in the management in Stage III and IV pressure ulcers and is urgent in the face of advancing cellulitis or sepsis.

Mechanical debridement, primarily using wet-to-dry gauze dressings, can be effective to further remove necrotic tissue. Hydrotherapy and wound irrigation can assist in debridement and soften the eschar, making mechanical debridement easier.

Both sharp and mechanical debridement are nonselective, and healthy tissue can be damaged while attempting to remove necrotic tissue. Moistening dressings prior to their removal decreases the damage to healthy cells, but is also less effective in debridement of necrotic tissue. Wet-to-dry dressings should only be used for debridement and discontinued once the wound bed is clean.

Enzymatic and autolytic debridement can be very effective in noninfected wounds.

14. The saying is "You can put anything on a pressure ulcer, except the patient, and it will heal." True?

Yes and no. The human body is amazing in its ability to heal itself, often in the face of continued injury or insult. However, scientific evidence demonstrates that many agents used historically in wound care actually delay healing and epithelialization. Povidone-iodine, hydrogen peroxide, acetic acid, and sodium hypochlorite, commonly used to cleanse wounds, are cytotoxic to human fibroblasts and delay wound healing. The cellular toxicity of these agents also exceeds their bactericidal potency.

15. What is the difference between the tried-and-true normal saline wet-to-dry dressings and the myriad of new-fangled wound dressings?

It is important to differentiate between "wet-to-dry" dressings and "wet-to-moist" dressings. Many times physicians order wet-to-dry dressings when they mean wet-to-moist. Normal saline wet-to-dry dressings should be used exclusively for debridement of necrotic wounds. However, wet-to-moist dressings, in which the dressing is changed before it dries out, can be used to maintain a clean, moist wound bed and have been used for years to heal pressure ulcers. It is hard to argue with success.

Both wet-to-dry and wet-to-moist dressings need to be changed every 6–8 hours, which can significantly increase costs of dressing materials and nursing care. Newer dressings can often be changed once a day or less. Regardless of the dressing chosen, the same principles apply—adequate cleansing and debridement of the wound, moist wound healing, and correction of underlying factors.

16. How does one know which type of dressing to choose?

Normal saline wet-to-dry dressings are especially beneficial for debridement of necrotic or infected wounds, but once the wound is clean, there are dressings, such as transparent membranes, hydrocolloids, hydrogels, alginate products, and foam dressings, that are better suited to providing a moist wound environment, are often easier to use, and require less nursing time. These dressings differ in properties such as degree of absorptive ability, oxygen permeability, and nonadherence to the wound bed, need for secondary dressings, patient comfort, and ease of use that distinguish one from the other and help determine which one would be the best alternative for a particular wound.

Properties and Common Uses of Five Major Classes of Wound-Care Products

	PROPERTIES	USES
Transparent membranes	Moist healing principle Semipermeable Allows O_2 exchange Prevents bacterial entry Promotes epithelial migration	Prevents shear and friction Stage I, II, and shallow III ulcers Clean, granulating, nondraining Autolysis Secondary dressing Change when leaks or excess fluid
Hydrocolloids	Occlusive barrier Forms gel with wound exudate Creates moist wound environment Prevents bacterial contamination Available in wafers, paste, powder, or granules	Stage I, II, III, and some IV ulcers Minimal to moderate exudating wounds Prevents shear and friction Secondary dressing Aids in liquefaction, nonsurgical debridement Change when leaks (if < 24 hr, try another dressing
Hydrogels	Water, polyethylene oxide or other compound Primary wound covering Provides moist wound environment Various absorption abilities Good for patient comfort Nonadherent to wound bed	Stage II, III, and some IV ulcers Burns Autolysis—softens eschar Granulating or necrotic wounds
Alginate dressings	Hydrophilic, nonwoven fiber converts to gel Calcium and sodium exchange Creates moist environment Nonadherent to wound Available in packing or sheets	Light to heavily draining wounds Stage II, III, and IV ulcers Burns, vascular ulcers, graft sites May be used with infected wounds Can pack deep wounds to fill deadspace
Foam dressings	Semipermeable, absorptive, nonwoven, polyurethane dressing Combines moist healing and absorbancy No dressing residue in wound Nonadherent to wound Thermal insulation Comfortable, trauma-free removal Can be used with topicals	Minimal to moderate draining wounds Donor sites Burns (1st and 2nd degree) Pressure ulcers Wound dehiscence Skin tears

Adapted from Cuttino C: Dermal Wound Management in Long Term Care Settings Conference. Houston, Texas, February 1994. King of Prussia, PA, Health Management Publications, Inc.

17. When are antibiotics indicated in the management of pressure ulcers?

When there is evidence of infection associated with the pressure ulcer. The problem is defining what constitutes an infection. Clearly, when there is evidence of sepsis, urgent care, including debridement and systemic antibiotics, is needed. However, in the absence of overwhelming infection, what is the best way to determine the need for antibiotics? Wound cultures are generally useless because all pressure ulcers are colonized with bacteria. The Agency for Health Care

Policy and Research recently suggested that wound cleansing and debridement will, in most cases, control colonization, purulent drainage, foul odor, and local inflammation. If a pressure ulcer is not healing after 2–4 weeks of optimal treatment, a 2-week trial of a broad-spectrum topical antibiotic may be helpful, e.g., silver sulfadiazine or triple antibiotic ointment. Systemic antibiotics are reserved for cases with evidence of osteomyelitis, cellulitis, or signs of systemic infection.

18. How is osteomyelitis underlying a pressure ulcer diagnosed?

Osteomyelitis underlying a pressure ulcer will impede wound healing and necessitate a very different approach to wound management. However, overdiagnosis of osteomyelitis may subject a patient to unnecessary treatments.

The gold standard for diagnosis of osteomyelitis is pathologic examination of a **bone biopsy**. Plain radiographs can be helpful, but changes on x-ray develop late in the course of osteomyelitis. Bone scans are rarely useful because of the high false-positive rate in the presence of a pressure ulcer. Lewis et al. reported that the combination of leukocyte count, erythrocyte sedimentation rate, and plain x-rays had a positive predictive value of 69% if all three are positive.

19. Is electrical stimulation or other adjuvant therapy useful in the management of pressure ulcers?

The role of adjuvant therapies in pressure ulcer care has a long and controversial history. The problem is lack of controlled trials using these forms of therapy. Of the adjuvant therapies, which include hyperbaric oxygen, electrical stimulation, growth factors, and other topical agents, only electrical stimulation has had adequate research and supporting evidence to warrant its recommendation.

Clinical trials using **electrical stimulation** have demonstrated an enhanced rate of pressure ulcer healing in chronic Stage III and IV pressure ulcers unresponsive to conventional treatment. It may also be useful for recalcitrant State II ulcers. Its therapeutic benefit is hypothesized to be due to increasing circulation as a result of electrical stimulation. Use of this form of therapy has been limited to a small number of research centers and is not yet widely accepted.

BIBLIOGRAPHY

1. Bergstrom N, Bennett MA, Carlson CE, et al: Treatment of Pressure Ulcers: Clinical Practice Guideline no 15. Rockville, MD, Agency for Health Care Policy and Research, 1994 [AHCPR publication no. 95-0652].
2. Darouiche RO, Landon GC, Klima M, et al: Osteomyelitis associated with pressure sores. Arch Intern Med 154:753–758, 1994.
3. Dinsdale SN: Decubitus ulcers: Role of pressure and friction in causation. Arch Phys Med Rehabil 55:147–154, 1974.
4. Hess CT: Wound care products: A directory. Ostomy/Wound Manag 40(3):70–94, 1994.
5. Kosiak M: Etiology of decubitus ulcers. Arch Phys Med Rehabil 42:19–29, 1961.
6. Krasner D, Kennedy LK, Rolstad BS, Roma AW: The ABCs of wound care dressings. Ostomy/Wound Manag 39(8):66–86, 1993.
7. Lewis VL, Bailey MH, Pulawski G, et al: The diagnosis of osteomyelitis in patients with pressure sores. Plast Reconstr Surg 81:229–232, 1988.
8. Linder RM, Morris D: The surgical management of pressure ulcers: A systematic approach based on staging. Decubitus 3(2):32–38, 1990.
9. National Pressure Ulcer Advisory Panel: Pressure ulcers prevalence, cost and risk assessment: Consensus development conference statement. Decubitus 2(2):24–28, 1989.
10. Panel for the Prediction and Prevention of Pressure Ulcers in Adults: Pressure Ulcers in Adults: Prediction and Prevention: Clinical Practice Guideline no. 3. Rockville, MD, Agency for Health Care Policy and Research, 1992 [AHCPR publication no. 92-0047].

92. THE DIABETIC FOOT

Heinz I. Lippmann, M.D., F.A.C.P.

1. Is loss of limb a real danger for a diabetic?

In the U.S., diabetes mellitus is the most important cause of lower-extremity amputation. Certainly, many diabetics (8 million diagnosed, 8 million undiagnosed in the U.S.) are at risk! Reliable statistics on the true incidence of diabetic amputations are unavailable, but an estimate of an 11% risk for a lower-extremity amputation by 25 years after the diagnosis of diabetes is largely accepted. This risk is 10–20 times higher than that for all other causes for amputations.[4] Many diabetic amputations could be prevented.

2. What basic pathophysiologic changes occur in diabetes that contribute to limb loss?

1. Peripheral neuropathies: motor, sensory, autonomic
2. Macrovascular arteriopathies: atherosclerosis obliterans, producing ischemia
3. Microangiopathies: involving arterioles and basement membranes, causing retinal damage, nephropathies, and reduced resistance to infections: do not cause significant limb ischemia[8]
4. Medial calcification (Mönckeberg's arteriosclerosis): only interferes with some diagnostic tests

Most of these complications are diagnosed from the history and clinical examination. Many are asymptomatic. None of these basic abnormalities per se threatens loss of limb. An intact skin covering the legs protects the limb, and strict blood sugar control retards the progression of the pathophysiologic changes that have developed.[2]

3. What structural and functional changes in the diabetic expose a limb to risk?

1. **Foot deformity** (intrinsic-minus foot), due to diabetic neuropathy, leads to overloading of small areas of the foot, resulting in calluses, inflamed bursae, abscesses, or plantar ulcers.[6]
2. **Sensory deprivation**, due to sensory neuropathy, reduces pain response to cutaneous injury, inflammation, pressure, and heat.[5]
3. **Dry skin**, due to autonomic neuropathy, leads to cracking and fissuring of skin, allowing entry of infectious agents.
4. **Tissue glycosylation**, which occurs with elevated blood glucose levels, interferes with normal healing of skin and weakens resistance to bacterial and fungal infections.[1]
5. **Retinopathy** interferes with visual control of balance.[7]
6. **Ischemia** causes intermittent claudication, curtails blood flow reserve, and lowers the threshold for pressure damage to the skin.
7. **Charcot foot**, a severely deformed foot with fractures, can lead to skin ulceration and osteomyelitis.[6]

Each of these 7 changes is **permanent** and may result in damage to viable skin. This hazard is overcome if the diabetic habitually inspects his or her feet, using a mirror for the soles or assistance in case of visual impairment. This self-supervised examination remains the best strategy to protect against loss of limb.

4. What sorts of foot deformities occur in diabetes?

A foot deformity termed the **intrinsic-minus** foot involves the intrinsic foot muscles and renders flexion of the metatarsophalangeal (MTP) joints and straightening of the toes difficult or impossible. This results in hammer toes and, by the patient's pulling the plantar fascia with the toes extended distally, in a heightened plantar arch. This alteration in foot architecture creates a small walking surface so that the foot is supported by only the protruding MTP joints and heel, reducing the normal ground-contact area of around 100 cm² to 10–20 cm². The overloaded areas gradually develop calluses, inflamed bursae, abscesses, or plantar ulcers. Proper shoewear can avert this complication.

Sensory deprivation in the foot may complicate this presentation. By reducing the response to pain and pressure, foot injuries develop from foreign bodies in the shoe, ingrowing toenails, and other painful stimuli.

5. Describe the Charcot foot.

The Charcot foot is a rare finding (0.16% of cases). The foot, unprotected by weak muscles, suffers stress or fatigue fracture from repetitive injury in any part of the foot, right through the tarsus. If such a foot, after healing, ulcerates at the overloaded rockerbottom, osteomyelitis may break up the foot. Charcot foot can mimic infection, and differentiation relies upon the sedimentation rate, improvement with casting, and radiographs.

6. What should diabetic patients be instructed to look for in their foot self-examinations?

Skin self-inspection searches for "hot spots," inflamed areas after overloading injuries, that are in danger of breaking down. They should note any fissures, cracks, discolored areas, ingrowing nails, lymphangitis, dryness, blisters, blabs, wetting areas, red or pale pressure points over protruding areas (the malleoli or bunions), foreign bodies in the shoes, unusual softening of the skin, or changing shape of toenails (subungual abscesses). This is admittedly a long list but becomes a daily routine after training. Such skin self-inspection has worked in a large number of diabetics and, combined with the special hygiene, has saved countless legs in jeopardy.[3]

7. Should there be any other precautions in the diabetic's daily habits?

The patient must not cut or file toenails. A podiatrist (or, if unavailable, a podiatric-trained family member) is needed. There is no benefit in removing calluses if the overload pressure in the shoe is not corrected.

Posterior pressure on the heel in bed is a hazard, especially for the ischemic leg. While the patient lies motionless during sleep for 1 hour, skin perfused by a vessel with reduced closing pressure may blister and get infected, beginning the struggle for limb survival. Heel protection must become a habit. Traditional poseys are of no value; they displace easily.

At the end of the day, the diabetic must walk slower and shorten the stride to protect against the heel pounding that people automatically do when fatigued. The diabetic needs instruction in recognizing a toenail abscess (paronychia, infection of the nailbed) or phlegmons, which cause a specific sensation at certain pressure points even in advanced neuropathy. Both complications require surgical intervention for drainage to safeguard the limb.

8. What are the safety rules for daily hygiene?

- Washing with soap and water, but not soaking which defats skin and causes dryness and cracking.
- Ensuring water is not warmer than 33° C (92° F), checked with a "bathroom" thermometer, to avoid burns, which endanger ischemic limbs.
- Using whirlpool baths only for specific indications, such as cleaning out or debriding necrotic material in a deep ulcer.
- Treating the skin, including the interdigital spaces, with an absorbable water-soluble cream, such as lanolin, olive oil, Eucerine, Nivea cream, or mink oil (not petroleum jelly or heavy mineral oil, which is not absorbed).

9. Explain the considerations for footwear in diabetics.[5]

The shoe and pedorthotic modifications should protect against extrinsic injury, distribute the body weight over as large an area as possible, and prevent edema, apart from cosmetic considerations. For most people, including diabetics, a shoe fits when it is felt enveloping the foot without pressing; however, the neuropathic foot needs to be compressed with higher forces to be felt, and hence, many diabetics purchase too tight or too pointed shoes, which cause trouble and decubiti.

A shoe for a person with an intrinsic-minus foot is open at the toes or is a high oxford to avoid pressure on the PIP joints of the hammer toes. Generally, all shoes worn on such a foot could be corrected by molded inlays or orthotics to expand the weight-bearing area. Such devices should be removable, since foot shapes change.

In early stages, an intrinsic-minus foot can be protected with a regular, medial counter-enforced oxford shoe with a **Denver heel**. In a more advanced deformity, a **metatarsal bar** is placed on the sole of the shoe. In a neuropathically deformed foot, customized shoes with molded insoles must usually be provided. Most custom shoes should have a strong medial counter, be constructed of soft leather, and relieve all protruding areas (e.g., hammer toes, bunions, exostoses, etc.). Such shoes should be glued or sewn and not nailed.

Diabetics should change shoes often, ideally twice a day, and inspect their shoes for pebbles or foreign bodies. After a transmetatarsal amputation, the forefoot stump is stressed during toe-break, when the distal shoe inlay impacts on it during walking. A steel plate or wooden board incorporated into the shoe sole prevents the toe break. Some amputation stumps at Chopart's and even at Lisfranc's levels are allowed to develop a contracted Achilles tendon and extreme plantarflexion of the stump. This unfortunate result requires professional orthotic adjustment for both lower extremities as the best of several therapeutic options.

10. What extrinsic events that may contribute to limb loss should a diabetic watch for?

The diabetic should be mindful of the skin of the limbs and protect them from irreversible damage. The injuries most threatening to the diabetic are, in order of frequency, burns, pressure ulcers, and those due to poor nail care. These account for 75% of cases of amputated limbs. Other causes include pebbles in shoes; fissured, dry, neglected skin; interdigital fungal infections; or other other noxious forces. Of course, unwelcome surprises, such as insect bites, poison ivy, or unexpected mechanical encounters with the environment call for a diabetic's alertness and judgment as to when to seek professional help.

BIBLIOGRAPHY

1. Brownlee M: Glycation and diabetic complications. Diabetes 43:836–841, 1993.
2. Diabetes Control and Complications Trial Research Group: The effect of intensive treatment of diabetes on the development and progression of long-term complications in insulin-dependent diabetes mellitus. N Engl J Med 329:977–986, 1993.
3. Eckman MH, Greenfield SH, Mackey WC, et al: Foot infections in diabetic patients. JAMA 273:712–719, 1995.
4. Humphrey LL, Palumbo PJ, Butters MA, et al: The contribution of non-insulin-dependent diabetes to lower-extremity amputation in the community. Arch Intern Med 154:885–892, 1994.
5. Lippmann HI: The foot of the diabetic. In Brodoff BN, Bleicher TJ (eds): Diabetes Mellitus and Obesity. Baltimore, Williams & Wilkins, 1982, pp 712–734.
6. Lippmann HI, Perotto A, Farrar R: The neuropathic foot of the diabetic. Bull NY Acad Med 52:1159–1178, 1976.
7. Uccioli L, Giacomini PG, Monticone G, et al: Body sway in diabetic neuropathy. Diab Care 18:339–344, 1995.
8. Vracko R: Skeletal muscle capillaries in nondiabetics: A quantitative analysis. Circulation 41:285–297, 1970.

93. METABOLIC BONE DISEASE

Charles E. Levy, M.D.

1. Which disorders are considered metabolic bone disease?

Metabolic bone disease refers to disorders of the skeletal system due to an alteration in bone cell function causing loss of skeletal integrity and strength. The major metabolic bone disease seen by physiatrists is osteoporosis, but this category also includes Paget's disease, osteomalacia, renal osteodystrophy, hyperparathyroidism, osteogenesis imperfecta, and osteopetrosis, among others.

2. What is peak bone mass? When is it achieved?

Peak bone mass (PBM), defined as the highest level of bone mass achieved as a result of normal growth, generally occurs between adolescence and age 30 years, with variation at specific skeletal sites. For example, PBM of the femoral neck is achieved in the 17th year, whereas the lumbar vertebrae reach their maximum mostly between ages 18–24. Bone mass of the other regions of interest either shows no difference in women between age 18 and menopause or it is maximal in 50-year-old women, indicating slow but permanent bone accumulation continuing at some sites up to the time of menopause. Bone mineral density is generally accumulated up through adolescence, after which it declines at variable rates depending on anatomic location.

3. What happens to PBM at menopause?

Starting around the fourth or fifth decade of life, bone mass declines at a rate of 0.3–0.5% per year. After menopause, this loss accelerates to up to 10 times the initial rate for a period of up to 5–7 years.

4. What is osteoporosis?

Osteoporosis is a disease of bone characterized by a reduction in bone mass that is caused by an imbalance between bone formation and bone resorption ultimately resulting in osteopenia. In osteoporosis, the ratio of hydroxyapatite mineral content to organic content is normal, but there is a reduction in total bone tissue. In contrast, in **osteomalacia** the amount of bone tissue is normal (or increased), but there is reduced mineral content to the organic component ratio, leading to a "softening" of bone. Osteoporosis has been defined by the World Health Organization as occurring when bone mineral density is > 2.5 SD below below the young adult mean. **Osteopenia**, likewise, is defined when bone mineral density falls between 1–2.5 SD below the mean.

5. What are the symptoms of osteoporosis?

Like many diseases associated with aging (e.g., hypertension), osteoporosis is largely asymptomatic until the occurrence of a catastrophic event. That event is likely to be a compression fracture of the low thoracic or lumbar vertebrae or a Colles' fracture of the wrist. While the initial pain of the typical compression fracture resolves in 4–6 weeks, an accumulation of compression fractures can lead to postural deformity (the kyphosis of the "dowager's hump") with accompanying chronic thoracic/low back pain, nuchal myalgia, and abdominal protrusion and gastrointestinal discomfort. In severe cases, restricted excursion of the thoracic cage predisposes to pulmonary insufficiency and pneumonia.

6. Is all osteoporosis the same?

No. It is important to break down osteoporosis into subcategories. First, one should distinguish localized versus generalized disease. **Localized osteoporosis** includes primary disorders, such as reflex sympathetic dystrophy and transient regional osteoporosis. Secondary causes of localized osteoporosis include immobilization, inflammation, tumor, and necrosis

Generalized osteoporosis includes primary and secondary forms. By far, the most common type of primary generalized osteoporosis is involutional osteoporosis, which can be further broken down into postmenopausal osteoporosis (type I) and age-associated osteoporosis (type II). Type I generally affects women between the ages of 50–65 years, while type II affects those over age 70. Finally, there is general osteoporosis that results from a secondary disease process (type III).

Classification of Osteoporosis

CLASSIFICATION	CLINICAL COURSE	REMARKS
Primary		
Involutional		
Type I (postmenopausal)	Affects women only within menopause, lasting 15–20 yrs	Predominantly trabecular bone loss in axial skeleton
Type II (age-associated)	Men or women over age 70	Proportional loss of trabecular and cortical bone
Idiopathic juvenile	Age 8–14, self-limited (2–4 yrs)	Normal growth; consider secondary forms
Idiopathic young adult	Mild to severe, self-limited (5–10 yrs)	
Secondary (type III)	Dependent on underlying cause	Usually reversible to some extent after treatment of the primary disease
Endocrine		
Gastrointestinal		
Bone marrow disorders		
Connective tissue disorders		
Malnutrition		
Lymphoproliferative diseases		
Medications		
Cadmium poisoning		
Others		
Regional		
Reflex sympathetic dystrophy	Three overlapping clinical stages: typical course lasts 6–9 mos, followed by spontaneous or assisted resolution	Radiographic changes may occur in first 3–4 wks, showing patchy demineralization of affected area; triple-phase bone scan shows increased uptake in involved extremity before radiographic changes; brief tapering dose of corticosteroids often warranted.
Transient regional osteoporosis	Localized, migratory, predominantly involves hip, usually self-limited (6–9 mos)	Rare; diagnosis by clinical suspicion, radiograph, and bone scan; treatment similar to that for reflex sympathetic dystrophy

7. Describe the history and physical exam for osteoporosis.

History and physical examination should be centered on assessing risk factors, such as nutritional insufficiencies, endocrine or gastrointestinal disease, alcoholism, medications known to affect bone (i.e., corticosteroids, certain anticonvulsants), and secondary amenorrhea (anorexia and extreme exercise). One should examine the body habitus for signs of anorexia, cushingoid appearance, hypogonadism, goiter, gynecomastia, and barrel chest of chronic obstructive pulmonary disease (COPD), perform lung auscultation for the distant breath sounds and wheezes of COPD, and examine for inflammatory disease.

8. What laboratory tests are warranted?
The medical workup is aimed at determining the cause and extent of osteoporosis.
- Serum chemistries, including calcium, phosphorus, protein, cholesterol, alkaline phosphatase, hepatic enzymes, renal function tests, and thyroid functions tests
- Complete blood count and erythrocyte sedimentation rate (ESR) (to rule out inflammatory processes and anemias associated with malignancies)
- Serum testosterone (in men) to rule out hypogonadism
- Urinalysis screens for proteinuria due to nephrotic syndrome and for low pH due to renal tubular acidosis
- 24-hour urine
- Serum parathyroid level and vitamin D levels
- Multiple myeloma is unlikely with normal serum protein electrophoresis, ESR, and hematocrit

9. How can bone mass be measured?
- **Roentgenographs:** relatively insensitive
- **Single photon absorptiometry** (1960s): requires water or gel immersion; typically measures density at the radius and the calcaneus
- **Dual photon absorptiometry** (1970s): study of the spine, hip, and whole body without immersion
- **Dual energy x-ray absorptiometry** (DEXA) (1980s): improved resolution, with shorter time of study and lower levels of radiation than dual photon absorptiometry. The preferred measure by most researchers and practitioners studying osteoporosis.
- **Quantitative computed tomography** (1980s): Separately measures cortical and cancellous bone on existing computed tomography instruments; measures true bone mineral density. However, radiation exposure is hundreds of times greater than for DEXA. Expensive.

10. List the four clinical indications for bone mass measurement.
According to the National Osteoporosis Foundation's Scientific Advisory Board, they are:
1. *To aid in the diagnosis of significantly lowered bone mass in estrogen-deficient women* as a guide for hormone replacement therapy.
2. *To aid in therapeutic and diagnostic decision-making for those with apparent compression fracture or roentgenographic osteopenia.* Even seemingly obvious vertebral compression fractures may actually represent old juvenile epiphysitis, positioning problems of the roentgenogram, or normal variations in vertebral body shape.
3. *To diagnose low bone mass for those on long-term glucocorticoid steroids.* Findings of significantly reduced bone mass may lead to reduction in dose.
4. *To identify candidates for parathyroid surgery* among those at risk for severe skeletal disease with asymptomatic primary hyperparathyroidism.

11. Who was Julius Wolff? What is Wolff's law?
Wolff was a professor of surgery at the University of Berlin who in 1892 published his famous monograph *The Law of Bone Remodeling*. The essential tenet of this work was that static stress to a bone—whether it be compression, tension, or shear—would cause bone to remodel along mathematically predictable lines. Wolff collaborated with a Professor Culman, a mathematician from Zurich, who developed a method of analyzing the structural stresses in various components of bridges, building frames, and cranes. To test Wolff's supposition, Culman assigned his students the task of drawing the stresses on a particular hypothetical crane, which, unbeknownst to the students, was shaped to resemble the human femur. The students' vectors closely resembled the trabeculae of the actual femur, thus confirming what was later called Wolff's Law. In essence, this law translates to the fact that mechanical use (weight-bearing) results in increased cortical bone mass and strength, while disuse leads to bone atrophy.

12. Describe the physical therapy and exercise considerations for osteoporosis.

Several studies confirm the fact that weight-bearing exercise improves bone mineral density. Aerobic low-impact exercises, such as walking and bicycling, are generally recommended. The height of the bicycle seat, saddle style, and handle bar height and style should be adjusted for an upright spinal alignment. Research also supports the contention that high-intensity strength training offers the multiple benefits of preservation of bone mineral density, improvement of muscle mass and strength, and maintenance of balance.

Although swimming is unlikely to improve bone mineral density, it provides chest expansion, spinal extension, and low-impact cardiopulmonary fitness, and therefore it has a place in an osteoporosis regimen. A home program of physical therapy should include deep breathing, back-extension exercises, pectoral stretching, isometric exercises to strengthen the abdomen, and avoidance of kyphosis.

13. Which back exercises should be avoided for those with postmenopausal spinal osteoporosis?

Spinal flexion exercises predispose osteoporotic women to vertebral compression fractures.

14. Why is bracing used for vertebral compression fractures?

Bracing can help acutely for pain relief, chronically to assist biomechanically compromised structures, and intermittently to allow participation in certain demanding activities.

- For the acute treatment of back pain due to a compression fracture, a brace can provide enough immobility to allow a patient to lessen the duration of bed rest. Bracing decreases spinal motion, allowing paraspinal muscles to cease painful guarding, and also provides a physical barrier to reinjury.
- For chronic back pain, bracing substitutes for weak muscles, reduces ligamentous strain, and offers some protection against the occurrence of new fracture. Patients are able to endure greater activity and achieve fuller independence.
- Occasionally, certain sports or recreational activities demand application of a brace, which is then removed when normal activity is resumed.

15. What bracing options are available?

1. The simplest brace is the **elastic binder**, which functions as a reminder to restrict motion and also increases intra-abdominal pressure.

2. Stepping up is the heat-moldable plastic thoracolumbar orthosis, which is shaped to the patient's contours and then applied in an elastic support, often fabricated by a physical therapist. This usually takes only minutes to fabricate and is generally a less-expensive option.

3. For greater control, an orthotist can fit a hyperextension thoracolumbosacral orthosis (TLSO), such as the Jewett and CASH (cruciform anterior sternal hyperextension) braces.

4. Further restriction may be obtained with a custom-molded plastic body jacket.

5. Posture-training supports consist of small pouches containing weights up to 2 lbs. The pouch, suspended by loops from the shoulders, is positioned just below the inferior angle of the scapula to counteract the tendency to bend forward and may be worn for 1 hour twice a day.

16. What other therapeutic options should be considered?

Home modifications can reduce the risk of falling. Elimination of throw rugs and application of nonskid tape on the outer edges of steps (of different colors if possible to aid those with poor visual acuity) can improve safety. Lighting dark hallways and rails at stairwells and in the bathrooms can blunt common household perils. Ramps can replace stairs. A transfer tub bench that straddles the bathtub with two legs in the tub and the remaining two legs positioned on the dry bathroom floor eliminates the need to step over the edge of the tub. An additional benefit is that the user can wash his or her lower limbs with less bending.

Work simplification is aimed at reduction of vertebral compressive forces. Proper body mechanics demands that heavy items are carried at waist height and close to the body. Repositioning desks, files, and telephones can spare trunk flexion. Pacing helps defer fatigue, as does alternating tasks that demand sitting with those that require standing. Wheeled carts of the proper height can decrease vertebral strain of carrying, as can a back pack. Rotating platforms (e.g., Lazy Susans) can decrease the need to reach, while a swiveling, wheeled office chair with a lumbar support can be adjusted to support and position the spine.

Electric can openers, knives, and mixers, lightweight cups and bowls, and levered door closures ease kitchen tasks. Long-handled reachers, shoehorns, sock aids, and sponges facilitate dressing and grooming.

17. What are the pharmacologic considerations in osteoporosis?

Drugs are used to achieve two goals: (1) pain control and/or (2) slowing or reversal of the underlying disease process.

18. Discuss the options for pain control for vertebral compression fractures.

Back pain due to a vertebral compression fracture usually resolves in 4–6 weeks. Bed rest may be helpful initially, but it should be of limited duration. Beyond 1 week, cardiovascular deconditioning, loss of strength, and further loss of bone density usually outweigh the benefit of pain avoidance. Modalities such as moist heat and massage may alleviate symptoms.

Nonsteroidal anti-inflammatory drugs (NSAIDs) are often helpful, although the physician must screen and monitor against the occurrence of peptic ulcer and renal diseases. Smaller doses are often appropriate for the elderly. Although **narcotics** may offer meaningful relief from pain, they often slow gastrointestinal motility, causing constipation, particularly in the elderly. Furthermore, there is some risk of drug dependence.

19. What role does calcitonin play in treatment of osteoporosis?

Calcitonin directly inhibits osteoclastic activity, reducing bone resorption; vertebral bone mass is increased. Some reports even show decreased fracture incidence. It may be administered subcutaneously, intramuscularly, or nasally. A high incidence of nausea, transient facial flushing, and inflammatory reaction is associated with injected calcitonin; this drops dramatically for nasal administration. Calcitonin exerts an analgesic effect for which it is often prescribed in the acute postfracture period. Concurrent adequate intake of vitamin D and calcium is essential.

20. What advantages does alendronate offer in comparison with the other bisphosphonates?

Bisphosphonates (etidronate, pamidronate, and alendronate) are phosphatase-resistant analogues of **pyrophosphates**, which are naturally occurring inhibitors of bone resorption. The bisphosphonates bind to hydroxyapatite, preventing its dissolution and impairing osteoclast function. As a result, there is a reduction in the frequency of osteoclast activation. The dosage of **etidronate** (Didronel) necessary to inhibit bone resorption unfortunately also impairs mineralization of newly synthesized bone matrix. To avoid this unwanted effect, it is typically dosed for 14 days every 3 months. **Alendronate** (Fosamax) has a much more favorable ratio of osteoclast suppression to bone mineralization inhibition. It is about 1000 times more potent than etidronate in terms of inhibiting bone resorption and therefore can be dosed daily. As is the case for calcitonin, calcium and vitamin D intake should be supplemented. Postmenopausal women with osteoporosis taking alendronate have shown increases in bone mineral density of the lumbar spine, femoral head and greater trochanter as well as a reduction in vertebral fractures.

21. Calcitonin and the bisphosphonates produce their effects by inhibiting osteoclasts, thus impairing bone resorption. Are there any agents that stimulate new bone formation?

Sodium flouride stimulates osteoblast proliferation and increases bone formation. Various formulations of flouride have been available in Europe for many years. Unfortunately, too much flouride can increase bone fragility. A slow-release form of sodium flouride, imbedded in wax, has been effective in decreasing the incidence of vertebral fractures and increased spinal bone mass in severely osteoporotic women. At the time of this printing, an advisory committee of the U.S. Food and Drug Administration has recommended approval of slow release sodium flouride for the treatment of osteoporosis, but this treatment still awaits official sanction.

22. What are codfish vertebrae?

Codfish vertebrae refer to a radiographic finding in osteoporosis. This deformity occurs when there is expansion of the intervertebral disks into the superior and inferior vertebral endplates, causing an exaggerated bioconcavity. Fuller Albright, a pioneer in metabolic bone disease, noted in 1948 that this bioconcavity resembled the vertebrae of codfish, which are naturally bioconcave. In order to remember this term, a codfish in profile can be imagined in the interspace between the vertebrae.

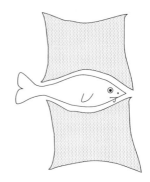

Radiographic findings in osteoporosis are nonspecific. Anterior vertebral compression fractures are common. Often, the external architecture of bone will be preserved, but mineral density is diminished. Loss of striations and a decrease in cortical thickness of the proximal femur are classic findings.

Codfish vertebrae. A representation of a lateral radiographic view of two vertebrae displaying an exaggerated bioconcavity. (Codfish is shown for illustrative purposes only. This is not ordinarily seen.)

23. What are the origins of the osteoblast and osteoclast?

The progenitors of both types of cells are located in bone marrow. **Osteoblasts** are members of a cell line derived from pluripotent mesenchymal stem cells called fibroblast colony-forming units (CFU-F). **Osteoclasts** arise from the hematopoietic granulocyte-macrophage colony-forming unit (CFU-GM).

24. What cytokines and colony-stimulating factors activate the development of osteoblasts and osteoclasts?

Osteoblasts	Osteoclasts
Interleukin-1	Interleukins I, 3, 6, and 11
Tumor necrosis factor	Granulocyte-macrophage colony-stimulating factor
Parathyroid hormone	Macrophage colony-stimulating factor
1,25-dihydroxyvitamin D3	Tumor necrosis factor
	Leukemia inhibiting factor
	Stem cell factor

25. How are estrogens and interleukin-6 connected in the pathophysiology of postmenopausal osteoporosis?

Estrogens inhibit the genetic transcription of interleukin-6. Therefore, loss of estrogens leads to greater amounts of interleukin-6, leading to increased numbers of osteoclasts. Ultimately, the homeostasis of bone formation/resorption is disrupted, favoring bone loss.

26. How does this apply to hypogonadal men?

Androgens exert a similar influence on interleukin-6 as estrogens.

27. What is coherence therapy? What does ADFR stand for?

Coherence therapy attempts to coordinate the normal sequence of bone remodeling throughout the body to allow strategic pharmacologic intervention. This intervention is aimed at limiting the resorption stage. It is also broken down into four phases, hence the acronym ADFR.

A—The **activation** stage is initiated with an agent such as phosphate, parathyroid hormone, thyroid hormone, 1,25-dihydroxyvitamin D_3, or growth hormone, which increases the number of remodeling units and coordinates their cycles (coherence).

D—**Depression** follows this stage wherein an agent such as etidronate, calcitonin, estrogen, or calcium is applied to reduce the amount of bone removed by osteoclasts.

F—Next comes the **free** stage, during which osteoblasts are left unimpeded to complete bone formation, usually for 2–3 months.

R—**Repetition** is the final stage, wherein the cycle is repeated. Typical durations range from 3–6 months, with the hope and expectation that a little more bone will be added with each cycle.

28. What are the typical dosages used in estrogen replacement?

Estrogen therapy in postmenopausal women leads to reduced rates of bone loss and fracture, as well as a reduced incidence of cardiovascular disease. Disadvantages are an increased risk of endometrial cancer (although this risk may be reduced when progesterone is added), possibly increased risk of breast cancer, and the resumption of menses. Bone mass measurement may be used to stratify risk: women whose bone mass is $\geq$ 1 SD above the young adult mean are relatively free from risk of fracture, although repeat measurement in 5 years may be warranted. Of course, reduction of cardiac risk by itself may be justification to start estrogen replacement.

Two types of 30-day regimens are commonly used in estrogen replacement: cyclic and continuous. The **cyclic** regimens include a resumption of menses. Estrogen, at 0.625 mg, is given daily for 25 days. This is combined with progesterone on days 12–25. Alternatively, estrogen can be taken for all 30 days with 5–10 mg of progesterone given daily for the first 14 days.

Likewise, there are two common **continuous** doses. For women without a uterus (i.e., hysterectomy), estrogen alone at 0.625/mg/day can be given, since there is no fear of endometrial carcinoma. Finally, 2.5 mg of daily progesterone can be added to the above schedule to provide protection against endometrial hyperplasia, while still avoiding the return of menses. The long-term safety and benefit of this schedule is still being evaluated.

29. How much calcium should be consumed daily by different age groups?

Optimal Calcium Requirements Recommended by the National Institutes of Health Consensus Panel

AGE GROUP	OPTIMAL DAILY INTAKE OF CALCIUM (mg)
Birth–6 mos	400
6 mos–1yr	600
1–5 yrs	800
6–10 yrs	800–1200
11–24 yrs	1200–1500
Men: 25–65 yrs	1000
Women: 25–50 yrs	1000
Postmenopausal women on estrogens:50–65 yrs	1000
Postmenopausal women not on estrogens: 50–65 yrs	1500
Men and women > 65 yrs	1500
Pregnant and nursing women	1200–1500

Dietary recommendations should be tailored to individual preferences. For example, 1 oz of Swiss cheese = 1 cup of milk = 1 cup of yogurt = 1 oz of calcium-enriched orange juice = approx 300 mg of calcium. For individual patients, a consultation with a dietician may be helpful. Others may be adequately served with educational pamphlets and charts. Calcium intake < 2000 mg/day is unlikely to be harmful.

30. How serious is the problem of hip fracture?

Hip fracture is a significant cause of morbidity and mortality in Caucasian women aged 50 years and above and, to a lesser extent, Caucasian men of similar age. Some 17.5% of these women will ultimately sustain a hip fracture, compared to 6% of men, and will account for a large percentage of the anticipated $45 billion in direct medical costs attributable to osteoporosis in the next 10 years.

31. Can any factors help predict who will sustain a hip fracture?

Caucasian postmenopausal women are at greatest risk. Furthermore, those with lower bone density are more likely to sustain a hip fracture. Poor self-rated health, a history of hyperthyroidism or maternal hip fracture, treatment with anticonvulsants, barbiturates, or long-acting benzodiazepines (half-life ≥ 24 hours), caffeine intake, and inactivity (< 4 hours on one's feet) raise the risk of hip fracture independent of bone mass. Findings on physical exam that are associated with fracture include inability to rise from a chair without using one's arms, resting tachycardia, poor depth perception, and poor perception of visual contrast. Taller, thinner women are also at increased peril.

BIBLIOGRAPHY

1. Cooper C, Barker DJ: Risk factors for hip fracture. N Engl J Med 332:814–815, 1995.
2. Cummings SR, Nevitt MC, Browner WS, et al: Risk factors for hip fracture in white women. N Engl J Med 332:814–815, 1995.
3. DeLisa JA (ed): Rehabilitation Medicine: Principles and Practice, 2nd ed. Philadelphia, J.B. Lippincott, 1993.
4. Downey JA, Myers SJ, Gonzalez EG, Lieberman JS (eds): The Physiological Basis of Rehabilitation Medicine, 2nd ed. Stoneham, MA, Butterworth-Henemann, 1994.
5. Favus MJ (ed): Primer on the Metabolic Bone Diseases and Disorders of Mineral Metabolism, 2nd ed. New York, Raven Press, 1993.
6. Grisso JE, Kelsey JL, Strom BL, et al: Risk factors for falls as a cause of hip fracture in women. N Engl J Med 324:1326, 1991.
7. Harris ST, Watts NB, et al: Four year study of intermittent cycle etidronate treatment of postmenopausal osteoporosis: Three years of blinded therapy followed by one year of open therapy. Am J Med 95:557–567, 1993.
8. Kattke FJ, Lehrmann JF (eds): Krusen's Handbook of Physical Medicine and Rehabilitation, 4th ed. Philadelphia, W.B. Saunders, 1990.
9. Manolagas SC, Jilka RL: Mechanisms of disease: Bone marrow, cytokines, and bone remodeling—Emerging insights into the pathophysiology of osteoporosis. N Engl J Med 332:305–311, 1995.
10. Matkovic V (eds): Osteoporosis. Phys Med Rehabil Clin North Am 6(2): 1995.
11. Matkovic V, Heany RP: Calcium balance during human growth: Evidence for threshold behavior. Am J Clin Nutr 55:992–996, 1992.
12. Wahner HW: Diagnostic procedures and new techniques [course handouts]. Presented at the 55th Annual Assembly, American Academy of Physical Medicine & Rehabilitation, 1993.
13. Watts NB: Osteoporosis: Methods to prevent fractures in patients at high risk. Postgrad Med 95:72–86, 1994.
14. Watts NB, Harris ST, et al: Intermittent cyclical etidronate treatment of postmenopausal osteoporosis. N Engl J Med 323:73–79, 1990.

XII. Therapeutics
A. General Principles

94. THERAPEUTIC PRESCRIPTION

Edgar L. Marin, M.D., and Andrea S. Coladner, D.O.

1. What is a prescription?

A prescription is a written formula for the preparation and administration of a therapeutic remedy. The physician, as the leader of the interdisciplinary team, "prescribes" and modifies rehabilitation therapeutics through guided consultation of allied professionals.

2. What attributes of a prescription help to improve its therapeutic efficacy?

Prescription of therapeutic exercises and modalities must be individually formulated and based on a logical and thorough understanding of a patient's medical, functional, and psychological profile. Prescriptions should serve as a helpful guide for therapists and must outline the basic objectives of a treatment program. Prescriptions must help to improve communications between the physician and other members of the PM&R team. Prescriptions must be written explicitly to prevent misunderstandings that might adversely affect the outcome of patient care.

3. List the basic components of a prescription in PM&R.

1. Identification of the discipline consulted (e.g., physical therapy, occupational therapy, speech)
2. Main diagnosis/secondary diagnoses
3. Impairments
4. Disabilities
5. Medical conditions affecting treatment, such as heart disease, chronic obstructive pulmonary disease, diabetes, seizure disorder, etc.
6. Goals (both short-term and long-term) and specific objectives of therapy
7. Specific therapeutic prescription for physical therapy, occupational therapy, speech therapy, respiratory therapy, etc.
8. Home exercise program if indicated
9. Precautions
10. Frequency of treatment (daily or two or three times weekly)
11. Duration of treatment (4 days, 2 weeks, 4 weeks)
12. Date of re-evaluation

4. What do we really want to achieve with the therapeutic prescription?

Relieve pain, improve function, and enhance quality of life.

5. List 10 categories of precautions that should be included when formulating a therapeutic prescription.

Cardiac	Skin insensitivity	Spine
Pulmonary	Impulsivity	Orthopedic (joint or bone instability
Falls	Incontinence	weight-bearing status)
Seizures	Hypoglycemic and diabetic	

6. What is meant by cardiac precautions?

Cardiac precautions are a set of explicit instructions written by a physician detailing pertinent signs, symptoms, and objective findings that may necessitate termination or modification of an exercise session. Cardiac precautions should be individualized and should ideally avoid being "generic." Examples of reasons to terminate an exercise session or modify it include:

1. Decrease in systolic blood pressure (SBP) of > 20 mmHg
2. Elevation of SBP or diastolic BP over parameters established for the patient
3. Elevations in heart rate (HR) greater than HR established by an exercise stress test
4. Elevation in HR > 80% of age-predicted maximal HR
5. Drop in HR > 10 bpm
6. Angina, shortness of breath, lightheadedness, fatigue

7. What details are required when writing a prescription for physical modalities, such as electrical stimulation, ultrasound, iontophoresis, hydrotherapy, or cold packs?

Areas to be treated
Duration
Goals
Intensity
Specific settings—amplitude, frequency, pulse width, waveform, current, voltage
Temperature range—heat/cold modalities
On/off cycles
Ionic material for iontophoresis

8. What general considerations are necessary in the exercise prescription for the cardiac patient?

Exercise must be prescribed in a manner similar to a drug prescription. The prescription should specify the type of exercise, intensity, duration, and frequency.

Type of exercise: It should be isotonic, rhythmic, and aerobic; should use large muscle groups; and should not involve a large isometric component. Walking, jogging, and stationary cycling are popular.

Intensity: It may be described as some percentage of the maximum attainable HR or oxygen consumption. The optimum level is 70–85% of maximum HR or 60–80% of maxVO_2.

Duration: This depends on the patient's level of fitness and the intensity of exercise. The usual duration when exercise is at 70% of maximum HR is 20–30 minutes at conditioning level.

Frequency: It is usually 3 days/week on alternate days. There is no contraindication to exercising every day, but the likelihood of musculoskeletal injury increases.

Format of exercise session: Start with a warm-up phase, follow by the training period, and finish with a cool-down phase. The warm-up phase increases joint readiness, opens up existing collateral circulation, and prevents sudden changes in peripheral resistance prior to the maximum contraction of the skeletal muscles required by the exercise. The cool-down period allows the gradual redistribution of blood from the extremities to other tissues and prevents the sudden reduction in venous return, thereby reducing the possibility of postexercise hypotension or syncope.

9. What are the stages of a progressive therapeutic exercise program for improving range of motion?

An exercise program will progress from:

1. Passive range of motion (ROM) when the patient has no active movement or if active movement is contraindicated
2. Active assistive ROM when the patient develops some movement or is allowed to perform active movement but requires assistance from the therapist to achieve full ROM
3. Active ROM when the patient is able to take the joint independently through its full range
4. Resisted exercise when full ROM is easily achieved (strengthening now becomes the therapeutic goal)

10. What are the steps leading to safe and independent ambulation?

Many patients consider ambulation as the primary goal of rehabilitation. The major elements of a gait program are:

1. Preambulation mat program to improve strength, coordination, and ROM; facilitate proprioceptive feedback; and develop postural stability and dynamic balance skills

2. Parallel bar progression for training in sit-to-stand transfers, balance, weight-shifting, appropriate gait pattern, and turning

3. Advanced parallel bar activities for increasing balance and strength under nonideal circumstances

4. Indoor progression for instruction and training in use of assistive devices: stair climbing; negotiating doors, thresholds, and ramps; and even falling techniques

5. Outdoor progression for instruction and training in use of assistive devices on outdoor and uneven terrain, crossing a street, and transferring in and out of a car or public transportation

11. When is it safe to prescribe passive stretching exercises of the fingers after hand surgery?

In tendon rehabilitation, stretching is usually contraindicated until 6 weeks postoperatively because connective tissue needs this interval to regain adequate tensile strength.

12. How are exercise training programs used in patients with neuromuscular diseases?

1. The exercise program is started early in the course of the disease.

2. It is restricted to individuals with slowly progressive or static disorders.

3. Submaximal resistive or high-repetition aerobic exercise is used.

Overwork, weakness, and further muscle degeneration are potential dangers in patients with rapidly progressive or far-advanced weakness.

13. Can a patient with multiple sclerosis (MS) and decubitus ulcers receive hydrotherapy (Hubbard tank) for cleansing of wounds?

No. Heat intolerance, which worsens symptoms, is extremely common in MS. Elevation of body temperature may block conduction along myelinated nerve tracks in MS patients. Any process that causes a rise in body temperature (hot water, warm environment, infection) increases this tendency for conduction block. Vigorous exercise, such as that performed during physical therapy, usually does not elevate body temperature, but it can if the therapy area is overheated or underventilated. Local irrigation of the wound may be more appropriate.

14. When can myositis ossificans develop?

Myositis ossificans can develop as a consequence of severe deep-muscle contusion, most frequently in the quadriceps. This type of heterotopic ossification may be precipitated by early injudicious stretching of an injured muscle that suffered significant hemorrhage. Heat, massage, and whirlpool treatments should not be used, as these therapies may initiate additional bleeding. Cryotherapy and electrical muscle stimulation, which facilitate resorption of hemorrhage, along with guarded movement for the first 24–48 hours, should be the first step taken to prevent myositis ossificans. Encapsulated hematomas should be evacuated whenever possible.

15. Which type of exercises should be avoided by osteoporotic patients?

Patients with osteoporosis should avoid **trunk flexion** exercises, because these seem to predispose the spine to compression fractures.

16. Is cervical traction helpful in the management of cervical radiculopathy?

Yes. The exact mechanism by which cervical traction is beneficial is unknown, but it may relieve pressure on the affected spinal nerve, at least temporarily.

17. Is there any contraindication to the use of cervical traction?

The obvious contraindications are fracture, instability, and tumor. It should be avoided in patients with known carotid artery stenosis or vertebral artery insufficiency.

18. **List the five important principles of fracture rehabilitation.**
   • All joints that do not require immobilization should be mobilized early to maintain function. For example, a patient with wrist fracture and a cast should perform ROM exercises of the shoulder to prevent adhesive capsulitis.
   • Gait training should start as soon as possible to avoid deconditioning. For lower-extremity fractures, assistive devices are usually necessary, since limitations in weight-bearing are common.
   • Mobilization of the injured area should begin when adequate fracture stability exists.
   • Local modalities should be used for pain control and reduction of muscle spasm.
   • Muscle strengthening of the involved area should begin as soon as fracture stability allows. It usually starts with isometric exercises, then progresses to isotonic strengthening when joint ROM has been regained, and finally involves resistive exercises when fracture healing and stability allow.

19. **In preparation for crutch walking, which muscles need strengthening?**
   Latissimus dorsi, triceps, biceps, quadriceps, hip extensors and abductors.

20. **Describe the general principles that apply to all techniques of stretching.**
   The body segments on each side of the joint to be stretched must be properly stabilized so that the maneuver is under complete control. The force must be applied in the precise direction that produces tension in the appropriate connective tissues. Prolonged moderate stretching is more effective than momentary vigorous stretching. Stretching must be held within the pain tolerance of the patient. During brief manual stretching, there may be pain when the stretch is applied, with relief of pain as soon as the stretch ceases. Prolonged stretching should remain within the patient's pain threshold to avoid tearing of blood vessels.

21. **During transfers, toward which side is the initial motion directed?**
   Most transfers are made toward the more normal or stronger side, regardless of the cause of muscle weakness.

22. **During stairs ambulation training, going up and down, which limb goes first?**
   Going up, the more normal or stronger side goes first. Going down, the weaker side goes first. "The good goes to heaven, the bad goes to hell" is a useful phrase to remember.

23. **Which physical therapy techniques are useful in managing slow initiation of movement in Parkinson's disease?**
   Multiple techniques, including proprioceptive neuromuscular facilitation, biofeedback, and neurodevelopmental techniques, have been used to facilitate movement. Training in a rhythmic pattern to music or with auditory cues such as clapping may help the patient in alternating motions required for activity, encouraging a more automatic pattern.

24. **Should passive exercise be prescribed in an acutely inflamed joint?**
   No, passive exercise should be avoided. Passive stretching to preserve or increase ROM should not be done if there is acute inflammation, because it may increase it. It also increases intra-articular pressure in the presence of joint effusion and has been associated with rupture of the joint capsule.

BIBLIOGRAPHY

1. DeLisa JA, Gans BM (eds): Rehabilitation Medicine: Principles and Practice, 2nd ed. Philadelphia, J.B. Lippincott, 1993.
2. Goodgold J: Rehabilitation Medicine. St. Louis, C.V. Mosby, 1988.
3. Hopkins HL, Smite HD (eds): Willard & Spackmans Occupational Therapy, 8th ed. Philadelphia, J.B. Lippincott, 1993.

4. Kottke FJ, Lehmann JF (eds): Krusen's Handbook of Physical Medicine and Rehabilitation, 4th ed. Philadelphia, W.B. Saunders, 1990.
5. O'Sullivan S, Schmitz TJ (eds): Physical Rehabilitation: Assessment and Treatment, 3rd ed. Philadelphia, F.A. Davis, 1994.

95. EXERCISE*

Richard W. Latin, Ph.D., L. Kay Thigpen, Ph.D., and Daniel Blanke, Ph.D.

AEROBIC POWER

1. What is aerobic capacity?

Aerobic capacity is the maximal capability to transport and utilize oxygen. Aerobic power is considered an important index of cardiovascular physical fitness.

2. How is aerobic capacity measured?

Maximal oxygen uptake, or VO_2max. The measure of VO_2max represents the maximal capabilities of the oxygen transport system and aerobic ATP resynthesis. VO_2max is usually expressed in ml of oxygen/kg body weight/min or in liters/min. Precise assessments of VO_2max require the metabolic analysis of expired gases while an individual is performing a maximal, incremental exercise test. However, many less accurate but simpler tests exist.

3. What are the guidelines related to an aerobic exercise program?

The guidelines proposed by the American College of Sports Medicine may be used to train individuals who are interested in health-related aerobic fitness.

Summary of ACSM Guidelines for the Quantity and Quality of Exercise Programs for Healthy Adults

COMPONENT	RECOMMENDATIONS
Frequency	3–5 days/week
Duration	20–60 min
Intensity	60–90% HRmax 50–85% VO_2max *or* 50–85% HRRmax
Mode	Any exercise using large muscle groups that is continuous and rhythmic in nature

HR = heart rate; HRR = heart rate reserve.

4. What are modes of aerobic exercise?

Aerobic exercises are those that use large muscle groups and that are continuous and rhythmic in nature. Examples of aerobic exercise are running, cycling, swimming, stair stepping, aerobic dance, and walking. Exercises that require heavy muscle contractions, such as weight training and sprinting, produce little change in VO_2max.

5. Does it matter which mode of exercise is used?

It depends on what the intent of training is. If a person is exercising for lifetime fitness, then the mode does not matter; if someone is training to improve a sport performance, it does. **Central**

* This chapter is excerpted from three chapters that appeared in *Sports Medicine Secrets*, with permission of the authors and the publisher, Hanley & Belfus, Inc., Philadelphia, Pennsylvania.

adaptations to exercise are relatively nondiscriminatory. Heart rate, stroke volume, and cardiac output may change regardless of the exercise task. In other words, the heart does not know what mode of exercise is being used—it simply knows that it must pump more blood. **Peripheral adaptations** to exercise modes are highly task-specific. Neuromuscular recruitment of specific motor units and appropriate blood flow shunts are essential to peripheral physiologic and biochemical adaptations. These changes allow for greater tissue utilization of oxygen and improvement of VO_2max.

STRENGTH TRAINING

6. Define strength.

Strength generally refers to a performance characteristic of muscle. It is the maximal force a muscle or muscle group can generate.

7. What are strength training, weight training, and resistance training?

Strength training refers to exercises designed to increase the maximal force that a muscle or muscle group can generate voluntarily. **Weight training** is a more specific term and refers to training with free or machine weights. **Resistance training** encompasses a wide range of training modalities for strength.

8. What type of exercise is most effective for gaining strength?

Exercises that require voluntary maximal muscular contractions. All types of muscular contractions (isometric, isotonic, and isokinetic) produce significant gains in muscular strength.

9. Describe isometric training.

Isometric training is the generation of muscular force with no visible joint movement. Isometric training occurs when external resistance is not overcome by internal force generation, as might occur when attempting to push open a locked door. Isometrics are most appropriate when joint motion is not wanted.

10. What is isotonic training?

Isotonic training is the generation of muscular force with visible joint movement at a variable speed but with constant external resistance. It encompasses free and machine weight training as well as exercises that use Thera-Band or similar devices and exercises that use the body's own weight as resistance (push-ups, sit-ups, etc.).

11. How does isokinetic training differ from isotonic training?

Isokinetic training is the generation of muscular force with visible joint movement that occurs at *constant speed* but with *variable external resistance*. Thus, a muscle can generate maximal force throughout its length-tension curve.

12. Are there any contraindications to isometric training?

Isometrics tend to elevate blood pressure more than do the other types of strength training and should be avoided by the elderly and others who are susceptible to hypertension. One of the other types of training would be more appropriate if a full-body or multiple-joint conditioning program were needed.

13. When is isotonic training indicated?

When strength gains throughout a joint's range of motion are desired.

14. When is isokinetic training appropriate?

Theoretically, isokinetic training is the most effective means of increasing muscle strength because it allows the muscle to generate maximal force throughout its length-tension curve. It is most beneficial during the early stages of rehabilitation. It is beneficial when the speed of training needs to resemble the higher speeds of contraction that would be unsafe to perform in isotonic training.

15. What physiologic adaptations occur in muscle tissue with resistance training?
Cellular adaptations occur that affect an individual's aerobic and anaerobic capabilities.

Adaptations to Resistance Training and Effect of Resistance Training on Anaerobic and Aerobic Metabolism

SYSTEM/VARIABLE	RESPONSE	METABOLISM	
		ANAEROBIC	AEROBIC
Bone			
Mineral content	Increase		
Cross sectional	No change		
Capillary Density			
H volume L intensity	No change		
L volume H intensity	Decrease		Decrease
Connective Tissue			
Ligament strength	Increase		
Tendon strength	Increase		
Collagen content	Increase		
Ratio of connective tissue to muscle	No change		
Fuel Stores			
ATP	Increase	Increase	
Phosphocreatine	Increase	Increase	
Glycogen	Increase	Increase	
Metabolic Enzymes			
Creatine kinase			
H volume L load	Increase	Increase	Increase
L volume H load	Decrease	Decrease	Decrease
Myokinase			
H volume L load	Increase	Increase	Increase
L volume H load	No change		
Phosphofructokinase			
H volume L load	Increase	Increase	
L volume H load	No change		
Lactate dehydrogenase			
H volume L load	No change		
L volume H load	No change		
Carbohydrate metabolism	Increase		Increase
Mitochondrial Density	Decrease		Decrease
Muscle			
Size	Increase	Increase	Increase
Number	No change		

16. How is bone affected by strength training?
Bone mineral content is increased by resistance training of high intensity and sufficient duration. However, studies have been unable to confirm changes in bone cross-sectional area due to strength training in humans.

17. What is meant by the terms "concentric" and "eccentric"?
Both terms describe types of muscular contractions, which may be isotonic or isokinetic. **Concentric** contractions occur when the muscle fibers are shortening, as in the lifting phase of a

bicep curl. **Eccentric** contractions occur when the muscle fibers are lengthening, as in the lowering phase of a bicep curl.

18. Is age a factor in response to resistance training?
No. All ages respond similarly to resistance training. Young and old alike increase in strength.

19. Are different programs needed for the extremes of age?
No. Muscular response to training is independent of age. The same protocols are appropriate regardless of age. Individuals (young, elderly, female, and sedentary) with less muscle mass need to lift less absolute weight, but as a percentage of their maximum, there is no difference.

FLEXIBILITY

20. What is flexibility?
Flexibility is the ability to move the joints of the body through the range of motion (ROM) for which they were intended. Each joint of the body is designed to allow a specific amount of motion. An individual lacks flexibility if he or she is unable to produce the amount of motion for which each joint is designed.

21. What is connective tissue?
Connective tissue is one of the most widely varied types of tissue and includes cartilage, bone, blood, and lymph. The connective tissue found in tendons, ligaments, intramuscular and extramuscular layers of fascia, and joint capsules is primarily composed of collagenous fibers arranged in a protein-polysaccharide ground substance. It possesses both elastic and plastic properties. This type of connective tissue is referred to as dense or **collagenous connective tissue**. Dense connective tissue exhibits high tensile strength and therefore is difficult to elongate. Because it is primarily responsible for limiting joint ROM, dense connective tissue is the target of flexibility training.

22. What is the range of motion expected at each joint?

Average Range of Joint Motion (In Degrees)

Shoulder		**Hip**	
Flexion	158	Flexion	113
Extension	53	Extension	28
Abduction	170	Abduction	48
Adduction	50	Adduction	31
Horizontal flexion	135	Horizontal flexion	60
Arm at side		Hip in flexion	
Internal rotation	68	Internal rotation	45
External rotation	68	External rotation	45
Arm in 90° abduction		Hip in extension	
Internal rotation	70	Internal rotation	35
External rotation	90	External rotation	48
Elbow		**Knee**	
Flexion	146	Flexion	134
Hyperextension	0	Hyperextension	10
Forearm		**Ankle**	
Pronation	71	Plantar Flexion	48
Supination	84	Dorsiflexion	18

(Table continued on following page.)

Average Range of Joint Motion (In Degrees) (Continued)

Wrist		**Hind foot**	
Extension	71	Inversion	5
Flexion	73	Eversion	5
Ulnar deviation	33	**Fore Foot**	
Radial deviation	19	Inversion	33
Thumb		Eversion	18
Abduction	58	**Great Toe**	
IP flexion	81	IP flexion	60
MP flexion	53	IP extension	0
MC flexion	15	MTP flexion	37
IP extension	17	MTP extension	63
MP extension	8	**2nd to 5th Toes**	
MC extension	20	DIP flexion	55
Fingers		PIP flexion	38
DIP flexion	80	MTP flexion	35
PIP flexion	100	Extension	40
MCP flexion	90	**Cervical Spine**	
DIP extension	0	Flexion	38
PIP extension	0	Extension	38
MCP extension	45	Lateral bending	43
		Rotation	45
		Thoracic and Lumbar Spine	
		Flexion	85
		Extension	30
		Lateral bending	28
		Rotation	38

From the American Academy of Orthopaedic Surgeons: Joint Motion: Method of Measuring and Recording. Chicago, AAOS, 1965.

23. What kinds of injuries are common as a result of lack of flexibility?

Individuals with limited flexibility are more susceptible to muscle strains because the connective tissue surrounding the joint limits the ROM and provides greater support for the joint. Specific limitations in flexibility may contribute to particular problems. Lack of adequate flexibility in the hamstrings is associated with pain in the low back, knee, and hip in exercisers. Lack of flexibility in the hand and wrist joints may contribute to repetitive motion syndrome or carpal tunnel syndrome.

24. What kinds of injuries are common as a result of too much flexibility?

Joint sprains. Because the connective tissue surrounding the joint has been elongated, it does not contribute as effectively to the stability of the joint. Excessive flexibility of a joint may contribute to osteoarthritis or joint pain.

25. How does one increase flexibility?

Several techniques of stretching can be used to increase flexibility safely and effectively. These include static stretching, static stretching with contraction of the antagonist (reciprocal inhibition), static stretching with contraction of the agonist (proprioceptive neuromuscular facilitation, PNF), and static stretching with contraction of the agonist followed by contraction of the antagonist (PNF). Individual exercises for each joint or area of the body should be performed using one or more of these techniques.

26. What is static stretching?

Static stretching is done by slowly moving the joint to the end of ROM and then holding the position for 5–60 sec. It is important when moving to the end of ROM to stop at the point of moderate discomfort and prior to pain. As a result of the slow movement, there is a reduced tendency to elicit the stretch reflex. Static stretch is therefore one of the safest techniques for increasing flexibility.

27. What is static stretching with contraction of the antagonist (reciprocal inhibition)?

Static stretching with contraction of the antagonist is done by slowly moving the joint to the end of ROM, then isometrically contracting the antagonist muscle group for 5–30 sec. This is the muscle group directly opposite the muscle being stretched. It is again important to move the joint just to the point of moderate discomfort and no farther. This technique enjoys all the benefits of static stretching with the added benefit of further reducing the tendency to elicit the stretch reflex by actively contracting the antagonist muscle group. By the action of reciprocal inhibition, there is a release of an inhibitory transmitter substance at the spinal cord to reduce the activity of the muscle being stretched.

28. What is static stretching with contraction of the agonist (PNF)?

Static stretching with contraction of the agonist is performed by slowly moving the joint to the end of ROM and then isometrically contracting the agonist muscle group for 5–30 sec. This is a contraction of the muscle group that is being stretched. No movement should occur in the muscle being stretched. The contraction must therefore be isometric. It is theorized that the isometric contraction of the muscle being stretched will relax the muscle, possibly through the action of the Golgi tendon organ, and therefore allow additional ROM at the joint. Minimally, the isometric contraction puts an additional stretch on the connective tissue surrounding the joint and therefore allows greater ROM.

29. Why is ballistic stretching not recommended?

Ballistic stretching is performed by using bouncing or jerking movements or momentum to force the joint beyond its normal ROM. The movements may be described as bobbing, swinging, or kicking movements. Although ballistic stretching can increase flexibility, it is not recommended because of its increased potential for injury. These forces can lead to muscle or connective tissue tears or bone avulsion.

30. What is the stretch reflex?

It is a protective reflex due to the action of the muscle spindles. When a muscle is stretched rapidly, especially at its greatest length, the muscle spindle sends a stimulus to the CNS, which in turn sends a stimulus back to the muscle. The muscle responds by contracting. The force of contraction is somewhat related to the speed of the stretch.

The purpose of this reflex is to protect the muscle and associated joints from injury by limiting the ROM of the muscle. The stretch reflex hampers flexibility training by actively contracting the muscle that is in the process of being elongated. Slow movements that reduce the intensity of the contraction and delay the activity of the stretch reflex until reaching maximum ROM are more desirable than fast movements that elicit the stretch reflex. Flexibility training that uses slow movements therefore reduces the incidence of injury.

31. Which techniques are recommended for a flexibility training program?

To improve flexibility, an individual should choose one of the techniques for performing flexibility exercises and then identify specific exercises for each joint. Flexibility exercises should be done daily or more than once per day. Contrary to exercises designed to increase strength, exercises to increase flexibility can be done safely as often as is convenient. Three to five repetitions of each exercise should be performed for best results. It is important that flexibility exercises be done regularly both to increase and maintain the desired joint ROM.

BIBLIOGRAPHY

1. Alter M: Science of Stretching. Champaign, IL, Human Kinetics, 1988.
2. American Academy of Orthopaedic Surgeons: Joint Motion: Method of Measuring and Recording. Chicago, AAOS, 1965.

3. American College of Sports Medicine: Guidelines for Exercise Testing and Prescription. Baltimore, Williams & Wilkins, 1995.
4. American College of Sports Medicine: Position statement on the recommended quantity and quality of exercise for developing cardiorespiratory and muscular fitness in healthy adults. Med Sci Sports Exerc 22:265, 1990.
5. Fleck S, Kraemer W: Designing Resistance Training Programs. Champaign, IL, Human Kinetics, 1987.

96. PHARMACOLOGIC AGENTS IN REHABILITATION

Nancy M. DeSantis, D.O., and Mark A. Young, M.D., F.A.C.P.

1. Name fifteen classes of drugs commonly prescribed by rehabilitation physicians.

Analgesics	Antihypertensives
Opioid agents	Antibiotics
Antispasmodics	Anticoagulants
Antispasticity drugs	Hypoglycemics
Anticonvulsants	Urologic agents
Psychopharmacologic agents	Gastrointestinal agents
Sedatives	Bone-acting agents
Corticosteroids	

2. What are the 2 most common types of analgesics used by rehabilitation physicians?

Acetaminophen: analgesic and antipyretic properties; few side effects. Overdose (usually in quantities > 10 gm/day) can lead to hepatic injury.

Nonsteroidal anti-inflammatory drugs (NSAIDs): anti-inflammatory, analgesic, and antipyretic properties; side effects include renal and GI effects; includes salicylate and nonsalicylated compounds.

3. Explain the mechanism of action of NSAIDs.

NSAIDs inhibit prostaglandin production usually by inhibiting the transformation of arachidonic acid to the stable prostaglandin. Unblocked, prostaglandins sensitize or excite the nociceptor (sensory nerve terminals of afferent A-delta and C-fibers), causing a change in local microcirculation that affects or stimulates release of substance P from nerve endings and results in mast cell degranulation and neurogenic inflammation. This leads to pain. NSAIDs are thought to work in chronic inflammatory states by accumulation within the inflamed tissue.

4. How is aspirin different from other NSAIDs?

All NSAIDs inhibit platelet aggregation and prolong bleeding time. Aspirin binds irreversibly, causing the platelet to remain ineffective for clotting for its entire lifespan of 7–12 days. Other nonacetylated salicylates do not have this property. The risk of a prolonged bleeding time is greater with the use of aspirin than with other NSAIDs.

5. Which lab parameters should be monitored for patients on NSAIDs?

Periodic renal and liver function tests
CBC for assessment of hemoglobin
Stool guaiac to detect GI bleeding
Urinalysis to assess for evidence of microscopic hematuria

6. What are the complications to the use of NSAIDs?

NSAIDs are contraindicated in patients in whom aspirin or other NSAIDs induce the syndrome of asthma, rhinitis, and nasal polyps; this reaction may be fatal. Serious GI toxicity, such as bleeding, ulceration, and perforation, can occur at any time and without warning. There is an increased risk of bleeding in those with a previous history of serious GI bleeding and in those with risk factors for peptic ulcer disease, such as alcoholism and smoking.

7. Explain the mechanism of action of the opiate compounds.

Opiates can bind with receptors in various sites:

1. In peripheral tissues, raising the stimulation threshold for pain at the nociceptive terminal. This inhibits release of substance P.
2. At the dorsal horn of the spinal cord (primary afferent for nociceptive information).
3. In the midbrain, brainstem, and thalamus (relay stations for ascending nociception).
4. In the limbic system and cortex (production of the emotional dimensions of pain).

8. What are the effects of opiates such as morphine?

Analgesia, drowsiness, mood changes, and mental clouding are common effects. At therapeutic levels, the painful stimulus may still be recognized but not perceived as painful.

9. What are the indications for the use of opiates like morphine?

Cardiac pain, pulmonary edema, postoperative pain, and cancer pain are common indications for opioid use. In general, severe, continuous dull pain, transmitted by C-fibers through the paleospinothalamic tract, is better controlled by opiates such as morphine than is intermittent sharp pain.

10. What are some common contraindications to the use of opiates?

Opiates should not be used for patients with COPD, emphysema, severe obesity, or cor pulmonale due to their respiratory depressant effects and blunting of the respiratory response to CO_2. Morphine causes increases in CSF pressure and should not be used in those with acute head injuries or suspected CNS diseases. Opiates are metabolized by the liver and should be used with caution in those with hepatic disease.

11. Are the antispasmodics the same as antispasticity drugs?

No, the antispasmodics are used as a short-term remedy to decrease muscular spasm arising from painful conditions and not neurologic dysfunction. Included in this category are cyclobenzaprine (Flexeril), methocarbamol (Robaxin), chlorzoxazone (Parafon Forte), carisoprodol (Soma), orphenadrine (Norflex). They are centrally acting agents that are sedating.

12. How do antispasticity medications work?

Dantrolene (Dantrium): works peripherally at the muscle fiber by affecting excitation-contraction coupling, thereby relaxing skeletal muscle contraction. Liver function testing should be performed frequently during treatment.

Baclofen (Lioresal): works centrally at the spinal level by inhibiting the release of excitory neurotransmitter. It is an analog of GABA.

Diazepam (Valium): exerts its effect on the CNS by potentiating the postsynaptic effects of GABA, an inhibitory neurotransmitter.

13. Name three categories of rehabilitation patients at risk for seizure development.

Cerebral trauma patients

Patients with space-occupying lesions

Patients with cerebral vascular accidents.

Seizure medications can be used both prophylactically as well as for treatment of seizure disorder. They typically need to be maintained within a therapeutic range.

14. Name the major anticonvulsant medications and their major indications.

Carbamazepine, phenobarbital, primidone, and **phenytoin** are indicated in generalized tonic-clonic seizures and partial seizures. **Ethosuximide** is indicated in absence seizures. **Diazepam** is indicated in partial seizures. **Valproic acid** is indicated in absence, myoclonic, tonic-clonic, akinetic, atonic, and photosensitive seizures. **Clonazepam** is indicated for akinetic, myoclonic, absence, and atonic seizures. **Phenytoin** is frequently used for prophylaxis during the first week after traumatic brain injury. The goal is to prevent secondary complications that are caused by seizures

15. What complications of antiseizure therapy must the rehab team be aware of?

Anticonvulsants can be associated with cognitive, behavioral, and perceptual dysfunction. Certain seizure medications (carbamazepine) can cause agranulocytosis, aplastic anemia and hyponatremia.

16. Which are the major sleep-inducing agents (sleepers) prescribed by physiatrists in inpatient settings?

Benzodiazepines: commonly used for short-term management of insomnia and for their anxiolytic effect. Examples include flurazepam (Dalmane), triazolam (Halcion), temazepam (Restoril). May induce psychological dependence.

Antihistamines: a relatively "safe" sedative that can be used for antiemetic, antipruritic, and antianxiety effects. Examples include diphenhydramine (Benadryl) and hydroxyzine (Atarax). Can cause increased agitation in brain-injured patients.

Barbiturates: associated with hypersensitivity reactions, respiratory depression, and other adverse reactions. Not recommended as treatment for insomnia.

Hypnotics: Chloral hydrate (Noctec) has minimal effect on the normal sleep cycle but can cause CNS depression.

Antidepressants: Selective serotonergic reuptake inhibitors (SSRIs). Zoloft may be effective for those individuals having difficulty with sleep initiation. Tricyclic antidepressants (Elavil) may be effective for patients who awaken frequently during the night. May cause hyponatremia.

17. What are the major classes of antihypertensives and their adverse effects?

Diuretics: can cause electrolyte and metabolic abnormalities, postural hypotension, and renal failure.

Calcium channel blockers (e.g., nifedipine, verapamil, and diltiazem): can cause dizziness and headaches; may increase digoxin level. Can cause reflex tachycardia.

ACE inhibitors (e.g., captopril, enalapril, and lisinopril): can cause nephritic syndrome and taste disturbance; may result in neuropathies. Hyperkalemia is a frequent side effect.

Central alpha agonist (e.g., guanabenz, methyldopa, clonidine): common side effects include sedation, dizziness, constipation, dry mouth.

Post-ganglion inhibitors (e.g., reserpine, guanethidine): can cause depression, diarrhea, orthostatic hypotension.

Beta blockers (e.g., atenolol, metoprolol, nadolol) are associated with congestive heart failure, decreased cardiac output, peripheral vascular disease, bradycardia.

Vasodilators (direct) (e.g., hydralazine, minoxidil): can cause reflex tachycardia, postural hypotension, headache, peripheral edema.

α_1-**Blockers** (e.g., prazosin, phenoxybenzamine): associated with headache and "first-dose hypotensive syncope."

18. What should the rehabilitation specialist know about hypoglycemic agents?

Insulin and oral hypoglycemic agents are two modes of pharmacologic treatment for the diabetic rehab patient. Insulin-dependent diabetics as well as non-insulin-dependent diabetics are at risk for developing hypoglycemic episodes. This tendency may be exacerbated in the rehab patient who has just started an accelerated exercise therapy program that changes insulin dosing requirements. **Hypoglycemia** is a frequent and very serious complication; its symptoms can include irritability, headache, anxiety, diminished arousal level, and, if left untreated, convulsions and death. For patients receiving oral hypoglycemic agents, GI effects and skin rash are common side effects, and their effects may be potentiated by monoamine oxidase inhibitors, probenicid, and NSAIDs.

19. What are the most common reasons for anticoagulation therapy in PM&R?
Deep venous thrombosis
Pulmonary embolism
Atrial fibrillation
Stroke resulting from cardiogenic embolus
Vertebrobasilar insufficiency
Arterial bypass graft surgery

20. Name 9 contraindications for anticoagulation treatment.

Active bleeding	Recent surgery
Gastric ulcers	Thrombocytopenia
Cerebrovascular accident/hemorrhage	Hemophilia
Pericarditis/endocarditis	Tumor metastasis
Pregnancy	Severe hypertension

21. Which are the most commonly prescribed categories of GI medications used in rehabilitation?
Antispasmodics/antidiarrheals: Should be prescribed only after etiology of diarrhea has been determined.
Antiemetics: Should be used with caution to avoid masking symptoms/signs of ileus or obstruction.
Laxatives/evacuants: Oral and rectal preparations to aid the regular passage of feces (not commonly prescribed).

BIBLIOGRAPHY

1. Backonja M, Fitzthum JE: Pharmacologic management of noncancer spinal pain syndromes. Spine State Art Rev 9:765–779, 1995.
2. Davidoff RA: Antispasticity drugs: Mechanism of action. Ann Neurol 17:107–116, 1985.
3. Fingl E: Laxatives and cathartics. In Gilman AG, et al (eds): The Pharmacologic Basis of Therapeutics, 6th ed. New York, Macmillan, 1980, pp 1002–1012.
4. Gualtieri CT: Neuropsychiatry and Behavioral Pharmacology. New York, Springer-Verlag, 1991.
5. Honig SM: Nonsteroidal anti-inflammatory drugs. In Tollison CA, Satterthwaite JR, Tollison JW (eds): Textbook of Pain Management, 2nd ed. Baltimore, Williams & Wilkins, 1994, pp 165–172.
6. Killian JM, Fromm GH: Carbamazepine in the treatment of neuralgia: Use and side effects. Arch Neurol 19:129–136, 1968.
7. Solomon GD: Analgesic medications. In Tollison CA, Satterthwaite JR, Tollison JW (eds): Textbook of Pain Management, 2nd ed. Baltimore, Williams & Wilkins, 1994, pp 155–164.
8. Weingarden SI: The gastrointestinal system and spinal cord injury. Phys Med Rehabil Clin North Am 3:765–781, 1992.
9. Young MA: Where all diseases meet: At physiatry. Medical Tribune, August 21, 1991.
10. Young MA, Ehrenpreis ED, Ehrenpreis M, Kirschblum S: Heparin-associated thrombocytopenia and thrombosis syndrome in a rehab patient. Arch Phys Med Rehabil 70:468–470, 1989.

XII. Therapeutics
B. Physical Modalities

97. THE PHYSICAL AGENTS

Jeffrey R. Basford, M.D., Ph.D.

1. What is a physical agent?

Physical agents are devices that use physical forces to produce beneficial therapeutic effects. In theory, any physical phenomenon—e.g., pressure, heat, cold, electricity, sound, or light—may be utilized. In practice, only heat, cold, water, ultrasound, shortwaves, and electricity are widely used.

Physical agents ares used as adjuncts to a therapy program. As such, they supplement, but do not replace, exercise, stretching, massage, education, and medical interventions.

2. Are physical agents new?

No. Heat, cold, pressure, light, and even electricity have been used for thousands of years to speed healing and lessen pain. Although newer agents, such as ultrasound, shortwaves, and electrical stimulation, have gained use, heat and cold remain the basis of most treatment.

3. What are the limitations of the physical agents?

Although each agent has unique characteristics, many ultimately rely on heat or cold to gain their effects. As a result, many share common restrictions on their use based on the amount of energy that can be added (heating) or taken away from (cooling) tissue. In particular, temperatures > 45–50°C (100–120°F) or < 0°C (32°F) can easily injure tissue. In practice, treatments involving these temperatures may be used for restricted portions of the body, but broader areas are treated less intensely.

HEAT AND COLD

4. How do physical agents alter tissue temperature?

The temperature of an object can be altered in only three ways:

1. **Conduction** is defined as the transfer of heat between two bodies in contact at different temperatures. Examples include hot packs and paraffin baths.

2. **Convection** also involves contact between two objects at different temperatures but also requires that one flow past the other. This flow maximizes the temperature gradient between the objects, so more intense heating and cooling are possible than by conduction alone. Whirlpool baths are an example.

3. **Conversive heating** utilizes the resistive properties of a material to convert nonthermal energy (e.g., sound and radio waves) to heat. Heat lamps and ultrasound diathermy use the dissipative properties of tissue to convert infrared light and sound to heat.

5. What forms of heat therapy are available?

Superficial and deep. Superficial agents heat the skin and subcutaneous tissues. Deep heating agents, also known as **diathermies**, heat more deeply and can raise temperatures to therapeutic levels at depths of 3.5–7 cm. Hot packs and heat lamps characterize the superficial agents, while ultrasound and shortwave typify the diathermies.

6. What forms of cold therapy (cryotherapy) are available?

Cold is produced by the relative absence of thermal energy. Because no devices can project a lack of energy, only superficial agents are available, such as ice packs.

7. What are five general indications for heat therapy? for cryotherapy?

Heat therapy
1. Analgesia
2. Muscle "spasm"
3. Hyperemia
4. Increasing collagen extensibility
5. Accelerating metabolic processes

Cryotherapy
1. Analgesia
2. Muscle "spasm"
3. Inflammation
4. Spasticity
5. Slowing metabolic activity

8. Name the contraindications to therapeutic heat.

Acute hemorrhage, inflammation, or trauma
Ischemia
Insensitivity

Malignancy
Inability to respond to pain
Atrophic or scarred skin
Bleeding dyscrasias

9. List four common superficial heating agents.

Hot packs, heat lamps, hot-water soaks, and paraffin baths.

10. Describe the use of hot packs.

Hot packs (such as Hydrocollator packs) consist of canvas bags filled with a silicon dioxide sand that can absorb many times its weight in water. The packs are hung on racks in water baths maintained at 70–80°C (168–175°F). During use, the packs are taken from the baths, excess water is drained off, and then they are wrapped in toweling or placed in an insulated cover. *Packs must be laid on, not under, the body* (see figure below). Packs can maintain therapeutically useful temperatures for 20–30 minutes.

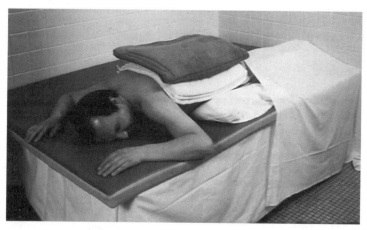

Hot pack treatment of the lower back. The pack is wrapped in an insulating cover and placed on, not under, the patient. (From Basford JR: Physical agents. In DeLisa JA, Gans BM (eds): Rehabilitation Medicine: Principles and Practice, 2nd ed. Philadelphia, J.B. Lippincott, 1993, pp 404–424, with permission.)

11. What should I know about heat lamps?

• While some heat lamps use special infrared (IR) heating elements, there is *no* proof that they are significantly more effective than other lamps. Ordinary incandescent light bulbs are much less expensive and release most of their energy as IR radiation. Thus, many clinics use these bulbs in their heat lamps.

- Most lamps act as "point sources," and their heating effectiveness decreases with the *square* of their distance from the body (the $1/r^2$ law).
- A reddish or brownish skin mottling (erythema ab igne) can result from heat use. The patient should be warned of this.
- In practice, most heat lamps in the home and clinic use 100–150 W incandescent light bulbs and are placed 50–75 cm from the body.

12. How are paraffin baths used?

Paraffin baths consist of 1:7 mixtures of mineral oil and paraffin maintained at about 52°C. Paraffin treatments commonly take one of three forms. **Dipping** is the most common method and involves placing the part to be treated (e.g., the hand) in the bath, removing it, pausing briefly to let the wax harden, and then repeating the cycle 10 times. The treated area is then covered with a plastic sheet and wrapped in an insulating material for about 20 minutes. **Immersion** provides a more vigorous heating than dipping and entails dipping the area into paraffin several times and then keeping it immersed for about 20 minutes. The third method uses a **brush** to paint paraffin onto portions of the body that cannot be easily placed in a bath.

Paraffin baths are widely used in patients with rheumatoid arthritis of the hands who find simpler treatments, such as hot soaks or contrast baths, ineffective. Paraffin baths also are used to treat contractures, particularly in the hands and in those with scleroderma. Paraffin baths are essentially filled with molten wax, so bath temperatures must be monitored carefully to avoid burns.

13. What are contrast baths and how are they used?

Contrast baths consist of two reservoirs filled with water, one warm (43°C) and one cool (16°C). Treatment typically begins with a 10-minute soak in the warm bath and then cycles between the warm and cool baths. Soaking durations vary but are often about 4 minutes in the warm bath and 1–2 minutes in the cool bath.

14. Why are contrast baths used?

Contrast baths are used primarily for their purported desensitization and vasogenic reflex effects. In practice, the hands and feet are the most common sites of treatment, usually in patients with rheumatoid arthritis and neuropathic or sympathetically mediated pain (reflex sympathetic dystrophy). Bath temperatures may be adjusted to the patient. In particular, the feet may be quite sensitive, and patients with sympathetically mediated pain may require less extreme initial temperatures.

15. Which superficial heating agent is the most beneficial?

No agent is clearly the most beneficial. In specific situations, there may be reasons to choose one agent over another, but the choice ultimately depends on patient and therapist preference.

16. When is cryotherapy appropriate? How is it performed?

Ice remains the mainstay of cryotherapy—ice packs, ice massage and ice slushes. Ice packs are probably the most common form of cryotherapy. Ice massage is frequently used for more intense treatment of localized areas of musculoskeletal pain, such as attachment syndromes (e.g., lateral epicondylitis). Ice slushes and whirlpools tend to be used mostly for motivated athletes who are willing to tolerate discomfort in the hopes of more rapid recovery. Chemical ice packs and vapo-coolant sprays have varying levels of use, the former for acute injuries and the latter in the "spray and stretch" treatment of trigger points. Ice use is enshrined in the RICE (rest, ice, compression, elevation) approach to the treatment of acute musculoskeletal injury, spasms, and chronic musculoskeletal pain.

17. What are some of the physiologic effects of cryotherapy?

Analgesia, vasoconstriction, and control of the swelling associated with acute injury come first to mind. In addition, spasticity can be reduced (if ice is applied sufficiently long to alter the muscle spindle), nerve conduction delayed, and metabolism slowed by cooling. Cryotherapy may produce longer-lasting effects than heat due to its vasoconstriction-related reductions in local blood flow.

18. Name the contraindications of cryotherapy.

Many of the contraindications for ice, like all physical agents, are relative. Thus, ice massage of a diabetic with neuropathy and atherosclerotic disease might be appropriate for trochanteric bursitis but not for a foot condition. The most common contraindications for ice include ischemia, Raynaud's syndrome, insensitivity, inability to respond to pain, cold allergy, and cold-induced pressor responses.

HYDROTHERAPY

19. What do I need to know about whirlpools?

Whirlpools use agitated water to produce convective heating or cooling, massage, and gentle debridement. Unit size, water temperature, agitation intensity, and solvent properties may all be adjusted to meet treatment goals. Water temperature is determined by the amount of the body submerged, the patient's health, and goals of treatment. A hand or limited portion of a limb with intact sensation may tolerate temperatures up to 45°C, but as more of the body is submerged, temperature should decrease—commonly to 40–41°C for immersion to the waist and 38–39°C if most of the body is submerged. Health is important, with an elderly diabetic patient being treated more cautiously than a young healthy athlete.

20. How are wounds treated with hydrotherapy?

Wounds treated with hydrotherapy typically have open areas with necrotic debris, adherent dressings, and/or contaminated or irregular surfaces. Wound sizes can range from small hand wounds to large, secondarily infected, healing abdominal wounds. Dehiscence is not a contraindication, and exposed omentum or intestinal tissues does not prevent treatment if bath temperature, osmolality, and agitation parameters are chosen carefully. Agitation is adjusted to match patient preferences and treatment goals. Patients with large wounds may be fearful that soaking the wound will be painful, but surprisingly, correctly adjusted baths are extraordinarily comfortable. Alternative hydrotherapy treatments are possible. When forceful debridement of large wounds is necessary, hand-held hoses and sprays may be used. Small wounds may be treated with commercial footbaths or handheld water jets, such as a WaterPik®.

21. How can solvent properties be manipulated? Why?

Warmed tap water (which is itself amazingly sterile) is usually used alone for hydrotherapy and debridement, but many solutes can be added. Gentle detergents and antiseptic solutions may be added in the hopes of improving debridement and wound cleansing. Salt can be dissolved in a bath to produce a normal saline (0.9% NaCl) solution to improve comfort and reduce concerns about hemolysis and water intoxication in patients with large wounds.

22. List five common indications for hydrotherapy.

1. Open, contaminated wounds
2. Contractures
3. Muscle spasm
4. Burns
5. Morbidly obese, immobilized patients who cannot be cleansed in another manner

ULTRASOUND

23. What is diathermy and what are the diathermy agents?

Diathermy means heating (*thermy*) through (*dia-*). Three diathermies have been used in the clinic: ultrasound, shortwave and microwave. All conversively heat tissue, sound being the energy source in the first case and electromagnetic energy in the latter. Microwave diathermy is now rarely used in therapy.

24. What are the important characteristics of ultrasound (US)?

US has all the characteristics of audible sound but is limited to frequencies above the nominal 20,000-Hz limit of human hearing. As such, US requires a medium for transmission and can be focused, reflected, or refracted. Although a wide range of frequencies are possible, the best trade-off between focusing properties and tissue penetration occurs at the 0.8–1.0-MHz frequencies found in most therapeutic US machines.

25. What effects does ultrasound have on the body?

Heating is the most important and best understood effect. **Nonthermal effects**, such as cavitation, media motion, and standing waves, also exist, but their therapeutic benefits are less understood. Cavitation, for example, produces bubbles which, by their forced oscillation and bursting, are capable of disrupting tissue. Small-scale media motion may occur from US exposure. Standing-wave patterns in a stationary US field produce fixed areas of elevated pressure and rarefaction that have been found in the laboratory to have physiologic effects.

26. How deep does ultrasound penetrate into tissue?

The depth of clinically beneficial heating depends on the power applied, nature of the tissue, direction of the beam, and frequency of US. For example, 50% of a US beam will penetrate 7–8 cm of fat but < 1 mm of bone. Direction is important in anisotropic tissue: a therapeutic US beam may penetrate 7 cm when travelling parallel to the fibers of a muscle, but only 2 cm when travelling perpendicularly. Frequency also has striking effects. Beam intensity in tissue may fall by about 85% as its frequency increases from 0.3 to 3.3 MHz. In practice, therapeutic US sources with frequencies of 0.8–1.0 MHz can produce 4–5°C temperature elevations at depths of 8 cm.

27. Where does the most intense heating take place during ultrasound treatment?

Ultrasound interacts with skin, fat, muscle, and bone during treatment. Heating occurs in all of these tissues due to beam attenuation but is most pronounced at tissue interfaces, where sound transmission discontinuities occur. **Bone–soft tissue interfaces** are where the most heating takes place. This tendency for bone–soft tissue heating provides support for the practice of avoiding US treatment in the vicinity of laminectomy sites.

28. How is ultrasound applied?

The skin is usually coated with mineral oil or an acoustic gel to provide optimal acoustic coupling. US is then applied by stroking the sound head (applicator) in circular motions. Irregular body surfaces are sometimes submerged in degassed water, and the slightly separated applicator is moved over the surface. US provides intense heating and requires the constant attention of the therapist. Treatments are relatively brief, 7–10 minutes.

29. What is phonophoresis?

In phonophoresis, medication is mixed with the acoustic coupling medium in the expectation that the US beam will "drive" the pharmacologically active substance into the tissue. Penetration depths depend on the particular substance involved, and significant amounts of drug are picked up by the subcutaneous circulation. Claims of penetration to depths of several centimeters have been made. Clinical studies with topical anesthetics, corticosteroids, phenylbutazone, and chymotrypsin have shown benefits, but more work is needed to establish the benefits of phonophoresis over injection or US alone.

30. What are some indications for therapeutic ultrasound?

COMMON	LESS ESTABLISHED
Contractures	Wound healing
Tendinitis	Herpes zoster
Musculoskeletal pain	Plantar warts
Degenerative arthritis	
Subacute trauma	

SHORTWAVE AND MICROWAVE

31. What is shortwave diathermy?

Shortwave diathermy (SWD) conversively heats tissue by exposing it to radio waves produced by a machine that is essentially a shortwave radio. Three frequencies—40.68, 27.12, and 13.56 MHz—have been allocated by the FCC for medical use in the United States, but 27.12 is the most commonly used. Typical treatments involve output powers of several hundred watts.

32. How is shortwave diathermy administered?

Energy is delivered to the body by either capacitive or inductive coupling. **Capacitive coupling** involves placing the portion of the body to be treated between two plates to which the shortwave output is applied (see figure below). The body thus acts as a dielectric (insulator) in a series circuit. Heating is most marked in high-impedance, water-poor tissues such as fat. **Inductive coupling**, on the other hand, uses the body as a receiver and induces eddy currents in the tissues in its field. The highest currents, and therefore the most intense heating, occur in low-impedance, water-rich tissues, such as muscle. In practice, temperature elevations of 4–6°C can occur at depths of 4–5 cm in muscles.

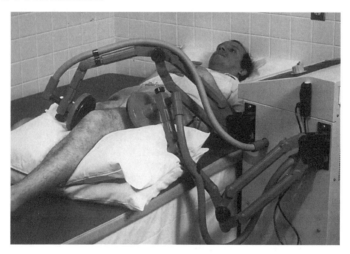

Capacitively coupled shortwave diathermy of the knee. The patient lies on an electrically nonconductive table. (From Basford FR: Physical agents. In DeLisa JA, Gans BM (eds): Rehabilitation Medicine: Principles and Practice, 2nd ed. Philadelphia, J.B. Lippincott, 1993, pp 404–424, with permission.)

33. Discuss the limitations and contraindications of shortwave diathermy.

Water and metal are excellent electrical conductors and potentially can cause burns if present in SWD fields. Therefore, jewelry is removed, and perspiration absorbed by toweling or pads. In theory, metal implants and sutures might produce "hot spots," so most people avoid SWD when these are present. General precautions, with varying degrees of theoretical or established concern, include the avoidance of treating pregnant women, the menstruating uterus, or patients with pacemakers, defibrillators, implantable pumps, or contact lenses.

34. What is microwave diathermy?

Microwave diathermy (MWD) is similar to shortwave diathermy in that electromagnetic waves are used to heat tissue. However, the FCC-approved frequencies for MWD are 915 and 2456 MHz, 30–100 times higher than those for SWD. MWD was relatively common in the past but is now rarely used, having been supplanted by US and SWD. However, it continues to have some medical use for localized hyperthermia.

35. What are the characteristics of microwave diathermy?

Microwave beams, due to their higher frequencies (short wavelengths), are much more directable than SWD fields. Because tissue penetration decreases as frequency increases, MWD tends to heat more superficially than SWD and often delivers a large proportion of its energy to subcutaneous tissue.

36. What are the contraindications to microwave diathermy?

The contraindications of heat and SWD apply. In addition, microwaves produce cataracts and selectively heat fluid-filled cavities. There are also some concerns about its effect on growing bones.

ELECTRICAL STIMULATION

37. What is TENS?

Transcutaneous electrical nerve stimulation (TENS) is a form of analgesia that uses superficial skin electrodes to apply small electrical signals to the body. Electrodes may be placed over peripheral nerves, nerve roots, and acupuncture points, as well as proximal to, distal to, over, and even contralateral to the areas of pain.

38. How does TENS produce analgesia?

A uniform mechanism is not well established. The "gate theory of pain," in which stimulation of large myelinated afferent fibers blocks the transmission of pain by small unmyelinated fibers at the level of the spinal cord, is often mentioned. While it seems plausible in many ways, this theory does not explain all aspects of TENS analgesia (e.g., prolonged pain relief following use, distal effects). Alteration of cerebrospinal endorphin concentrations is reported following TENS treatment (particularly for low-frequency TENS) but is difficult to correlate with therapeutic response.

39. Describe the characteristics of a TENS unit.

TENS units are usually programmable and small enough to fit in a pocket. Typically, they consist of a battery, one or more signal-generators, and two pairs of output electrodes. Although clear benefits of one waveform over another are difficult to establish, a wide variety of continuous and modulated (pulsed, burst, ramped, etc.) signals are available. In practice, signal amplitudes are usually < 100 mA, pulse rates < 200 HZ, and pulse widths < 300 μsec. Biphasic and asymmetric waveforms are usually chosen, as they seem to be the most comfortable and should limit any tendencies for a single polarity to produce electrolysis and skin irritation.

40. How many distinct TENS settings are possible?

In theory, an infinite number; in practice, two. "**High**" (or conventional) TENS uses barely perceptible signal intensities with frequencies typically of 60–80 Hz. "**Low**" TENS uses larger-amplitude, low-frequency signals (< 4–8 Hz) that may be uncomfortable.

41. When is TENS therapy prescribed?

TENS is not a curative modality and should be used only in the absence of more effective alternatives. A unit may cost the patient $90 a month to rent and $1000 to purchase, so the decision to prescribe one requires careful assessment. Frequently, several therapy sessions are needed to establish electrode placement, stimulator settings, and benefits. Ideally, the unit can be used at home for a day or so before a final judgment is made. If the condition being treated has been refractory to other treatment and TENS's benefits are significant, rental is reasonable. Purchase is not considered until several months of stable, consistent use with continued benefits have been documented.

42. Is TENS effective?

Systematic assessment of TENS's effectiveness is difficult due to the subjective nature of pain, varying study designs, diverse parameter choices (stimulation frequency, waveform, electrode placement, etc.), and the differing conditions evaluated. Studies in postsurgical, obstetric, and general musculoskeletal settings find benefits ranging from placebo levels (25–30%) to 95%. Other studies have reported elevated cutaneous perfusion and temperature in patients with neuropathy, accelerated wound healing and elevated pain thresholds following treatment. In the end, success is sporadic and seems to depend on the individual patient.

43. List seven common uses for TENS.
1. Diabetic neuropathic pain
2. Post-traumatic pain
3. Postsurgical pain
4. Peripheral nerve injury
5. Chronic musculoskeletal pain
6. Phantom limb pain
7. Sympathetically mediated pain (reflex sympathetic dystrophy, causalgia)

44. List six contraindications for TENS use.
1. Stimulation over the carotid sinuses
2. Cardiac pacemakers (controversial)
3. Pregnancy (although the risk from distal treatment seems small)
4. Inability to report effects or discomfort
5. Atrophic skin
6. Allergies to the electrodes or gels

45. What is iontophoresis?
Electric fields can accelerate the movement of charged atoms or molecules (ions) through the skin. Iontophoresis, operating on this principle, uses charged electrodes (positive or negative) to drive medically active, charged (polar) substances into the skin. Any charged or polar substance can theoretically be iontophoresed, and medications have included lidocaine, iodine, salicylate, gentamicin, cefoxin, and silver.

46. What is iontophoresis used for?
Iontophoresis is an effective treatment of hyperhidrosis of the hands, feet, and axilla. It has also been used to deliver antibiotics to poorly vascularized tissue such as cartilage, to produce local anesthesia, to speed wound healing, and to treat musculoskeletal pain. Although there is evidence that treatment can be effective, many feel that an injection can provide higher concentrations of an active medication with more speed and less difficulty.

47. What is low-intensity electrical stimulation?
TENS is one form of low-intensity electrical stimulation. In addition, a variety of milliampere and even microampere current generators have been studied for > 30 years. Although benefits are well established in the treatment of nonhealing fractures, their use for other indications such as wound healing remains mostly investigational.

48. Can electrical stimulation increase muscle strength?
Electrical stimulation can be used to maintain muscle bulk and strength, but there is little evidence that it can strengthen healthy active muscle more effectively than exercise alone. Applications of this technique are relatively limited: maintaining strength in immobilized limbs and training of paretic muscles following stroke or peripheral nerve or spinal injury.

49. What is functional neuromuscular stimulation?
Functional neuromuscular stimulation (FNS), also known as functional electrical stimulation (FES), utilizes electrical stimulation to provide functional use of paretic muscles. Stimulation may be done in conjunction with orthotics and may involve the complex programming and stimulation of many muscles. Theoretically, FNS might benefit any neuromuscularly impaired individual, but in practice, limitations imposed by its complexity, cost, reliability, electrode positioning, donning, and safety have restricted its use. Foot-drop orthoses and exercise and ambulation devices for spinal cord injury are the best known applications of this approach. With time,

FNS may supply simple and unobtrusive help for people with stroke and other neurologic deficits.

50. What is interferential current?

Electrical waves that differ slightly in frequency but are otherwise identical can interact with each other and produce product waveforms with frequencies equal to the sum or differences of the original waves. Interferential current machines take advantage of this fact to generate waves at different frequencies—e.g., 2,000 and 2,040 Hz—which can penetrate tissue without discomfort. Pairs of electrodes associated with each wave are placed so that the waves cross at the area to be treated. The waves *interfere* at this crossing point and produce a "difference" wave (here, 40 Hz—in the clinical situation, only the low-frequency "difference" waves are important) which can be used to produce TENS effects or stimulate muscle contraction.

PRESSURE

51. How are pneumatic pumps used?

Numerous pneumatic devices are available with varying cycling modes (e.g., fixed or associated with heart beat) and construction (e.g., single or multicompartment). These pumps are often effective in controlling edema but should be used only if elevation and compressive wraps alone are ineffective. Pressure settings depend on the device but are often set between the venous and arterial pressures. Treatment durations are prolonged, sometimes involving hours per day. Between treatments, the limb is kept elevated and wrapped in compressive dressings. There are also many reports that pneumatic pumping can improve arterial perfusion in the distal extremities, but their value and usage are still under investigation.

52. What do I need to know about using compressive garments?

Compressive garments are measured once limb edema has been minimized. Pressures are maximal at the wrist or ankle and lessen proximally in a graduated manner. Garments are specified by their maximal pressures (e.g., 20, 30, 40, and at times, ≥ 50 mmHg). Stocking pressures and style (e.g., calf-high, thigh-high, leotard) are dictated by edema severity and the patient's ability to doff and don the stocking. Most lower-extremity stockings are in the 30–40-mmHg range with allowances made for sensation, perfusion, and patient compliance.

53. List six common indications for compression garments.

1. Treated deep venous thrombosis
2. Venous incompetence
3. Postmastectomy edema
4. Edema due to congestive heart failure
5. Lymphedema
6. Orthostatic blood pressure resistant to medical treatment (garments must be thigh-length or leotard to be effective)

54. List four contraindications to pneumatic pumping.

Active deep venous thrombosis, cellulitis, severely compromised perfusion, or severely impaired sensation.

55. What are some simple rules of thumb about compressive garments?

- Use the shortest garment possible.
- Thigh-length garments slide down the leg without the use of straps or adhesive.
- Men tend to resist leotards.
- Garments are more effective with slender people.
- Heavy people are difficult to fit comfortably.
- Most patients can be fit with off-the-shelf garments.

TRACTION

56. What are the indications for traction?
The most widely accepted indication for traction is radicular pain. Many also consider traction useful for paraspinal muscle relaxation and for sources of pain in which a widening of the intervertebral spaces might be helpful.

57. What parameters should be specified for traction?
Position
    Body (sitting or supine)
    Spine (cervical spine in 20–30° flexion)
Technique (e.g., manual, weight, mechanical)
Force (usually > 12 kg)
Duration
Form (continuous or intermittent)
Adjunct modalities and exercise

58. List the contraindications for traction.
1. Ligamentous instability
2. Radiculopathy of unclear etiology
3. Acute injury
4. Rheumatoid arthritis
5. Metastatic bone disease
6. Vertebrobasilar atherosclerotic disease
7. Spinal infection (e.g., Pott's disease, disc space infection)
8. Patient misgivings
9. Increased pain through traction

LASERS

59. What is the role of laser therapy in physical medicine?
Low-intensity laser irradiation has been used for 30 years to promote wound healing and to lessen pain and speed recovery from musculoskeletal injury. Many devices have been used, but most have powers < 100 mW and utilize red (632.8 μm) or infrared (820–904 μm) wavelengths. Irradiation produces striking effects on cellular processes, immune function, and collagen formation in the laboratory. Unfortunately, translation of these findings into the clinic has been difficult. Despite widespread use in Europe and Asia, laser therapy has not yet gained FDA approval for clinical use in the United States.

BIBLIOGRAPHY

1. Ali J, Yaffe CS, Serratte C: The effect of transcutaneous electric nerve stimulation on postoperative pain and pulmonary function. Surgery 89:507–512, 1981.
2. Balmaseda MT, Fatehi MT, Koozekanani SH, Lee AL: Ultrasound therapy: A comparative study of different coupling media. Arch Phys Med Rehabil 67:149–152, 1986.
3. Basford JR: Low intensity laser therapy: Still not an established clinical tool. Lasers Surg Med 16:31–42, 1995.
4. Basford JR: Physical agents. In DeLisa JA, Gans BM (eds): Rehabilitation Medicine: Principles and Practice, 2nd ed. Philadelphia, J.B. Lippincott, 1993, pp 404–424.
5. Chantraine A, Ludy JP, Berger D: Is cortisone iontophoresis possible? Arch Phys Med Rehabil 67:38–40, 1986.
6. Downing DS, Weinstein A: Ultrasound therapy of subcranial bursitis: A double blind trial. Phys Ther 66:194–199, 1986.
7. Ebersold MJ, Laws ER, Stonnington HH, Stillwell GK: Transcutaneous electrical stimulation for treatment of chronic pain: A preliminary report. Surg Neurol 4:96–99, 1975.
8. Franchimont P, Juchmes I, Lecomite J: Hydrotherapy—Mechanisms and indications. Pharmacol Ther 20:79–93, 1983.
9. Hunt JW: Applications of microwave, ultrasound, and radiofrequency heating. Natl Cancer Inst Monogr 61:447–456, 1982.
10. Knight KL: Cryotherapy: Theory, Technique and Physiology. Chattanooga, TN, Chattanooga Corp., 1985.

11. Lehman JF, de Lateur BJ: Diathermy and superficial heat, laser and cold therapy. In Krusen's Handbook of Physical Medicine and Rehabilitation, 4th ed. Philadelphia, W.B. Saunders, 1990, pp 283–367.
12. Lundeberg T: The pain suppressive effect of vibratory stimulation and transcutaneous electrical nerve stimulation (TENS) as compared to aspirin. Brain Res 294:201–209, 1984.
13. Matsen FA, Questad K, Matsen AL: The effect of local cooling on postfracture swelling: A controlled study. Clin Orthop 109:201–206, 1975.
14. Melzack R, Jeans ME, Stratford JG, Monks RC: Ice massage and transcutaneous electrical stimulation: Comparison of treatment for low back pain. Pain 9:209–217, 1980.

98. TRACTION, MANIPULATION, AND MASSAGE (The Rack, the Crack, and the Smack)

Steven R. Hinderer, M.D., M.S., P.T., and Steve R. Geiringer, M.D.

1. What physiologic effect(s) does traction have?

Most studies have concluded that elongation of the cervical spine, of 2–20 mm, can be achieved with 25 lbs or more of tractive force. Ten pounds is needed to counterbalance the weight of the head (less in some persons, more in others). It is proposed that prolonged pull on the cervical spine with adequate force leads to fatigue of cervical paraspinal muscles, which is potentially of therapeutic value when muscle spasm is present.

It has been less consistently demonstrated that traction on the lumbar spine also causes elongation when the effects of friction are overcome by adequate pull or a split table. Retraction of herniated disc material is another potential effect of lumbar traction.

2. What techniques are available for applying traction? Or, for the more sadistic readers, how many ways can you hang someone? There are five.

Manual—cervical traction performed by the physician or therapist, usually to gauge the effectiveness of mechanical or motorized methods of application

Mechanical—administered using a pulley and free weight system

Motorized—mechanical traction applied by a motorized system, administered in continuous or intermittent periods

Gravity—hanging upside down

Autotraction—uses a specially designed device that self-administers lumbar traction by pulling with the arms

3. Describe the two modes of mechanical traction.

Mechanical traction can be administered at home using a pulley and free weight system. Home cervical traction units typically consist of a bag filled with 20 lbs or more of water or sand and a pulley system mounted on top of a door. Improper head or neck position, along with inadequate weight (< 20 lbs) are the most common reasons home cervical traction fails. Initial instruction and weekly follow-up by the therapist or physician greatly improve the chances for success.

Administration of continuous or intermittent (timed on and off periods) mechanical traction applied with a motorized device is commonly limited to physical therapy clinical settings, due to the need for close monitoring of position and its effect on symptoms. Most patients tolerate greater forces of pull with intermittent administration. It is common to prescribe mechanical traction initially in the treatment course, and, if benefit ensues, to continue treatment with a home unit.

4. For which patients is gravity traction recommended?

Gravity (inversion) traction was marketed extensively a few years ago. Its theoretical basis is that body weight, when inverted (by hanging upside down), will distract the lumbar spine.

Numerous side effects have been reported, including persistent headaches, blurred vision, petechiae, and numerous musculoskeletal complaints. Along with the potential implications of contraindications associated with these symptoms, one should probably reserve this method for use only with nonhuman primates having back pain.

5. What parameters need to be specified in a prescription of traction?

Positioning

Intermittent or continuous administration

Amount of pull

Duration

Other modalities to be used concurrent to traction also should be specified and may include methods to facilitate muscle relaxation, which is essential to maximize the therapeutic effects from traction. Hotpacks are most commonly prescribed.

6. Discuss positioning.

Positioning is a key element of a traction prescription. For **cervical traction**, specification of sitting or supine should be based on patient comfort in different positions. If cervical traction is being administered to relieve symptoms of nerve root compression, 20–30° of flexion will optimally open the intervertebral foramina. Less flexion is required for treatment of muscle spasm in the absence of radicular symptoms.

The supine position with 90° of hip and knee flexion is the most common position for **lumbar traction** so that the lumbar lordosis is maximally reduced with the low back well supported on the traction table and the spine in a relatively flexed position to facilitate optimal vertebral separation.

7. When is intermittent traction prescribed? When continuous?

It is thought that a greater force of pull can be tolerated with intermittent as opposed to continuous administration. Selection is based on the desired therapeutic effect. If distraction of the spine is desired to open neural foramina or retract herniated disc material, then the greater forces of pull that can be tolerated by intermittent application are more desirable. If the goal is muscle relaxation, then it may be more beneficial to provide the prolonged stretch of continuous traction.

8. How much pull is usually used and for how long?

The amount of pull should be specified in the traction prescription. For cervical spine distraction, forces > 25 lbs need to be achieved, but forces > 50 lbs probably do not provide any additional advantage. Forces above 50 lbs are required with lumbar traction to achieve posterior vertebral separation, and forces > 100 lbs are required for anterior separation. The countertraction on the chest and shoulders to provide tractive forces over 100 lbs is often poorly tolerated by patients.

The duration of treatment sessions is usually specified as 20 minutes. Studies seem to support that therapeutic effects are achieved over this time period.

9. What are the contraindications to prescribing or administering traction?

The potential for cervical ligamentous instability, as might occur with rheumatoid arthritis, achondroplastic dwarfism, Marfan syndrome, or previous trauma, are *absolute* contraindications. Cervical extension during traction should be avoided, especially in the presence of vertebrobasilar insufficiency. Documented or suspected tumor in the region of the sine, osteopenia, infectious process of the spine or surrounding soft tissue, and pregnancy are *absolute* contraindications. Old age is a *relative* contraindication due to degenerative spine changes.

10. What is manipulation?

A dictionary definition is "to control or change, especially by artful or unfair means to achieve a desired end." While this definition has nothing to do with PM&R, it is certainly something we all have or will experience in our professional careers. More appropriately, spinal manipulation is an application of forces to the muscles, tendons, ligaments, joints and capsules, bones, and cartilage of the vertebral column, which has as a major goal the restoration of normal spinal motion and the elimination of pain secondary to disturbed biomechanics.

11. Isn't manipulation dangerous?

There are few risks with the application of spinal manipulation. No complications have been reported in the literature regarding isometric or articulatory treatment techniques. The most severe complications following manipulation were associated with cervical thrust techniques, in which the neck was extended during the procedure resulting in vascular compromise of the vertebrobasilar system or spinal cord. These complications are quite rare, given the frequency with which thrust manipulation procedures are performed.

12. When would you choose to implement manipulation in a patient's treatment program?

Spinal manipulative therapy is potentially useful in all biomechanical pain problems of the pelvis, back, and neck, e.g., pelvic asymmetries and vertebral rotations.

13. What skills does a physiatrist need to perform manipulation therapy?

By the dictionary definition of manipulation, it depends on how artful or unfair your adversary is. For spinal manipulation, though, the physiatrist must have at least palpatory diagnostic skills, which generally requires participation in a several-day CME course. Palpatory skills enable the physician to write a prescription for the specific body part with biomechanical dysfunction to be treated, the motion(s) to be restored, the technique(s) of treatment to be used, and the frequency and duration of treatment. Referral is usually made to a physical therapist with specific training in manipulation skills. With basic palpatory skills, the physician can then monitor progress of therapy and determine an appropriate endpoint.

Acquisition of competent treatment skills for manipulation requires several months of training and sufficient time in one's practice to provide therapy to patients, which is usually beyond the practical limits of available time for most physiatrists.

14. When is manipulation contraindicated?

Articulation techniques (mobilization or low-velocity/high-amplitude):

Vertebral malignancy	Multiple adjacent radiculopathies
Infection of inflammation	Vertebral bone diseases
Cauda equina syndrome	Vertebral bony joint instability
Myelopathy or spondylosis	(fractures, dislocations)
	Rheumatoid disease in the cervical region

Thrust techniques (high-velocity/low-amplitude, adjustment, impulse). The above contraindications as well as the following:

Spinal deformity or anomalies	Spondyloarthropathies
Systemic anticoagulation	Inactive rheumatoid disease
(disease-related or	Ligamentous joint instability
pharmacologic)	Congenital laxity syndromes
Severe diabetes	(Marfan's or Ehlers-Danlos)
Atherosclerosis	Aseptic necrosis
Severe degenerative joint disease	Local aneurysm
Vertigo or symptoms of	Osteomalacia
vertebrobasilar disease	Osteoporosis

Isometric techniques (e.g., muscle energy): None

15. When is a massage medium required?

A massage medium is used to reduce friction over the skin. Examples include mineral oil, glycerin, coconut oil, cocoa butter, Nivea cream, and baby powder. Such media are used when the massage is intended for edema reduction, relaxation/sedation, or relief of muscle spasm/tightness. When the massage is used to loosen or stretch scar tissue, fascia, or subcutaneous tissue, no medium is used, allowing the therapist to gain purchase on and move appropriate tissue structures.

16. What are the physical parameters of massage that can be altered depending on the desired therapeutic effect?

Components of Massage

THERAPEUTIC INTENT	RATE AND RHYTHM	PRESSURE	DIRECTION	DURATION
General relaxation/ sedative effect	Slow speed, even rhythm	Light to medium	Trunk: follow direction of muscle fibers Extremities: cen-tripetal	Depends on size of area to be treated; full back massage, 10 min minimum
Decrease muscle spasm/tightness	Slow speed, even rhythm	Begin light, move to deeper movements, end light	Parallel to direction of muscle fibers Deep circulation over trigger points	Depends on size of area to be treated, e.g., low back or neck and upper back, 10 min
Reduce edema	Slow speed, even rhythm	Moderate to deep	Centripetal; treat proximal seg-ment first	Depends on size of area
Loosen/stretch fascia	Slow to mod-erate speed, even rhythm	Moderate	All directions	Depends on size of area
Prevent or break up adhesions in liga-ments, tendons, and muscles	Moderate speed, even rhythm	Heavy	Perpendicular to direction of fibers	15 min/involved structure
Stretch scar of skin and subcu-taneous tissue	Moderate speed, even rhythm	Moderate to heavy	Circular and all directions	5 min minimum

From Geiringer et al: Traction, manipulation, and massage. In DeLisa JA, Gans B (eds): Rehabilitation Medicine: Principles and Practice, 2nd ed. Philadelphia, J.B. Lippincott, 1993.

17. What are commonly used techniques of therapeutic massage?

Classical massage involves stroking and gliding movements (**effleurage**), kneading (**petrissage**), and percussion (**tapotement**). Stroking, gliding, and friction movements are helpful for locating areas of muscle spasm or focal pain. Stroking can help produce muscle relaxation in locations where spasm exists. Kneading techniques are performed on muscle and subcutaneous tissue for the purposes of muscle relaxation, improving circulation, and reducing edema. Percussion is primarily used for chest therapy in conjunction with postural drainage. It is also sometimes used on the temporal regions of unwitting residents to facilitate clearer thought processes.

Deep **friction massage** is used to prevent adhesions in acute muscle injuries and to break up adhesions in subacute and chronic injuries. Deep friction is applied transverse across the muscle fiber, tendon, or ligament.

Soft-tissue mobilization is a forceful massage of the muscle-fascial system element and differs from most massage in that it is done with fascia and muscle in a stretched position rather than relaxed or shortened. It is particularly effective as an adjunct to passive stretching for reduction of contractures.

Myofascial release has been defined as "a hands-on technique that applies prolonged light pressure in specific directions into the fascia system." It is applied in conjunction with passive ROM with the purpose of stretching focal areas of muscle/fascial tightness.

Accupressure is the application of sustained deep pressure over trigger points, as defined by Travell. Accupressure is often done in conjunction with application of other therapeutic modalities to the trigger points (e.g., ice, ultrasound, electrical stimulation).

18. Are there any contraindications to massage?

Yes, there can be potential harm from massage. It is contraindicated over malignancies, open wounds, thrombophlebitis, and infected tissues. Peripheral nerve compression from hematoma formation has been reported when accupressure was applied too vigorously.

BIBLIOGRAPHY

1. Bourdillon JF: Spinal Manipulation, 3rd ed. New York, Appleton-Century-Crofts, 1983.
2. Bridger RS, Ossey S, Gourie G: Effect of lumbar traction on stature. Spine 14:82–90, 1989.
3. Cyriax JH: Textbook of Orthopaedic Medicine: Treatment by Manipulation, Massage and Injection, 10th ed. London, Bailliere-Tindall, 1982.
4. Geiringer SR, Kincaid CB, Rechtien JR: Traction, manipulation, and massage. In DeLisa JA, Gans BM (eds): Rehabilitation Medicine: Principles and Practice, 2nd ed. Philadelphia, J.B. Lippincott, 1993.
5. Gianakopoulos G, Waylonis GW, Grant PA, et al: Inversion devices: Their role in producing lumbar distraction. Arch Phys Med Rehabil 66:100–102, 1985.
6. Greenman PE: Principles of Manual Medicine. Baltimore, Williams & Wilkins, 1989.
7. Onel D, Tukzlaci M, Sari H, Demir K: Computed tomographic investigation of the effect of traction on lumbar disc herniations. Spine 14:82–90, 1989.
8. Sherman DG, Hart RG, Easton JD: Abrupt change in head position and cerebral infarction. Stroke 12:2–6, 1981.
9. Travell J: Myofascial Pain and Dysfunction. Baltimore, Williams & Wilkins, 1983.
10. Twomey LT: Sustained lumbar traction: An experimental study of long spine segments. Spine 10:146–149, 1985.

99. FUNCTIONAL ELECTRICAL STIMULATION

Peter H. *Gorman,* M.D., M.S.

1. What is functional electrical stimulation (FES)?

FES is the technique of applying safe levels of electric current to activate the damaged or disabled nervous system. FES is sometimes referred to as functional neuromuscular stimulation or neuromuscular electrical stimulation. Neuromuscular electrical stimulation, depending on one's perspective, can be considered a more general or more specific term, since it includes use for both therapeutic and functional purposes but excludes use in sensory systems, such as cochlear prostheses.

2. Is FES a new technique?

Yes and no. While modern FES is a relatively recent technology, the use of electricity for medicinal purposes dates back to the beginning of the Christian era. Electrical discharges of the torpedo fish were used for treatment of headache and gout in the year 46 AD. With the advent of electrical generators and storage devices (i.e., capacitors) in the 18th century, practitioners reported on the involuntary contraction of muscle and touted the use of electrical charges to cure paralytic disease.

3. Describe the mechanism of electrical excitation of neural tissue.

Both nerve and muscle cells have excitable membranes with internal negative resting potentials. When an external electric field is applied to a nerve via two electrodes (at least two electrodes are always needed to complete an electrical circuit), depolarization of the axon below the cathode, or negative electrode, occurs. As the potential decreases under the cathode, the membrane becomes more permeable to Na^+ ions, which in turn causes further depolarization of the nerve. This "voltage-gated channel" for Na^+ ions is responsible for the generation of the all-or-none action potential if the electrical stimulation is sufficient to reach a threshold value. A separate voltage-gated K^+ channel is responsible for subsequent repolarization of the nerve.

4. What does Ohm's law have to do with clinical use of FES?

For a given voltage, current is inversely proportional to the resistance of the medium through which the current is flowing (i.e., voltage = current $\times$ resistance, or $V = IR$). Since larger diameter axons have lower resistance, more current flows through them, and they therefore are preferentially activated by externally applied electrical stimuli. In addition, Ohm's law is important in understanding electrode properties. Electrodes with high impedance (resistance) require greater applied voltages to achieve the same current levels.

5. Do FES systems for muscle activation stimulate nerve or muscle?

Motor units are activated electrically by depolarization of motor axons or their terminal nerve branches at the neuromuscular junction. A muscle can be directly depolarized by electrical current, but the amount of current necessary for this to occur is considerably greater than that for the nerve. Therefore for practical purposes, FES systems stimulate nerves, not muscles.

6. What happens to FES-stimulated muscles over time?

Just like muscles undergoing voluntary exercise, FES-stimulated muscles change morphologically and physiologically. Type II glycolytic fibers convert to type I oxidative fibers over weeks to months, depending on the intensity and frequency of stimulation. This phenomenon is associated with changes in vascular supply and increases the fatigue resistance of the muscle. One question that remains incompletely answered is how much FES exercise is adequate to achieve fiber conversion and allow for functional use. This is important clinically as one sets up exercise protocols.

7. What are the clinical applications of FES in physical therapy practice?

1. Muscle strengthening
2. Improvement in ROM
3. Facilitation and re-education of voluntary motor function
4. Orthotic training, functional movement
5. Inhibition of spasticity or muscle spasm

8. What parameters are set by the rehabilitationist when using FES?

1. **Pulse amplitude** (in milliamps) and **duration** (in microseconds) determine the size of individual pulses provided. As either is increased above threshold, spatial recruitment of additional motor units occurs, thereby increasing muscle force output.

2. **Pulse frequency** determines the rate at which the muscle will fire. For most applications, it is desirable to have a fused or tetanic contraction of muscle, which generally occurs at 20–30 Hz (cycles per second).

3. **Waveforms** available for use in FES include monophasic, asymmetric biphasic, or symmetric biphasic. Monophasic stimulation is generally not appropriate for long-term FES.

4. The **duty cycle** (on/off time) is the percentage of time that the stimulator is on. The greater the duty cycle, the more profound the problem with muscle fatigue, since the time of rest is reduced.

9. What are the contraindications to FES?

While there are no **absolute** contraindications for use of FES, patients with a cardiac demand pacemaker should be approached with extreme caution. Electrical stimulation applied anywhere on the body has the potential to interfere with the sensing portion of the demand pacemaker. **Relative** contraindications include patients with cardiac arrhythmias, congestive heart failure, pregnancy, electrode sensitivity, or healing wounds (muscle stimulation may adversely move healing tissues).

10. What conditions may benefit from FES technology?
Paralysis, spasticity, and cardiovascular deconditioning
Neurogenic bowel, bladder, and sexual dysfunction resulting from spinal cord injury, stroke, multiple sclerosis, or closed head injury
Epilepsy, scoliosis, tremor, restoration of hearing, and restoration of vision
Pain control (TENS), iontophoresis, and wound healing

11. What are the uses of FES in spinal cord injury?
Therapeutic uses: Muscle strengthening and cardiac conditioning. Possible other benefits include improvement in venous return from the legs, reduction of osteoporosis, improvement in bowel function, and psychological benefits.

Functional uses: Standing, walking, hand grasp (and release), bladder, bowel and sexual function, respiratory assist, and electroejaculation for fertility.

12. Explain the rationale behind use of FES-induced exercise in patients with spinal cord injury (SCI).
Persons with SCI are generally forced to become more sedentary. Paralysis is compounded by impaired autonomic nervous system function, which limits the cardiovascular response to exercise, especially in individuals with lesions above T5. Muscle bulk, strength, and endurance all decrease after SCI, and muscle fibers convert primarily to anaerobic metabolism after injury. Paralysis of intracostal musculature reduces vital capacity. In addition, there is reduced peripheral circulation, lean body mass, and bone density and an altered endocrine response.

13. What types of systems are available for therapeutic electrical stimulation in persons with SCI?
The most common system for lower-extremity FES exercise is the **bicycle ergometer**. This computer controlled FES exercise ergometer uses six channels and surface electrodes to sequentially stimulate quadriceps, hamstring, and glutei bilaterally. Some systems also include the capacity for simultaneous voluntary arm-crank exercise by paraplegics, permitting **hybrid exercise**.

14. What benefits can be anticipated in subjects involved in FES bicycle ergometry?
Cardiac capacity and muscle oxidative capacity both improve with FES ergometry. Some subjects can train with FES ergometry up to a similar aerobic metabolic rate (measured by peak VO_2) as achieved in the able-bodied population. Electrical exercise also increases peripheral venous return and fibrinolysis, and in one study, FES in conjunction with heparin therapy was more effective in preventing deep venous thrombosis than heparin alone. There are limits to the cardiovascular benefits of FES ergometry, however, especially in those with lesions at or above T5. In those patients, there is loss of supraspinal sympathetic control, which in turn limits the body's ability to increase heart rate, stroke volume and cardiac output.

15. What about FES for standing and walking in paraplegia?
There are at least 17 laboratories worldwide investigating the use of FES for lower-extremity standing and walking in paraplegia, using several different approaches. Hybrid approaches, such as the **reciprocating gait orthosis** (RGO), use both mechanical bracing and surface FES. Specifically, FES hip extension on one side provides contralateral leg swing through the RGO mechanism. Quadriceps stimulation then provides knee lock.

Only one surface FES walking system is FDA-approved for use in the U.S. The **Parastep System** (Sigmetics, Inc.) uses the triple flexion response elicited by peroneal nerve stimulation as well as knee and hip extensor surface stimulation to construct the gait cycle. The patient controls the gait with switches integrated into a rolling walker (which is also needed for stability and safety).

Implantable lower-extremity FES has also been developed to aid in activating deep musculature. Both percutaneous electrodes and implantable stimulator-receivers with epimysial or intramuscular electrodes have been tested, although neither is currently available commercially. Major problems with maintenance of the many percutaneous electrodes (48 electrodes in one system) needed to stimulate reciprocal gait have made this system impractical for widespread use.

16. What about FES for restoration of hand grasp in tetraplegia?

Tetraplegic hand grasp systems have focused on the C5 and C6 level SCI populations. Patients with C4 level injury, and therefore no biceps or deltoid strength, have participated in limited laboratory investigations of FES systems. Patients injured at the C7 and lower levels have multiple voluntary active forearm muscles (e.g., brachioradialis, extensor carpi radialis longus and brevis, pronator teres) which can be used to motor new functions without sacrificing current function by means of tendon transfer surgery.

Physiologically, patients considered for implantable hand grasp systems need to have adequate motor innervation of forearm and hand muscles to allow for FES grasp synthesis. Best results occur with motivated people who have good social support systems to reinforce use.

17. What are the components of the implantable FES hand grasp system? How does it work?

The Neuroprosthetic Hand Grasp System, also known as the Freehand System, initially developed at Case Western Reserve University, consists of (1) an external joint position transducer/controller, (2) a rechargeable programmable external control unit (ECU), and (3) an implantable 8-channel stimulator/receiver attached via flexible wires to epimysial disc electrodes. The user controls the system through small movements of either the shoulder or wrist. The joint position transducer, which operates somewhat like a computer joystick, is typically mounted on the skin from sternum to contralateral shoulder or across the ipsilateral wrist, and senses these movements. The ECU uses this signal to proportionally control hand grasp and release. Communication between the ECU and the implantable stimulator, which is located in a surgical pocket created in the upper chest, is through a radio frequency coupling. The system can be programmed through a personal computer interface by a trained therapist to individualize the grasps as well as the shoulder control for each patient.

Future improvements in quadriplegic hand grasp systems will likely include implantable controllers, closed loop feedback, proximal muscle control (i.e., triceps and/or biceps) in C4 and C5 subjects, and bilateral implementation of grasp in C6 level tetraplegics.

18. Are bladder stimulation systems effective in spinal cord injury?

Electrical stimulation to control bladder function after suprasacral SCI has been under investigation for several decades. In Great Britain, Brindley et al. have had the most experience and success with S2–4 anterior sacral nerve root stimulation in combination with posterior rhizotomy. This system is surgically implanted through lumbar laminectomy and employs either epidural or intradural electrodes. Pulsed stimulation is used to take advantage of the differences between activation of the slow response smooth musculature of the detrusor and activation of the fast-twitch striated sphincter musculature. This produces short spurts of urination but can result in nearly complete bladder emptying. The sacral anterior root stimulators also improve bowel care (i.e., increased defecation, reduced constipation), and approximately 60% of men can also produce penile erection with the device.

19. Are electroejaculation programs an accepted treatment for infertility?

Yes, at several specialized centers around the country. Originally developed within veterinary medicine, electroejaculation provides a mechanism by which men with SCI can father children. Electrically stimulated rectal probes are used to produce seminal emission. After serial electroejaculation procedures, the quality of the semen produced (as measured by sperm count, motility, and morphology) generally improves to the point where artificial insemination or in vitro fertilization is possible. Because of the great deal of coordination required to achieve successful pregnancies with this technique, multidisciplinary expertise is required for establishment of a fertility center for these couples.

20. Describe the role of FES in respiratory assistance.
   In a high-level quadriplegic, usually injured at C1 or C2, the use of the phrenic pacemaker has become a standard part of the clinical armamentarium and an alternative to chronic ventilator dependence. Those with lower injuries (i.e., C3 and C4) may have phrenic nerve denervation precluding the use of phrenic pacing. In these patients, intracostal muscle stimulation has been tried with limited success.

21. What about stroke?
   The development of FES applications in stroke has been less dramatic than that seen in SCI, although some of the original FES-assisted gait studies were done in hemiplegia. In one major rehabilitation center in Slovenia today, greater than half of all patients are treated with some form of FES during their stroke rehabilitation course. In the U.S., the use of FES in stroke is certainly not as prominent. A recent study has indicated that FES can be used to reduce shoulder subluxation and arm functional recovery in hemiplegia.

22. Is there a role for FES in multiple sclerosis or cerebral palsy?
   Electrical stimulation, especially spinal cord (dorsal column) stimulation for spasticity management and for pain management, has been tried in patients with **multiple sclerosis.** The Therapeutic Claims Committee of the International Foundation of Multiple Sclerosis Societies has stated that there is no clear indication for the use of FES in patients with MS.
   In modern practice, children with **cerebral palsy** are treated with surface electrical stimulation for improvement in ROM and facilitation or reduction of spasticity just like any other clinical diagnostic group referred to the physical therapy clinic. Implanted cerebellar stimulation, once popular in some circles, is no longer done.

BIBLIOGRAPHY

1. Baker LL, McNeal DR, Benton LA, et al: Neuromuscular Electrical Stimulation: A Practical Guide, 3rd ed. Downey, CA, Rancho Los Amigos Medical Center, 1993.
2. Brindley GS, Rushton DN: Long-term follow-up of patients with sacral anterior root stimulator implants. Paraplegia 28:469–475, 1990.
3. Faghri PD, Rodgers MM, Glaser RM, et al: The effects of functional electrical stimulation on shoulder subluxation, arm function recovery, and shoulder pain in hemiplegic stroke patients. Arch Phys Med Rehabil 75:73–79, 1994.
4. Glaser RM: Physiology of functional electrical stimulation-induced exercise: Basic science perspective. J Neurol Rehabil 5:49–61, 1991.
5. Glenn WWL, Brouillette RT, Dentz B, et al: Fundamental considerations in pacing of the diaphragm for chronic ventilatory insufficiency: A multi-center study. Pacing Clin Electrophysiol 11:2121–2127, 1988.
6. Keith MW, Lacey SH: Surgical rehabilitation of the tetraplegic upper extremity. J Neurol Rehabil 5:75–87, 1991.
7. Nathan RH, Ohry A: Upper limb functions regained in quadriplegia: A hybrid computerized neuromuscular stimulation system. Arch Phys Med Rehabil 71:415–421, 1990.
8. Peckham PH, Creasey GH: Neural prostheses: Clinical applications of functional electrical stimulation in spinal cord injury. Paraplegia 30:96–101, 1992.
9. Ragnarsson KT, Pollack SF, Twist D: Lower limb endurance exercise after spinal cord injury: Implications for health and functional ambulation. J Neurol Rehabil 5:37–48, 1991.
10. Yarkony GM, et al: Neuromuscular stimulation in spinal cord injury: I. Restoration of functional movement of the extremities. Arch Phys Med Rehabil 73:78–86, 1992.

Additional Resource: Additional information about many of the emerging technologies within the FES field can be obtained from: FES Information Center, 11000 Cedar Avenue, Cleveland, Ohio 44106-3052. Telephone: (800) 666-2352 or (216) 231-3257.

100. TRANSCUTANEOUS ELECTRICAL NERVE STIMULATION (TENS)

Norman Shealy, M.D., Ph.D., Saul Liss, Ph.D., Stanley H. Kornhauser, Ph.D., and Charles Cannizzaro, M.D., P.T.

1. What is TENS?

TENS is a form of electrical analgesia whose mechanism of action is based partially on the gate theory of pain popularized by Melzack and Wall in 1965. That theory explains TENS analgesia as resulting from a blocking mechanism via non-nociceptive receptors carrying the TENS signal on faster-conducting, myelinated fibers, inhibiting the nociceptive stimuli caused by smaller, myelinated, slower A-delta and small, unmyelinated C-fibers in subthalamic nuclei. It is also postulated that TENS effects are partially secondary to release of endogenous opiates (neuropeptides), possibly endorphins in higher CNS centers and enkephalins in the dorsal horns of the spinal cord.

TENS is a single therapeutic modality and is best utilized as part of a comprehensive individualized rehab program.

2. Is there an optimal waveform employed in the use of TENS for pain management?

Some studies claim that there is a stronger endorphin release at low-frequency (< 10Hz), high-amplitude stimulation than with higher-frequency (60–100 Hz), lower-intensity stimulation ("conventional" TENS), but experimental findings are mixed.

3. What other effects besides analgesia have been noted with the use of TENS?

Although these effects are controversial and results remain poorly confirmed, some authors report TENS affecting vasodilatation in subjects with chronic skin ulcers, diabetes neuropathy, and Raynaud's phenomena. Low-frequency TENS has been reported to raise pain thresholds, but pain thresholds are not altered or increased according to other authors. The relative effects of low- and high-frequency TENS are not well understood and may be related to the intensity of the stimulation.

4. What applications are commonly used for TENS in pain management?

TENS is appropriate in the treatment of both acute and chronic pain, with varying success ranging from placebo rates of approximately 30% to 80–95%. The reasons for the difference in outcomes may be multifactorial, depending on differences in stimulating parameters, electrode placement, type and duration of pain, concurrent medication, previous treatment, choice of controls, length of follow-up, and patient expectations.

Applications of TENS

Migraine headache treatment	Neck pain
Migraine headache prophylaxis	Shoulder pain
Tension headache	Elbow pain
Sinus headache	Back pain
Tic doloreux	Leg pain (diabetic neuropathy)
Temporomandibular joint pain	Pain associated with multiple sclerosis
Postherpetic facial neuralgia	Carpal tunnel syndrome pain
Relaxation (stress reduction)	Postoperative pain
Reflex sympathetic dystrophy	Arthritic pain
Spasticity reduction	Phantom limb pain
Depression symptom reduction	Finger pain
Drug detoxification	Shingles pain (intercostal)
Anxiety symptom reduction	Decubitus ulcer
Insomnia symptom reduction	Gastroenterologic pain

5. Is there an optimal placement of TENS electrodes on the skin?

Stimulation parameters and patterns of electrode placement remain more an art than a science. Generally, a painful area is "sandwiched" between a pair or pairs of electrodes. (Most TENS units have dual-channel capability with independent stimulation parameter settings for each pair of electrodes.) However, electrodes can be placed paravertebrally or proximal and distal to a nerve feeding a site of pain. Some applications are placed over acupuncture sites on the body or auricular points via small clip electrodes as a form of electroacupuncture.

6. Does one know immediately whether a TENS placement provides adequate analgesia?

A single session usually will not indicate the success or failure of a TENS application. The patient usually requires at least an overnight trial or even several days to establish efficacy. A reasonable period of evaluation (1 week) also allows elimination of placebo effect as well as optimization of stimulation parameters, such as pulse width, duration, and intensity.

Too often, TENS may be considered a failure, not for lack of physiologic effect, but for lack of adequate patient instruction, less-than-optimal electrode placement montage or stimulation parameter setting, or failure of the clinician to get a detailed description from the subject on what effect was derived and the patient's opinion as to the success of the trial.

7. Is TENS used continuously for pain management when it has been determined to be beneficial in a subject?

No optimal utilization time of TENS has been determined. Usage is individualized and usually is determined with an adequate trial-and-error period.

High-frequency TENS ("conventional" TENS, 60–100 Hz) is applied at barely perceptible levels to two to three times the sensory threshold and can usually be tolerated for many hours daily. Low-frequency TENS (~0.5–10 Hz) usually involves stronger intensities at three to five times the sensory threshold and is comfortably tolerated for 20–30 minute periods for several short sessions daily. An often-used approach is to initiate TENS therapy at high-frequency levels and then switch to low-frequency only if the higher frequency is not effective. Most patients find the low-frequency uncomfortable at the higher intensity and additionally complain of the annoying perception of "beating."

8. What is the key to successful use of TENS?

Reported success rates vary from placebo levels at ~30% to as high as 80–95%. Studies often are not comparative due to many variables. If TENS is to be successful, it directly reflects the patience, time, and anatomical knowledge of the therapist. TENS should never be employed solely in the treatment of low back pain. The Quebec Task Force concluded that decreased pain relief has been demonstrated, but the sole use of TENS has not been shown to accelerate return to work or to a usual level of function. TENS contributes most effectively to a carefully developed comprehensive rehab program with close physiatric monitoring.

9. What are the contraindications for TENS use?

TENS should best be viewed as an ancillary device utilized for the symptomatic control of pain to facilitate exercise training and functional restoration.

• Avoid TENS in the presence of a pacemaker, particularly a demand one.
• Placement over the carotid sinus may produce a vasovagal response.
• Safety in pregnancy has not been established.
• Skin sensitivity to the electrode or tape may occur but is sometimes avoidable with skin barrier preparation.

10. What are the precautions for TENS?

1. TENS should be used with caution for undiagnosed pain syndromes in which the etiology has not been established.
2. TENS is less effective for pain of central origin than pain of peripheral origin.
3. TENS devices should be used only under the supervision of a physician.
4. TENS devices should be kept out of reach of children.

BIBLIOGRAPHY

1. Mannheimer J, Lampe G: Pain and TENS management. In Mannheimer J, Lampe G (eds): Clinical Transcutaenous Electrical Nerve Stimulation. Philadelphia, F.A. Davis, 1985, pp 7–27.
2. Spitzer W, et al: Scientific approach to the assessment and management of activity-related spinal disorders: A monograph for clinicians: Report of the Quebec Task Force on Spinal Disorders. Spine 12(suppl):S1–S57, 1987.

101. ACUPUNCTURE

John Giusto, M.D., and Joseph M. Helms, M.D.

1. What is acupuncture?

Acupuncture is the use of fine needles inserted through the skin at various points on the body to treat illnesses of all kinds. The basic idea is that the stimulation provided by the needles is assistive to the body's mechanisms of physiologic regulation and repair.

2. When did acupuncture begin? Where?

Acupuncture is a traditional treatment that dates back some 2,000 years in China. As a tradition it has spread to other cultures, being adapted to local needs and customs. As a medical art, it has evolved with the passage of time. Acupuncture has been used for 1,500 years in Japan and 200 years in Europe but has only been used to any significant extent in the U.S. for 25 years. Comparatively recent developments include the use of electrical stimulation and treatments solely based on neuroanatomic principles.

3. What can acupuncture treat?

The clinical literature of **controlled trials** includes treatment of low back pain, headaches, arthritic pain, extremity pain, postoperative pain, respiratory problems, urologic problems, and substance abuse. **Uncontrolled reports** include claims of effective application in almost every discipline of medicine.

4. How big are the needles, and how deep do they go?

Acupuncture needles are much thinner than needles to draw blood or give injections. They are available in sizes from 30–36 gauge. The needles are usually 1–1.5 inches long but range from 0.5–5 inches for special applications. The depth of insertion depends on the type of treatment and location of the point as well as the size of the patient. Most points on the extremities are needled to a depth of 0.25–0.5 inch, while points on the low back are routinely needled 1–1.5 inches. Points on the buttocks may require insertion of 3 inches or more.

5. How many needles are used in a treatment?

The usual range is 10–20 needles in any given treatment. Often fewer needles (5–10) are used in the initial treatment of someone who has not had acupuncture before. Many needles (25–40) may be used when superficial (< ⅛ inch) needling techniques are employed to treat large areas of chronic myofascial pain.

6. Does it hurt?

There may be a pinching sensation when the needle first breaks the skin. This sensation is minimized through the use of proper insertion techniques or guide tubes. Most patients report a mild but deep ache lasting for several seconds when the acupuncture needle reaches the depth of the point. Occasionally, fleeting, sharp, or electric sensations occur when a sensory nerve is stimulated. These are not dangerous and do not last.

7. How many treatments are needed, and how often are they given?

A typical course of treatments will number 6–12, with the first 2–4 treatments done twice weekly, the next 4–6 done weekly, and the remainder at 2–4-week intervals. While some recent problems (< 3 months' duration) can be resolved in as few as 3 visits, most long-standing conditions (> 1 year's duration) need a full course of 10–12 sessions. A reasonable clinical trial would be 6 treatments; it is unlikely that significant results will be obtained if there has not been a response in this period.

8. What effects can one expect after receiving acupuncture?

The most common effect after the first few treatments is a global feeling of euphoria and mild disorientation that can last several hours. It is more pronounced after the use of electrical stimulation and is attributed to endorphin release.

At times patients experience intermittent residual achiness at the points that were needled. This achiness rarely lasts > 12 hours and can be relieved with nonprescription analgesics.

With respect to the underlying condition, there are three possible treatment outcomes—no response, improvement, or worsening. The last response, treatment aggravation, is not necessarily a bad sign. Often, it is simply the result of too vigorous or too extensive an input. It should not last > 3 days and may be addressed with anti-inflammatory or analgesic medications, including prescription strength drugs.

9. Have studies been done to show the analgesic effects of acupuncture?

Acupuncture for purposes of analgesia is one of the most thoroughly researched areas in medicine. Animal and human experiments started in China in the 1960s and since have been pursued in Europe and the United States.

Two types of analgesia have been identified. One is **endorphin-dependent** and is induced by manual twirling of the needle or electrical stimulation that is of low frequency (2–4 Hz) and high intensity (> 10 mA). Characteristics of this response include slow onset with peak response at 30 minutes; long duration with effects usually lasting many hours; potentiation, with a second treatment in a few hours having a greater effect than the first one; cumulative effects after several treatments; and systemic reactions.

The other type of acupuncture analgesia is **monoamine-dependent** and is induced by electrical stimulation that is of high frequency (> 70 Hz) and relatively low intensity (< 10 mA). Its characteristics include rapid onset and local/segmental effects only.

10. How is the brain stimulated by acupuncture?

As summarized by B. Pomeranz:

"Acupuncture actuates nerve fibers (type II and type III) in the muscle which send impulses to the spinal cord and activate three centers (spinal cord, midbrain, and hypothalamus-pituitary) to cause analgesia. The **spinal** site uses enkephalin and dynorphin to block incoming messages with stimulation at low frequency, and other transmitters (perhaps GABA) with high-frequency stimulation. The **midbrain** uses enkephalin to activate the raphe descending system, which inhibits spinal cord pain transmission by a synergistic effect of the monoamines, serotonin, and norepinephrine. The midbrain also has a circuit which bypasses the endorphinergic links at high-frequency stimulation. Finally, at the third center, the **hypothalamus-pituitary**, the pituitary releases beta-endorphin into the blood and CSF to cause analgesia at a distance (e.g., the midbrain). Also, the hypothalamus sends long axons to the midbrain and via beta-endorphin activates the descending analgesia system. This third center is not activated at high frequency, only a low-frequency stimulation."

11. Has research shown any other effects?

There also has been research on the circulatory and autonomic influences of acupuncture. Inserting a needle into a muscle in spasm dilates the blood vessels in that muscle via a reflex action involving sympathetic nerve fibers. Needles inserted into paravertebral muscles result in dilitation of blood vessels in peripheral spastic ischemic muscles at the same segmental level through a somato-autonomic reflex whose center is located in the contralateral anterior hypothalamus. Both the local and segmental needling result in decreased muscle spasm in the symptomatic area. A generalized decrease in peripheral sympathetic tone also has been noted after acupuncture. The above findings may help explain thermographic studies that show a normalizing increase in the temperature of chronic pain areas from acupuncture treatments given local or distant to the painful site. Also of note are studies on tissue healing that have found a measurable current of injury emanating from acupuncture points after needling. This current has been shown to modulate neurohormonal activity and activates tissue-repair mechanisms.

12. How effective is acupuncture?

Effectiveness of Analgesia for Chronic Pain	
Placebo	30–35%
Sham acupuncture	33–50%
(needles inserted in wrong location)	
True acupuncture	55–85%
Morphine	70%

13. Explain the physiology of acupuncture's effectiveness in myofascial pain.

Myofascial pain syndromes of neuropathic origin seem to be uniquely qualified for acupuncture therapy. C. Chan Gunn has introduced a physiologic theory of these syndromes and developed a specialized form of intramuscular needle stimulation to treat them. **Neuropathic pain** is distinguished by either chronic dysesthetic or deep, aching pain in the absence of ongoing injury or inflammation. This pain is typically accompanied by sensorimotor and autonomic manifestations, such as disuse supersensitivity (hyperexcitability, increased susceptibility, and super-reactivity), vasomotor changes (decreased temperature), sudomotor changes (increased sweating), pilomotor changes (goosebumps), and trophedema (local subcutaneous edema caused by increased tone in lymphatic vessel smooth muscle and increased blood vessel permeability).

Gunn considers the most common cause of neuropathic pain in any location to be **spondylosis** of all gradations. This phenomenon increases with age because of an accumulation of minor and sometimes major injuries to a segment. If neuropathy arises from pressure on a nerve root, the stage is set for a vicious cycle: neuropathy (radiculopathy) leads to pain and spasm in segmentally innervated muscles, including paraspinal muscles, both directly and indirectly from supersensitivity to minor trauma. The spasm in the paraspinal muscles compresses the intervertebral disc and narrows the intervertebral foramina, which further compresses the nerve root and worsens the neuropathy. Increased pressure on facet joints can also cause arthralgia, i.e., **facet syndrome**. Even in solitary peripheral lesions, there often is asymptomatic segmental paraspinal muscle spasm precipitating or aggravating the symptomatic peripheral neuromuscular dysfunction.

The key to treating neuropathic dysfunction is to release the muscle spasm, especially in the deep paraspinal muscles, and desensitize the involved nerves by reflex-stimulation. Acupuncture seems to be uniquely qualified for safely accessing the anatomic locations involved in myofascial pain of neuropathic origin while addressing the causative physiologic mechanisms. It should be noted that if fibrotic changes have replaced most striated muscle tissue so that spasm can no longer be considered a major component of the pain syndrome, acupuncture is unlikely to be of benefit. Extreme fibrosis would be evidenced by a lack of "needle grasp."

14. Is acupuncture safe? What about risks of infection, pneumothorax, and other complications?

Infection is an extremely rare consequence of acupuncture treatment. There have been only two reported incidences of hepatitis transmission in the U.S. literature, both by nonphysicians reusing unsterilized needles. Acupuncture needles are stainless steel and should be sterile. Care should be taken not to insert the needle through areas of cellulitis. Sterile skin preparation is only necessary for deep needling or for needling of the ear, groin, or rectal areas.

Pneumothorax is an infrequent complication. Deep needling of the thoracic cage and hilar areas is discouraged. The small size of the acupuncture needles makes a significant pneumothorax unlikely in any case.

While **ecchymoses** are occasionally seen, significant **hematomata** are not. This is probably because of the torpedo shape of an acupuncture needle, as opposed to the beveled cutting edge of a hypodermic needle. The needle shape is also probably responsible for the lack of enduring damage to nerves or other tissues and structures.

One phenomenon to be aware of is **"needle shock."** It is a vasovagal response to needling that may occur in initial treatments. It responds readily to standard maneuvers.

15. Are there any contraindications to acupuncture?

Contraindications to acupuncture are similar but less restrictive than those for injection techniques: overlying cellulitis, severe coagulopathy, and anticoagulation out of control. Therapeutic anticoagulation does not in general present any difficulties, although ecchymoses are more common. Vigorous or deep needling and repetitive needle-pecking techniques should be avoided.

Pregnancy is not a contraindication to acupuncture. Certain points, however, are avoided on practical or theoretical grounds, such as points overlying the pregnant uterus and those stimulating the lumbosacral nerve plexes.

Contraindications to **electrical stimulation** of acupuncture needles are the same as those for electrical stimulation in general: stimulation of the thorax in patients with pacemakers, pregnancy (safety not established), and carcinoma (unknown effects).

16. Is there any standardized training in acupuncture?

There are not yet nationally recognized standards for physician training in acupuncture. Each state establishes its own requirements for licensure, and those requirements vary widely. The most comprehensive training available for physicians is given through the Office of Continuing Medical Education, UCLA School of Medicine. It is a 200-hour CME I program entitled "Medical Acupuncture for Physicians." Shorter courses are offered at other teaching centers. It should be noted that licensed nonphysician acupuncturists are not generally familiar with the principles and techniques of medical acupuncture.

17. Where does one find a qualified practitioner?

The most important resource for general information and referrals to qualified practitioners is:
American Academy of Medical Acupuncture (AAMA)
5820 Wilshire Boulevard
Los Angeles, CA 90036
Tel: 213-937-5514 (general information) or 800-521-5016 (referrals)
Fax: 213-937-0959

18. How many acupuncture points are there? Where are they located?

There are 361 classically described channel points and almost as many nonchannel points. General anatomic characteristics of acupuncture points include:
- Proximity to the neurovascular hilus of the muscle, probably equivalent to motor or trigger points
- Passage of peripheral nerves through bone foramina
- Penetration of deep fascia by peripheral nerves
- Bifurcation points of peripheral nerves
- Nerve plexes
- Sagittal plane where superficial nerves from both sides of the body meet
- Areas of dense fibrous connective tissue that are richly innervated
- Suture lines of the skull

As all of the above points generally show a decrease in electrical resistance when compared to the surrounding tissue, especially when they are tender to palpation, any point of lowered electrical resistance can be considered a potential acupuncture point.

19. What are the most common problems treated by acupuncture in outpatient pain management?

The most common problem is pain of > 3 months' duration that has not responded to pharmacologic, surgical, or traditional physical therapies. By location, low back and neck/shoulder pain are the most common, followed by appendicular joint pains and headaches. By physiologic pathology, myofascial mechanisms are the most common, followed by inflammatory and degenerative processes.

20. What are the main techniques of acupuncture treatment for musculoskeletal problems?

Apart from the use of electrical stimulation, there are three major forms of treatment for musculoskeletal disorders distinguished by the location and depth of needle insertion:

1. In the **surface technique**, many needles are employed and a repetitive pecking motion is utilized to free up palpable restrictions in the superficial fascia of entire zones of the body.

2. **Intramuscular needling** is used for treating skeletal muscle spasm anywhere in the body.

3. **Deep needling** of fascia or even periosteum is used when these tissues or adjacent neurovascular structures are implicated in the pain syndrome, e.g., by tenderness to palpation or analysis of pain distribution patterns.

One highly effective method for treating recalcitrant chronic pain combines elements from all three techniques. In its purest form, peripheral and paravertebral points are needled to address dermatomal, myotomal, and splanchnotomal pain-generation mechanisms.

21. How is electrical stimulation used?

Electrical stimulation can be used with intramuscular or deep needling techniques. For most chronic pain problems, treatment is begun at low frequencies (2–4 Hz) at an intensity that is strong enough to be felt but is not uncomfortable. If there is no satisfactory response after two to three treatments, intermediate (10–30 Hz) and then high (75–200 Hz) frequencies may be tried. Some stimulation devices allow for an alternation of stimulation frequencies at intervals of a few seconds, presumably to prevent accommodation and tolerance. Usually alternating 2 Hz and 15 Hz can help if low-frequency treatment alone has not been successful. More acute problems or flare-ups of chronic conditions may be treated solely with high-frequency stimulation, a combination of low followed by high-frequency stimulation, or alternating low- and high-frequency stimulation.

22. What is the role of ear acupuncture?

In acupuncture, the ear is considered a microsystem, an area of the body that registers and can be used to treat pathology occurring anywhere in the body. (For justification of this claim, see Helms and Oleson in the bibliography.) Clinically, the ear can be needled as an entire treatment in itself, especially in needle-sensitive patients, or used to reinforce the body acupuncture treatment. Points on the ear generally are located with the aid of a point-locating device that detects areas of decreased resistance (increased conductivity) with respect to the surrounding skin. Ear points commonly are used in treatment protocols for substance abuse management.

23. How can acupuncture be integrated into the therapeutic armamentarium of the physiatrist?

Acupuncture can be seen as lying on a continuum of available treatment options. In terms of increasing invasiveness, we might consider the following order: conventional physical therapy modalities, acupuncture, therapeutic injections, and then surgery. For electrical stimulation procedures, the following breakdown may be useful: transcutaneous electrical nerve stimulation (TENS), interferential current, neuromuscular stimulation (NMS), and then electro-acupuncture.

One method of integration is to simply proceed across the spectrum, increasing the invasiveness if the starting treatment regimen is not successful. Another method is to follow the continuum in the opposite direction as part of an effort at progressive rehabilitation and decreased reliance on invasive procedures.

BIBLIOGRAPHY

1. Greenman PE: Principles of Manual Medicine. Baltimore, Williams & Wilkins, 1989.
2. Gunn CC: Treating Myofascial Pain: Intramuscular Stimulation (IMS) for Myofascial Pain Syndromes of Neuropathic Origin. Seattle, University of Washington, 1989.
3. Helms JM: Acupuncture Energetics: A Clinical Approach for Physicians. Berkeley, Medical Acupuncture Publishers, 1995.
4. Lee MHM, Liao SJ: Acupuncture in physiatry. In Kottke FJ, Lehmann JF (eds): Krusen's Handbook of Physical Medicine and Rehabilitation. Philadelphia, W.B. Saunders, 1990.
5. Ng LKY, Katims JJ, Lee MHM: Acupuncture: A Neuromodulation Technique for Pain Control. In Aronoff GM (ed): Evaluation and Treatment of Chronic Pain, 2nd ed. Baltimore, Williams & Wilkins, 1992, pp 291–298.
6. Oleson TD, Kroening RJ, Bresler DE: An experimental evaluation of auricular diagnosis: The somato-topic mapping of musculoskeletal pain at ear acupuncture points. Pain 8:217–229, 1980.
7. Pomeranz B: Scientific basis of acupuncture. In Stux G, Pomeranz B: Acupuncture: Textbook and Atlas. Heidelberg, Springer-Verlag, 1987, pp 1–34.
8. Seem M: The New American Acupuncture: Acupuncture Osteopathy: The Myofascial Release of the Bodymind's Holding Patterns. Boulder, CO, Blue Poppy Press, 1993.
9. Travell JG, Simons DG: Myofascial Pain and Dysfunction: The Trigger Point Manual. Baltimore, Williams & Wilkins, 1983.
10. Travell JG, Simons DG: Myofascial Pain and Dysfunction: The Trigger Point Manual: Vol 2. The Lower Extremities. Baltimore, Williams & Wilkins, 1992.
11. Walsh NE, Dumitru D, et al: Treatment of the patient with chronic pain. In DeLisa J (ed): Rehabilitation Medicine: Principles and Practice. Philadelphia, J.B. Lippincott, 1988, pp 708–864.

102. LOCAL INJECTIONS FOR MUSCLE SPASTICITY (NERVE BLOCKS)

Thomas J. Cava, M.D.

1. What are the clinical indications for local injection techniques to reduce spasticity?

Spasticity that is localized, that is unresponsive to stretching, modalities, or systemic medications, and that interferes with mobility, sleep, or ADLs. Specific indications include risk of contracture, limitation in positioning, orthosis fitting, and facilitation of serial casting.

2. What are most common diagnoses of patients treated with local injections for spasticity?

Upper motor neuron lesions, which include stroke, head injury, multiple sclerosis, spinal cord injury, and cerebral palsy.

3. Which drugs are locally injected to treat patients with spasticity?

Phenol (carbolic acid) is commonly prepared in a 6% aqueous solution for adults and 3% for pediatric injection. It has been injected in peripheral nerve and intramuscular nerve blocks since the 1960s.

Ethyl alcohol is prepared in concentrations of 35–100%. Though it has been injected to treat spasticity since the 1950s, recent literature regarding its use in treating spasticity is limited.

Botulinum toxin type A (BTX), the most significant new drug in the treatment of localized muscle spasticity, is one of the most potent pharmacologic toxins known to man—6 million times more toxic than snake venom! BTX is produced by the anaerobic bacterium *Clostridium botulinum* and is injected in minute qualities referred to as biologic units. BTX has been used in the past decade with dramatic results when injected intramuscularly to treat strabismus, blepharospasm, and cervical dystonia (torticollis). In the past several years, its effectiveness in the treatment of limb muscle spasticity has become established.

4. How do these agents work to reduce spasticity?

Each has a different specific mechanism of action, but their final effects is **chemodenerva-tion**, or the chemical disconnection of a nerve from the muscle that it innervates. This results in a localized, focal muscle relaxation. Phenol and alcohol are neurolytic agents which cause imme-diate axonal lipid extraction. BTX is a potent neurotoxin which inhibits the release of acetyl-choline at the neuromuscular junction (NMJ) via a complex mechanism of action.

5. What is so complex about the action of BTX?

Plenty. There are three steps involved in BTX-mediated muscle paralysis: **binding** to the cholinergic, presynaptic nerve terminal; **internalization** into the acetylcholine vesicle; and **inhi-bition** of neurotransmitter release into the synapse. BTX cleaves the synaptic fusion protein, SNAP-25, thereby preventing the "chemical handshake" that occurs when the acetylcholine vesi-cle docks and fuses to the presynaptic membrane. Without acetylcholine, the propagation of the action potential is terminated, resulting in a partial muscle paralysis.

6. With such complex pharmacology, accurate treatment dose must be important?

The treatment dose varies with each agent and is dependent on the type of block, size of muscle or nerve injected, degree of spasticity reduction desired, and toxicity profile of the drug chosen.

For the procedure of **phenol nerve block** (phenol neurolysis), a dose of 1–10 ml of 5% aque-ous solution is typically injected. For phenol motor point block (phenol intramuscular neuroly-sis), a total dose of 1–15 ml is commonly given in multiple 0.2–0.5-ml perineural injections. The recommended maximum total dose per treatment sessions is 1 gm, which is equivalent to 20 ml of 5% solution. Phenol has systemic toxicity at doses > 8.5 gm, which can cause seizures, CNS depression, and cardiac failure.

Alcohol nerve blocks and motor point blocks (intramuscular alcohol wash) are performed less commonly than those with phenol and BTX, and typical doses injected range from 1–30 ml of a 45–100% solution of ethanol. **BTX** dosage is altogether different than dosing the other agents.

7. How is dosage of botulinum toxin determined?

BTX dosage is measured in units of **potency** instead of quantity. The amount of BTX required to kill 50% of a colony of female, Swiss-Webster mice is referred to as the LD_{50} in mice and is equal to 1 mouse unit. While no PM&R residents have yet volunteered for the human LD_{50} study, the extrapolated lethal dose in humans is **3,000 units**! Typical treatment doses are 30–40 units/muscle for small, distal limb muscles and 100–300 units/muscle for large proximal muscles. General recommendations set a maximum dosage of 400 units/treatment session, which is an order of magnitude below the estimated LD_{50} in humans. Pediatric dosage guidelines are emerging.

8. How is BTX supplied?

In the U.S., BTX is available in 100-unit vials of lyophilized toxin which must be reconsti-tuted with sterile, preservative-free, 0.9% sodium chloride solution. BTX is an FDA-approved drug for treatment of strabismus, blepharospasm, and related focal dystonias. A 1990 NIH con-sensus statement also determined BTX as safe and effective for the treatment of cervical torticollis, spasmodic dysphonia, and writer's cramp, but its use in these conditions, as well as in spasticity, remains unlabeled. With proper training, physicians may use BTX in appropriate patients to manage spasticity. Extensive clinical studies since 1989 have demonstrated its therapeutic safety and effectiveness in patients with spastic hypertonia.

9. Describe the technique for intramuscular neurolysis with the injection of phenol.

Skin surface stimulation is used to identify sites that produce low threshold muscle twitches. These motor points are marked and prepared with betadine and alcohol for sterile injection. A 27-gauge teflon-coated cathode simulator needle is attached by flexible tubing to a 3–5-ml syringe containing 5% aqueous phenol. The cathode is attached to a stimulator with the following set-tings: a square wave pulse duration of 0.1 ms, a pulse rate of 1 Hz, and a stimulus intensity of 0.2–30 mA. The motor nerve is located with needle advancement and maximization of muscle twitch response. Stimulus intensity is then reduced and needle placement refined to produce the largest twitch with the lowest amperage (0.5–1 mA). The syringe should be aspirated to avoid intravascular injection, and phenol is injected, 0.1–0.5 ml at a time. The needle is twisted or the position adjusted to redirect the dose if the muscle twitch does not disappear. The process is repeated at multiple motor points until the desired clinical effect is achieved.

10. How does the procedure for BTX and alcohol injection differ?

BTX must be reconstituted with preservative-free normal saline. Because minute quantities are injected, a tuberculin syringe is needed for measurement. A needle stimulation technique may be used to identify and confirm the designated muscle belly; however, precise motor point identification by reduction of stimulus intensity is not necessary. The onset of action of BTX is not immediate and typically occurs in 12–72 hours. The procedure for alcohol is similar to phenol injection.

11. How do you choose which muscle(s) to inject?

Carefully. Clinical and functional examination is indispensable, and gait lab analysis is at times advantageous. Careful attention to the balance of forces about the involved joint is critical. Hypertonic muscles should be chosen if spasticity limits function. Potential benefits may include spasm and pain relief, prevention of joint contracture, improved gait, improved seating position, improved perineal hygiene, potential for greater voluntary antagonist muscle activity, and improved ADLs. Clinical success can be quantitated with the Modified Ashworth Scale, hand-held myometry, goniometry, and gait analysis.

12. What are the advantages of BTX injection in the treatment of spasticity?

- BTX is locally applied
- Effect can be titrated withe stepwise, incremental dosing
- BTX affects only motor function
- No risk of sensory dysesthesias
- Effect is sustained but reversible
- Procedure is relatively quick to perform
- Patient tolerance is excellent

13. How long does the effect of the injections last?

The duration of action varies with the agent injected, dosage, anatomic localization, and severity of spasticity. Phenol blocks typically last from 3–6 months, although longer periods have been reported in unblinded studies. Alcohol blocks have been reported to last for 1–36 months, but clinical consensus is that alcohol generally has a shorter duration of action than phenol. The duration of action of BTX is 3–6 months. Comprehensive physical therapy and occupational therapy programs after the blocks may optimize functional outcome.

14. Can spasticity return after the block?

Yes. Indirect evidence suggests that reinnvervation of the muscle occurs by axon terminal sprouting. This sprouting begins in a few days and eventually reverses the paralysis over subsequent months. The blocks typically allow greater movement, permitting better success with stretching and new functional routines. If new capabilities are regularly exercised, spasticity may have less severe effects despite reinnervation.

15. What are the side effects of injections for spasticity?

A potential side effect of all spasticity injections is **loss of motor function**, which is dependent on the affected muscle spasticity. Each agent has its own adverse effect profile. **Phenol** may cause sensory dysesthesias when injected into mixed sensory-motor nerves, but this is rarely reported in its use in motor point blocks. It may also cause transient muscle swelling, induration, and tenderness. **Alcohol** may cause hyperemia and a transient burning sensation. The most common side effects of **BTX** are transient injection site edema or erythema. An infrequent side effect (2%) is the formation of anti-botulinum toxin antibodies. While this presents no adverse clinical effects, it may render a patient a nonresponder to future treatment. Antibody formation has been reported in treatment of patients with cervical dystonia and strabismus but not yet in limb spasticity.

16. Name some common specific procedures for each of the major agents.

Phenol

Obturator nerve, musculocutaneous nerve, and tibial nerve blocks

Gastrocnemius, posterior tibialis, biceps and triceps motor point blocks

Alcohol

Tibial nerve block

Gastrocnemius, soleus, and biceps motor point blocks

Botulinum toxin

Biceps, wrist flexor, and finger flexor injections in the upper extremities

Adductor, quadriceps, gastrocnemius, tibialis posterior, and toe flexor injections in the lower extremities

17. What are the contraindications to local injections for spasticity?

Absolute contraindications

Allergy to the proposed agent

Infection of inflammation at the planned injection site

Pregnancy

Relative contraindication

Coagulopathy

Specific precautions for BTX injection

Preexisting disorders of the neuromuscular junction

Concurrent use of aminoglycosides or other drugs that may potentiate neuromuscular blockade

BIBLIOGRAPHY

1. American Academy of Neurology, Therapeutics and Technology Assessment Subcommittee: The clinical usefulness of botulinum toxin-A in treating neurologic disorders. Neurology 40:1332–1336, 1990.
2. Brin MF: Interventional neurology: Treatment of neurological conditions with local injections of botulinum toxin. Arch Neurol 54(suppl):1–23, 1991.
3. Cava TJ: Botulinum toxin management of spasticity in upper motor neuron lesions. Eur J Neurol 2(suppl 3):57–60, 1995.
4. Cosgrove AP, Graham HK: Botulinum toxin-A in the management of children with cerebral palsy. J Bone Joint Surg (B) 74(suppl):135–136, 1992.
5. Glenn MB: Nerve blocks. In Whyte J (ed): The Practical Management of Spasticity in Children and Adults. Philadelphia, Lea & Febiger, 1990, pp 227–259.
6. Halpern DM, Meelhysen FE: Phenol motor point block in the management of muscular hypertonia. Arch Phys Med Rehabil 47:659–644, 1966.
7. NIH Consensus Development Statement: Clinical use of botulinum toxin. Arch Neurol 48:1294–1298, 1991.
8. Snow BJ, et al: Treatment of spasticity with botulinum toxin: A double-blind study. Ann Neurol 28:512–515, 1990.
9. Yablon SA, Agana BT, Ivanhoe CB, Boake C: Botulinum toxin in severe upper extremity spasticity among patients with traumatic brain injury: An open-labeled trial. Neurology 45: 1995.

XII. Therapeutics
C. Orthotics and Prosthetics

103. UPPER-LIMB ORTHOSES

John B. Redford, M.D., Abna A. Ogle, M.D.,
and Richard C. Robinson, M.D.

1. What is an orthosis?

An orthosis is an external apparatus worn to restrict or assist movement. An orthosis can be used to transfer load from one area to another.

2. State three general reasons why orthotics are prescribed.

S = support
A = alignment
P = protection

The mnemonic SAP highlights the three cardinal broad indications for the orthotic prescription. By supporting, aligning, and protecting body parts, orthotics can enhance the function of movable body regions and prevent or correct deformities. Orthotics can be used to enhance functionality.

3. State four functions of upper limb movement that must be considered in the orthotic prescription.

1. **Reach:** Primarily accomplished by shoulder and elbow positioning and function. Severe loss of shoulder function is devastating to reach, yet hard to treat with orthoses.

2. **Carry:** The action of transporting a load. Orthotic substitutions are of little consequence.

3. **Prehension pattern:** All the functional aspects of holding objects in the hand. This aspect is very important in orthotic prescription and follow-up.

4. **Release:** Active digital extension accompanied by relaxation of digital flexors. This is an essential reverse action in all prehensile function, and it may need special orthotic attention.

4. They say that monkeys cannot use their hands like humans. What does that mean?

Hook prehension (such as carrying a suitcase) or **cylindrical grasp** (such as grabbing a rail) are tasks monkeys can do as easily as humans. However, only humans have an opposable thumb, and so monkeys cannot compare with humans for fine motions such as **fingertip pinch**, **lateral pinch** (holding a key), and **palmar prehension** (three jaw chuck prehension or opposition between the thumb and second and third digits). Monkeys cannot be baseball pitchers; they cannot hold balls well because they lack **spherical grasp**. These observations imply that for any hand orthosis to work—in conjunction with hand therapy—it must restore these unique human functions as closely to normal as possible.

5. The patient asks, "What are upper limb splints good for?"

1. To rest the body part so that the patient does not hurt inflamed joints or further injure muscles, ligaments, or fractured bones

2. To prevent contractures; i.e., to prevent patients from losing adjoining joint motion as the result of untreated burns, injury to nerves, or spasticity

3. To correct deformity; in conjunction with surgery and occupational or physical therapy, a splint will be formed to keep the treated parts on a stretch

4. To promote exercise for recovery of weak muscles or to correct muscle imbalances; splints are worn to strengthen certain key muscles

5. To substitute for lost function; if the patient has lost a certain muscle action, it may be partly restored or retrained with an orthosis.

6. How do static and dynamic orthoses differ?

Static orthoses keep underlying segments from moving. Often, they are simply used to rest body parts, but in some cases they can substitute for lost joint function (e.g., an orthotic thumb post makes the thumb rigid to oppose the fingers).

Dynamic orthoses move; they have external or internal power sources and encourage restoration and control of joint movements. External power means providing motion primarily by elastics, springs, or, rarely, pneumatic or electrical systems; internal power means providing motion through action of another body part, such as using wrist extension or a shoulder motion via harness and cable to operate finger grasp and release. The prescription should always indicate which motion a dynamic orthosis is to assist: for example, the phrase *finger flexion assist* would be part of the prescription for an orthosis to restore prehension.

7. How long should patients expect to wear an orthosis?

Generally no more than a month or two. Most upper limb orthoses are to be worn only during postoperative recovery or until the useful effects of medication, physical modality, or exercise to improve mobility and strength evidently have overcome the acute problem. At first, orthoses are applied 2–3 hours once or twice a day. Gradually, patients wear them longer, depending on the condition. Some are worn mainly at night.

8. When are upper limb orthoses most likely to be used?

Indications include:

Trauma and surgery

    Tendon repair

    Postreconstructive surgery (Dupuytren's contracture release)

    Joint injuries

    Nerve injuries

Painful disorders (rheumatoid arthritis, carpal tunnel syndrome)

Improve function after disease (poststroke, neuromuscular disease, peripheral nerve disorders)

9. What are static shoulder orthoses?

We rely so much on free unrestricted motion for shoulder function that static orthoses to immobilize fractures of the upper arm can only be used for short periods. Effective immobilization is hard to achieve unless the orthosis applies most of the force through the longitudinal axis of the upper arm and combines this with a force in the frontal plane to hold the humerus into the glenoid cavity.

Most varieties of static or partly dynamic shoulder slings do not really perform well biomechanically. Many orthoses tried for the subluxed paralyzed shoulder, a frequent sequela of stroke, do help to relieve pain but do little to promote function. An **airplane splint** holds the arm out like a wing. It is designed to promote healing of fractures or immobilizing the shoulder in abduction after reconstructive surgery or injury. However, it is an example of a good mechanical or orthotic idea, but a bad human interactive idea, because patients tolerate them so poorly. Nevertheless, an airplane splint may be the only useful device to prevent an axillary burn from causing a contracture or to ensure healing of a shoulder fusion.

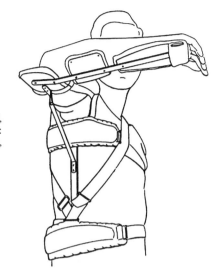

Airplane splint. A static shoulder orthosis. (From Long C, Schutt AH: Upper limb orthotics. In Redford JB (ed): Orthotics Etcetera, 3rd ed. Baltimore, Williams & Wilkins, 1986, pp 198–277, with permission.)

10. Is a ballbearing feeder used to feed patients ballbearings?

No. Ballbearing feeder is an old name for the dynamic shoulder orthosis called a **balanced forearm orthosis** (BFO). This device attaches to the upright of a wheelchair and supports the forearm with a freely moving rod located beneath the forearm trough. The BFO works to modify the effects of gravity so that persons confined to a wheelchair and with slight use of the shoulder or elbow (Grade 2 at least in area muscles) may be more functional in a wheelchair. A BFO is not useful unless some hand function remains and the patient really wants to feed himself or do other activities requiring reach. An occupational therapist must make the necessary adjustments before conducting training. The patient should have a trial of a dynamic overhead sling suspension orthosis before applying the BFO because the sling is much easier to set up and use for evaluation.

11. What are some purposes of elbow orthoses?

Elbow orthoses are used most commonly to **reduce flexion contractures**, employing a static type with hinged bars attached by Velcro to the upper arm and forearm cuffs. Single-axis elbow joints can be sequentially adjusted to extend the elbow further. A tension spring to extend the elbow joint dynamically, or a turnbuckle applied between the upper arm and the lower forearm cuffs, can provide steady stretch to reduce the contracture. Less commonly, a static or dynamic orthosis is used to **reduce an extension contracture**. Dynamic elbow orthoses are rarely used to substitute for muscle loss, such as lost elbow flexion, because they lack cosmetic appeal and are just not very effective.

12. What special problems must be considered when splinting the wrist or hand?

1. After any surgery or injury to the hand, it will swell. Unless this **edema** is properly approached, joints may become stiff as a result of the subsequent overactivity of fibroblasts. It has been said, "Hand therapy is behavior modification of fibroblasts during the healing response." As part of this hand therapy, you do not want hand splints applied incorrectly during recovery. Orthoses may aggravate edema. Their use must be carefully monitored, especially in patients with limited cognition or inappropriate emotional reactions to using splints.

2. The hand has great **sensibility**, and any sensory loss results in significant effects on function. Unfortunately, sensory loss is very common. Its extent must be mapped carefully and orthotic pressure over insensate areas kept to a minimum. Because the hand is the organ of touch, the orthosis must be designed to avoid blocking sensation to critical areas, such as the fingertips. The hand is so sensitive that fitting must be exact; any discomfort will result in rejection of the orthosis.

3. There is a multiplicity of joints in the hand. It may be necessary to make an orthosis that immobilizes one or more joints to allow movement in others. Deciding how to do this requires good judgment and wide experience with the various materials needed for fabrication. A good example is the MCP (metacarpophalangeal) block orthosis: The MCP joints are held in flexion to block the action of the long finger extensors and allow the proximal (PIP) and distal interphalangeal (DIP) joints to extend.

13. What is a SEWHO?

Upper limb orthoses are all named for the parts that they incorporate, and these are then usually abbreviated. Some examples are:

Shoulder/elbow/wrist/hand orthosis—SEWHO
Wrist/hand orthosis—WHO
Hand orthosis—HO
Finger orthosis—FO

14. Hand therapists, like all specialists, have their own language. Define some of the more common terms.

1. **Assist:** Any dynamic component designed to provide a certain motion.
2. **Block or stop:** Any part of an orthosis designed to block a given motion as in the MCP block orthosis. The block is sometimes in the form of a lock (e.g., an elbow lock).
3. **C-bar:** A C-shaped strip of plastic or metal applied in the thumb/index finger webspace to prevent thumb adduction against the palm.
4. **Dorsal wrist/hand orthosis** (*WHO*): An orthosis applied to the superior surface of the hand and wrist; it contrasts with the more common palmar or volar WHO.
5. **Finger deviation splint:** A hand orthosis with components to prevent abduction or adduction of the fingers, as incorporated in splints for the rheumatoid arthritic hand to prevent ulnar drift. Whether they really help prevent drift is controversial.
6. **Opponens bar:** A component for positioning the thumb, such as a bar outside the thumb to prevent it from extending.
7. **Opponens splint:** An orthosis that holds the thumb in opposition to the fingers; sometimes described as "short" (below the wrist) or "long" (incorporating the wrist and hand).
8. **Outrigger:** A component applied above or below an orthosis to provide a platform from which various dynamic components can pull against the digits with elastics and cuffs or springs.
9. **Splint:** A commonly used synonym for orthosis. The word seems to be most commonly used in reference to the hand.

15. How should you order and classify orthoses for the wrist and hand?

The easiest way to describe a hand orthosis is to state whether it is static or dynamic and the main area it encompasses or immobilizes. In any orthosis, the prescriber should also say if it is to mobilize, assist, or apply traction to a certain joint or movement.

Common Kinds of Hand Orthoses

Wrist orthosis	Ends in the palm
Wrist/hand orthosis	Ends over digits
Wrist/thumb orthosis	Extends into webspace of thumb
Wrist/MCP orthosis	Extends just distal to PIP crease
Forearm/wrist/finger orthosis	Many variations, but must end on fingers
Hand orthosis	Starts below the wrist
Thumb orthosis	Incorporates the thumb in some way
Finger orthosis	One finger only
Tenodesis orthosis	A special class of orthosis prescribed mainly in tetraplegic patients, employing the natural tendency for the fingers to close when the wrist is extended and open when it is flexed

16. Making splints is expensive. Why not just buy off-the-shelf orthoses?
Many static splints and a few dynamic ones can be prefabricated and kept in stock. A common WHO, for example, is the Futuro line of products. However, like army clothing designed to fit everyone but really fitting no one, prefabricated orthoses may produce unexpected problems if poorly fitted. Custom-made orthoses used to be more expensive when they were made from metal or polyester resins. Almost all now are made from low-temperature thermoplastic and take much less time to make than the older aluminum or epoxy resin ones. Hands differ so much in size, shape, and even innervation that only custom-made orthoses can be used in many situations.

BIBLIOGRAPHY

1. Carcis D, Lamb J, Johnson: Upper limb orthoses. In Bowker P, Condie DN, Bader DL, Pratt DJ (eds): Biomechanical Basis of Orthotics Management. Oxford, Butterworth-Heineman, 1993, pp 191–218.
2. Irani KD: Wrist and hand orthoses. Phys Med Rehabil State Art Rev 1:137–160, 1987.
3. Long C, Schutt AH: Upper limb orthotics. In Redford JB (ed): Orthotics Etcetera, 3rd ed. Baltimore, Williams & Wilkins, 1986, pp 198–277.
4. Malick MH: Manual on Dynamic Hand Splinting with Thermoplastic Materials, 3rd ed. Pittsburgh, American Rehabilitation Education Network, 1982.
5. Schutt AH: Upper extremity and hand orthotics. Phys Med Rehabil Clin North Am 3:223–241, 1992.
6. Shurr DG, Cook TM: Upper-extremity orthotics. In Shurr DG, Cook TM (eds): Prosthetics & Orthotics. East Norwalk, CT, Appleton & Lange, 1990, pp 173–181.
7. Rose GK: Hand and wrist orthoses, elbow orthosis, shoulder. In Rose GK (ed): Orthotics: Principles & Practice. London, William Heinemann Medical Books, 1986, pp 97–116.

104. LOWER-LIMB ORTHOTICS

Jay Schechtman, M.D., and Kristjan T. Ragnarsson, M.D.

1. What are the indications for use of an ankle-foot orthosis (AFO) to improve a patient's gait?
1. Mediolateral instability at the ankle
2. "Foot drop," passive plantarflexion in swing phase
3. "Foot drop" at heal strike due to weak ankle dorsiflexors
4. Weak push-off at late stance phase

2. What requirement must the patient meet in order to use an AFO effectively?
1. Knee extension strength of > 3/5
2. Stable limb size without fluctuating edema for use of a plastic AFO
3. Skin pressure tolerance and patient compliance with skin checks

3. What are posterior and anterior stops on an AFO?
Anterior and posterior stops are used to control ankle dorsiflexion and plantarflexion on a jointed AFO. A posterior stop limits plantarflexion; an anterior stop limits dorsiflexion following mid-stance. Limiting dorsiflexion at the ankle allows less knee flexion moment during stance and stabilizes it. A posterior stop is helpful when moderate spasticity is present to control plantarflexion spasms and to prevent equinus deformity from developing.

4. How is the AFO altered to stabilize the knee?
An AFO can be adjusted to alter the forces that are transmitted from ground reaction through the closed kinetic chain of the limb to the knee. When the AFO is set into plantarflexion, the knee is provided with a stabilizing extension moment during stance in foot-flat and push-off. The opposite result can occur if the AFO is set in dorsiflexion, causing a destabilizing knee flexion movement at heel strike.

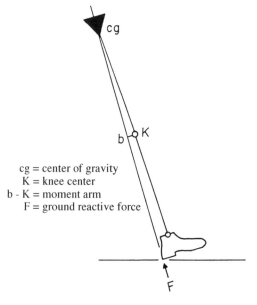

cg = center of gravity
K = knee center
b - K = moment arm
F = ground reactive force

Knee bending moment at heel strike. (From Lehmann JF: The biomechanics of ankle foot orthoses: Prescription and design. Arch Phys Med Rehabil 60:200–207, 1979; with permission.)

5. Which type of AFO is used when clonus is present at the ankle?

When a patient has severe clonus at the ankle, the foot should usually be locked in a **solid AFO**. In a patient with significant spasticity, an AFO with any form of spring action may permit movement to trigger and perpetuate clonus.

6. What is a spiral brace? How does it work?

A spiral brace is a thermoplastic AFO that is made in a spiral design to control both dorsiflexion and plantarflexion. The spiral winds around the patient's calf from the medial footplate in a full spiral to the anterior tibial area at the level of the tibial condyles. The spiral unwinds with weight-bearing to allow plantarflexion. When the body weight is removed, the spiral rewinds and provides a dorsiflexion assist.

A **hemi-spiral brace**, in contrast, has only a half-spiral winding up the leg from the lateral footplate and provides a better control of equinus and varus forces at the ankle; i.e., it limits inversion and plantarflexion.

The spiral brace uses the **three-point pressure system** common to all orthotics to provide eversion and inversion control at the ankle. Spiral braces are most useful in patients with flaccid weakness of all the ankle muscles (i.e., both dorsiflexors or plantarflexors), but these orthoses are contraindicated in the presence of significant spasticity.

7. What is a floor-reaction orthosis?

The biomechanics of the floor-reaction orthosis are based on the same principles that were discussed regarding AFOs and knee stability (see Question 4), because in essence the floor reaction orthosis is an AFO with the footplate set in slight plantarflexion. The extension moment created by plantarflexing the orthosis is transferred to the patellar tendon by a band of material on the top of the orthosis. The extension moment helps to stabilize the knee. Floor reaction orthoses are prescribed to help with knee extension in patients who have at least fair (3/5) quadriceps motor strength.

8. What is a Klenzack joint?

Klenzack ankle joints are (or were) used in a jointed metal AFO. The joint has a spring assist for ankle dorsiflexion. This brace should generally not be used in the presence of significant spasticity, as the spring may amplify clonus.

9. Explain the considerations necessary when ordering an AFO.

A patient who has weakness of the ankle dorsiflexors without spasticity or mediolateral instability can be prescribed a plastic AFO. A posterior-leaf-spring AFO, however, provides limited mediolateral stability and does not compensate for weak plantarflexors. If the patient has both weak dorsiflexors and plantarflexors with no or very little spasticity, the most appropriate orthoses would be a custom-molded plastic AFO with an anterior trimline cut just anterior to malleoli. To provide maximal mediolateral stability, toe pick-up and push-off require the use of a solid ankle double-upright AFO with a T-strap medially for eversion control and laterally for inversion control. For a person with mild spasticity and a tendency for equinus, a hemi-spiral AFO or a plastic AFO with a posterior trimline could suffice.

10. Does prophylactic knee bracing prevent knee injuries in football?

There is some controversy on this issue. A study of college football players at West Point found a statistically significant decline in medial collateral injuries in defensive players who used prophylactic knee braces. A larger study on NCAA collegiate football players actually showed more knee injuries in those using prophylactic knee orthoses. Currently, it appears that there is no compelling evidence to recommend prophylactic knee bracing to football players.

11. What should be checked when a patient receives a new AFO?

If the orthosis is jointed, the anatomical ankle joint which runs through the malleoli should be in the same axis as the orthotic joint. In stance, the knee should be fully extended and the sole of the shoe should be flat on the floor. In swing, there should be adequate toe clearance. The knee should flex slightly immediately following heel strike.

12. Which type of orthosis is used in Legg-Calvé-Perthes disease?

Legg-Calvé-Perthes disease is a childhood disorder with avascular necrosis of the capital femoral epiphysis. The goal of bracing in this disorder is to maintain the femoral head completely within the acetabulum in order to maintain its sphericity. Both plaster casts and orthoses of different designs, such as the Toronto, Newington, and Atlanta Scottish Rite orthoses, have been used to place the **hip in hyperabduction and external rotation**. It is not necessary to remember the names of all the different designs of such orthoses, as long as the hyperabduction concept is understood.

13. What type of orthosis is used for persons with spina bifida who are community ambulators?

Persons with spina bifida who can ambulate successfully in the community, generally must be intact, to at least the L3 neurologic level, and have fair (3/5) quadriceps strength. The child should be braced in bilateral solid AFO. It is unwise to extend the orthoses to the knee, as the child may not be able to advance the limb with the knee locked in extension. An assistive device for balance is often needed.

14. Should you prescribe knee-ankle-foot orthoses (KAFOs) for a patient with thoracic paraplegia?

Clinical experience has shown that few persons with thoracic paraplegia use KAFOs (long leg braces) for functional ambulation. This has been attributed to the high energy expenditure and the slow speed of such gait. A study of persons with high thoracic paraplegia using Scott-Craig KAFOs to ambulate has shown that energy expenditure was similar regardless of the exact neurologic level. These individuals were found to decrease the energy expenditure by decreasing ambulation speed in order to reach a comfortable power output level.

There are, however, significant psychologic and functional benefits for persons who achieve the ability to be able to stand erect and perform some ADLs upright. There may also be considerable physiologic benefits from regularly assuming the standing position and performing the physical exercise associated with KAFOs (swing-to or swing-through) ambulation. Therefore, KAFOs should not be denied to a person based only on the SCI level and the poor prospects for functional ambulation. However, the person with paraplegia must be advised that KAFOs are only an adjunct to, and not a replacement for, the wheelchair as primary means of locomotion.

15. Why is ambulation with bilateral KAFOs and pair of crutches so much more energy-consuming than wheelchair propulsion?

Ambulation requires moving the center of gravity up and down as well as side to side, and along with it the whole weight of the body. Bilateral KAFO ambulation requires lifting the limbs with shoulder depressors and swinging them forward while on crutches. This tripod or swing-through gait is energy-consuming. A wheelchair translates the center of gravity horizontally and in a straight line without the energy cost associated with moving the center of gravity vertically or laterally.

16. What is the difference between the reciprocating gait orthosis (RGO) and other types of hip-knee-ankle foot orthoses (HKAFO)?

The RGO is designed to include a custom-molded pelvic girdle with a thoracic extension (as required by the patient for balance) which is attached with ballbearing hip joints to bilateral KAFO components. The unique characteristic mechanism consists of two cables with conduits that translate hip extension movement on one side into hip flexion on the other. The RGO is usually used with a walker and infrequently crutches. The unloaded limb is thereby advanced forward with forces transmitted from the loaded side, thus providing a "reciprocating" gait. Experimental work continues to focus on enhancement of ambulation efficiency with functional electric stimulation (see Chapter 99).

17. Can orthotics correct in-toeing in children?

In-toeing in children may be caused by metatarsus adductus, internal tibial torsion, and/or femoral anteversion. In-toeing due to any of these causes generally improves or resolves as the child grows older and rarely causes long-term impairment or disability. Orthoses, such as Dennis-Browne splints, are no longer recommended for this condition.

18. How are shoes modified to correct leg-length discrepancy?

Minor leg-length discrepancies of up to ½ inch may be left uncompensated or are corrected by placing ¼-inch heel pads inside the heel only of the shoe. Any lift > ½ inch should be added externally to both the heel and sole of the shoe. The outer sole elevation should be approximately half of the heel elevation and taper forward from the ball of the shoe to the toe.

ACKNOWLEDGMENT

The authors are grateful to H. Richard Lehneis, Ph.D., for his review of the manuscript and comments.

BIBLIOGRAPHY

1. Dietz FR: Intoeing—Fact, fiction and opinion. Am Fam Phys 5:1249–1259, 1994.
2. Douglas R, Larson PF, D'Ambrosia R, McCall RE: The LSU reciprocating gait orthosis. Orthopaedics 6:834–839, 1983.
3. Lehneis HR: Plastic spiral ankle-foot orthoses. Orthotics Prosthetics 28:3–13, 1974.
4. Lehmann JF: Biomechanics of ankle-foot orthosis: Prescription and design. Arch Phys Med Rehabil 60:200–207, 1979.
5. Merkel KD: Energy expenditure in patients with low, mid, or high thoracic paraplegia using Scott-Craig knee-ankle-foot orthoses. Mayo Clin Proc 60:165–168, 1985.
6. Ragnarsson KT: Lower extremity orthotics, shoes, and gait aids. In DeLisa JA, Gans BM (eds): Rehabilitation Medicine: Principles and Practice, 2nd ed. Philadelphia, J.B. Lippincott, 1993, pp 307–329.
7. Sitler M, Ryan J, Hopkinson W, et al: The efficacy of a prophylactic knee brace to reduce knee injuries in football: A prospective, randomized study at West Point. Am J Sports Med 18:310–315, 1990.
8. Stauffer ES, Hussey RW: Spinal cord injury: Requirements for ambulation. Arch Phys Med Rehabil 54:544–547, 1973.
9. Teitz CC, Hermanson BK, Kronmal RA, Diehr PH: Evaluation of the use of braces to prevent injury to the knee in collegiate football players. J Bone Joint Surg 69A:2, 1987.

105. UPPER-LIMB PROSTHESES

Anthony S. Salzano, M.D.

1. What is the most common congenital upper-extremity limb deficiency?

A unilateral, short below-elbow deficiency, with absence of the forearm, wrist, and hand.

2. What is the prevalence of upper-limb amputations among all amputees in the U.S.?

Approximately 10% of all amputations involve the upper limb, most frequently below the elbow. The ratio of lower- to upper-extremity amputations is 6:1.

3. Describe the most common upper-extremity prosthetic patient.

A male, 20–50 years old, who has suffered a traumatic injury to his right arm.

4. At what age should an infant with a congenital limb deficiency be fitted with an upper-extremity prosthesis?

From 3–6 months of age, when the child begins to sit and needs the arms for prop support. At first, a passive-type prosthesis is provided; active components are added as motor landmarks are reached.

5. How are upper-extremity amputations classified?

For below-elbow amputations, the length of the stump remaining below the elbow is measured from the medial epicondyle of the humerus to the end of the longer residual bone (the radius or ulnar). For above-elbow amputations, the length of the stump remaining above the elbow is measured from the tip of the acromion to the end of the residual humerus. This length is expressed as a percentage of the distance from the acromion to the lateral humeral epicondyle of the sound limb.

Figure from Kottke FJ, Lehmann JF (eds): Krusen's Handbook of Physical Medicine and Rehabilitation, 4th ed. Philadelphia, W.B. Saunders, 1990; with permission.

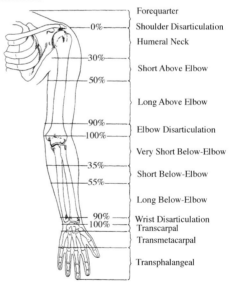

6. Why is it so important to preserve as much of the limb as possible during surgical amputation?

The longer the residual upper limb, the greater the potential power source to control the prosthetic components. A longer limb also preserves more joint proprioception.

7. What are the goals of upper-extremity stump care?

To control swelling and promote shrinkage by compression bandaging, and to prevent joint contractures, especially of the shoulder. The stump usually is bandaged for 6–8 weeks before prosthetic fitting.

8. What is the foremost goal of the pre-prosthetic training period?

To help the patient achieve functional independence in ADL skills using the remaining normal arm. This promotes self-esteem and encourages the patient to realize that he or she can accomplish more than was thought possible prior to training.

9. What are the essential goals of prosthetic training?

During early prosthetic training, the patient wears the prosthesis for short periods of time, usually not longer than 15 minutes. Skin integrity is carefully monitored. The amputee progresses from learning to put on (don) and to take off (doff) the prosthesis, to executing and controlling ROM of the prosthetic joints, to developing basic essential prehension movements. The final step is learning terminal-device dexterity in various elbow and shoulder positions.

Bilateral amputees must have one functional prosthesis as soon as possible; ideally, this should be provided to the dominant limb.

10. What requirements must an amputee meet before he or she can be fitted with a permanent upper-extremity prosthesis?

1. The stump must be free of edema and skin breakdown for comfortable fitting.

2. The patient must have adequate active ROM and motor strength to operate the prosthetic control system.

3. The patient must demonstrate adequate cognitive ability to participate successfully in prosthetic training.

11. Name the most important things to keep in mind when developing the prescription for an upper-extremity prosthesis.

Function and comfort, rather than cosmesis. The patient's vocational and avocational habits must be evaluated to determine the combination of components that will best meet his or her needs—the requirements of a farmer who operates heavy equipment will differ substantially from those of a housewife.

12. After receiving the permanent prosthesis, when should the amputee be seen for follow-up visits?

Usually within 4–6 weeks. But this depends on several factors, including how well the patient functions at home, and whether medical problems develop, such as phantom limb pain, neuroma, diminished joint mobility, bony overgrowth, and—the most common problem—skin complications such as blisters, ulcers, infections, or stasis eczema.

13. What are the essential components of every prescription for a functional upper-limb prosthesis?

Socket, suspension system (cuffs and harness), control system (cables for a body-powered prosthesis, batteries for an externally-powered prosthesis), and terminal device (hook or hand). Depending on the level of amputation, a wrist unit, elbow hinge or unit, and shoulder component might also be needed. A nonfunctional or cosmetic prosthesis is usually indicated when the patient is unable to operate a functional prosthesis for his or her level of amputation.

14. Name the most commonly prescribed components of a below-elbow prosthesis.

Voluntary opening (VO) split hook, friction wrist, double-walled plastic laminate socket, flexible elbow hinge, single-control cable system, biceps or triceps cuff, and figure-eight harness.

15. Name the most commonly prescribed components of an above-elbow prosthesis.

VO split hook, friction wrist, double-walled plastic laminate socket, internal-locking elbow, dual-control cable system, and figure-eight harness.

16. What is the purpose of the terminal device?

To provide prehension. The human hand is capable of six types of prehension: lateral, palmar, tip, cylindrical grasp, spherical grasp, and hook or snap. The terminal device replaces the types of prehension that allow the amputee to perform ADL skills either with one device or, at most, with two.

17. What are the advantages of a hook terminal device? Of a prosthetic hand?

Normal lateral prehension or pinch is grasping an object between the pad of the thumb and the lateral surface of the index finger. The **hook** provides this function and is better suited for tasks requiring manual dexterity. It is lighter in weight and easier to maintain, and its less cumbersome construction facilitates visual cues.

Normal palmar prehension, or three-jaw chuck pinch, is grasping an object between the pad of the thumb and the pads of the index and middle fingers. The **prosthetic hand** provides this function and can be used to grasp larger objects and rounded ones. It also provides better cosmesis.

The selection of a hook or a prosthetic hand is determined by the needs and preferences of the amputee.

18. What is the most commonly used terminal device?

The Dorrance VO split hook. This device was patented in 1912 by D.W. Dorrance, who was a bilateral upper-extremity amputee. Prior to this "split" hook, terminal devices were actually hooks and provided no prehension at all.

19. What functions do wrist units provide?

Both the friction and locking types of wrist units serve as the attachment point for the terminal device, and thus, they do not function as true wrist joints. They provide passive pronation and supination which the patient controls by using the normal hand to rotate the wrist.

20. Explain the advantages of the epicondyle suspension prosthesis (Muenster-type below-elbow prosthesis).

Used with very short below-elbow amputations, the socket of this prosthesis is set at 30° of elbow flexion. Since this shortens the lever arm during flexion movements, it requires much less effort to operate. Because the socket is securely fitted above the humeral epicondyles, a high degree of retention is attained without the use of suspension devices, such as elbow hinges, cuffs, or pads.

21. Name the three basic types of below-elbow hinges. What are their indications?

Flexible, rigid, and step-up hinge. The selection of the type of hinge depends on the level of amputation and on the functional status of the residual limb. A long below-elbow amputee will use the **flexible hinge**; the short below-elbow amputee requires more stability and needs the **rigid hinge**. When the below-elbow stump is very short and flexion is severely limited, the gear arrangement of the **step-up hinge** permits the socket to flex through a greater range than the residual elbow joint would otherwise allow. Keep in mind that with short below-elbow stumps, the supracondylar suspension prosthesis is often a good alternative to hinges.

22. How does the amputee operate the body-powered upper-extremity prosthesis?

An amputee is trained to perform coordinated body movements that transmit tension along a cable system that slides inside one or more flexible housings. The stainless-steel cable is attached proximally to the harness and distally to the terminal device. With an above-elbow prosthesis, the cable is also attached to the elbow unit.

An amputee with a below-elbow prosthesis uses a single-control system (Bowden control system) to operate the terminal device through coordinated arm flexion and shoulder abduction.

An amputee with an above-elbow or very short below-elbow prosthesis needs a dual-control system (fair-lead system) in which arm flexion operates the terminal device and controls forearm flexion, and arm extension operates the elbow lock. When the elbow is locked between 90–135°, the terminal device is operated by biscapular abduction (shoulder shrug).

23. Why is the figure-eight harness the most commonly used? What are some other types?
It provides the widest range of everyday activities with the least restrictions of the body.

Other harness types meet more specific requirements of an amputee. The **figure-nine harness**, for example, affords more freedom of movement and is used in the supracondylar prosthesis. The **triple-control system harness**, which separates terminal-device operation from forearm flexion and replaces the dual-control system, is useful for people with above-elbow amputations. The **modified shoulder saddle harness** provides a larger weight-bearing area and permits the amputee to lift heavy objects without transmitting excessive pressure to the sound axilla.

24. How does the myoelectric-type prosthesis work?
When this type of prosthesis is worn by a patient with an upper-extremity amputation, surface electrodes housed in the socket are brought into contact with muscles that have been trained to contract and to generate a minimum signal of 10 μV. This voltage, which is amplified 20,000–40,000 times, activates a rechargeable nickel-cadmium battery that then operates the small reversible electric motors in the terminal device and prosthetic joints.

25. What is the value of the myometric evaluation?
This evaluation uses a myotester to measure the action potentials of the amputee's stump muscles and to determine whether the muscles are capable of activating the surface electrodes of the prosthesis that operate the terminal device.

26. What particular difficulties does a patient with a shoulder disarticulation or forequarter amputation face?
These patients have no residual stumps and therefore cannot easily mobilize their shoulder girdle strength to operate the control systems. In the forequarter amputation (interthoracoscapular amputation), the problem is even more difficult, since there is no residual shoulder girdle. Thus, an amputee must expend great effort and be highly motivated to operate a body-powered shoulder disarticulation prosthesis.

27. What are the essential components of the body-powered shoulder disarticulation prosthesis?
This appliance, also called the active prehensile arm, consists of the terminal device, wrist unit, forearm section, elbow unit, arm section, and shoulder section. All are operated by shoulder girdle movements.

BIBLIOGRAPHY

1. Nader EHM (ed): Otto Bock Prosthetic Compendium—Upper-Extremity Prostheses. Berlin, Schliele & Schon GmbH, 1990.
2. New York University Post-Graduate Medical School: Upper-Limb Prosthetics, 1986.
3. Schmidl H: Protesi per arto superiore. Riv Chir Mano 20(1):53–58, 1983.

106. GAIT DEVIATIONS AND LOWER-LIMB PROSTHESES

Norman Berger, M.S.

1. What do I need to know to observe deviations and analyze their causes?

The most important prerequisite is a thorough understanding of normal gait, including directions and ranges of joint motions, the phasic action of muscles in controlling these motions, and the significance of gravity and inertia as determinants of joint motion and muscular activity. These concepts require consideration of the center of gravity, the force line through the extremity, ground reaction forces, and imposed moments around joints. Also helpful is an understanding of the prosthesis and its components, particularly the influence of prosthetic alignment on pressure distribution within the socket and on joint motion.

2. Which joint should be observed primarily when evaluating the gait of a transtibial (below-knee) amputee?

The prosthetic-side knee joint during stance phase. Since most transtibial amputees retain essentially normal muscular control of the hip and knee, there is no reason for swing phase to be compromised. During stance phase, however, both stability and forward progression must be maintained while walking over a prosthetic foot-ankle component. Problems are often evident as abnormalities in knee joint motion. A word of advice—sagittal plane knee motions are best seen from the side, while frontal plane motions are best seen from the rear. Be sure to get both views.

3. When watching the knee joint from the side, what specifically should be looked for?

When a nonamputee walks at a comfortable speed (approx 80 m/min), the knee flexes about 15° between heel strike and foot-flat. At the slower comfortable walking speed of the unilateral transtibial amputee, the knee flexes only about 10° following heel strike. The observer must note whether the knee flexion on the amputated side is significantly more or significantly less than the expected 10°.

4. If there is significantly more, what might cause this excessive knee flexion?

Heel cushion or bumper too hard or too stiff: Normally, as a result of ankle plantarflexion and knee flexion, the ball of the foot descends to the floor very quickly after heel strike. However, if plantarflexion is restricted by too hard a prosthetic heel, the knee will flex excessively (> 10°) after heel strike to allow the forefoot to reach the floor rapidly and gracefully. Also, an overly hard or stiff heel will not absorb the impact force as the prosthetic heel strikes the floor. Absorption must then be accomplished by rapid and excessive flexion of the knee.

Foot in dorsiflexion: If the foot is attached to the shank in an excessive dorsiflexed position, the ball of the foot is so far from the floor at heel strike that it cannot descend to foot-flat without excessive knee flexion.

Socket too far forward over the foot: The force transmitted through the socket (Force A) and the reaction force from the floor (Force B) constitute a force couple which tends to rotate the prosthesis in the clockwise direction around the heel as a fulcrum. Clearly, the farther forward of the heel the socket force occurs, the greater will be the moment causing the clockwise rotation. This rotation will be seen by the observer as an abrupt and excessive flexion of the knee immediately after heel strike. Also, the quadriceps, which is eccentrically contracted at this time to prevent knee buckling, will contract much more forcefully to resist the increased flexion moment. Fatigue and overloading may result. Also, it is important to remember that as the quadriceps contracts to control the flexing knee, pressure and shear between the socket and residual limb increase dramatically, particularly at the anterior-distal tibia. No wonder that this area is a common site of discomfort and complaint.

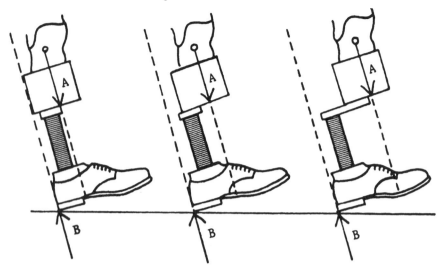

Knee flexion contracture, uncompensated: If the tibial remnant is flexed on the femur because of tight hamstrings, the socket of an uncompensated prosthesis will be considerably forward of the foot. An increased knee flexion moment, excessive knee flexion, and increased anterior-distal tibial pressure will all be present. If the residual limb is short and the contracture is not large, the prosthetist can move the foot forward underneath the socket. The shorter the residual limb, the greater the degree of contracture that can be accommodated by this compensating realignment.

5. What happens to gait during late-stance phase?
At heel off, the body's center of gravity passes over the metatarsophalangeal (MTP) joints, and the knee, which had been extending, begins to flex. If the weight of the body were to pass over the MTP joints too soon (e.g., if the foot were very short), the resulting early loss of anterior support would allow the knee to flex prematurely, and the body would drop fairly abruptly until arrested by heel strike on the other side. Note that the last three causes discussed above each have the effect of moving the weight forward with respect to the foot. Thus, the distance that the weight must travel forward before anterior support is lost is minimized, and premature knee flexion and "drop off" will likely be seen in the latter part of stance phase.

6. If there is too little or no knee flexion, what might cause this deviation?
Heel cushion or bumper too soft or too flexible: The soft heel absorbs so much of the floor reaction force that little remains to cause knee flexion.

Prosthetic foot in excessive plantarflexion: The foot reaches the floor too quickly after heel strike, with no need for knee flexion to contribute to the process.

Socket too far posterior over foot: The clockwise rotation of the prosthesis (flexion moment) produced by the force couple is reduced as the socket force moves closer to the floor reaction. In fact, if the force transmitted through the socket is coincident with the floor reaction force, there would be no flexion moment at all.

Quadriceps weakness: Supporting body weight over a flexed knee is possible only if the quadriceps is sufficiently powerful to prevent the knee from buckling. The individual with weak knee extensors avoids the danger of collapse by walking over a fully extended knee; with gluteus maximus largely responsible for maintaining knee extension against the knee flexion moment normally present at heel strike.

Anterior-distal tibial discomfort: Increased pressure between the anterodistal tibia and the socket stems primarily from the activity of the quadriceps controlling the rate and extent of knee flexion after heel strike. To alleviate any resulting discomfort, the amputee may develop a habit of holding the knee in full extension. Thus, the gait may be the same as the weak quadriceps pattern, even though examination reveals normal strength. Differentiation between these two causes requires muscle testing, residuum and socket inspection for evidence of high-pressure injury, and careful questioning of the patient.

7. When observing the transtibial amputee from the rear to see frontal plane knee motion, what specifically should you see?

Excessive lateral thrust, i.e., a fairly sudden lateral motion of the socket that occurs at about midstance. This lateral thrust results from an alignment in which the supporting foot on the floor is medial to the force line extending through the weight-bearing socket. The foot is excessively "in-set." The resulting force couple tends to rotate the prosthesis laterally, so that the medial socket brim presses in against the stump (increases pressure), and the lateral socket brim moves away from the stump (decreases pressure).

Considering that the medial side of the residuum is quite tolerant of pressure (medial tibial flare) and that the lateral side is quite sensitive to pressure (fibular head), this would seem to be an excellent arrangement. And it is! The foot should be slightly medial to the socket. But, if the foot is excessively "in-set," an excessive lateral thrust results. The observer will see this lateral motion, the amputee may complain of discomfort on the medioproximal aspect, and skin and lateral collateral knee ligaments may be damaged.

8. Describe the gait of the transfemoral (above-knee) amputee.

As compared to the transtibial amputee, the transfemoral amputee walks more slowly, expends more energy, is more likely to use a cane or other supports, and exhibits more deviation from a normal pattern. These are among the consequences of loss of the anatomic knee.

To be more specific, the loss of the quadriceps necessitates a fully extended or stable prosthetic knee throughout stance phase to avoid the danger of buckling under weight-bearing. Maintaining full extension requires strength of the gluteus maximus, prosthetic alignment that brings the force line anterior to the knee very early in stance enhancing stability, a relatively soft prosthetic heel to absorb heel strike impact and limit the knee flexion moment, and in some cases, special knee unit designs that inhibit or prevent flexion.

During swing phase, the quadriceps normally functions to accelerate the foot forward immediately after toe-off, while the hamstrings act to decelerate the foot prior to heel strike. In the absence of these muscular controls, both the speed and direction of the swinging shank are difficult for the amputee to regulate.

9. What are the more common deviations seen when observing the above-knee amputee from the rear?

Lateral trunk bend
Abducted gait (wide walking base)
Circumduction
Whips, medial or lateral

10. Describe the mechanics and causes of lateral trunk bend.

As soon as the sound limb lifts off the floor and begins its swing phase, the pelvis tends to drop or dip on the unsupported side. The hip abductors on the prosthetic, stance-phase side contract strongly to control the pelvic dip. In the absence of hip abductor strength, the trunk must lean toward the prosthetic side to counteract the instability toward the swing-phase side (**Trendelenburg sign**). Among the conditions that interfere with pelvic control by the hip abductors and thus are causes of lateral trunk bend are:

1. Weak hip abductors

2. Hip abduction contracture or abducted socket. The effectiveness of the shortened hip abductors is considerably reduced.

3. Poor fit of lateral socket wall. When the gluteus medius contracts, it exerts force at both its origin and its insertion, i.e., on the pelvis and femur. For it to stabilize the pelvis, the femur must be prevented from moving. This is the primary function of the lateral socket wall, which must fit intimately and accurately to prevent femoral abduction.

4. Lateral-distal femoral discomfort. If femoral abduction against the lateral wall results in discomfort, the amputee may adopt a lateral trunk bend to reduce pressure.

11. What are the causes of abducted gait (wide walking base)?
In this deviation, the prosthetic foot is held away from the midline throughout the gait cycle. The major causes include:

Perineal discomfort. When the amputee experiences pain in the crotch area, the prosthesis is abducted to move the medial socket brim away from the sensitive spot.

Prosthesis too long. It is difficult for the long prosthesis to clear the floor during swing phase and to be placed directly under the hip during stance phase. Both problems are solved by holding the prosthesis out to the side.

Abduction contracture, uncompensated

12. How does circumduction manifest?
This swing-phase deviation is characterized by a laterally curved line of progression, i.e., the prosthesis is swung out to the side but brought back to the midline for the next heel strike. Amputees who are fearful of stubbing the toe adopt this maneuver to ensure that the prosthetic foot clears the floor. Because prosthetists rarely fabricate a prosthesis of excessive length, it becomes necessary to examine the patient for conditions that create a "functionally long" prosthesis:

1. Foot in plantarflexion: toe tends to scuff floor.

2. Socket too small: residuum cannot enter fully.

3. Inadequate suspension: socket slips down during swing.

4. Insufficient or no knee flexion during swing because the knee unit includes a manual lock, excessive friction, or too tight an extension aid.

5. Amputee is reluctant to flex the knee during swing because of poor balance, insecurity, or fear.

13. What are whips? Why do they occur?
A whip is a sudden, abrupt rotation of the prosthesis that occurs at the end of stance phase, as the knee is flexed to begin swing. If the prosthetic heel is seen to move medially, a **medial whip** is noted, while lateral rotation of the heel denotes a **lateral whip**.

Mechanically, flexion and extension of the prosthetic knee (i.e., motion of the shank and foot) can take place only in a plane perpendicular to the knee axis. Thus, for the shank to swing along a sagittal line, the knee axis must be perpendicular to that line. If the knee axis were externally or internally rotated, the shank could only swing diagonally. Keeping this in mind, major causes of whips are:

1. Improper alignment of the knee axis: An externally rotated axis produces a medial whip, because at initial flexion of the knee, the prosthesis rotates to a position perpendicular to the axis. Similarly, an internally rotated axis produces a lateral whip.

2. Flabby, weak musculature that rotates freely around the femur. The prosthesis rotates with this underlying soft tissue unless a suspension component, such as a Silesian bandage, is used as a rotation control mechanism.

14. Which deviations in the gait of the above-knee amputee are best observed from the side?
Short step on sound side
Uneven heel rise
Terminal impact

15. What causes a short step on the sound side?

1. Hip flexion contracture: In order for the sound limb to take a normal length step, the prosthetic side must assume a hyperextended position. When a hip flexion contracture prevents this, the sound side step-length must decrease.

2. Insufficient socket flexion: In the presence of any restriction of hip extension range, the socket should be aligned in compensatory flexion so that the prosthesis may still reach a position of hyperextension though the femur cannot. Whether this can be accomplished depends on the degree of extension limitation and the length of the residuum. The shorter the residual limb, the more compensatory socket flexion can be introduced.

3. Pain, insecurity, fear: Discomfort from an ill-fitting socket or fear of balancing on an insensate, jointed stilt will cause the amputee to spend as little time as possible in prosthetic stance phase. Body weight is shifted quickly back to the sound side, which has taken a rapid, short step so as to be prepared to accept the weight.

16. Describe the mechanics of uneven heel rise.

Normally, the quadriceps is responsible for limiting knee flexion in early swing. Without a quadriceps, the transfemoral amputee must depend on resistance to motion provided by the prosthetic knee unit through friction mechanisms, pneumatic or hydraulic cylinders, or extension aids. If these produce too little resistance to motion, there will be excessive heel rise in early swing as the knee flexes too much. Conversely, if there is too much resistance to motion, there will be insufficient heel rise as the knee flexes too little.

17. How do you recognize terminal impact?

Toward the end of swing phase, the hamstrings are responsible for decelerating the rapidly moving shank, i.e., controlling the rate of knee extension. Without hamstrings, the transfemoral amputee must depend again on resistance to motion from the prosthetic knee unit. If there is too little resistance from the friction or cylinders, the forward inertia will swing the shank forward too quickly and produce a forceful impact into full extension—clunk!

A small amount of terminal impact is often considered useful and beneficial by the above-knee prosthesis wearer. The impact provides important feedback information, signaling that the knee is fully extended and that it is now safe to put the prosthesis on the floor and transfer body weight to it. This is a good example of the general proposition that gait deviations are seldom accidents but habitual compromises that make the amputee reluctant to walk without them.

BIBLIOGRAPHY

1. Berger N: Analysis of amputee gait. In Bowker JH, Michael JW (eds): Atlas of Limb Prosthetics, 2nd ed. St. Louis, Mosby, 1992, pp 371–379.
2. Kapp S, Cummings D: Transtibial amputation: Prosthetic management. In Bowker JH, Michael JW (eds): Atlas of Limb Prosthetics, 2nd ed. St. Louis, Mosby, 1992, pp 453–478.
3. Murray MP, Drought AB, Kory RC: Walking patterns of normal man. J Bone Joint Surg 46A:335, 1964.
4. Perry J: Normal gait. In Bowker JH, Michael JW (eds): Atlas of Limb Prosthetics, 2nd ed. St. Louis, Mosby, 1992, pp 359–369.
5. Saunders JB, Inman VT, Eberhart HD: Major determinants in normal and pathological gait. J Bone Joint Surg 35A:543, 1953.
6. Schuch CM: Transfemoral amputation: Prosthetic management. In Bowker JH, Michael JW (eds): Atlas of Limb Prosthetics, 2nd ed. St. Louis, Mosby, 1992, pp 509–533.

107. SPINAL ORTHOSES

John B. Redford, M.D., Abna A. Ogle, M.D., and Richard C. Robinson, M.D.

1. What is a spinal orthosis?

The name *orthosis* derives from the Greek word meaning *making straight*. Spinal orthoses or braces are appliances used in an attempt to correct and support the spine. Their use has been extensively documented in human history, predating Christ until the present day.

2. What does the functional unit consist of in the human spine?

Two vertebral bodies, their articulating joints, and an interposed fibroelastic disc. The human spine is an aggregate of superimposed segments, each segment being a self-contained functional unit, with the sum total of all the units forming the vertebral column.

3. List the three principal functions of the vertebral column.

1. Protect the spinal cord and its nerve roots
2. Absorb axial compressive forces
3. Provide a base for mobility of the human skeleton

4. What is the purpose of a spinal orthosis?

1. Prevention and correction of deformities
2. Reduction of axial loading
3. Stabilization of a vertebral segment
4. Relief of pain by limiting motion or weight-bearing
5. Improvement of spinal function
6. Provision of effects such as heat, massage, and kinesthetic feedback

5. How do spinal orthoses work?

Spinal orthoses, when applied to the body, exert forces on the spine. This is accomplished in one or more of the following ways:

Three-point pressure system: (see figure)

Fluid compression: When the brace encompasses the trunk, it forms a semirigid cylinder surrounding the vertebral column. This results in an increase in intra-abdominal pressure, which measurably decreases intervertebral disc pressure, and decreases shearing forces across the lowest functional units.

Irritant: The brace is constructed so that the wearer is forced into the desired posture to avoid discomfort (kinesthetic feedback).

Skeletal fixation: The scientific basis for orthotic use is well delineated in the correction of certain progressive spine deformities. However, as orthopedic surgery has advanced, the use of external corrective devices has declined. They are commonly used in nonsurgical musculoskeletal complaints, such as back or neck strains. It is in this arena that empirical evidence is incomplete. However, clinical experience and patient report provide justification for their continued use.

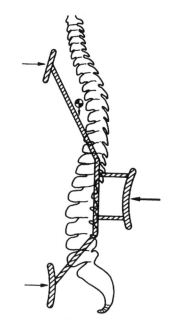

Three-point pressure system as applied in a hyperextension TLSO.

6. What are the potential complications of spinal orthoses?
1. Loss of skin integrity due to compressive forces
2. Weakening of axial muscles
3. Soft-tissue contractures
4. Increased movement at the ends of immobilized segments
5. Physical and psychological dependence
6. Osteopenia

7. There are so many different orthoses, how can I remember their names?
There is a bewildering variety of devices, several even sporting the name or hometown of the creator. To avoid confusion and aid in classification of braces, the American Academy of Orthopaedic Surgeons and the American Academy of Prosthetists and Orthotists together have devised a uniform naming system.

The orthosis is named for the segments of the body and/or spine that it covers. Thus, a CO is a cervical orthosis covering only the neck. A CTO is a cervicothoracic orthosis encompassing the neck and thoracic spine.

8. What does LSO refer to?
Lumbosacral orthosis.

Commonly Used Spinal Orthoses

Cervical orthosis	CO
Cervicothoracic orthosis	CTO
Cervicothoracolumbosacral orthosis	CTLSO
Thoracolumbosacral orthosis	TLSO
Lumbosacral orthosis	LSO
Sacroiliac orthosis	SIO

9. How do I choose an orthosis?
The spinal segments have very different characteristics. The specific complaint, anatomic pathology, as well as the unique properties of the spinal segment must be considered when recommending an orthosis.

10. Describe the possible movement in the cervical spine.
The cervical segment is the most mobile portion of the spine. It is capable of movement in three planes: flexion and extension; lateral rotation; and side bending.

Most cervical rotation occurs between C1 and C2. The greatest amount of flexion and extension is between C5 and C6. Because of extensive innate mobility, the cervical spine is very difficult to immobilize or stabilize.

11. Your patient has an acute but uncomplicated cervical strain. What orthosis do you prescribe?
The **soft collar** is probably the most commonly used orthosis. It is made of a firm foam covered with cotton and fastened posteriorly with Velcro. It is usually prescribed for **cervical muscle strain**. It provides little restriction of cervical movement (only reduction of flexion and extension by approximately one-fourth, and virtually no reduction of lateral bending or rotation) but allows soft tissues to rest, provides warmth to strained muscles, and reminds the patient to avoid extremes of neck movement.

12. When is a Philadelphia collar used?
This type of cervical orthosis provides more restriction to movement than does the soft collar, but less than a halo vest or custom-made plastic CTO. The Philadelphia collar is made of a foam reinforced by firm thermoplastic material. It has an anterior and posterior portion that conform to the chin and occiput.

A Philadelphia collar is frequently prescribed **after cervical surgery** when very strict neck immobilization is not necessary. It may also be used in cases with **cervical ligament rupture** and in some relatively **stable cervical spine fractures**. It provides more limitation in flexion and extension and side-bending than a soft collar but does not significantly limit rotation. Patients frequently complain of feeling hot and sweaty under this collar, but it is generally well-tolerated.

13. What is a halo vest orthosis?

This CTO consists of two parts: The halo portion is a circular band of steel attached to the skull via metal screws. Adjustable rods connect the halo to a vest that encircles the trunk. This device provides the most rigid fixation of the cervical spine and is the orthosis most widely used in **cervical fractures**. Some intervertebral movement is still possible, however, as evidenced by the "snaking" phenomenon (slight movement between the individual cervical segments, which can be seen on plain films of the neck). This brace makes possible early mobilization and rehabilitation of the patient following spinal surgery, while maintaining a stable spine.

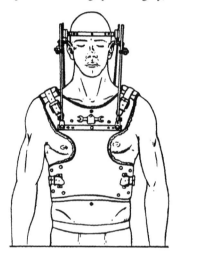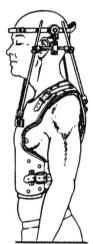

Halo vest orthosis, front and side views.

14. When are thoracic orthoses used?

The thoracic spine is the most stable and least mobile portion of the spine. It owes its stability, at least in part, to the thoracic cage with its connecting ribs and sternum. Problems such as **compression fractures, fracture-dislocations**, and **scoliotic** or **kyphotic** deformities of the spine are the most common reasons for prescriptions of this orthosis. It is important to know that to limit motion in one segment of the spine, the orthosis must extend proximally and distally to adjacent segments.

15. What braces are used for thoracic deformities?

For low thoracic scoliosis, there appears to be a real and predictable effect from bracing. For mid and high thoracic scoliosis, the efficacy of corrective orthoses remains debatable. Idiopathic or paralytic scolioses are amenable to surgery. Milwaukee bracing for progressive spinal curvature is a complex system of dynamic bracing. The pressure and discomfort necessary for correcting posture is frequently so great as to diminish compliance in use of the brace.

The **Taylor brace** is prescribed for counteracting kyphosis. It has high thoracic uprights and shoulder straps. These straps must be tightened (often to the discomfort of the patient) to provide adequate antideformity forces.

The **CASH** (cruciform anterior spinal hyperextension) **orthosis** is also used to decrease kyphosis. It has an anterior cross-bar with pads at the four ends of the cross. This orthosis adjusts posteriorly with straps held closed with Velcro. It is lightweight and easy to put on but may require frequent repositioning.

The **Jewett** (hyperextension TLSO) **orthosis** uses the three-point system to facilitate thoracic hyperextension. The two anterior pads are positioned over the sternum and pubic symphysis, while the third opposing posterior pad lies over the thoracolumbar junction. It does not limit spine rotation but is fairly comfortable to wear and more easily adjusted than the CASH orthosis.

16. How is a painful nondisplaced thoracic compression fracture treated?

There is clinical experience that orthoses can alleviate acute pain, but no scientific evidence exists of how this may occur. Short-term use of a brace is acceptable in the first 7–10 days following a fracture. The patient should also receive back protection and posture education, as well as trunk-strengthening exercises.

17. How are unstable thoracic fractures treated?

Surgery is usually indicated, but postoperative bracing may be recommended by the surgeon.

18. When are lumbosacral orthoses used?

They are frequently prescribed for **uncomplicated low back pain** but are primarily used for support and immobilization of the spine after **trauma** or **surgery**. Application of these orthoses for low back pain is controversial. Some clinicians cite the lack of consistent scientific evidence to support their use, especially in chronic low back pain. Others would agree with their limited use during high-impact activities, along with patient education and an exercise program.

19. There are so many LSOs on the market. How can I choose appropriately?

One way to keep straight the ever-increasing multitude of LSOs is to consider them in order from the least to the most immobilizing:

1. **Corsets** provide the least restriction in spinal movement. These can be made of canvas or elasticized material and can be reinforced with metal or plastic stays or even a thermomolded plastic pad. Corsets are more comfortable than rigid metal orthoses, such as the chair-back brace, and achieve lumbar support by increasing intra-abdominal pressure. They also provide some warmth to extensor muscles of the spine and can remind the wearer to avoid extremes of movement.

2. **Spinal braces**, reinforced with rigid metal bars and rigid plastic jackets, are more restrictive than corsets and vary in length: the greater the length, the more immobilizing the effect. An example is the short flexion jacket (Raney orthosis) that has been advocated by some for preventing extension in the lumbar spine; it is used in low back pain, particularly that caused by spondylolisthesis. This orthosis is made of thermomolded plastic anterior and posterior parts, fastened with Velcro. The anterior portion presses into the abdomen, causing increased intra-abdominal pressure. The forced flexion of the lumbar spine may also alleviate pressure in the posterior elements of the vertebral column.

3. **Lumbosacral spicas** provide the most effective way of immobilizing the lower lumbar spine. They are made of thermomolded plastic extending from 2 cm below the inferior angle of the scapulae to the sacrum. A unilateral side piece is extended distally, usually immobilizing the hip in 15–20° of flexion. Investigation of lumbosacral movements has demonstrated that the lower lumbar vertebrae are best immobilized when there is fixation of the pelvis (via the extended thigh piece). This orthosis is useful for postoperative immobilization and unstable lower spine fractures.

BIBLIOGRAPHY

1. Fisher SV: Spinal orthoses: In Krusen's Handbook of Physical Medicine and Rehabilitation, 4th ed. Philadelphia, W.B. Saunders, 1990, pp 593–601.
2. McLain RF, Karol L: Conservative treatment of the scoliotic and kyphotic patient. Arch Pediatr Adolesc Med 148:646–665, 1994.
3. Nachemson AL: Orthotic treatment for injuries and disease of the spinal column. Phys Med Rehabil State Art Rev 1(1):11–24, 1987.
4. Sypert GW: External spinal orthotics. Neurosurgery 20:642–649, 1987.

XIII. The Future of PM&R

108. PROFESSIONAL ORGANIZATIONS FOR THE PHYSIATRIST

Leon Reinstein, M.D.

1. Why join a professional organization?

Fortunately or unfortunately, physicians today do not practice medicine in a vacuum. Instead, they practice in a fishbowl. All around today's practicing physiatrist is an alphabet soup of organizations that will directly impact on your future practice in PM&R. Membership in these organizations allows you to "grow professionally" throughout your career.

2. What is the largest organization of physiatrists?

With more than 4,300 members, the **American Academy of Physical Medicine and Rehabilitation** (AAPM&R) is the largest organization of physiatrists. Founded in 1938 and headquartered in Chicago, the AAPM&R provides its members with educational materials, scientific meetings and courses, legislative advocacy and national affairs, and physiatric practice management and copublishes the *Archives of Physical Medicine and Rehabilitation*.

The AAPM&R has three major categories of membership: Fellow, Associate, and Affiliate. A **Fellow** is a diplomate of the American Board of PM&R. An **Associate** member has passed Part I of the board examination. An **Affiliate** member is a full-time resident in training in an approved residency program. If you join only one professional organization, this is the one.

3. Is there an organization for "Academic" physiatrists?

The **Association of Academic Physiatrists (AAP)**, founded in 1967 and headquartered in Indianapolis, is the national organization of physiatrists who are affiliated with medical schools. It has more than 1,000 members. The AAP promotes the advancement of teaching and research in PM&R within an academic environment. It holds an annual meeting focusing on academic physiatric research, education, and administration and publishes the *American Journal of Physical Medicine and Rehabilitation*.

The AAP also has three major categories of membership: Diplomate, Associate, and Resident. A **Diplomate** member must hold an academic faculty appointment as a physiatrist in a North American medical school or a full-time teaching position in a nonuniversity affiliated residency program, as well as be a diplomate of the American Board of PM&R. An **Associate** member must be actively engaged in the training of physicians and/or students in the specialty of PM&R. A **Resident** member must be actively engaged in a training program leading to admissibility to the certifying examination of the American Board of PM&R.

4. Is there an organization of physiatrists and nonphysiatrists interested in rehabilitation?

The American Congress of Rehabilitation Medicine (ACRM), founded in 1923 and headquartered in Skokie, Illinois, is the multidisciplinary association of medical rehabilitation professionals. It has more than 1,700 members, including physiatrists, other physicians, allied health professionals, administrators, and educators. It seeks to promote through education, advocacy, and membership services the art, science, and practice of interdisciplinary rehabilitation care for persons with or at risk of functional limitation. The ACRM holds an annual educational and scientific meeting and co-publishes the *Archives of Physical Medicine and Rehabilitation*. An active member of the ACRM has a baccalaureate degree in a medical rehabilitation discipline or a related field.

5. What is the American Board of Physical Medicine and Rehabilitation?

Established in 1947 and headquartered in Rochester, Minnesota, the American Board of Physical Medicine and Rehabilitation (ABPM&R) administers certifying and re-certifying examinations in PM&R to physicians. The **Part I written examination** is taken upon satisfactory completion of an approved residency in PM&R. The **Part II oral examination** is taken following satisfactory completion of the written examination and 1 year of clinical practice in PM&R.

6. Does Board certification ever expire?

Board certification in PM&R is now time-limited. Ten years after initial certification and for each 10 years thereafter, you must obtain re-certification. Requirements for re-certification include evidence of 500 hours of continuing medical education during the 10 years, and satisfactory completion of an open-book, take-home written examination. The first re-certification examination will be given in the year 2000.

7. Does the ABPM&R also certify residency programs?

No. Accreditation of residency programs in PM&R is the responsibility of the **Residency Review Committee (RRC) for Physical Medicine and Rehabilitation**. In 1994, there were 71 PM&R residency programs in the United States with full accreditation.

8. What about the American Association of Electrodiagnostic Medicine (AAEM)?

Founded in 1953 and also headquartered in Rochester, Minnesota, the AAEM has 3,800 members, about half of whom are physiatrists, the other half being neurologists. Its primary goal is to increase the quality of care for patients with disorders of muscle and the central and peripheral nervous systems by contributing to steady improvements in electrodiagnostic methods. The AAEM holds an annual educational and scientific meeting and publishes *Muscle and Nerve*. In 1987, it established the American Board of Electrodiagnostic Medicine (ABEM) as an independent credentialing body in electrodiagnostic medicine.

9. What about the American Medical Association (AMA)?

The AMA is the largest medical organization in the world. Forty-two percent of American physicians belong to it. It publishes *JAMA: The Journal of the American Medical Association*, nine specialty journals, and *American Medical News*. It holds educational and scientific meetings throughout the year. All of the state medical societies and many specialty societies are represented in its House of Delegates, which determines AMA policy. The AMA has a major presence in Washington, DC, and provides physician advocacy at the national level.

10. My rehab facility is having a CARF survey. Do I need to be concerned?

CARF is the **Commission on Accreditation of Rehabilitation Facilities**. It is the rehab equivalent of the Joint Commission on Healthcare Organizations, which accredits all hospitals in the United States.

CARF reviews agencies and organizations that serve people with physical disabilities and accredits specific programs based on its detailed, published standards. Obtaining CARF accreditation is not just good PR—many insurers and some states *require* CARF accreditation to permit a facility to identify itself as a rehabilitation facility. So when you hear "CARF is coming," attend the mock reviews sessions and pay attention.

11. What about NARF (rhymes with CARF)?

NARF stands for the **National Association of Rehabilitation Facilities**. Founded in 1969, this organization changed its name to the **American Rehabilitation Association** (ARA) several years ago. It is headquartered in Washington, DC, and includes over 900 rehabilitation facilities. ARA serves its member facilities by spearheading changes in public policy, developing educational and training programs, and promoting research. It also provides networking and communications opportunities. It's basically a trade association of rehabilitation facilities.

12. What is PASSOR?

No, it's not the Jewish holiday occurring around Easter time (that's Passover). This is the new kid on the block. PASSOR is the **Physiatric Association of Spine, Sports, and Occupational Rehabilitation**. It was founded in 1993 as a council of the AAPM&R to foster the growth of the specialty of physiatry in research, education, and the physiatric practice of musculoskeletal medicine. It has an annual educational and scientific program in conjunction with the annual meeting of the AAPM&R.

13. Any others?
1. American Society of Handicapped Physicians (318-283-4436)
2. Society for Disability Studies (510–549-6520)
3. American Spinal Cord Injury Association (404-355-9772)
4. World Rehabilitation Fund (212-340-6062)
5. National Center for Medical Rehabilitation Research (301-402-2242)

109. THE REHABILITATION INFORMATION SUPERHIGHWAY: WHERE TO NEXT?

Gary Fisher and Kurt Gold, M.D.

1. How can informatics improve patient care?

Just as functional outcome analysis can assist in deciding which patients should receive what level of care, so too can the computers assist in generation of therapy protocols and schedules, differential diagnosis and literature review, vital sign tracking, functional progress evaluations, discharge planning and reporting.

2. How can informatics help with PM&R research?

In addition to literature surveillance, enhanced communication improves prospects for multi-center studies. Centers recruiting patients for intervention trials can submit inclusion criteria to a central server, enabling remote collaborating sites to match protocols with patients likely to benefit via study participation.

3. How can informatics help with education?

College by e-mail is common. Interactive educational software can be used for continuing medical educational credits. The American Academy of Physical Medicine and Rehabilitation (AAPM&R) recently inaugurated the "EMG Case of the Month" via e-mail. On-line informational resources are rapidly expanding. Televideo applications can reveal microsurgery's narrow focus to much wider audiences. Videolog and CD-ROM may already be more efficient for "one-on-one" instruction than traditional lecture hall or laboratory settings. Indeed, medical education by modem may become the way training is done.

Brain Injury Resources on the Internet*

WWW RESOURCES	URL ADDRESS (WWW LOCATION)	TYPE OF SITE
Center for Neuro Skills: Traumatic Brain Injury	http://www.neuroskills.com/~cns/injury.html	Clinical site
The Neuroscience Center (NSC) of Indianapolis	http://www.inetdirect.net/nsc/	Clinical site
The Brain Injury Association (TBIA) of Connecticut	http://www.connix.com/~dpyers/cttbia.html	Organization
Ohio Valley Center (OVC) for Head Injury Prevention and Rehabilitation	http://beetle.marion.ohio-state.edu/ovchome/ovc.html	Organization
TBI-SPRT listserv	http://www.tile.net/tile/listserv/tbisprt.html	Support group
TBI Support Group	http://www.ibmpcug.co.uk/~copernic/tbi2.htm	Support group
Traumatic Brain Injury Update, Univ of Washington	http://weber.u.washington.edu/~reh/tbi/	Education and information
Brain Injury, Disability Services	ttp://disserv.stu.umn.edu/ag-s/3-8.html	Education and information
The ABI/TBI Information Project	http://www.sasquatch.com/tbi/	Education and information
TPN Brain Map	http://www.sasquatch.com/tpn/brainmap.html	Education and information (image)
The Traumatically Brain Injured and the Law	http://seamless.com/talf/txt/brain.html	Education and information (legal)
Neurorehabilitation	http://www.elsevier.nl/catalogue/SAI/130/04000/04290/525015/	Journal
The Journal of Cognitive Rehabilitation	http://www.inetdirect.net/nsp/	Journal
The Journal of Vocational Rehabilitation	http://www.elsevier.nl/catalogue/SAI/130/04000/04290/525014	Journal

* A good (summary outline) Universal Resource Locator (URL) Internet address for brain injury is: http://griffin.vcu.edu/html/pmr/trowland/brainref.html

4. How do I get on the rehabilitation information superhighway?

Participate in AAPM&R's Informatics Special Interest Group (call 312-464-9700, ext. 283, for information), explore local e-mail resources and begin using what works for you.

ACKNOWLEDGMENT

Appreciation is expressed to Dr. Todd Rowland, M.D., of the Medical College of Virginia for providing information on AAPM&R's Medical Informatics S.I.G. and Internet references.

BIBLIOGRAPHY

1. Glowniak JV, Bushway MK: Computer networks as a medical resource: Accessing and using the Internet. JAMA 271:1934–1939, 1994. (See also Goldwein JW et al. and reply.JAMA 272:1898, 1994.)
2. Heinemann AW, Hamilton B, Linacre JM, et al: Functional status and therapeutic intensity during inpatient rehabilitation. Am J Phys Med Rehabil 74:315–326, 1995.
3. Schatz BR, Hardin JB: NCSA Mosaic and World Wide Web: Global hypermedia protocols for the Internet. Science 265:895–901, 1995.
4. Tilleson SJ: Chart Notes [software review]. JAMA 273:878–883, 1995.

110. EPILOGUE

Joel A. DeLisa, M.D., M.S.

Physiatry was born in 1947 in response to the challenge to help disabled citizens reach their maximum potential. The recent workforce study by Lewin-VHI demonstrated that there is still a shortage of physiatrists and that this will continue into the foreseeable future. There are approximately 5000 board-certified physiatrists in practice.

This is an exciting and challenging time to be a physiatrist. The advances in basic sciences have resulted in a better understanding of disease processes, better diagnostic tools, and better treatment modalities. Nerve regeneration, implantable bionic parts, gene transplantation, tailored drugs, microsurgery, robotics, and computers offer major advances that will have direct consequences on physiatry.

However, future advances are tempered by health care costs. The nation appears to be moving very quickly toward the managed-care model of medical practice. There are predictions that this form of managed care with capitation will dominate health care service delivery. As managed-care organizations mature and have to deal with larger and generally older populations, they may tend to value the use of physiatry to treat a higher incidence of musculoskeletal and serious impairment problems prevalent in these patients. Physiatrists, because of their ability to manage the overall treatment of many of the payers' costliest cases, may be in demand. Since patient care will be viewed in longitudinal rather than episodic perspectives, our specialty may be the model for rest of medicine. How these managed-care systems use physician extenders and to what extent, as well as where as we are with respect to the "gate-keeper," will determine much of the demand for our clinical services.

Our specialty is in the process of analyzing whether physiatrists should have the option of being primary care physicians or principal providers for the severely disabled. Our patients are asking us to assume this role, but many physiatrists prefer the specialist role and believe that this broader knowledge base required may exceed the capacity of a physician to assimilate it. How we make the decision will have a significant effect on our workforce demand. Another priority we need to address is teaching rehabilitation to students and residents destined for careers in primary care. If we decide to undertake this, we will need to significantly increase our academic faculty.

There are also threats to the field: (1) Significant cuts in graduate medical education may erode the number of residents we train. This could be especially harmful to the clinical and research fellowships that have been so carefully nurtured over the past 5 years. (2) We are still trying to develop the specialty's research base. As research funding decreases and overall competition for grants increases, we have to be creative in developing additional funding sources.

Another area of concern is the possible splitting of the specialty into two parts, physical medicine and rehabilitation. Economic pressures may try to force this split but hopefully it will not occur. The functional approach, with unique exercise physiology, therapeutic heat and cold as well as other modalities training, and our holistic, team-oriented approach have served patients well. These skills are needed by all physiatrists.

Physiatry needs to be actively involved in organized medicine, to advocate legislation that protects our patients and provides for them a continuum of care that is cost-effective as well as high quality. We need to hone our administrative and managerial skills to be flexible and to understand the changing health care delivery system. We need to be creative enough to add new services/products but to always build in evaluation tools to be able to measure the outcome of our patients' treatment. The future offers many opportunities, and the challenges can bring our hopes and dreams to fruition.

Reference: Lewin-VHI: Physical Medicine and Rehabilitation Workforce Study: The Supply and Demand for Physiatrists. Chicago, IL, American Academy of PM&R, Sept. 1995.

INDEX

Page numbers in **boldface type** indicate complete chapters.